Gastroenterological Surgery

Gastroenterological Surgery

Editor: John Youngman

AMERICAN
MEDICAL PUBLISHERS
www.americanmedicalpublishers.com

AMERICAN
MEDICAL PUBLISHERS
www.americanmedicalpublishers.com

Cataloging-in-Publication Data

Gastroenterological surgery / edited by John Youngman.
p. cm.
Includes bibliographical references and index.
ISBN 979-8-88740-129-4
1. Gastrointestinal system--Surgery. 2. Digestive organs--Surgery.
3. Surgery, Operative. I. Youngman, John.
RD540 .G37 2023
61743--dc23

American Medical Publishers,
41 Flatbush Avenue,
1st Floor, New York,
NY 11217, USA

ISBN 979-8-88740-129-4 (Hardback)

Contents

Preface

Gastrointestinal surgery is a surgical method used for the treatment of diseases associated with the digestive system. The parts of the body involved in digestion are stomach, small intestine, large intestine, liver, gallbladder, pancreas and rectum. There are several gastrointestinal conditions, like appendicitis, diverticular disease, gallbladder disease, hernia, inflammatory bowel disease and rectal prolapse, which can be treated through gastrointestinal (GI) surgery. This surgery can be either open GI surgery or minimally invasive surgery depending on the health condition of the patient. Minimally invasive surgery involves smaller incisions and camera to view inside the body. Nephrectomy, foregut surgery, adrenalectomy and splenectomy are some common types of minimally invasive GI procedures. Open GI procedures such as abdominal surgery, Nissen fundoplication and Whipple procedure are performed with larger incisions, which leads to larger scars, more pain and takes a longer time for recovery. This book includes some of the vital pieces of work being conducted across the world, on various topics related to gastrointestinal surgery. Medical professionals and students actively engaged in this field will find it full of crucial and unexplored concepts.

This book is the end result of constructive efforts and intensive research done by experts in this field. The aim of this book is to enlighten the readers with recent information in this area of research. The information provided in this profound book would serve as a valuable reference to students and researchers in this field.

At the end, I would like to thank all the authors for devoting their precious time and providing their valuable contribution to this book. I would also like to express my gratitude to my fellow colleagues who encouraged me throughout the process.

Editor

1

Role of surgical resection and its alternative local therapy for pulmonary metastasis of colorectal cancer

Hiroomi Ogawa[1] | Toshiki Yajima[1,2] | Makoto Sohda[1] | Ken Shirabe[1] | Hiroshi Saeki[1]

[1]Department of General Surgical Science, Graduate School of Medicine, Gunma University, Maebashi, Japan

[2]Department of Innovative Cancer Immunotherapy, Graduate School of Medicine, Gunma University, Maebashi, Japan

Correspondence
Hiroshi Saeki, Department of General Surgical Science, Graduate School of Medicine, Gunma University, 3-39-22 Showa-machi, Maebashi 371-8511, Japan.
Email: h-saeki@gunma-u.ac.jp

Abstract

We reviewed surgical and alternative treatments for pulmonary metastasis of colorectal cancer, focusing on recent reports. The standard treatment for pulmonary metastasis of colorectal cancer is pulmonary resection, if resectable, despite the fact that the metastasis is hematogenous to distant organs. Guidelines in several countries, including Japan, have described pulmonary resection as a useful option because of the favorable long-term prognosis reported in various studies pertaining to pulmonary resection. The indications for pulmonary resection have been reviewed in several studies; additionally, the number of metastases, pretreatment carcinoembryonic antigen value, and disease-free interval from the primary resection to pulmonary recurrence have been proposed. However, no consensus has been reached to date. Contrastingly, recent advances in chemotherapy have remarkably improved the outcome of distant metastases, indicating that it is time to reconsider the significance of local treatment, including pulmonary resection. In addition to surgical resection, minimally invasive therapies, such as stereotactic body radiation therapy and radiofrequency ablation have been developed as local treatments for pulmonary metastases, and their long-term results have been reported. Prospective controlled trials and large-scale data analyses are needed to determine the best local treatment for pulmonary metastases and to find the appropriate indication for each treatment.

KEYWORDS

colorectal cancer, pulmonary metastasis, pulmonary resection, radiation therapy, radiofrequency ablation

1 | 1. INTRODUCTION

Colorectal cancer is one of the most common cancers in the world, along with breast, pulmonary, and prostate cancers.[1] In Japan, the number of patients with colorectal cancer is increasing annually. Recently, it has been observed that approximately 153,000 people suffer from colorectal cancer, and approximately 50,000 individuals die due to colorectal cancer each year.[2,3] Although the relative 5-y survival rate for colorectal cancer in Japan is approximately 71.4%,[4] the survival rate varies greatly depending on the stage at the time of diagnosis. Colorectal cancer often metastasizes to the liver and lungs. Pulmonary metastases are the second most common metastatic malignancies following liver metastases.[5] Metastases have been reported to occur in 19% of patients undergoing radical resection.[6]

There are several reports on the treatment of metastatic colorectal cancer, and the development of chemotherapy in recent years has particularly been remarkable. Over the last decade, treatments for metastatic colorectal cancer have made great strides, with the overall survival improving from 5 mo in 1993 to more than 30 mo.[7,8]

In contrast, there have been several reports on the local treatment for metastatic lesions, and numerous studies on the usefulness of surgical resection have been reported. Accordingly, the main guidelines worldwide now state that the resection of resectable lesions for metastatic colorectal cancer should be considered.[9,10] Additionally, the Japanese guidelines for the treatment of colorectal cancer state that multidisciplinary treatments, such as systemic chemotherapy, surgical resection, and radiation therapy should be considered.[11] However, a number of questions remain unanswered, including the usefulness, indications, timing, and order of treatment for resection and other treatments for liver and pulmonary metastases.

Numerous reports have focused on the pulmonary metastasis of colorectal cancer, and several prognostic factors have been proposed. Most reports have examined pulmonary resection; however, almost all reports were retrospective studies, and few were prospectively randomized. Based on these retrospective studies, pulmonary resection has been regarded as the standard treatment for resectable tumors.

Although pulmonary resection is a representative local treatment, radiation therapy and ablation therapy have recently been developed as local treatments to replace pulmonary resection.[12,13] These have also achieved important results as new treatment options.

This review focuses on the recent reports highlighting the usefulness of surgical resection and alternative treatments as local treatments for pulmonary metastases of colorectal cancer.

2 | 2. SURGICAL TREATMENT

2.1 | Resection of pulmonary metastases

There has been much debate about the survival benefits of pulmonary resection for pulmonary metastases of colorectal cancer. Although no conclusions have been reached regarding the life-prolonging effect of pulmonary resection, resection is said to be the only curative treatment; in fact, radical resection for pulmonary metastases has improved the 5-y survival rate.[14,15] According to the annual report of the Japanese Association for Thoracic Surgery, resection for metastatic lung tumors was performed in 8950 patients, of whom 4240 patients had pulmonary metastases from colorectal cancer.[16] According to a report by Murakawa, pulmonary resection for pulmonary metastases of colorectal cancer has doubled every 10 y.[17]

According to the European Society for Medical Oncology (ESMO) guidelines,[9] systemic therapy is the standard treatment for colon cancer metastasis. Contrastingly, local treatment should be considered as an option only according to the disease site, treatment goal, and patient factors, such as comorbidity and age. The National Comprehensive Cancer Network (NCCN) guidelines[10] recommend chemotherapy and resection for liver and pulmonary metastases; however, the guidelines recommend chemotherapy and immunotherapy for multiple organ metastases. Although both guidelines have some restrictions on surgery, there are no clear criteria for surgical resection. This is due to the lack of appropriate randomized clinical trials that prospectively considered surgical resection for pulmonary resection. Nevertheless, pulmonary resection is recognized as the standard treatment for resectable pulmonary metastases because some retrospective studies have shown good survival after pulmonary resection. Several retrospective studies have shown an overall 5-y survival rate of approximately 32.4%–43% after pulmonary metastasis resection,[18–20] and a meta-analysis reported a 5-y survival rate of 27%–68%.[21] In some cases, long-term survival is considered curative. Unfortunately, pulmonary recurrence can occur after pulmonary resection, for which repeat resection has been reported as a useful treatment. Hishida et al[22] reported that pulmonary recurrence after resection was found in 24.1% (216/898) of patients, and repeat resection resulted in a 5-y survival rate of 75.3% in a nationwide survey in Japan. They reported that patients who underwent repeat pulmonary resection had better outcomes than other patients, suggesting that pulmonary resection may be a promising curative treatment at this time. However, Menna et al[23] reported that there was no significant difference between repeat and single pulmonary resection, suggesting that there are limitations to repeat pulmonary resection. Further studies are needed to determine the patients who benefit from repeat pulmonary resection. In the Japanese guidelines, it was reported that the 5-y survival rate for pulmonary resection was 46.7% and the cumulative 5-y relapse-free survival rate was 33.7%, while the 5-y survival rate for non-resected cases was 3.9%, based on a multicenter aggregate project study by the Japanese Society for Cancer of the Colon and Rectum (JSCCR).[24,25] The 5-y survival rate for pulmonary metastases without resection was considered to be 0%, at least 5% or less in the past.[21,25] On the other hand, several retrospective studies on pulmonary resection cases have reported the above-mentioned good treatment results, demonstrating the superiority of resection. There was a small report in 1980 that determined that there was no difference in the survival among 12 patients with resectable pulmonary metastases, who did not undergo resection and 70 patients who did.[26] However, it was a small-scale, old study. It is difficult to refer to the results because the medical treatment situation was completely different from that of the present.

A large multicenter prospective clinical trial was planned in Europe to resolve this situation. The Pulmonary Metastasectomy in Colorectal Cancer (PulMiCC) trial was a prospective framework for assigning patients with resectable pulmonary metastases of colorectal cancer to those who underwent metastatic resection and those who did not.[27] However, the study was discontinued prematurely due to delayed accumulation of cases. Therefore, the originally set statistical analysis has not been performed; however, an update summarizing the results of 93 randomized cases was recently reported.[28] Notably, the 4-y survival rate and median survival time of the pulmonary resection group and the nonresection group (control arm) were almost similar (resection group vs. control group = 44% vs. 47%, 3.5 y vs. 3.8 y). Although the study lacked statistical significance, it has a certain clinical value.

No other prospective trials have compared pulmonary resection with nonresection. In contrast, a large retrospective study examining the National Cancer Database (NCDB) has recently been reported.[29] Of the 600,000 patients with colorectal cancer enrolled in the NCDB, 7217 patients with pulmonary metastases alone were examined, of which 3.63% underwent primary resection, pulmonary resection, and chemotherapy, while 14.7% of the patients were untreated. The overall 5-y survival rate for pulmonary metastases alone was 16.7%, while the 5-y survival rate for patients who underwent resection of primary and metastatic lesions and chemotherapy was the best, at 44.52%. However, the prognosis was 24.48% with resection of the primary lesion and chemotherapy, 10.36% with resection of the primary lesion alone, and 9.22% with chemotherapy alone, suggesting that the prognosis was not extremely poor even without pulmonary resection. This indicates that good outcomes are likely to be selected only for patients with limited disease and for a small proportion of patients receiving the treatment.

In another population-based study, data from the Surveillance, Epidemiology, and End Results Program of the National Cancer Institute in the United States were used to extract 807 patients with simultaneous pulmonary metastases from 217,068 colorectal cancer patients.[30] Based on the analyses, although pulmonary resection was better for the overall survival and cancer-specific survival when unadjusted, pulmonary resection did not benefit the overall survival or cancer-specific survival when adjusted by the propensity score and inverse probability-weighted adjustment.

Table 1 shows the major recent reports investigating the long-term survival of patients who underwent pulmonary resection and those who did not.[28,30-33] Although the 5-y overall survival rate of pulmonary resection tends to be better in retrospective studies, the survival rate of nonsurgery is also worthy of comparison.

The prognosis of patients with pulmonary metastases from colorectal cancer has been gradually prolonged in recent reports, regardless of pulmonary resection. This may be due to advances in systemic chemotherapy and improvements in diagnostic imaging techniques, such as the spread of thin-slice computed tomography (CT) and positron emission tomography (PET), which has resulted in a more accurate diagnosis and reduced oversight of micrometastases.

2.2 | Prognostic factors and indication for surgery

Metastatic resection of colorectal cancer is not performed in all cases, but in approximately a quarter or a fifth of the cases.[34] The indications for pulmonary resection were first described by Thomford et al[35] in 1965. According to the Japanese guidelines,[11]

TABLE 1 Major recent reports investigating the long-term survival of pulmonary resection and nonsurgery

Author	Year	Recruitment period	Study design	Registries	Number of patients		Survival of surgery group			Survival of nonsurgery group			P-value	HR (CI)
					Surgery	Nonsurgery	3y OS (%)	5y OS (%)	MST (y)	3y OS (%)	5y OS (%)	MST (y)		
Milosevic M, et al[28]	2020	2010-2016	Randomized controlled trial	Multicenter	46	47	—	36.4	3.5	—	29.6	3.8	—	—
Siebenhüner AR, et al[30]	2020	2010-2015	Retrospective cohort	National registry	144	663	60.0	—	3.5	44.0	—	2.7	.024	0.73 (0.56-0.97)
			(propensity score adjusted)		77	125	58.9	—	3.4	51.0	—	3.1	.348	0.79 (0.47-1.31)
Davini F, et al[31]	2020	2010-2016	Retrospective cohort	Single center	210	—	74.0	54.0		—	—	—	—	—
Rapicetta C, et al[32]	2019	2000-2016	Retrospective cohort	Single center	344	—		61.9		—	—	—	—	—
Margalit O, et al[33]	2019	2000-2014	Retrospective cohort	National registry	—	4498	—	—	—	—	—	1.4	—	—

Abbreviations: 3y, 3 year; 5y, 5 year; CI, confidence interval; HR, hazard ratio; MST, median survival time; OS, overall survival.

the criteria for pulmonary resection are: (a) the patient should be capable of tolerating the surgery; (b) the primary tumor has been controlled or can be controlled; (c) the metastatic lung tumor can be completely resected; (d) there are no extrapulmonary metastases or they can be controlled; and (e) the function of the remaining lung will be adequate; however, specific eligibility criteria are not specified. Although numerous studies have been published using the data on survival after surgical resection of pulmonary metastases, identifying the best prognostic factors remains an unsolved problem.

Previous reports have listed high carcinoembryonic antigen (CEA) levels, disease-free interval (DFI) from primary resection to metastasis, number of metastases, and hilar mediastinal lymph node metastasis as the prognostic factors. A multicenter retrospective study in Japan showed that a DFI of <2 y, presence of extrathoracic lesions, high CEA level, three or more pulmonary metastases, and age >70 y were significantly associated with poor prognosis.[36] To date, numerous studies have reported that high CEA levels before pulmonary resection correlate with a poor prognosis. However, the cutoff value is not clear, and the CEA value alone is not a criterion as an indication for resection.

Regarding DFI, Yokoyama et al[37] identified short DFI (<24 mo) and N2 of the primary lesion as risk factors for recurrence after pulmonary resection, but not for survival. Other reports have similarly identified DFI as a risk of recurrence; however, a cutoff for DFI was reported as 36 mo by Davini et al,[31] while it was determined to be 12 mo by Rapicetta et al.[32] It is a convincing theory that DFI is a predictor of prognosis, as shorter DFI are expected to be biologically more malignant. However, the cutoff period has not yet been established because there is a great deal of variability in the optimal period.

Several studies have been conducted on the effect of the number of pulmonary metastases on prognosis. Although Pfannschmidt et al[18] reported that patients with up to four lung metastases showed a significantly better overall survival compared with patients with more than four metastatic lesions, most reported that the patients eligible for pulmonary resection had a single metastasis, based on the results that a single metastasis had a better prognosis.[20,24,38] On the other hand, Yokoyama et al[37] pointed out that the number of metastases did not become a prognostic factor, and proposed that the recent advances in thin-slice CT images and the development of chemotherapy have had a major impact on the results. The same opinion has been proposed in a meta-analysis by Gonzalez et al,[21] and with the recent increase in the ability of CT images, we may have to be careful in interpreting the results of previous reports.

The presence of hilar/mediastinal lymph node metastases in several reports has been reported to lead to a poor prognosis.[21,39] However, some studies have reported that it does not affect the prognosis.[31] It is considered that the small number of objects has been a limitation in previous analyses, because dissection of the hilar/mediastinal lymph nodes is not a routine procedure in the pulmonary resection for pulmonary metastases. The surgical indications for pulmonary metastasis with hilar/mediastinal lymph node metastases and their effects on the prognosis of lymph node dissection are still controversial.

Regarding the prognosis of patients with pulmonary metastases with a history of hepatectomy, a meta-analysis and a systematic review in 2013 showed that a history of hepatectomy was not associated with an increased risk of death.[21] Contrastingly, a subsequent large-scale meta-analysis confirmed a history of liver metastases as a poor prognostic factor for pulmonary resection.[40] However, in the same study the survival rates were comparable between heterogeneous and simultaneous liver and lung metastases. Although these reports are meta-analyses and have a large number of cases, the interpretation of these results must be carefully performed due to the conspicuous heterogeneity of the patient background. Notably, the history of hepatectomy or the presence of concurrent liver metastases does not appear to be a contraindication for surgery for pulmonary metastases at this time. Additionally, these two meta-analyses identified other poor prognostic factors. Gonzalez et al[21] found that short DFI, lymph node infiltration, multiple metastases, and high CEA values were poor prognostic factors. In addition to the above four factors, Zabaleta et al[40] identified three factors with positive resection margins, large tumor diameters, and a history of liver metastasis as poor prognostic factors.

Davini et al[31] recently conducted a retrospective cohort study concerning resection margins and reported that shorter margins correlate with poorer prognoses, with distances of 2 cm or more having the best prognosis. Pulmonary-sparing surgery, such as the wedge resection, is desirable if possible, considering pulmonary recurrence after pulmonary resection. However, since it is a prerequisite to secure a sufficient margin for resection, further discussions including surgical procedures, such as wedge resection and anatomical resection, and approach methods such as open surgery or video-assisted thoracic surgery are necessary.

2.3 | Perioperative chemotherapy

The recurrence rates after the resection of pulmonary metastases of colorectal cancer have been reported to be high,[31,41] and recurrence after pulmonary resection remains a concern. Although the effectiveness of various additional chemotherapies has been investigated to reduce recurrence, no studies have prospectively examined preoperative and postoperative chemotherapy. To date, it is debatable whether perioperative chemotherapy contributes to prolonged survival before and after resection of pulmonary metastases from colorectal cancer.

Several retrospective studies and reviews have reported that perioperative chemotherapy improves the prognosis.[31,42,43] However, recent meta-analyses have reached different conclusions. Li and Qin[44] performed a meta-analysis of eight studies and found perioperative chemotherapy to be a prognostic factor for favorable overall survival, while Zhang et al[45] analyzed 18 studies and concluded that postoperative chemotherapy did not provide a significant survival benefit. On the other hand, Rapicetta et al[32] reported that neither preoperative chemotherapy nor postoperative chemotherapy improved the prognosis, and that survival was slightly worse in those who received chemotherapy than in those who did not, although the difference was not significant. This may reflect the fact that postoperative chemotherapy is administered in high-risk cases. It is notable that not only do the conclusions vary by study, but all of these are retrospective studies and have different patient backgrounds; thus, these conclusions should be interpreted carefully. In addition, since the regimen is diverse in every report, it is necessary to conduct a well-controlled prospective study to investigate which drug is effective, for how long, and when to perform it.

3 | 3. ALTERNATIVE LOCAL THERAPY

Stereotactic body radiation therapy (SBRT) and radiofrequency ablation (RFA) have recently attracted attention as local treatments that could replace surgical resection. These therapies meet the standards required for local treatment in terms of the feasibility for patients with poor lung function, lung preservation, and repeatability. A Danish national statistical survey reported an increase in the number of minimally invasive SBRT and RFA treatments for liver and pulmonary metastases over the last 14 y.[46] Of these, surgical resection demonstrated a higher survival rate than SBRT or RFA, while multivariate analysis showed no significant difference. These treatment selection criteria are not the same, and it is generally considered that RFA/SBRT be selected for patients who are not eligible for surgical resection. No clinical trial has directly compared these three modalities.

3.1 | 3.1. Stereotactic body radiation therapy

SBRT provides an accurate irradiation of lesions and minimal radiation exposure to surrounding normal tissues, making it an alternative treatment option for metastatic resection. SBRT is recommended when surgery cannot be considered, even with the ESMO or NCCN guidelines. In Japanese guidelines, SBRT should be considered when surgery is not tolerated, primary lesions and extrapulmonary metastases are controlled, and the number of metastatic lung tumors is within 5 cm is 3 or less.

Choi et al[12] conducted a meta-analysis of 14 studies and examined 495 patients who underwent SBRT for pulmonary metastases. The 5-y overall survival (OS) rate was 43.0%, the local control rate was 61.8%, and the adverse events of grade 3 or higher were observed in 2.2%. This is comparable to the reports of retrospective trials of pulmonary metastasis resection and the prospective randomized study (PulMiCC) mentioned above. The fact that the results were comparable to resection in this study, which included many cases that were not indicated for pulmonary resection, suggests that SBRT is a candidate for alternative treatment. In contrast, the local control rate after SBRT for pulmonary metastases from colorectal cancer has been reported to be worse than that for pulmonary metastases from other primary sites.[47] As another treatment option, Takahashi et al[48] showed that carbon ion radiotherapy (CIRT) could achieve a good local control rate for lung metastases from colorectal cancer without serious side effects, and patients with single lung metastases from colorectal cancer are the best candidates for CIRT.

However, the average number of metastases per patient treated with SBRT and CIRT was 1.4 and 1, respectively, and the therapeutic effect of multiple lesions was unknown. As mentioned above, assuming that the number of pulmonary metastases suitable for pulmonary resection is one, SBRT and CIRT are not only an alternative treatment but also a sufficiently powerful treatment option. However, the treatment targets of these therapies are still limited.

3.2 | 3.2. Radiofrequency ablation

RFA has been widely used in the last decade as a local treatment alternative to surgical treatment. In an international study in 2004, RFA was reported as a useful minimally invasive tool for local treatment with low mortality and complications. Long-term survival for RFA treatment has also been reported, with a median OS of 52 mo in a recent report, compared to 33–50 mo in the past.[49,50] A systematic review of 903 patients in eight studies summarized that RFA is a safe and effective treatment for pulmonary metastases of colorectal cancer, with 5-y survival rates ranging from 20%–54% and serious complications from 0.5%–8%.[13]

Since RFA is less invasive than surgical resection and is advantageous for lung preservation, it is considered a suitable treatment for cases in which surgery is not indicated or repeated treatment is expected. However, Hiyoshi et al[49] reported that ≥15 mm is an independent poor prognostic factor, which limits its indications as an alternative to surgical treatment. In addition, most retrospective studies are mixed cohorts of surgical resection and other local treatments and systemic chemotherapy, and there have been insufficient analyses of the oncologic prognosis of RFA alone. Therefore, several authors have stated that prospective randomized controlled trials are required.

Recently, alternatives to RFA, such as microwave ablation and cryoablation, have been developed and reported to be effective in local control; however, there is not yet enough evidence for them to be useful in clinical practice.[51,52]

4 | 4. COMMENTS

In the past, resection was considered the only effective treatment for pulmonary metastases; in fact, some guidelines such as NCCN and ESMO also recommend resection. The Japanese guidelines also weakly recommend resection. However, numerous reports in recent years have cast doubt on this stereotype.

SBRT is beginning to show results that are less toxic to patients in poor condition and leads to long-term survival. Although RFA is restricted in its indications due to tumor size and other factors, it offers the advantage of local control, such as the ability to perform repeated treatments. Resection, SBRT, and RFA are still local treatments for pulmonary metastases. From that point of view, it is understandable that these outcomes are similar.

Recent chemotherapy has made rapid progress, and the development and progress of various chemotherapies have made it possible to significantly extend survival. Currently, several patients achieved long-term survival without surgery. If distant metastasis is considered a systemic disease, the underlying treatment is systemic therapy, that is, chemotherapy. Given that these local therapies act on some of the diseases, it is evident that chemotherapy is a major factor in determining the ultimate survival. The PulMiCC trial is a notable suggestion, albeit a discontinued trial.

Although the survival benefits of pulmonary resection for pulmonary metastases from colorectal cancer are controversial, it is true that some patients will benefit from long-term survival or cure from pulmonary resection of pulmonary metastases. Local treatment needs to be sought for its potential to be an extremely effective tool for a more optimized patient population.

Well-controlled prospective trials that directly compare resection with these treatments are not yet sufficient. However, in this era of advanced chemotherapy, the time may no longer allow us to continue to advocate resection as the only curative strategy. It is time for us to build a new strategy for the next era.

ACKNOWLEDGMENT

We thank Editage (www.editage.com) for editing the draft of this article.

REFERENCES

1. Siegel RL, Miller KD, Jemal A. Cancer statistics, 2020. CA Cancer J Clin. 2020;70(1):7–30.
2. Cancer Registry and Statistics. Cancer Information Service, National Cancer Center, Japan (Vital Statistics of Japan).
3. Cancer Registry and Statistics. Cancer Information Service, National Cancer Center, Japan (Ministry of Health, Labour and Welfare, National Cancer Registry).
4. Monitoring of cancer incidence in Japan - survival 2009-2011 report. Tokyo: Center for Cancer Control and Information Services, National Cancer Center; 2020.
5. Disibio G, French SW. Metastatic patterns of cancers: results from a large autopsy study. Arch Pathol Lab Med. 2008;132(6):931–9.
6. Elferink MA, de Jong KP, Klaase JM, Siemerink EJ, de Wilt JH. Metachronous metastases from colorectal cancer: a population-based study in North-East Netherlands. Int J Colorectal Dis. 2015;30(2):205–12.
7. Scheithauer W, Rosen H, Kornek GV, Sebesta C, Depisch D. Randomised comparison of combination chemotherapy plus supportive care with supportive care alone in patients with metastatic colorectal cancer. BMJ. 1993;306(6880):752–5.
8. Loupakis F, Cremolini C, Masi G, Lonardi S, Zagonel V, Salvatore L, et al. Initial therapy with FOLFOXIRI and bevacizumab for metastatic colorectal cancer. N Engl J Med. 2014;371(17):1609–18.
9. Van Cutsem E, Cervantes A, Adam R, Sobrero A, Van Krieken JH, Aderka D, et al. ESMO consensus guidelines for the management of patients with metastatic colorectal cancer. Ann Oncol. 2016;27(8):1386–422.
10. National Comprehensive Cancer Network. NCCN guidelines for colon cancer, version 2.2017 [updated 2017 Mar; cited 2020 Dec 31]. Available from https://www.nccn.org
11. Hashiguchi Y, Muro K, Saito Y, Ito Y, Ajioka Y, Hamaguchi T, et al. Japanese Society for Cancer of the Colon and Rectum (JSCCR) guidelines 2019 for the treatment of colorectal cancer. Int J Clin Oncol. 2020;25(1):1–42.
12. Choi HS, Jeong BK, Kang KM, Jeong H, Song JH, Ha IB, et al. Tumor control and overall survival after stereotactic body radiotherapy for pulmonary oligometastases from colorectal cancer: a meta-analysis. Cancer Res Treat. 2020;52(4):1188–98.
13. Lyons NJ, Pathak S, Daniels IR, Spiers A, Smart NJ. Percutaneous management of pulmonary metastases arising from colorectal cancer; a systematic review. Eur J Surg Oncol. 2015;41(11):1447–55.
14. Riquet M, Foucault C, Cazes A, Mitry E, Dujon A, Le Pimpec Barthes F, et al. Pulmonary resection for metastases of colorectal adenocarcinoma. Ann Thorac Surg. 2010;89(2):375–80.
15. Vatandoust S, Price TJ, Karapetis CS. Colorectal cancer: metastases to a single organ. World J Gastroenterol. 2015;21(41):11767–76.
16. Shimizu H, Okada M, Tangoku A, Doki Y, Endo S, Fukuda H, et al. Thoracic and cardiovascular surgeries in Japan during 2017: annual report by the Japanese Association for Thoracic Surgery. Gen Thorac Cardiovasc Surg. 2020;68(4):414–49.
17. Murakawa T. Past, present, and future perspectives of pulmonary metastasectomy for patients with advanced colorectal cancer. Surg Today. 2021;51(2):204–11.
18. Pfannschmidt J, Muley T, Hoffmann H, Dienemann H. Prognostic factors and survival after complete resection of pulmonary metastases from colorectal carcinoma: experiences in 167 patients. J Thorac Cardiovasc Surg. 2003;126(3):732–9.
19. Saito Y, Omiya H, Kohno K, Kobayashi T, Itoi K, Teramachi M, et al. Pulmonary metastasectomy for 165 patients with colorectal carcinoma: a prognostic assessment. J Thorac Cardiovasc Surg. 2002;124(5):1007–13.
20. Zampino MG, Maisonneuve P, Ravenda PS, Magni E, Casiraghi M, Solli P, et al. Lung metastases from colorectal cancer: analysis of prognostic factors in a single institution study. Ann Thorac Surg. 2014;98(4):1238–45.
21. Gonzalez M, Poncet A, Combescure C, Robert J, Ris HB, Gervaz P. Risk factors for survival after lung metastasectomy in colorectal cancer patients: a systematic review and meta-analysis. Ann Surg Oncol. 2013;20(2):572–9.
22. Hishida T, Tsuboi M, Okumura T, Boku N, Ohde Y, Sakao Y, et al. Does repeated lung resection provide long-term survival for recurrent pulmonary metastases of colorectal cancer? Results of a retrospective Japanese Multicenter Study. Ann Thorac Surg. 2017;103(2):399–405.
23. Menna C, Berardi G, Tierno SM, Andreetti C, Maurizi G, Ciccone AM, et al. Do repeated operations for recurrent colorectal lung metastases result in improved survival? Ann Thorac Surg. 2018;106(2):421–7.
24. Watanabe K, Nagai K, Kobayashi A, Sugito M, Saito N. Factors influencing survival after complete resection of pulmonary metastases from colorectal cancer. Br J Surg. 2009;96(9):1058–65.
25. Hirosawa T, Itabashi M, Ohnuki T, Yamaguchi N, Sugihara K, Kameoka S, et al. Prognostic factors in patients undergoing complete resection of pulmonary metastases of colorectal cancer: a multi-institutional cumulative follow-up study. Surg Today. 2013;43(5):494–9.
26. Åberg T, Malmberg K-Å, Nilsson B, Nõu E. The effect of metastasectomy: fact or fiction? Ann Thorac Surg. 1980;30(4):378–84.
27. Treasure T, Farewell V, Macbeth F, Monson K, Williams NR, Brew-Graves C, et al. Pulmonary metastasectomy versus continued active monitoring in colorectal cancer (PulMiCC): a multicentre randomised clinical trial. Trials. 2019;20(1):718.

28. Milosevic M, Edwards J, Tsang D, Dunning J, Shackcloth M, Batchelor T, et al. Pulmonary metastasectomy in colorectal cancer: updated analysis of 93 randomized patients – control survival is much better than previously assumed. Colorectal Dis. 2020;22(10):1314–24.
29. Zhang GQ, Taylor JP, Stem M, Almaazmi H, Efron JE, Atallah C, et al. Aggressive multimodal treatment and metastatic colorectal cancer survival. J Am Coll Surg. 2020;230(4):689–98.
30. Siebenhüner AR, Guller U, Warschkow R. Population-based SEER analysis of survival in colorectal cancer patients with or without resection of lung and liver metastases. BMC Cancer. 2020;20(1):246.
31. Davini F, Ricciardi S, Zirafa CC, Romano G, Alì G, Fontanini G, et al. Lung metastasectomy after colorectal cancer: prognostic impact of resection margin on long term survival, a retrospective cohort study. Int J Colorectal Dis. 2020;35(1):9–18.
32. Rapicetta C, Lococo F, Davini F, Carleo F, Kauppi J, Di Stefano TS, et al. Is adjuvant chemotherapy worthwhile after radical resection for single lung metastasis from colorectal cancer? A multicentric analysis evaluating the risk of recurrence. Front Oncol. 2019;9:763.
33. Margalit O, Shacham-Shmueli E, Lawrence YR, Yang Y-X, Reiss KA, Golan T, et al. Lung metastasis predicts better prognosis in metastatic colorectal cancer with mutated KRAS. Clin Colorectal Cancer. 2019;18(3):e300–7.
34. Li CL, Tang DR, Ji J, Zang B, Chen C, Zhao JQ. Colorectal adenocarcinoma patients with M1a diseases gain more clinical benefits from palliative primary tumor resection than those with M1b diseases: a propensity score matching analysis. World J Clin Cases. 2020;8(15):3230–9.
35. Thomford NR, Woolner LB, Clagett OT. The surgical treatment of metastatic tumors in the lungs. J Thorac Cardiovasc Surg. 1965;49(3):357–63.
36. Okumura T, Boku N, Hishida T, Ohde Y, Sakao Y, Yoshiya K, et al. Surgical outcome and prognostic stratification for pulmonary metastasis from colorectal cancer. Ann Thorac Surg. 2017;104(3):979–87.
37. Yokoyama S, Mitsuoka M, Kinugasa T, Hashiguchi T, Matsumoto R, Murakami D, et al. Survival after initial lung metastasectomy for metastatic colorectal cancer in the modern chemotherapeutic era. BMC Surg. 2017;17(1):54.
38. Cho JH, Kim S, Namgung MI, Choi YS, Kim HK, Zo JI, et al. The prognostic importance of the number of metastases in pulmonary metastasectomy of colorectal cancer. World J Surg Oncol. 2015;13:222.
39. Iida T, Nomori H, Shiba M, Nakajima J, Okumura S, Horio H, et al. Prognostic factors after pulmonary metastasectomy for colorectal cancer and rationale for determining surgical indications: a retrospective analysis. Ann Surg. 2013;257(6):1059–64.
40. Zabaleta J, Iida T, Falcoz PE, Salah S, Jarabo JR, Correa AM, et al. Individual data meta-analysis for the study of survival after pulmonary metastasectomy in colorectal cancer patients: A history of resected liver metastases worsens the prognosis. Eur J Surg Oncol. 2018;44(7):1006–12.
41. Guerrera F, Mossetti C, Ceccarelli M, Bruna MC, Bora G, Olivetti S, et al. Surgery of colorectal cancer lung metastases: analysis of survival, recurrence and re-surgery. J Thorac Dis. 2016;8(7):1764–71.
42. Guerrera F, Falcoz PE, Renaud S, Massard G. Does perioperative chemotherapy improve survival in patients with resectable lung metastases of colorectal cancer? Interact Cardiovasc Thorac Surg. 2017;24(5):789–91.
43. Nakajima J, Iida T, Okumura S, Horio H, Asamura H, Ozeki Y, et al. Recent improvement of survival prognosis after pulmonary metastasectomy and advanced chemotherapy for patients with colorectal cancer. Eur J Cardiothorac Surg. 2017;51(5):869–73.
44. Li Y, Qin Y. Peri-operative chemotherapy for resectable colorectal lung metastasis: a systematic review and meta-analysis. J Cancer Res Clin Oncol. 2020;146(3):545–53.
45. Zhang C, Tan Y, Xu H. Does adjuvant chemotherapy improve the prognosis of patients after resection of pulmonary metastasis from colorectal cancer? A systematic review and meta-analysis. Int J Colorectal Dis. 2019;34(10):1661–71.
46. Boysen AK, Spindler K-L, Høyer M, Mortensen FV, Christensen TD, Farkas DK, et al. Metastasis directed therapy for liver and lung metastases from colorectal cancer – a population-based study. Int J Cancer. 2018;143(12):3218–26.
47. Takeda A, Kunieda E, Ohashi T, Aoki Y, Koike N, Takeda T. Stereotactic body radiotherapy (SBRT) for oligometastatic lung tumors from colorectal cancer and other primary cancers in comparison with primary lung cancer. Radiother Oncol. 2011;101(2):255–9.
48. Takahashi W, Nakajima M, Yamamoto N, Yamada S, Yamashita H, Nakagawa K, et al. Carbon ion radiotherapy for oligo-recurrent lung metastases from colorectal cancer: a feasibility study. Radiat Oncol. 2014;9:68.
49. Hiyoshi Y, Miyamoto Y, Kiyozumi Y, Sawayama H, Eto K, Nagai Y, et al. CT-guided percutaneous radiofrequency ablation for lung metastases from colorectal cancer. Int J Clin Oncol. 2019;24(3):288–95.
50. Zhong J, Palkhi E, Ng H, Wang K, Milton R, Chaudhuri N, et al. Long-term outcomes in percutaneous radiofrequency ablation for histologically proven colorectal lung metastasis. Cardiovasc Intervent Radiol. 2020;43(12):1900–7.
51. Prud'homme C, Deschamps F, Moulin B, Hakime A, Al-Ahmar M, Moalla S, et al. Image-guided lung metastasis ablation: a literature review. Int J Hyperthermia. 2019;36(2):37–45.
52. Yuan Z, Wang Y, Zhang J, Zheng J, Li W. A meta-analysis of clinical outcomes after radiofrequency ablation and microwave ablation for lung cancer and pulmonary metastases. J Am Coll Radiol. 2019;16(3):302–14.

2

Clinical impact of the triple-layered circular stapler for reducing the anastomotic leakage in rectal cancer surgery: Porcine model and multicenter retrospective cohort analysis

Ryota Nakanishi[1] | Yoshiaki Fujimoto[2] | Masahiko Sugiyama[2] | Yuichi Hisamatsu[1] | Tomonori Nakanoko[1] | Koji Ando[1] | Mitsuhiko Ota[1] | Yasue Kimura[1] | Eiji Oki[1] | Tomoharu Yoshizumi[1]

[1]Department of Surgery and Science, Graduate School of Medical Sciences, Kyushu University, Fukuoka, Japan

[2]Department of Gastroenterological Surgery, National Hospital Organization Kyushu Cancer Center, Fukuoka, Japan

Correspondence
Ryota Nakanishi, Department of Surgery and Science, Graduate School of Medical Sciences, Kyushu University, Maidashi 3-1-1, Higashi-ku, Fukuoka, 812-8582, Japan.
Email: naka12030930@gmail.com

Abstract

Aim: To investigate the impact of the triple-layered circular stapler compared with the double-layered circular stapler on anastomotic leakage after rectal cancer surgery.

Methods: The bursting pressure was compared between porcine ileocolic anastomoses created using a double- or triple-layered stapler. We also retrospectively analyzed the incidence of severe anastomotic leakage in 194 patients who underwent colorectal anastomosis using a double- or triple-layered circular stapler during rectal cancer resection performed in two cancer centers between January 2015 and April 2021.

Results: In the porcine model, the bursting pressure was higher in anastomoses created using the triple-layered stapler than the double-layered stapler (end-to-end anastomosis: 26.4 ± 6.2 mm Hg vs 14.5 ± 4.3 mm Hg, $P = .0031$; side-to-side anastomosis: 27.7 ± 5.0 mm Hg vs 18.0 ± 2.9 mm Hg, $P = .0275$). Intersectional leakage occurred in 41% and 83% of anastomoses created using the triple- or double-layered stapler, respectively ($P = .0821$). In the clinical cohort, the double- and triple-layered stapler was used in 153 and 41 patients, respectively. The incidence of anastomotic leakage was lower for anastomoses created using the triple-layered stapler vs the double-layered stapler (0.0% vs 5.8%, $P = .0362$). In multivariate analysis, the factors independently associated with a lower incidence of anastomotic leakage were female sex (odds ratio: 0.16, 95% confidence interval: 0.01-0.90, $P = .0354$) and triple-layered stapler usage (odds ratio: 0.00, 95% confidence interval: 0.00-0.96, $P = .0465$).

Conclusion: Anastomoses created using a triple-layered circular stapler had high bursting pressure, which might contribute to a lower incidence of anastomotic leakage after rectal cancer surgery.

KEYWORDS
anastomotic leak, colorectal surgery, postoperative complications, rectal neoplasms, surgical instruments

1 | INTRODUCTION

In rectal cancer surgery, the most common major postoperative complication is anastomotic leakage (AL).[1,2] A systematic review and meta-analysis showed that AL after anterior resection for rectal cancer has a negative effect on local recurrence and long-term survival.[3,4] AL is also associated with permanent stoma development, fecal incontinence, and reduced sexual activity, which negatively affect patients' long-term quality of life.[5-7] Furthermore, AL greatly increases the medical costs.[8] Based on investigations in large patient cohorts, the reported incidence of AL after rectal resection varies from 6.3% to 13.7%.[9-12] Some techniques or procedures to prevent AL have been reported, but further improvement is needed.

Recently, the EEA™ Circular Stapler with Tri-Staple™ Technology (tri-EEA) (Medtronic Japan, Tokyo, Japan) was released as the first triple-layered circular stapler, which is expected to decrease the incidence of AL. The tri-EEA has three rows of staples that vary in height, whereas the previously released EEA™ Circular Stapler with DST Series™ Technology (EEA) (Medtronic Japan) deploys two rows of uniform-height staples.[13] In the tri-EEA, the staples closest to the lumen have the shortest height to provide the greatest occlusion and barrier to leaks and bleeding. The second and third rows, each incrementally higher, contribute strength to the closure line. To the best of our knowledge, no study has evaluated the impact of the tri-EEA on the anastomotic bursting pressure and incidence of AL in a clinical cohort compared with EEA.

This study was performed to compare the bursting pressure of anastomoses created using the tri-EEA vs the EEA in a porcine model and to evaluate whether the incidence of AL in a multicenter clinical cohort was lower after rectal cancer surgery using the tri-EEA than the EEA.

2 | METHODS

2.1 | Porcine model

Commercially available small intestine and colon specimens from healthy 6-month-old Japanese domestic pigs weighing 100 to 110 kg were used in this study, which was conducted in full accordance with the principles of the Helsinki Institutional Review Board for animal studies. End-to-end anastomosis using the double-stapling technique (DST) was performed as previously described.[14] The colon was closed and cut with a linear stapler using the Signia™ Stapling System (Tri-Staple™ 60-mm purple cartridge; Medtronic Japan). The small intestine was fitted with a 3-0 Polysorb™ (Medtronic Japan) purse-string suture around the open stump. The anvil head of the circular stapler (EEA or tri-EEA) was placed at the edge of the stump, and the anvil shaft was secured. The instrument of the circular stapler was inserted through the open stump of the colon and advanced to the closed stump. The colon wall was penetrated by the center rod of the instrument just beside the colonic closure line. The anvil shaft and the center rod were joined and closed, and the instrument was activated and removed. After anastomosis, it was confirmed that the mucosal layer, muscular layer, and serosa layer were detected without any defect in the entire circumference of both rings that were attached to the instrument.

The side-to-side anastomosis was performed as previously described.[14] The anvil head was inserted through the open stump of the small intestine and advanced to the closed stump. The tip of the anvil head was penetrated through the antimesenteric site 2 cm from the closed stump so that the linear staple line and the anvil head did not overlap. The instrument of the circular stapler was inserted into open stump of the colon and advanced to the closed stump. The center rod was brought through the colonic wall 2 cm from the closed stump so that the linear staple line and the circular staple line did not overlap. The anvil shaft and center rod were then joined and closed, and the instrument was activated and removed. The completion of both rings was confirmed as described for the end-to-end anastomosis.

An anastomotic bursting pressure test was performed after the completion of each anastomosis. Both stumps that were not anastomosed were clamped, and a sensor cord was inserted inside the anastomotic site. Air leakage was monitored by placing the specimen in a water-filled basin and observing the water to detect escaped air bubbles. When air leakage began, the bursting pressure was measured using an electronic manometer (PG-100N-102GP; Nidec Copal Electronics, Tokyo, Japan). The leakage site was evaluated to determine whether it was located at the intersection. All experiments were performed in accordance with relevant institutional and national guidelines and regulations for the care and use of animals.

2.2 | Patients and specimens

A retrospective multicenter study was performed across two comprehensive cancer centers (Kyushu University and National Hospital Organization Kyushu Cancer Center). Of 536 consecutive patients who underwent surgical resection of rectal malignancies and colorectal anastomosis between January 2015 and April 2021, we analyzed 194 patients who underwent colorectal anastomosis using the EEA or the tri-EEA. We excluded patients in whom other instruments were used for anastomosis, such as the PROXIMATE™ intraluminal stapler (Johnson & Johnson, Tokyo, Japan) or the ECHELON CIRCULAR™ Powered Stapler (Johnson & Johnson) (n = 326), and those who received preoperative chemoradiotherapy (n = 16). The clinicopathological background data were extracted from the database at each hospital. All patients, except those with bowel obstruction, underwent mechanical bowel preparation with magnesium citrate and sennoside on the day before surgery. Surgical procedures were performed or supervised by expert colorectal surgeons qualified by the Endoscopic Surgical Skill Qualification System of Japan,[15] each of whom had performed more than 200 laparoscopic colorectal operations.

2.3 | Rectal resection and colorectal anastomosis

The inferior mesenteric artery was clipped and cut at the root, and the left colic artery and inferior mesenteric vein were clipped and cut at the same level. The marginal vessels were preserved. Tumor-specific mesorectal excision was performed. After clamping the rectum on the anal side of the tumor, the anal canal was washed thoroughly through the anus. The rectum was cut using the Signia™ Stapling System (Tri-Staple™ 60-mm purple cartridge). After removing the specimen through the abdominal incision, the anastomosis was performed. End-to-end anastomosis was performed using the DST as previously described.[16] Side-to-side anastomosis was performed using a previously described method.[17] We previously reported that the side-to-side anastomosis was a safe and useful procedure in anastomosis after rectal resection.[18] In this study, the type of anastomosis was selected at the surgeon's discretion, and there was no specific indication for each procedure. If the surgeon intended to perform side-to-side anastomosis for very low anterior resection, side-to-end anastomosis was sometimes selected because the stump of the rectum was too short to anastomose to the side wall. Therefore, side-to-end anastomoses were performed with intersection of the circular and linear staple lines of the remnant rectum. After division of the patients according to whether such intersections were present, we included side-to-end anastomosis in the end-to-end anastomosis group. An air leak test was performed after each anastomosis, and it was confirmed that no anastomoses had an air leak. Reinforcement was performed at the surgeon's discretion regardless of the leak test result or the anastomosis type. The reinforcement was not always performed at the intersection; some surgeons performed it only at the non-intersection site. A closed drain was placed behind the anastomotic site in all cases. A transanal drainage tube was placed when considered necessary by the surgeon.

2.4 | Postoperative management

Oral intake started on postoperative day 3, and the transanal tube was removed on the same day. The intra-abdominal drain was removed on postoperative day 4. Postoperative complications that occurred during hospitalization and within 90 days after surgery were extracted and classified using the Clavien-Dindo (CD) system. If patients developed postoperative complications such as fever, abdominal and/or pelvic pain, or elevated inflammatory markers, radiological examinations (computed tomography [CT] and/or transanal enema examination) were performed. AL was diagnosed when a communication between the intra- and extraluminal compartments caused by a defect of the intestinal wall integrity at the anastomosis was detected by CT and/or transanal enema examination.[19] In this study, we focused on AL requiring active therapeutic interventional drainage, transanal drainage, or reoperation (CD grade ≥3). The site of leakage was determined by identification of the defect on CT or endoscopy. If AL was detected, reoperation was performed

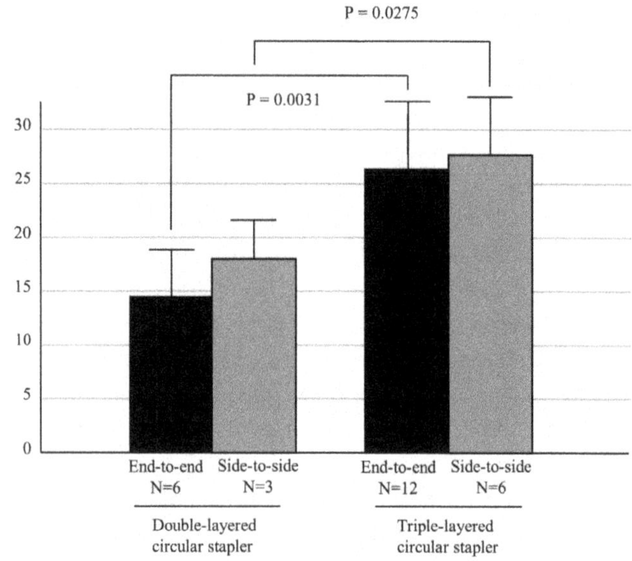

FIGURE 1 Bursting pressure of anastomoses created using the double- or triple-layered circular stapler. Black bars: end-to-end anastomoses; grey bars: side-to-side anastomoses

in patients who had no covering stoma, and interventional drainage or transanal drainage was performed in patients who had a covering stoma. We considered reoperation if the infection could not be controlled by drainage. In patients who underwent covering ileostomy, AL was examined not only during hospitalization and within 90 days after surgery but also after stoma closure (however, no patients in this study developed AL after stoma closure).

2.5 | Statistical analysis

Continuous variables were analyzed using the Mann-Whitney U-test, while categorical valuables were analyzed with Pearson's χ^2 test or Fisher's exact test, as appropriate. A P value of <.05 was considered significant. Statistical analysis was performed using JMP® software version 10.0.2 (SAS Institute).

3 | RESULTS

3.1 | Impact of the triple-layered circular stapler on anastomotic bursting pressure in a porcine model

The bursting pressure was measured in a total of 27 anastomoses. End-to-end anastomosis (using the DST) was performed six times using the EEA and 12 times using the tri-EEA. Side-to-side anastomosis was performed three times using the EEA and six times using the tri-EEA. As shown in Figure 1, the bursting pressure was significantly higher in anastomoses created using the tri-EEA than in those created using the EEA, regardless of the type of anastomosis (end-to-end anastomosis: EEA 14.5 ± 4.3 mm Hg vs tri-EEA 26.4 ± 6.2 mm Hg, P =.0031; side-to-side anastomosis: EEA

18.0 ± 2.9 mm Hg vs tri-EEA 27.7 ± 5.0 mm Hg, *P* =.0275). Among the end-to-end anastomoses, the leakage was located at the intersection site in five of six anastomoses created using the EEA (83%) and in five of 12 anastomoses created using the tri-EEA (41%); however, this difference was not significant (*P* =.0821).

3.2 | Patient characteristics and short-term outcomes

The patient characteristics are summarized in Table 1. The median age was 66 years, 55% were male, and the median body mass index was 21.9 kg/m^2. One hundred and eighty-eight patients had rectal cancer, five had neuroendocrine tumors, and one had an endometrial stromal sarcoma. Among the total cohort, the EEA was used in 153 patients (EEA group) and the tri-EEA was used in 41 patients (tri-EEA group). The prevalence of more advanced rectal cancer (stage III-IV) was higher in the tri-EEA group than in the EEA group (20% vs 1%, *P* <.0001). There were no significant differences between the two groups in other characteristics, including age (*P* =.6976), sex (*P* =.8912), body mass index (*P* =.9763), history of diabetes mellitus (*P* =.2169), preoperative chemotherapy (*P* =.3988), tumor location (*P* =.4058), and maximum tumor diameter (*P* =.6131).

The intraoperative characteristics and short-term outcomes are summarized in Table 2. Compared with the EEA group, the tri-EEA group had a longer operation time (278 minutes vs 227 minutes, *P* =.0042), lower prevalence of laparoscopic surgery (0% vs 7%, *P* =.0270), higher prevalence of side-to-side anastomosis (17% vs 6%, *P* =.0328), and lower prevalence of 25-mm circular stapler usage (0% vs 64%, *P* <.0001). There were no significant differences between the two groups in intraoperative characteristics, such as the prevalence of low anterior resection (61% in the EEA group vs 51% in the tri-EEA group, *P* =.2396) and the use of a transanal tube (86% in the EEA group vs 95% in the tri-EEA group, *P* =.0897). The two groups had similar short-term outcomes, including the postoperative hospital stay (14 days in the EEA group vs 14 days in the tri-EEA group, *P* =.4757) and incidence of all postoperative complications (CD grade ≥3) (8% in the EEA group vs 2% in the tri-EEA group, *P* =.1731). The incidence of AL (CD grade ≥3) was significantly lower in the tri-EEA group than in the EEA group (0.0% vs 5.8%, *P* =.0362).

3.3 | Risk factors for anastomotic leakage

The results of the univariate and multivariate analyses are described in Table 3. In univariate analysis, the factors significantly correlated

TABLE 1 Patients' background

Characteristics	Total N = 194	EEA group N = 153	tri-EEA group N = 41	P value
Age (years), median (IQR)	66 (56.75-71.25)	66 (56.5-71)	67 (56.5-73)	.6976
Gender, No.(%)				
Male	107 (55)	84 (55)	23 (56)	.8912
Female	87 (45)	69 (45)	18 (44)	
Body mass index (kg/m^2), median (IQR)	21.9 (19.6-24.7)	21.8 (19.7-24.5)	22.1 (19.4-24.9)	.9763
Diabetes mellitus yes, No. (%)	12 (6)	11 (7)	1 (2)	.2169
Preoperative chemotherapy yes, No. (%)	13 (7)	9 (6)	4 (10)	.3988
Location, No. (%)				
High rectum	85 (44)	67 (44)	18 (44)	.4058
Middle rectum	83 (43)	68 (44)	15 (37)	
Low rectum	26 (13)	18 (12)	8 (20)	
Pathological stage[a], No. (%)				
I	58 (31)	49 (33)	9 (23)	<.0001
II	53 (28)	41 (28)	12 (30)	
III	68 (37)	57 (39)	11 (28)	
IV	9 (5)	1 (1)	8 (20)	
Maximum tumor diameter (mm), median (IQR)	35 (25-55)	35 (25-53)	40 (29.5-57.5)	.6131
Histologic grade, No. (%)				
Well/moderately differentiated	187 (96)	147 (96)	40 (98)	.7565
Poorly differentiated	1 (1)	1 (1)	0 (0)	
Others[b]	6 (3)	5 (3)	1 (2)	

Abbreviations: BMI: body mass index; EEA, EEA™ Circular Stapler with DST Series™ Technology; IQR, interquartile range; Tri-EEA, EEA™ Circular Stapler with Tri-Staple™ Technology.

[a]Only for rectal cancer patients.

[b]Five neuroendocrine tumor and one endometrial stromal sarcoma.

TABLE 2 Intraoperative characteristics and short-term outcomes

Characteristics	Total N = 194	EEA group N = 153	tri-EEA group N = 41	P value
Duration of operation (min), median (IQR)	237.5 (191.5-301.75)	227 (186-298)	278 (220-341)	.0042
Bleeding (g), median (IQR)	15 (8-30)	15 (10- 30)	15 (5.5-33)	.6967
Intraoperative transfusion, yes, No. (%)	3 (2)	2(1)	1(2)	.6218
Procedure, No. (%)				
Open	10 (5)	10 (7)	0 (0)	.0270
Laparoscopy	184 (95)	143 (93)	41 (100)	
Surgery, No. (%)				
Anterior resection	79 (41)	59 (39)	20 (49)	.2396
Low anterior resection	115 (59)	94 (61)	21 (51)	
Covering stoma, yes, No. (%)	47 (24)	34 (22)	13 (32)	.2181
Type of anastomosis, No. (%)				
End-to-end/Side-to-end	178 (92)	144 (94)	34 (83)	.0328
Side-to-side	16 (8)	9 (6)	7 (17)	
Size of circular stapler (mm), No. (%)				
25	99 (51)	98 (64)	0 (0)	<.0001
28	95 (49)	55 (36)	41 (100)	
Transanal tube, yes, No. (%)	171 (88)	132 (86)	39 (95)	.0897
Postoperative hospital stay (day), median (IQR)	14 (11-19)	14 (11-19)	14 (11.25-24)	.4757
Postoperative complication (CDC≥3), No. (%)				
None	181 (93)	141 (92)	40 (98)	.1731
Present	13 (7)	12 (8)	1 (2)	
Anastomotic leakage (CDC≥3), No. (%)				
None	185 (95)	144 (94)	41 (100)	.0362
Present	9 (5)	9 (6)	0 (0)	

Abbreviations: CDC, Clavien-Dindo Classification; EEA, EEA™ Circular Stapler with DST Series™ Technology; IQR, interquartile range; Tri-EEA, EEA™ Circular Stapler with Tri-Staple™ Technology.

with AL were male sex (*P* =.0247), low anterior resection (*P* =.0444), and the use of the EEA (*P* =.0362). In multivariate analysis adjusted for these factors, the use of the tri-EEA for anastomosis was independently associated with the absence of AL (hazard ratio [HR] [95% confidence interval (CI)]; 0.00 [0.00-0.96], *P* =.0465), while male sex was independently associated with AL (HR [95% CI]; 6.40 [1.12-120.90], *P* =.0354).

3.4 | Details of patients who developed anastomotic leakage

The details of the nine patients with AL are summarized in Table 4. Eight of nine patients were male, and eight had undergone low anterior resection. Three patients had a covering stoma after low anterior resection. All nine patients had a transanal tube. The anastomosis had been performed in an end-to-end fashion with the EEA in all nine patients. The leak was located at the intersection site in six patients and a site other than the intersection in three patients.

4 | DISCUSSION

In this porcine model study and the retrospective clinical cohort analysis, we evaluated the impact of the tri-EEA on the anastomotic strength compared with the previously used EEA. In the porcine model, the anastomoses created using the tri-EEA had significantly higher bursting pressure than those created using the EEA. Furthermore, in the clinical cohort, the patients in whom the tri-EEA was used had a significantly lower incidence of AL than those in whom the EEA was used. Use of the tri-EEA was independently associated with the absence of AL. The present study is the first to demonstrate that triple-layered anastomosis was superior to double-layered anastomosis in patients who underwent rectal resection for rectal malignancies.

Previous studies have shown that the intrarectal pressure measured using high-resolution manometry is 80 mm Hg during simulated defecation and up to 200 mm Hg during squeezing.[20,21] In addition, the peak intrarectal pressure is higher in males than in females, which might contribute to male sex being a reported risk factor for AL.[11,21,22] Although these intrarectal pressures are

TABLE 3 Univariate and multivariate analysis for anastomotic leakage

Variable	Univariate analysis		Multivariate analysis	
	HR (95%CI)	*P* value	HR (95%CI)	*P* value
Sex				
Male vs Female	6.95 (1.24-130.22)	.0247	6.40 (1.12-120.90)	.0354
Age				
≤65 year vs >65 years	0.86 (0.21-3.36)	.8297		
BMI				
≤25 kg/m^2 vs >25 kg/m^2	0.57 (0.14-2.79)	.4543		
Location				
High rectum vs middle/low rectum	0.35 (0.05-1.50)	.1659		
Pathological Stage[a]				
I-II vs III-IV	0.55 (0.13-2.13)	.3769		
Maximum tumor diameter				
≤50 mm vs >50 mm	0.40 (0.08-1.86)	.2371		
Surgery				
Anterior resection vs low anterior resection	0.17 (0.01-0.96)	.0444	4.68 (0.11-1.24)	.0911
Covering stoma				
No vs yes	0.62 (0.16-3.05)	.5281		
Type of anastomosis				
Side-to-side vs end-to-end/side-to-end	0.00 (0.00-5.44)	.2076		
Size of circular stapler				
25 vs 28	0.47 (0.10-1.85)	.2869		
Stapler, No. (%)				
Tri-EEA vs EEA	0.00 (0.00-0.86)	.0362	0.00 (0.00-0.96)	.0465

Abbreviations: BMI, body mass index; CI, confidence interval; EEA, EEA™ Circular Stapler with DST Series™ Technology; HR, hazard ratio; Tri-EEA, EEA™ Circular Stapler with Tri-Staple™ Technology.
[a]Only for rectal cancer.

much higher than the anastomotic bursting pressure in our porcine model, the anastomotic bursting pressure in patients who undergo low anterior resection reportedly becomes much higher at 3-6 months after surgery.[23] Because high intrarectal pressure during defecation can lead to AL, we usually advise patients to maintain soft stool and avoid excess force during defecation for at least 1-2 months after surgery. This gap between the intrarectal pressure and the anastomotic bursting pressure is effectively bridged by the placement of a transanal tube and reinforcing sutures, especially in patients with risk factors such as a short distance from the anastomosis to the anus, male sex, and advanced tumor stage.[24,25] Our study suggests that the higher anastomotic bursting pressure resulting from the use of the tri-EEA may also be effective in preventing AL.

Other than anastomotic strength and intrarectal pressure, it has been reported that the blood flow and tension at the anastomotic site are important factors related to AL.[26-29] A recently proposed technology with which to evaluate the blood flow is indocyanine green fluorescence-guided visualization, and the clinical significance of this method has been reported.[29,30] Some studies have shown that high ligation of the inferior mesenteric artery is associated with a higher risk of AL, although this finding is controversial.[31,32] We do not routinely use indocyanine green fluorescence-guided visualization, and we clip the inferior mesenteric artery at the root, unless the patient has severe arteriosclerosis on CT, because low ligation sometimes leads to tension at the anastomotic site. Selective mobilization of the splenic flexure is an established method for reducing the tension at the anastomotic site.[26,27] We usually perform splenic flexure mobilization when there seems to be tension at the anastomotic site. As a result, our overall incidence of AL was 4.6% (9/194), which is lower than that reported in previous studies with large patient cohorts.[9-12] However, some previous single-institutional retrospective studies have reported very low incidences of AL[22,33]; these institutions would have undertaken their own preventative measures to achieve these low incidences. Because AL is caused by multiple factors, every conceivable precautionary measure should be undertaken to reduce the incidence of AL.

End-to-end anastomosis (using the DST) is often used for anastomosis after rectal resection. Endoscopic evaluation of patients with AL after anastomosis using the DST has shown that AL often occurs at the intersection of the anastomosis lines of the circular stapler and linear stapler.[14] Our porcine model study also showed

TABLE 4 Details of patients with anastomotic leakage

No.	Sex	Age	BMI	Location	Preoperative chemotherapy	Pathological Stage	Surgery	Covering stoma	Type of anastomosis	Transanal tube	EEA/tri-EEA	Site of leakage
1	F	24	14.5	Middle rectum	None	IIIB	LAR	None	End-to-end	Present	EEA	Not intersection
2	M	87	20.5	Middle rectum	None	IIIB	LAR	None	End-to-end	Present	EEA	Intersection
3	M	64	29.0	Middle rectum	None	IIIA	LAR	Present	End-to-end	Present	EEA	Intersection
4	M	62	21.6	Upper rectum	None	IIIB	LAR	None	End-to-end	Present	EEA	Intersection
5	M	81	24.4	Middle rectum	None	II	LAR	Present	End-to-end	Present	EEA	Intersection
6	M	61	28.5	Middle rectum	None	II	LAR	None	End-to-end	Present	EEA	Intersection
7	M	75	20.9	Lower rectum	None	I	LAR	None	End-to-end	Present	EEA	Not intersection
8	M	67	27.1	Middle rectum	None	II	LAR	Present	End-to-end	Present	EEA	Not intersection
9	M	69	19.6	Upper rectum	None	IIIA	AR	None	End-to-end	Present	EEA	Intersection

Abbreviations: AR, anterior resection; BMI, body mass index; EEA, EEA™ Circular Stapler with DST Series™ Technology; F, female; LAR, low anterior resection; M, male; Tri-EEA, EEA™ Circular Stapler with Tri-Staple™ Technology.

that five of six anastomoses created with the EEA were ruptured at the intersection. In our clinical cohort study, the intersection was ruptured in six of nine patients with AL, and the EEA had been used in all nine of these patients. This finding indicates the presence of a structural weakness at the intersection of anastomoses created with the EEA via the DST. In contrast, less than half of the anastomoses created with the tri-EEA in our porcine model were ruptured at the intersection. Although the difference in the incidence of rupture at the intersection between the EEA and tri-EEA groups was not significant, our results might suggest that the tri-EEA reduces the vulnerability of the intersection. In our porcine model, the anastomoses created with the tri-EEA had a significantly higher bursting pressure than those created with the EEA, even in side-to-side anastomoses that have no intersection. This implies that the use of triple-layered stapler leads to higher bursting pressure at the circular anastomosis line than the use of the double-layered stapler. Side-to-side anastomosis reportedly produces a superior bursting pressure than that produced by end-to-end anastomosis.[18] Although it is possible that the use of the side-to-side anastomosis technique affected the incidence of AL in the present study, the univariate and multivariate analyses did not prove that side-to-side anastomosis had a significant impact on the development of AL. Finally, we observed no AL in any patients in the tri-EEA group. This suggests that AL after colorectal anastomosis with the tri-EEA might be rare in appropriately managed cases.

The operation time was longer in the tri-EEA than in the EEA group. However, in the multivariate analysis adjusted for the factors significantly correlated with the operation time in the univariate analysis, a longer operation time (>300 minutes) was significantly associated with the tumor location (Rb vs RS/Ra; HR, 2.38; 95% CI, 1.01-5.67; P =.0498), but not male sex (P =.2316) or the device used for the anastomosis (P =.4050) (data not shown). This analysis showed no direct relationship between the device used and the operation time.

Our study has some limitations. First, the animal experiments on anastomosis strength were not intracorporeal, and were performed using the colon and small intestine of pigs. We chose to perform extracorporeal experiment so not to be influenced by other factors than the devise (the tri-EEA or the EEA), such as the preparation status, the blood flow, or the wall thickness of the intestine. Regarding the wall thickness, the rectum usually lacks serosa and has thick muscle layers. Therefore, our animal model did not specifically reflect the actual situation in clinical practice. However, the aim of our animal study was to compare the strength of anastomoses created using the tri-EEA vs the EEA, and we successfully proved the superiority of anastomoses created using the tri-EEA. Second, the sample size was relatively small. Although our multicenter study analyzed about 200 patients with rectal cancer, only nine patients had AL. Third, our study is subject to the selection bias inherent in observational retrospective studies. Neoadjuvant chemoradiotherapy is used to reduce the incidence of local recurrence, but it may cause tissue edema, fibrosis, and even necrosis.[34] There was a meta-analysis examining the influence of the neoadjuvant chemoradiotherapy to

AL, and the authors concluded that neoadjuvant radiotherapy did not increase the incidence of AL.[35] However, the *P* value was marginal (Odds ratio = 1.24, 95%CI; 0.97-1.58, *P* =.08), and we thought it was still controversial. So, we excluded the patients who underwent neoadjuvant chemoradiotherapy. The impact of the tri-EEA on the anastomosis strength in patients who undergo neoadjuvant chemoradiation therapy warrants further investigation. As shown in Tables 1 and 2, the tri-EEA group had higher prevalence of more advanced rectal cancer, laparoscopic surgery, side-to-side anastomosis, and use of the 28-mm circular stapler. Although advanced tumor stage is reportedly a risk factor for AL,[11] the tri-EEA group had a lower incidence of AL. In this study, nine patients had stage IV rectal cancer (Table 1). All of these patients underwent total mesorectal excision with D3 lymph node dissection, and we do not believe that it affected the outcome. Because only 10 patients underwent open surgery, and because all patients who had AL underwent laparoscopic surgery, we could not statistically analyze the impact of laparoscopic surgery on our results. The incidence of AL was associated with the use of the tri-EEA, even when open surgery was excluded (0.0% in the tri-EEA group vs 6.3% in the EEA group, *P* =.0307). We used the tri-EEA with a circular stapler size of 28 mm, while the EEA was used with 25-, 28-, and 31-mm circular staplers; therefore, the size of the circular stapler was 28 mm in all patients in the tri-EEA group. None of these factors were risk factors for AL in our univariate and multivariate analyses. Further prospective studies are necessary to confirm the clinical significance of anastomosis using the tri-EEA.

5 | CONCLUSIONS

This animal model and multicenter retrospective study revealed that anastomoses created with the tri-EEA had higher bursting pressure than those created with the EEA, and that anastomoses created with the tri-EEA were associated with a lower incidence of AL. Our study indicated that the use of the tri-EEA leads to safer rectal surgery, suggesting that the indications for covering stomas might need to be reevaluated.

AUTHOR CONTRIBUTIONS

Each person listed as an author or coauthor meets all four criteria listed in the Author Guideline of Annals of Gastroenterological Surgery.

REFERENCES

1. Hallbook O, Sjodahl R. Anastomotic leakage and functional outcome after anterior resection of the rectum. Br J Surg. 1996;83(1):60–2.
2. Rullier E, Laurent C, Garrelon JL, Michel P, Saric J, Parneix M. Risk factors for anastomotic leakage after resection of rectal cancer. Br J Surg. 1998;85(3):355–8.
3. Ma L, Pang X, Ji G, Sun H, Fan Q, Ma C. The impact of anastomotic leakage on oncology after curative anterior resection for rectal cancer: a systematic review and meta-analysis. Medicine (Baltimore). 2020;99(37):e22139.
4. Yang J, Chen Q, Jindou L, Cheng Y. The influence of anastomotic leakage for rectal cancer oncologic outcome: a systematic review and meta-analysis. J Surg Oncol. 2020;121(8):1283–97.
5. Kverneng Hultberg D, Svensson J, Jutesten H, Rutegård J, Matthiessen P, Lydrup M-L, et al. The impact of anastomotic leakage on long-term function after anterior resection for rectal cancer. Dis Colon Rectum. 2020;63(5):619–28.
6. Marinatou A, Theodoropoulos GE, Karanika S, Karantanos T, Siakavellas S, Spyropoulos BG, et al. Do anastomotic leaks impair postoperative health-related quality of life after rectal cancer surgery? A case-matched study. Dis Colon Rectum. 2014;57(2):158–66.
7. Midura EF, Hanseman D, Davis BR, Atkinson SJ, Abbott DE, Shah SA, et al. Risk factors and consequences of anastomotic leak after colectomy: a national analysis. Dis Colon Rectum. 2015;58(3):333–8.
8. La Regina D, Di Giuseppe M, Lucchelli M, Saporito A, Boni L, Efthymiou C, et al. Financial impact of anastomotic leakage in colorectal surgery. J Gastrointest Surg. 2019;23(3):580–6.
9. Paun BC, Cassie S, MacLean AR, Dixon E, Buie WD. Postoperative complications following surgery for rectal cancer. Ann Surg. 2010;251(5):807–18.
10. Kang CY, Halabi WJ, Chaudhry OO, Nguyen V, Pigazzi A, Carmichael JC, et al. Risk factors for anastomotic leakage after anterior resection for rectal cancer. JAMA Surg. 2013;148(1):65–71.
11. Park JS, Choi G-S, Kim SH, Kim HR, Kim NK, Lee KY, et al. Multicenter analysis of risk factors for anastomotic leakage after laparoscopic rectal cancer excision: the Korean laparoscopic colorectal surgery study group. Ann Surg. 2013;257(4):665–71.
12. Watanabe T, Miyata H, Konno H, Kawai K, Ishihara S, Sunami E, et al. Prediction model for complications after low anterior resection based on data from 33,411 Japanese patients included in the National Clinical Database. Surgery. 2017;161(6):1597–608.
13. Medtronic.com. [internet]. Available from: https://www.medtronic.com/covidien/en-us/products/surgical-stapling/eea-circular-stapler.html
14. Ikeda T, Kumashiro R, Taketani K, Ando K, Kimura Y, Saeki H, et al. Endoscopic evaluation of clinical colorectal anastomotic leakage. J Surg Res. 2015;193(1):126–34.
15. Akagi T, Endo H, Inomata M, Yamamoto H, Mori T, Kojima K, et al. Clinical impact of Endoscopic Surgical Skill Qualification System (ESSQS) by Japan Society for Endoscopic Surgery (JSES) for laparoscopic distal gastrectomy and low anterior resection based on the National Clinical Database (NCD) registry. Ann Gastroenterol Surg. 2020;4(6):721–34.
16. Kuroyanagi H, Akiyoshi T, Oya M, Fujimoto Y, Ueno M, Yamaguchi T, et al. Laparoscopic-assisted anterior resection with double-stapling technique anastomosis: safe and feasible for lower rectal cancer? Surg Endosc. 2009;23(10):2197–202.
17. Oki E, Ando K, Saeki H, Nakashima Y, Kimura Y, Hiyoshi Y, et al. The use of a circular side stapling technique in laparoscopic low anterior resection for rectal cancer: experience of 30 serial cases. Int Surg. 2015;100(6):979–83.
18. Ando K, Kuriyama N, Fujimoto Y, Jogo T, Hokonohara K, Hu Q, et al. New anastomosis technique to prevent anastomotic leakage in laparoscopic anterior resection for rectal cancer, especially upper rectal cancer. In Vivo. 2020;34(6):3533–8.
19. Rahbari NN, Weitz J, Hohenberger W, Heald RJ, Moran B, Ulrich A, et al. Definition and grading of anastomotic leakage following anterior resection of the rectum: a proposal by the International Study Group of Rectal Cancer. Surgery. 2010;147(3):339–51.
20. Dinning PG, Carrington EV, Scott SM. The use of colonic and anorectal high-resolution manometry and its place in clinical work and in research. Neurogastroenterol Motil. 2015;27(12):1693–708.
21. Attari A, Chey WD, Baker JR, Ashton-Miller JA. Comparison of anorectal function measured using wearable digital ma-

nometry and a high resolution manometry system. PLoS One. 2020;15(9):e0228761.
22. Akiyoshi T, Ueno M, Fukunaga Y, Nagayama S, Fujimoto Y, Konishi T, et al. Incidence of and risk factors for anastomotic leakage after laparoscopic anterior resection with intracorporeal rectal transection and double-stapling technique anastomosis for rectal cancer. Am J Surg. 2011;202(3):259–64.
23. Dulskas A, Samalavicius NE. Usefulness of anorectal manometry for diagnosing continence problems after a low anterior resection. Ann Coloproctol. 2016;32(3):101–4.
24. Choy KT, Yang TWW, Heriot A, Warrier SK, Kong JC. Does rectal tube/transanal stent placement after an anterior resection for rectal cancer reduce anastomotic leak? A systematic review and meta-analysis. Int J Colorectal Dis. 2021;36(6):1123–32.
25. Maeda K, Nagahara H, Shibutani M, Ohtani H, Sakurai K, Toyokawa T, et al. Efficacy of intracorporeal reinforcing sutures for anastomotic leakage after laparoscopic surgery for rectal cancer. Surg Endosc. 2015;29(12):3535–42.
26. Kennedy R, Jenkins I, Finan PJ. Controversial topics in surgery: splenic flexure mobilisation for anterior resection performed for sigmoid and rectal cancer. Ann R Coll Surg Engl. 2008;90(8):638–42.
27. Marsden MR, Conti JA, Zeidan S, Flashman KG, Khan JS, O'Leary DP, et al. The selective use of splenic flexure mobilization is safe in both laparoscopic and open anterior resections. Colorectal Dis. 2012;14(10):1255–61.
28. You X, Liu Q, Wu J, Wang Y, Huang C, cao G, et al. High versus low ligation of inferior mesenteric artery during laparoscopic radical resection of rectal cancer: a retrospective cohort study. Medicine (Baltimore). 2020;99(12):e19437.
29. Yanagita T, Hara M, Osaga S, Nakai N, Maeda Y, Shiga K, et al. Efficacy of intraoperative ICG fluorescence imaging evaluation for preventing anastomotic leakage after left-sided colon or rectal cancer surgery: a propensity score-matched analysis. Surg Endosc. 2021;35(5):2373–85.
30. Watanabe J, Ishibe A, Suwa Y, Suwa H, Ota M, Kunisaki C, et al. Indocyanine green fluorescence imaging to reduce the risk of anastomotic leakage in laparoscopic low anterior resection for rectal cancer: a propensity score-matched cohort study. Surg Endosc. 2020;34(1):202–8.
31. Kang J, Choi G-S, Oh JH, Kim NK, Park JS, Kim MJ, et al. Multicenter analysis of long-term oncologic impact of anastomotic leakage after laparoscopic total mesorectal excision: the Korean laparoscopic colorectal surgery study group. Medicine (Baltimore). 2015;94(29):e1202.
32. Hajibandeh S, Hajibandeh S, Maw A. Meta-analysis and trial sequential analysis of randomized controlled trials comparing high and low ligation of the inferior mesenteric artery in rectal cancer surgery. Dis Colon Rectum. 2020;63(7):988–99.
33. Yamaguchi T, Kinugasa Y, Shiomi A, Sato S, Yamakawa Y, Kagawa H, et al. Learning curve for robotic-assisted surgery for rectal cancer: use of the cumulative sum method. Surg Endosc. 2015;29(7):1679–85.
34. Geisler D, Marks J, Marks G. Laparoscopic colorectal surgery in the irradiated pelvis. Am J Surg. 2004;188(3):267–70.
35. Hu MH, Huang RK, Zhao RS, Yang KL, Wang H. Does neoadjuvant therapy increase the incidence of anastomotic leakage after anterior resection for mid and low rectal cancer? A systematic review and meta-analysis. Colorectal Dis. 2017;19(1):16–26.

3

Essential updates 2020/2021: Colorectal diseases (benign)—Current topics in the surgical and medical treatment of benign colorectal diseases

Hiroshi Sawayama | Yuji Miyamoto | Naoya Yoshida | Hideo Baba

Department of Gastroenterological Surgery, Graduate School of Medical Sciences, Kumamoto University, Kumamoto, Japan

Correspondence
Hideo Baba, Department of Gastroenterological Surgery, Graduate School of Medical Sciences, Kumamoto University, 1-1-1, Honjo, Chuo-ku, Kumamoto 860-8556, Japan.
Email: hdobaba@kumamoto-u.ac.jp

Abstract

The development of new drugs for inflammatory bowel disease (IBD) is remarkable, and treatment strategies using multiple agents and various techniques are required; however, the treatment strategy is likely to be complex. Therefore, appropriate evaluation of traditional surgical treatment strategies and accurate knowledge of the efficacy and limitations of novel treatments are required. Total infectious complications were found to be associated with the use of corticosteroids and anti-tumor necrosis factor-α agents, but not with immunomodulators, anti-integrin agents, and 5-aminosalicylic acid. Regarding surgical procedures for IBD, conceived anastomosis methods, including Kono-S for Crohn's disease stenosis, are associated with better outcomes than conventional techniques. Autologous cell transplantation for Crohn's fistulae has been shown to have a favorable outcome. Diverticulitis is increasing and will be treated more frequently in the future. Risk factors for the incidence of diverticulitis and differences in pathogenesis according to right or left side diverticulitis have been reported. Antibiotic therapy may be omitted for uncomplicated diverticulitis. Moreover, regarding surgical procedures, both bowel resection and anastomosis are associated with favorable short-term outcomes, higher stoma closure rate, and superior medical economy compared to Hartmann's procedure. Risk factors for recurrence after diverticulitis surgery may provide better postoperative follow-up. In this review, we explore the current topics of colorectal benign diseases, focusing on IBD and diverticulitis, based on clinical trials and meta-analyses from 2020-2021. This review consolidates the available knowledge and improves the quality of surgical procedures and perioperative management for IBD and diverticulitis.

KEYWORDS
Crohn's disease, diverticulitis, inflammatory bowel disease, surgery, ulcerative colitis

1 | INTRODUCTION

Inflammatory bowel disease (IBD) and diverticular disease are treated with a combination of medical and surgical therapy. The treatment and perioperative management of IBD and diverticulitis are major concerns among surgeons owing to the frequency and complexity of treatment and the severity of these diseases in clinical practice.

Currently, there are more than 1 million patients with IBD in the United States and 2.5 million in Europe, with substantial costs for health care.[1] Ulcerative colitis (UC) and Crohn's disease (CD) are two of the most common types of IBD. Infliximab was approved for the treatment of UC by the Food and Drug Administration in 2005 in the United States. Although the number of patients hospitalized for ulcerative colitis increased by over 70% in a nearly linear trend, the rate of patients who underwent total proctocolectomy decreased from 111.1 to 77.1 per 1000 UC admissions between 2002 and 2013, according to the Nationwide Inpatient Sample database. However, the majority of total proctocolectomies (69%) were performed within 24 hours of hospital admission.[2] The development of recent medical therapeutic agents for IBD has been remarkable; however, in many cases, surgical treatment is still required.

Diverticulitis and diverticular bleeding require medical treatment for colon diverticulosis. Moreover, diverticular disease-related mortality increased in 58 nations from 1994 to 2016; during this period, the relevant mortality rate increased in 57% of nations, whereas it decreased in only 7% Mortality associated with diverticular disease is increasing worldwide.[3] Surgical treatment for diverticulitis is likely to increase in the future.

Benign colorectal disease from 2018 to 2019 was reviewed in this journal.[4] Several clinical trials and meta-analyses have revealed novel treatment strategies and outcomes of these treatments developed in 2020. In the present review, newly determined characteristics, prognostic markers, non-operative management, and surgical treatment strategies optimal for IBD and diverticulitis are reviewed in accordance with articles published in the last 2 years (2020-2021) (Figure 1).

2 | IBD

2.1 | Association between IBD and other diseases

Arthritis, uveitis, pancreatitis, primary sclerosing cholangitis, and erythema nodosum are extraintestinal complications associated with IBD. Other diseases accompanying IBD have been reported in previous meta-analyses (Table 1). Inflammatory resorption of alveolar bones is caused by polymicrobial biofilm-mediated disease. Moreover, inflammatory processes are similar in periodontitis and IBD; the presence of periodontitis was associated with IBD, and periodontitis was strongly associated with both CD and UC.[5] The prevalence of cutaneous symptoms, pyoderma gangrenosum, psoriasis, and herpes zoster infection was frequently revealed to be accompanied by IBD.[6,7] Patients with IBD had an increased risk of

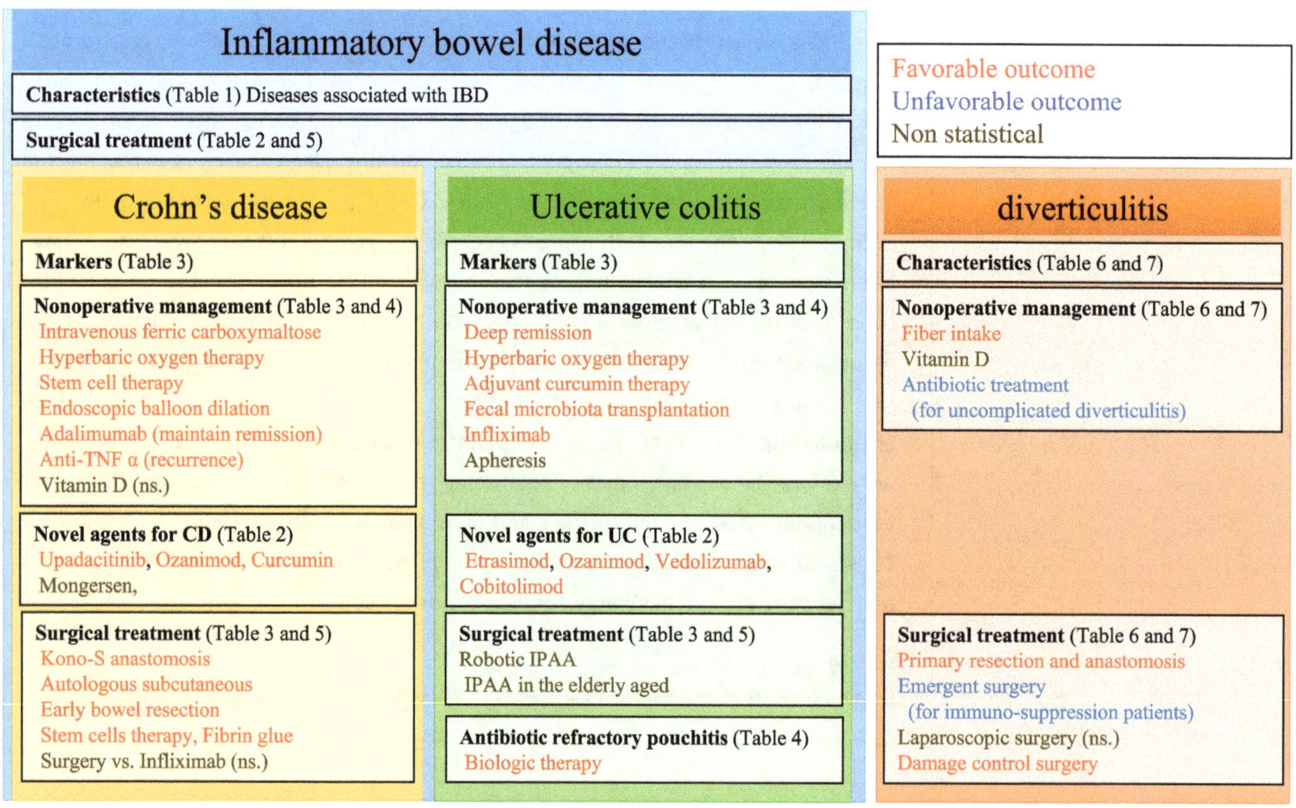

FIGURE 1 Summary of key articles on clinical trials and meta-analyses of inflammatory bowel disease and diverticulitis

TABLE 1 Meta-analyses of characteristics and markers inflammatory bowel disease

Focus	Main results	Reference
Periodontitis	The association between periodontitis and UC: present (OR 5.37)	*BMC Oral Health.* 2020 Mar 12;20(1):67
Periodontitis	The relation between periodontitis and IBD: OR: 2.10 (CD 1.72, UC: 2.39)	Biomed Res Int. 2021 Mar 12;2021:6692420
Periodontal disease (PD)	The presence of PD was associated with IBD: OR: 2.78 (CD: 3.41, UC 3.98)	*Acta Odontol Scand.* 2021 Jul;79(5):344-35
Pyoderma gangrenosum (PG)	The incidence of PG in IBD: 0.4 to 2.6%. PG was associated with female gender (RR: 1.33), CD (RR: 1.19), erythema nodosum (RR: 9.28), and ocular extra-intestinal manifestation (RR: 4.55)	Dig Dis Sci. 2020 Sep;65(9):2675-2685
Psoriasis	The prevalence of psoriasis: CD 3.6% and UC 2.8%.	*J Crohns Colitis.* 2020 Mar 13;14(3):351-360
Herpes zoster (HZ) infection	Risk of HZ infection: CD: RR: 1.74 (steroid users RR: 1.78). UC: RR: 1.40 (steroid users RR: 1.99, anti-TNFα users RR: 2.29) IBD patients with high risk of HZ infection may benefit from an HZ vaccine	*Eur J Clin Microbiol Infect Dis.* 2020 Feb; 39(2):219-227
Rheumatoid arthritis	The association between IBD and the risk of RA: higher risk of RA among patients with IBD: RR 2.59 (CD, RR: 3.14, UC, RR: 2.29)	*BMC Gastroenterol.* 2020 Jun 17;20(1):192
Elderly onset (EO) and adult onset (AO) IBD	EO = AO: 5-year risk of surgery, overall exposure to corticosteroids EO < AO: exposure to immunomodulators, biologic agents	*Clin Gastroenterol Hepatol.* 2020 Oct;18(11):2437-2447
Anxiety and depression	Anxiety symptoms: 32.1%, depression symptoms: 25.2% CD > UC: anxiety symptoms (OR 1.2), depression symptoms (OR 1.2)	*Lancet Gastroenterol Hepatol.* 2021 May;6(5):359-370
Opioid use	Prevalence of opioid use: outpatients setting 21%, hospitalized 62% female (RR 1.20), depression (RR 1.99), substance abuse (RR 4.67), prior surgery (RR 2.33), biologic use (RR 1.36), steroid use (RR 1.41)	*Clin Gastroenterol Hepatol.* 2021 May;19(5):895-907.e4.

infection due to immune system dysregulation associated with the use of corticosteroids, immunosuppressant drugs, and anti- tumor necrosis factor (TNF)α. The risk of herpes zoster infection increased in CD (Risk ratio [RR]: 1.74, steroid users RR: 1.78) and UC (RR: 1.40, steroid users RR: 1.99, anti-TNFα users RR: 2.29). Patients with IBD with a high risk of HZ infection may benefit from an HZ vaccine.[8] Skin lesions are likely to be associated with IBD, and when treating patients with IBD, it is important to carefully examine the skin condition.

Anxiety and depression are commonly experienced by patients with IBD. The prevalence of corresponding symptoms was 32.1% and 25.2%, respectively, and the incidence of such was higher in patients with CD than in those with UC.[9] Moreover, these symptoms were associated with CD-related surgery, the Crohn's disease activity index, and corticosteroid use in patients with CD.[10] Patients with IBD often experience anxiety and depression during the perioperative period, and appropriate psychological care may be beneficial in these patients.

2.2 | Novel agents for IBD

The development of novel therapeutics for IBD is remarkable, so much so that it is difficult for general surgeons to understand all of them. The perioperative impact of these drugs will be discussed later; here, we enumerate novel therapeutic agents that were reported from 2020 to 2021. The results of the clinical trials are summarized in Table 2. Table S1 presents a summary of the approval status of novel agents.

The effects and tolerability of upadacitinib (a selective Janus kinase 1 inhibitor),[11] ozanimod (targeting sphingosine-1-phosphate receptor subtypes 1 and 5),[12] and mongersen (antisense oligodeoxynucleotide to Smad7)[13] have been reported in clinical trials for CD.

Novel agents for UC, including etrasimod (selective sphingosine 1-phosphate receptor modulator),[14] ozanimod,[15] vedolizumab (inhibits the gut-selective α4β7 integrin),[16] cobitolimod (activates Toll-like receptor 9),[17] and budesonide (systemic corticosteroids)[18] were reported from 2020 to 2021.

TABLE 2 Novel agents for inflammatory bowel disease

Agents	Target	Endpoints	Main results	Reference
Crohn's disease				
Upadacitinib	Janus kinase 1 inhibitor	Clinical remission (16 wk) and endoscopic remission (12 wk)	Endoscopic (not clinical) remission increased	*Gastroenterology.* 2020 Jun;158(8):2123-2138.e8
Ozanimod	Sphingosine-1-phosphate receptor subtypes 1 and 5	Endoscopic Score for Crohn's Disease (SES-CD) from baseline to 12 wk	The mean change SES-CD: 2.2, endoscopic, histological, clinical improvements	*Lancet Gastroenterol Hepatol.* 2020 Sep;5(9):819-828
Mongersen	Antisense oligodeoxynucleotide to Smad7	Clinical remission CD Activity Index score <150 (12 wk)	NS	*Am J Gastroenterol.* 2020 May;115(5):738-745
Ulcerative colitis				
Etrasimod	Sphingosine 1-phosphate receptor modulator	Improvement in modified MCS (etrasimod vs placebo)	Etrasimod favorable ($P = 0.009$) endoscopic improvement: 41.8% vs 17.8%	*Gastroenterology.* 2020 Feb;158(3):550-561
Ozanimod	Sphingosine-1-phosphate receptor subtypes 1 and 5	Induction and maintenance therapy (ozanimod vs placebo)	Clinical remission (18.4% vs 6.0%, $P < .001$), maintenance (37.0% vs 18.5%, $P < .001$)	*N Engl J Med.* 2021 Sep 30;385(14):1280-1291
Vedolizumab	Inhibits the gut-selective α4β7 integrin	Maintenance treatment, intravenous vedolizumab vs placebo groups	Clinical remission: 46.2%, 42.6%, and 14.3%, respectively	*Gastroenterology.* 2020 Feb;158(3):562-572
Cobitolimod	Activates Toll-like receptor 9	The proportion of clinical remission	Cobitolimod: 21% vs placebo: 7% (OR 3.8)	*Lancet Gastroenterol Hepatol.* 2020 Dec;5(12):1063-1075

A meta-analysis showed that anti-TNF-α agents prevented endoscopic recurrence (RR: 0.34) but not clinical recurrence (RR: 0.60, not significant [n.s.]). Patients receiving anti-TNFα therapy experienced more adverse effects than those who were not (RR: 1.75).[19] Curcumin, as an adjuvant treatment for mesalamine, was proven to be effective in inducing clinical remission (odds ratio [OR]: 5.2), endoscopic remission (OR: 5.7), and endoscopic improvement (OR: 17.1), and was shown to be safe in UC.[20]

2.3 | Non-drug treatment for IBD

Hyperbaric oxygen (HBO) and endoscopic balloon dilation are typical treatments for bowel obstruction caused by adhesion and stenosis, respectively. The favorable effects of these treatments on the symptoms associated with IBD are described below (Table 3 and 4).

A previous study reported patients with UC who were hospitalized for acute flares and were treated with HBO. The patients who responded to HBO treatment on day 3 required less rehospitalization or colectomy than non-responders (0% vs 66%).[21] Moreover, patients with CD (n = 20) with high perianal fistula(s) who failed to respond to conventional treatment were treated with HBO, and the rates of clinical response and clinical remission were 60% and 20%, respectively.[22] In a meta-analysis, the response rate of HBO was 83.2% in UC and 81.9% in CD, while complete healing of the fistula was noted in 47.6% of fistulizing CD cases.[23]

Endoscopic balloon dilation for small intestinal strictures in CD was evaluated in a previous meta-analysis. The technical success rate of endoscopic balloon dilation was 94.9%, major complication rate was 5.3%, symptom recurrence rate was 48.3%, and rate of re-dilation or surgery was 38.8% and 27.4%, respectively.[24]

The safety and efficacy of fecal microbiota transplantation (FMT) for the treatment of *Clostridioides difficile* infections have been reported.[25] The intestinal flora plays an important role in the progression of UC. FMT has been shown to change the production of mucosal-associated invariant T cell cytokines.[26] In a meta-analysis, the safety and effectiveness of FMT for treating UC was reported.[27] Reportedly, FMT did not have a sustained effect on the treatment of UC patients unless the administration was repeated and prolonged.[28] The efficacy of FMT depends on microbial interactions between the donor and recipient strains.[29] The interactions between bacterial and metabolic pathways are also associated with the induction of remission.[30] Future studies are needed so that a sustained therapeutic effect can be obtained after FMT treatment in UC patients.

2.4 | Surgical management for IBD

In patients with CD, stenosis and fistula are the main indications for surgery. The optimal time for surgery and surgical procedures are the main concerns of surgeons (Table 3 and 5). The effects of laparoscopic ileocecal resection and infliximab were similar to

TABLE 3 Clinical trials of inflammatory bowel disease

Factor	Endpoints	Main results	Reference
Markers of inflammatory bowel disease			
Disease activity miR-320a levels	Appropriate clinical disease indices and endoscopic scoring systems	MiR-320a expression (peripheral blood) are associated with the clinical and endoscopic disease activities of IBD	*Clin Transl Gastroenterol.* 2020 Mar;11(3):e00134
Response to infliximab in CD	Predicting mucosal healing	Oncostatin M can predict the outcome of infliximab treatment. (AUC = 0.91)	*Aliment Pharmacol Ther.* 2020 Jul;52(2):284-291
Vedolizumab	Variables response to vedolizumab (against the $\alpha4\beta7$ integrin heterodimer)	Markers associated with vedolizumab -induced clinical remission: CD: IL17A, TNF, CXCL1, CCL19, UC: G-CSF and IL7	*Clin Gastroenterol Hepatol.* 2021 Mar;19(3):503-510.e1
Anxiety/depression	The risk factors of anxiety/ depression in IBD	CD: CD-related surgery and CDAI/ depression in IBD UC: corticosteroid use	*Sci Rep.* 2021 Jan 14;11(1):1440
Microbial factors	Maintenance of remission	Favorable: Lac unfavorable: Enterobacteriaceae (OR 6.35) Lachnospiraceae family (OR 0.47)	*Gut Microbes.* 2020 Nov 1;11(6):1713-1728
Faecal calprotectin (Fcal)	Prediction of postoperative recurrence after ileocolonic resection (CD)	Fcal variation: predictor of early endoscopic postoperative recurrence AUC = 0.73, sensitivity = 64.7%, specificity = 87.5%	*Dig Liver Dis.* 2020 Jul;52(7):740-744
Nonoperative treatment for IBD			
HBO for chronic antibiotic-refractory pouchitis (CARP)	The efficacy and safety of HBO for CARP	mPDAI symptom score: 3.19 to 1.91 mPDAI endoscopy scores: 2.34 to 1.29 improving CARP	*Inflamm Bowel Dis.* 2021 Jun 15;27(7):965-970
Nonoperative treatment for Crohn's disease			
Oral Sucrosomial® Iron	Intravenous ferric carboxy -maltose (FMC) vs Sucrosomial® Iron (SI)	FCM = SI: Hemoglobin, Iron (4, 8, 12 wk) FCM > SI: Ferritin levels	*Nutrients.* 2021 Feb 12;13(2):608
Vitamin D	Endoscopic recurrence (26 wk)	Vitamin D vs placebo (58% vs 66%, NS)	*Clin Gastroenterol Hepatol.* 2021 Aug;19(8):1573-1582.e5
Hyperbaric oxygen therapy (HBO)	Efficacy, safety, and feasibility of HBO in CD	Clinical response: 60% Clinical remission: 20%	*Aliment Pharmacol Ther.* 2021 Mar;53(5):587-597
Nonoperative treatment for ulcerative colitis			
Deep remission (a tight control strategy)	Major adverse outcomes that indicate CD progression	Favorable: deep remission CD endoscopic index of severity scores below 4, with no deep ulcerations or steroid use	*Gastroenterology.* 2020 Jul;159(1):139-147
HBO 2.4 atmospheres (90 min)	Day 3 responders: 5 days vs 3 days of HBO	HBO favorable: low rates of re-hospitalization, colectomy at 3 mo (0% vs 66%)	*Aliment Pharmacol Ther.* 2020 Sep;52(6):955-963
Fecal microbiota transplantation (FMT)	T regulatory and mucosal associated invariant T (MAIT) cell populations	Changes in MAIT cell cytokine production were observed in cFMT	*BMC Gastroenterol.* 2021 Jul 8;21(1):281
Apheresis selective removal of leukocytes	Clinical remission (Mayo score ≤2) at 12 mo	Apheresis: 46.6%, control: 36.4% (NS)	*J Gastroenterol.* 2020 Apr;55(4):390-400
Cannabis 80 mg tetra -hydrocannabinol	Lichtiger disease activity index, CRP, calprotectin, Mayo endoscopic score and QOL	Cannabis favorable: Lichtiger index, QOL Cannabis = placebo: Mayo endoscopic score	*PLoS One.* 2021 Feb 11;16(2):e0246871

(Continues)

TABLE 3 (Continued)

Factor	Endpoints	Main results	Reference
Surgical treatment for Crohn's disease			
Surgery vs Infliximab	Need for surgery or repeat surgery or anti-TNF therapy	Treatment effect was similar Laparoscopic ileocecal resection: not successful	*Lancet Gastroenterol Hepatol*. 2020 Oct;5(10):900-907
Kono-S anastomotic methods	Kono-S vs stapled ileocolic side-to-side anastomosis Endoscopic recurrence (ER)	22.2% in the Kono-S group and 62.8% in the Conventional group presented an ER	*Ann Surg*. 2020 Aug;272(2):210-217
Autologous subcutaneous adipose tissue	Clinical and radiographic healing at 6 mo	All patient: reduction in the size of fistula tracts 3 of 5: cessation of drainage None: complete healing	*Inflamm Bowel Dis*. 2020 Apr 11;26(5):670-677
Autologous adipose-derived stem cells	The closure of fistulas at months 3, 6, and 12	Healing rate (3, 6, 12m): the observation vs control, 90.9% vs 45.5%, 72.7% vs 54.5%, and 63.6% vs 54.5%, respectively (NS)	*Stem Cell Res Ther*. 2020 Mar 17;11(1):124
Allogeneic mesenchymal stem cells	Follow-up 1 y after the procedure	Perianal abscess (15%), complete closure (69%)	*Dis Colon Rectum*. 2021 Mar 1;64(3):328-334
Allogeneic mesenchymal stromal cells	Fistula closure using bone marrow-derived mesenchymal stromal cells	Fistulas with closure at 24 wk were still closed after 4 y	*J Crohns Colitis*. 2020 Jan 1;14(1):64-70
Fibrin glue	The rate of complete clinical remission at 1 y	Complete clinical remission (1 y): 45.4%	*Gastroenterology*. 2021 Feb;160(3):710-719.e2

Abbreviations: ACU, area under the curve; OR, odds ratio; TNF: tumor necrosis factor.

those reported in a retrospective study (n = 134).[31] However, the incidence of relapse in patients with ileocolonic CD (n = 1863) after early bowel resection was compared to that after initial therapy, and the overall (OR: 0.53) and surgical relapse (OR: 0.47) were lower in patients who underwent early bowel resection than in those who received initial medical therapy. Moreover, the requirement for maintenance biologic therapy (OR: 0.24) was lower in patients who received early bowel resection than in those who received initial medical therapy.[32] The incidence of relapse after strictureplasty was also compared to that of bowel resection for patients with CD. The results demonstrated that strictureplasty alone increased disease recurrence compared to bowel resection (hazard ratio [HR]: 1.61), and the morbidity rate was not significantly different between the two groups.[33] Antimesenteric cutback end-to-end isoperistaltic anastomosis, known as Sasaki-W anastomosis, has been reported as a novel hand-sewn anastomotic technique for CD.[34] In a previous randomized control trial (RCT), Kono-S anastomosis, antimesenteric functional end-to-end handsewn anastomosis, were performed for the stenosis of the patients with CD, and the endoscopic recurrence was 22.2% in the Kono group and 62.8% in the conventional group (n = 79).[35] In a previous meta-analysis, the surgical outcomes of Kono-S were found to be 0% for surgical recurrence and 5% for endoscopic recurrence.[36] Kono-S anastomosis yields a favorable outcome with increasing evidence, hence may be considered an optimal procedure for CD stenosis.

Fistula formation in CD is an intractable disease that is difficult to treat. The injection of allogeneic or autologous tissue is a promising new treatment for perianal fistulas in CD. Panes et al[37] reported the efficacy and safety of allogeneic adipose-derived mesenchymal stem cells in the treatment of complex perianal fistulas in CD. Additionally, the effects of the injection of autologous adipose tissue as a treatment modality for fistulas were reported in a cohort of CD patients in 2019.[38] Further trials on autologous tissue implantation have been attempted for fistulas in patients with CD in phase 1 trials and RCTs. Autologous subcutaneous,[39] adipose-derived,[40] and allogeneic mesenchymal stem cells,[41] as well as bone marrow-derived mesenchymal stromal cells,[42] were harvested in these trials, and the results suggested that such treatments for fistulas may be effective and feasible (Table 3). In a meta-analysis (n = 1252), the stem cell treatment group had a higher rate of fistula healing than the placebo group (61.8% vs 40.5%, OR: 2.21).[43]

The number of patients admitted for UC is increasing; however, the number of surgeries per admission is decreasing.[2] Colonic perforation, life-threatening bleeding, and toxic megacolon remain key indicators for emergency surgery, regardless of therapeutic advancements. Biologic agents have been used in patients with severe ulcerative colitis who are refractory to steroid therapy. Patients who are refractory to steroid therapy and infliximab are recommended for surgery.[44] Even when control is achieved with drugs, the problem of carcinogenesis remains. This poses a significant issue, particularly since the prognosis of UC patients with colorectal cancer is worse than that of colorectal cancer patients without UC.[45]

Song et al reported that elderly onset ulcerative colitis (EOUC) was increasing. In a Korean study, the 10-year cumulative colectomy rate was significantly higher in the EOUC than in the NEOUC group. The EOUC patients also had a higher mortality rate.[46] In Japan, it was reported that patients with EOUC had more advanced inflammation, were more likely to be hospitalized, had greater corticosteroid

TABLE 4 Meta-analyses of nonoperative treatment for inflammatory bowel disease

Focus	Endpoints	Main results	Reference
Nonoperative treatment for inflammatory bowel disease			
Sleep quality	The relation between sleep quality and disease activity	Subjective sleep quality and disease activity (OR 3.52), sleep efficiency and disease activity (OR 4.55)	*Sleep Med.* 2020 Nov;75:301-308
Iron supplementation	Ferric carboxymaltose (FCM), iron isomaltoside (IIM), iron sucrose (IS), oral iron (OI)	Response rates with FCM, IIM, IS, OI: 81%, 74%, 75%, 69% FCM: the most cost-effective	*Adv Ther.* 2021 Jan;38(1):660-677
Hyperbaric oxygen therapy (HBO)	Response rate and complete healing of fistula	Response rate of HBO, UC: 83.2%, CD: 81.9%, the complete healing of fistula: 47.6%	*Eur J Gastroenterol Hepatol.* 2021 Apr 19
Antibiotic refractory pouchitis	The safety and efficacy of various biological agents for antibiotic refractory pouchitis	Clinical improvement: IFX 71.4%, ADA 58.2%, VDZ 47.9%, remission: IFX 65.7%, ADA 31%, VDZ 47.4%	*J Clin Gastroenterol.* 2021 Jul 1;55(6):481-491
Nonoperative treatment for ulcerative colitis			
Adjuvant curcumin therapy	Clinical and endoscopic remission	Clinical remission (OR 5.18) Endoscopic remission (OR 17.05) Clinical improvement (OR 4.79 NS)	*J Gastroenterol Hepatol.* 2020 May;35(5):722-729
Infliximab (IFX) vs cyclosporine and tacrolimus (TAC)	Short-term remission, short-term, colectomy rate	IFX favorable: lower short-term (OR 0.59), 1 y colectomy rate (OR 0.53), 3 y colectomy rate (OR 0.41)	*Medicine.* 2020 Oct 30;99(44):e22894
Faecal microbiota transplantation (FMT)	Safety and effectiveness of treating UC	Efficacy: FMT favorable (OR 2.29) Multiple donors delivered (OR 2.76) Side effects: NS	*Int J Colorectal Dis.* 2020 Jun;35(6):1025-1034
Nonoperative treatment for Crohn's disease			
Adalimumab	Failure to maintain clinical remission in people with quiescent CD	Adalimumab: 59% vs placebo: 86% Adalimumab is an effective therapy for maintenance of clinical remission	*Cochrane Database Syst Rev.* 2020 May 16;5(5):CD012877
Anti-tumor necrosis factor (TNF) α	Preventing endoscopic and clinical recurrence	Endoscopic recurrence (RR 0.34) clinical recurrence (RR 0.60, NS) AEs with anti-TNF therapy (RR 1.75)	*J Gastroenterol Hepatol.* 2021 Apr;36(4):864-872
Stem cell therapy	CD activity index	Reduce: CD activity index, CD endoscopic index of severity, simplified endoscopy score for CD	*Stem Cell Res Ther.* 2021 Aug 18;12(1):463
Placebo	The rate of response to placebo endoscopic assessment of CD activity	Response: 16.2%, remission 5.2% lower rates of response to placebo increased concentration of CRP	*Clin Gastroenterol Hepatol.* 2020 May;18(5):1121-1132.e2
Endoscopic balloon dilation	Small intestinal strictures in CD evaluate endoscopic balloon dilation	Technical success: 94.9%, efficacy: 82.3%, complications: 5.3%, rec.: 48.3% (re-dilated: 38.8%, surg.: 27.4%)	*Aliment Pharmacol Ther.* 2020 Oct;52(7):1104-1116

use, and were more likely to require surgical treatment for UC than NEOUC patients.[47]

Ileal pouch-anal anastomosis (IPAA) was selected for patients who required total proctocolectomy. In recent years, the number of elderly patients undergoing the said procedures for UC has increased (age >50 years). The overall 30-day morbidity and mortality rates after surgery for elderly patients were 47.3% and 1.3%, respectively. Neither short- nor long-term functional outcomes were significantly different between patients aged 50-65 years and elderly patients (age >65 years).[48] However, the general condition, organ function, anorectal function, and activities of daily living (ADL) were impaired in the EOUC patients.[49] It is therefore important to select an appropriate procedure.

Proximal stoma diversion is commonly constructed when IPAA is performed. Anastomotic strictures and pouch failures have been shown to be more common in diverted patients than in non-diverted patients, but re-operation was more frequently required in non-diverted patients. However, this meta-analysis contained only one RCT; more evidence-based research is therefore desirable to exclude selection bias.[50] Retrospective studies showed that postoperative stoma outlet obstruction, a complication after stoma construction, occurred in 7.0%-16.9% of IBD patents who underwent IPAA. Maximum stoma drainage volume, loop ileostomy, and body mass index (≥22.2) are risk factors for stoma outlet obstruction, and thick rectus abdominis is associated with recurrent stoma outlet obstruction.[51,52]

TABLE 5 Meta-analyses of surgical treatment for inflammatory bowel disease

Focus	Endpoints	Main Results	Reference
Surgical treatment for inflammatory bowel disease			
Urgent surgeries vs elective surg.	Overall postoperative complications (30d)	Urgent surgery: ~ 40% increase in overall complication (RR: 1.43) Mortality and readmission rates: NS	*Int J Colorectal Dis*. 2021 Feb;36(2):253-263
Robotic vs laparoscopic IPAA	Complications and quality of life outcomes	NS	*Int J Colorectal Dis*. 2021 Jul;36(7):1345-1356
Rectal stump management	Mortality, complications, Pelvic stump dehiscence	Mortality: 1.7%, wound infection 11.3% Stump leak: 4.9%, pelvic abscess / sepsis 5.7%	*Tech Coloproctol*. 2020 Jul;24(7):671-684
IPAA (CD vs UC)	Complications, functional outcome	CD unfavorable: pouch fistulae (OR 6.08), strictures (OR 1.82), failure, (OR 5.27) CD = UC: pouchitis	*J Crohns Colitis*. 2020 Mar 13;14(3):418-427
IPAA	Outcomes following IPAA with and without proximal stoma diversion	Non-diverted favorable: Anastomotic strictures (OR 0.40), pouch failures (OR 0.54), diverted favorable: Re-operation (OR 2.51)	*Int J Colorectal Dis*. 2021 Apr;36(4):657-669
IPAA in the elderly aged >50 years	Perioperative safety and long-term functional success	The overall morbidity and mortality rates (30 d): 47.3% and 1.3% Functional outcomes 50-65 vs >65 years: NS	*Colorectal Dis*. 2021 Aug;23(8):2062-2074
Bariatric surgery	Adverse events, change in medications	Early/late adverse events: 15.9%/16.9% IBD medications: decrease 45.6%, increase 11%, no change 57.6%	*Obes Surg*. 2020 Oct;30(10):3872-3883
Bariatric surgery	Wound infection, Clavien-Dindo grade >II and IBD exacerbation	Wound infection (4.1%), CD grade >II (2.0%) and IBD exacerbation (4.3%). Bariatric surgery is safe in patients with IBD	*Clin Obes*. 2020 Dec;10(6):e12405
Bariatric surgery	Quality of life	Half of patients had decrease in their IBD medications after bariatric surgery	*Obes Surg*. 2020 Oct;30(10):3872-3883
Postoperative infectious complications	IBD medications on the risk of postoperative infections within 30 d	Corticosteroids (OR 1.70), immunomodulators (OR 1.29 NS), anti-TNF (OR 1.60), anti-integrin (OR 1.04 NS), 5-ASA (OR 0.76 NS)	*Cochrane Database Syst Rev*. 2020 Oct 24;10(10):CD013256
Preoperative anti-TNF	Overall, infectious, and noninfectious postoperative complications	Use of anti-TNF agents increases in postoperative complications: overall (OR 1.13), infectious (OR 1.44), noninfectious (OR: 1.44)	*Eur J Gastroenterol Hepatol*. 2021 Jun 1;33(6):799-816
Vedolizumab	Overall and infectious postoperative complication rates	Overall complications: NS Infectious complications: NS	*South Med J*. 2021 Feb;114(2):98-105
Vedolizumab (VDZ)	Postoperative complications	Overall complications (OR 1.25 NS) VDZ favorable: infection (OR 0.49) VDZ unfavorable: SSI (OR 2.97), ileus (OR 2.16), mucocutaneous separation (OR 4.69)	*Int J Colorectal Dis*. 2021 Oct;36(10):2081-2092
Surgical treatment for ulcerative colitis			
Predict colectomy	Prognostic factors (predict colectomy)	Pediatric Ulcerative Colitis Activity Index score, hemoglobin, hematocrit, albumin, family history of UC, extraintestinal manifestations, disease extension over time	*Gastroenterology*. 2021 Jan; 160(1):378-402.e22

TABLE 5 (Continued)

Focus	Endpoints	Main Results	Reference
Two-stage restorative colectomy	Complication rates (modified 2-stage, classic 2-stage, 3-stage approaches)	Pediatric pts: modified 2-stage approaches leak rates higher, adult cohorts: modified 2-stage approaches lower leak rates	*Int J Colorectal Dis*. 2020 Oct; 35(10):1817-1830.
Surgical treatment for Crohn's disease			
Kono-S anastomosis	Recurrence (rec.), complications	Surgical rec. 0%, endoscopic rec. 5%, ileus 3%, small bowel obstruction 4%, anastomotic leak 1%, postoperative infection 10%	*Surg Today*. 2021 Apr;51(4):493-501
IPAA	Long-term functional outcomes The pouch failure rate	Mean 24-h stool frequency: 6.3 bowel movement, overall pouch failure rate:15%, no risk factors for pouch failure were identified	*Dis Colon Rectum*. 2021 Mar 1;64(3):355-364
Surgery vs initial medical therapy	Early bowel resection (EBR) relapse rate, Newcastle-Ottawa and Jadad scales	EBR favorable: overall/surgical relapse (OR 0.53/0.47), requirement biologic therapy (OR 0.24), RFS, (OR 0.62), morbidity (NS)	*Int J Colorectal Dis*. 2020 Mar;35(3):501-512
Strictureplasty (SPX)	Recurrence-free survival SPX vs bowel resection (BR)	SPX alone increased disease recurrence than BR (HR 1.61) No difference in morbidity	*Int J Colorectal Dis*. 2020 Apr;35(4):705-717
Stem cells therapy	The efficacy and safety for CD fistula Stem cell therapy vs placebo	Stem cell group favorable: fistula healing (61.8% vs 40.5%, OR 2.21) the treatment-related adverse events (RR 0.58)	*Stem Cell Res Ther*. 2021 Jan 7;12(1):32
Risk of recurrence (rec.)	Risk of clinical, surgical and endoscopic (ES) rec. in positive resection margins, granulomas or plexitis	Positive resection margins: clinical/ surgical /ES rec. (RR 1.26/1.87/ND), Granulomas: clinical/surgical /ES rec. (RR 1.31/1.37/NS), Plexitis: ES/ clinical rec (RR: 1.31/NS)	*Clin Gastroenterol Hepatol*. 2021 Mar;19(3):451-462
Rate of recurrence	Postoperative recurrence (POR)	TNF-α agents (1 y) endoscopic, clinical, surgical POR: 21.7, 13.1, 3.8%, 5-y rec. rate: endoscopic, surgical rec.:84.2%, 17.5%	*J Dig Dis*. 2021 Jul;22(7):399-407

Ileal pouch-anal anastomosis is a safe procedure for EOUC patients; however, anorectal function and ADL should be considered when determining whether to perform the procedure. Further studies are needed to determine how to construct the diverting stoma.

2.5 | Perioperative managements for patients with IBD

Patients with IBD are often immunosuppressed before surgery, therefore requiring careful perioperative management. A meta-analysis examined the combined data from 68 published studies and identified the association between IBD medication and infectious complications within 30 days after surgery for IBD. Most patients were 18 years or older, and both men and women participated. The patients were divided into five groups based on their IBD medications (corticosteroids, anti-TNFα agents, immunomodulators, anti-integrin agents, and 5-ASA); the patients in these groups were compared with those who were not taking medications. Total infectious complications were associated with the use of corticosteroid (OR: 1.70) and anti-TNFα agent (OR: 1.60); however, they were not associated with the use of immunomodulators (OR: 1.29), anti-integrin agents (OR: 1.04), or 5-ASA (OR: 0.76).[53] The patients treated with vedolizumab (VDZ) showed a decrease in the incidence of infectious complications (OR: 0.49), but the risks of surgical site infection (SSI) (OR: 2.97), superficial SSI (OR: 2.24), and ileus (OR: 2.16) increased. The reason for the decreased risk of infectious complications may be that VZD suppresses intestinal inflammation by inhibiting the interaction between MAdCAM-1 and α4β7 and preventing T cells from entering the intestinal mucosal system. The suppression of intestinal inflammation by VDZ reduces postoperative infectious complications, whereas excessive immunosuppression may be the cause of postoperative SSI.[54]

Vitamin D is commonly deficient in patients with CD and the risk of CD-related surgery increases in patients with lower serum vitamin D levels. However, the incidence of postoperative endoscopic or clinical recurrence of CD in patients who underwent ileocolonic resection was not found to be significantly different between patients who received postoperative treatment with high-dose vitamin D and those who received placebo.[55]

In Crohn's disease, the treatment strategy emphasizes the preservation of intestinal function. Although Crohn's disease rarely leads to short bowel syndrome, some cases of this condition are unavoidable.[56] Teduglutide, a glucagon-like peptide-2 (GLP-2) analog, has been approved in Japan for the treatment of short bowel syndrome. Teduglutide promotes improved intestinal absorption function and reduces the need for long-term intravenous support, which is difficult to manage.[57]

Pouchitis is a common complication after total proctocolectomy with IPAA, and if it persists (≥3 episodes/y) despite antibiotic treatment, is considered as chronic antibiotic refractory pouchitis (CARP). The efficacy and safety of treatment with infliximab (IFX; n = 22), adalimumab (ADA; n = 42), and vedolizumab (VDZ; n = 144) were evaluated in a meta-analysis. Clinical improvement rates after treatment with IFX, ADA, and VDZ were 71.4%, 58.2%, and 47.9%, respectively, and the clinical remission rates were 65.7%, 31%, and 47.4%, respectively.[58] Biologic therapy is effective in the treatment of CARP. Moreover, HBO has been reported as an effective therapy for CARP in a meta-analysis (Tables 3 and 4).[59]

3 | DIVERTICULITIS

3.1 | Characteristic diverticulitis in a recent study

In the United States, the first incidence rate of diverticulitis was 2.9% between February 2015 and February 2020. The risk factors for the incidence of diverticulitis were being male, elderly (age >65 years), and Caucasian.[60] Low physical activity, overweight and obesity,[61] smoking, appendectomy, proton-pump inhibitors, and non-steroidal anti-inflammatory drug use[62] are other established risk factors for diverticular disease. The risk of developing such was reduced by high fiber intake. Individuals consuming fiber (30 g/d) have a 41% risk reduction compared to those with low fiber intake.[63]

The right- and left-sided acute colonic diverticulitis has different characteristics. Right-sided diverticulitis affects younger, male (OR: 1.33), and taller patients with a lower body mass index. Smoking (OR: 2.23), alcohol consumption (OR: 1.85), and comorbidity (OR: 0.21) were also associated with right-sided diverticulitis. Further, it has a more favorable outcome with lower risk of complications, less frequent emergency surgery, recurrence, and length of hospital stay (Table 6 and 7).[64,65]

TABLE 6 Clinical trials of diverticulitis and diverticular disease

Factor	Endpoints	Main results	Reference
Characteristics			
Right side vs left side diverticulitis	Clinical features	Right side: younger, male, tall, lower BMI, less advanced Hinchey stages, shorter hospital stays, less recurrent	*Sci Rep.* 2020 Feb 28;10(1):3754
Nonoperative treatment			
Vitamin D vs placebo	Time to diverticular disease hospitalization from randomization	Vitamin D: 1.4% and placebo: 1.5% (NS)	*Clin Nutr.* 2021 Mar;40(3):839-843
Antibiotic treatment vs placebo	Treatment effect	Antibiotic treatment = placebo: length of hospital stay, adverse events, readmission, intervention, inflammation markers, pain	*Clin Gastroenterol Hepatol.* 2021 Mar;19(3):503-510.e1
Surgical treatment			
Primary anastomosis (PRA) vs Hartmann's procedure (HP)	Costs and cost -effectiveness	PA favorable: overall costs: PAR vs HP (€20 544 vs €28 670), incremental cost-effectiveness: €-39 094 cost-utility: €-101 435	*Br J Surg.* 2020 Nov;107(12):1686-1694
PRA vs HP	Long-term outcomes and quality of life (QoL)	PA favorable: general QoL (EQ-VAS), EQ-5D index scores, PA = HP: GIQLI (intestine-specific QOL)	*Int J Colorectal Dis.* 2021 Oct;36(10):2159-2164
Surgery or not	QoL at 5-year follow-up	Surgery favorable: potential to improve quality of life	*Ann Surg.* 2020 Aug;272(2):284-287
Damage control surgery (DCS)	Rate of stoma at discharge and at 6 mo	DCS 8.3% vs conventional treatment 57% (at discharge), DCS 0% vs conventional treatment 42% (at 6 mo)	*World J Surg.* 2020 Dec;44(12):4098-4105
Hartmann's reversal	Factors of morbidity and mortality of Hartmann's reversal	Low albuminemia, renal failure, coronary artery disease, corticosteroids	*Sci Rep.* 2020 Feb 27;10(1):3643

TABLE 7 Meta-analyses of diverticulitis and diverticular disease

Focus	Endpoints	Main results	Reference
Characteristics			
Right-sided diverticulitis	Characteristic, comorbidity, recurrence (rec.)	Younger, male, smoking, alcohol consumption, less comorbidity, lower rec., less emergency surgery, shorter length of hospital stays	*Colorectal Dis.* 2020 Dec;22(12):1908-1923
Left-sided acute diverticulitis	Disease severity, risk of recurrence according to age	Young = elder: need emergency surgery or drainage, recurrence	*Eur J Gastroenterol Hepatol.* 2020 May;32(5):547-554
Preventive medicine Fiber intake	The risk of diverticular according to dietary fiber intake, fiber subtypes	Risk reduction: 23/41/58% (Fiber intake 20/30/40 g/d). Cereal/fruit/vegetable fiber per 10 g/d (RR 0.74/0.56/0.80)	*Eur J Nutr.* 2020 Mar;59(2):421-432
Nonoperative treatment			
Conservative treatment for uncomplicated right-side diverticulitis	Treatment failure, ES at rec for uncomplicated right-sided diverticulitis	Treatment failure: 2.5%, rec. rate: 10.9%, complicated diverticulitis at rec: 4.4%, emergency surgery at rec: 9.0%	*Int J Colorectal Dis.* 2021 Aug;36(8):1791-1799
Observation vs Antibiotic treatment for uncomplicated diverticulitis	Rates of ongoing diverticulitis, rec., complicated diverticulitis, sigmoid resection	NS Observational management of uncomplicated AD is safe	*Br J Surg.* 2020 Jul;107(8):1062-1069
Intravenous antibiotics for Right-sided diverticulitis (Hinchey I/II)	Rec. rate, morbidity associated with rec.	Rec. rate: 12% (nonoperative management is safe and feasible) required urgent surgery at the time of first rec.: 9.9%	*Dis Colon Rectum.* 2020 Oct;63(10):1466-1473
Nonoperative management for sigmoid complicated diverticulitis with abscess	Relapse rate at 30 d, rec. of AD	Relapse rate: 18.9%, rec. of AD: 25.5% (distant abscess: 51% vs pericolic abscess: 18%)	*Langenbecks Arch Surg.* 2020 May;405(3):277-281
Nonoperative management for complicated diverticulitis with abscess	Treatment failure (time intervals: 1986-2000, 2000-2010, 2010-)	Treatment failure rate at 90 days: 16.4%, (1986-2000:19.2%, 2000-2010:18.6%, 2010-: 15.3%, NS)	*Int J Colorectal Dis.* 2021 Jul;36(7):1367-1383
Surgical treatment			
Primary anastomosis (PRA) vs Hartmann's procedure (HP)	Mortality, morbidity, stoma reversal after surgery for Hinchey III or IV diverticulitis	PRA favorable: stoma reversal, reversal-related morbidity, PRA = HP: mortality, morbidity, reintervention rates	*Int J Colorectal Dis.* 2020 Aug;35(8):1371-1386
PRA vs HP	Mortality, morbidity after surgery for Hinchey III or IV diverticulitis	NS	*Arq Bras Cir Dig.* 2021 Jan 15;33(3):e1546
PRA vs HP for perforated diverticulitis with generalized peritonitis	Stoma rate, 30-day mortality, overall mortality, major complications	PRA favorable: stoma rate, overall mortality, major complications, PRA = HP: 30-day mortality	*Tech Coloproctol.* 2020 Jun;24(6):527-543
Open vs laparoscopic surg. (LS) for diverticulitis with colovesical fistula	Operative time, stoma rates, complications, mortality	Open = LS: operative time, stoma rates, leakage, SSI, mortality, LS favorable: postoperative complications, length of stay	*ANZ J Surg.* 2021 Sep; 91(9):E570-E577.
Open vs LS emergency surgery for complicated diverticulitis	Mortality, morbidity, severe complications, and reoperation rates	Open = LS: postoperative mortality, morbidity, severe complications, and reoperation rates	*Medicine.* 2020 Oct 2;99(40):e22421
Damage control surgery for complicated diverticulitis	Leakage, mortality	Major leakage: 4.7%, overall mortality: 9.2%	*Int J Colorectal Dis.* 2021 May;36(5):867-879
Surgery for immune-suppressed patients	Mortality	Elective surgery: immunosuppressed = immunocompetent patients, emergent surgery: immunocompetent patients favorable	*Am J Surg.* 2021 Jan;221(1):72-85

3.2 | Treatment approach for diverticulitis

Patients with uncomplicated acute diverticulitis are commonly treated with antibiotics; however, in recent RCTs, this has been omitted for acute uncomplicated diverticulitis, which is characterized by elevated body temperature, inflammatory parameters, except for sepsis, and any sign of complications, such as abscess, free air, or fistula on computed tomography. Moreover, an earlier study demonstrated that the median hospital stay duration, adverse events, and hospital readmission were not significantly different during antibiotic treatment and observation.[66] In a 1-year follow-up of patients with uncomplicated diverticulitis, the rates of ongoing, recurrent, and complicated diverticulitis and undergoing sigmoid resection were not significantly different during antibiotic treatment and observation.[67] These results provide evidence for the omission of antibiotics in patients with uncomplicated acute diverticulitis.

In cases of recurrent diverticulitis or persistent symptoms, the choice between surgery and conservative treatment is an important concern. The failure rates of nonoperative management for acute diverticulitis with complicated abscesses is 16.4%, and the failure rates have not significantly decreased in the last 30 years.[68] The failure rate of percutaneous drainage as a nonoperative management for patients with pelvic abscess was three times higher than that for pericolic abscesses.[68,69] Hence, surgical treatment should be considered for abscesses in areas distant from colonic diverticulitis.

The aim of diverticulitis surgery is to treat acute inflammation and symptoms, and improve quality of life (QOL). A previous study compared elective sigmoid resection and conservative management in patients who had ongoing abdominal complaints for >3 months and/or frequently recurring left-sided diverticulitis of >2 episodes in 2 years. The Gastrointestinal Quality of Life Index of the patients after sigmoid resection was higher than that after conservative treatment.[70] Colonic resection for recurrent diverticulitis improved QOL, and these data are helpful in determining the indications for bowel resection.

3.3 | Surgical procedure for diverticulitis

The major concerns of acute diverticulitis surgery are associated with bowel resection. These factors were analyzed in meta-analyses and RCTs (Table 6 and 7).

Primary anastomosis (PRA) and nonrestorative resection (NRR), which are defined as end colostomy or diverting transverse colostomy without resection, respectively, were selected as emergency surgeries. The morbidity rates after PRA did not differ from those after NRR; however, postoperative morbidity rates of stoma closure surgery were significantly lower in PRA (12%) than in NRR (27.2%) (OR: 0.31). The non-reversal rate of stoma in PRA (16%) was lower than that in NRR (35.5%) (OR: 0.37).[71] Moreover, PRA was associated with better short- and long-term outcomes than NRR.

Further, it is important to establish whether PRA or Hartmann's procedure (HP) should be selected when performing colonic resection for acute diverticulitis. PRA has favorable rates of stoma reversal (PRA, 80.3%; HP, 62.1%; OR, 2.62) and reversal-related morbidity (PRA, 11.9%; HP, 27%; OR, 0.33). The mortality (PRA 5%, HP 6.4%, OR: 0.83, n.s.), morbidity (PRA 50.6%, HP 49.5%, OR: 0.99, n.s.), and reintervention rates (PRA 7.4%, HP 7.5%, OR: 0.90, n.s.) did not differ between PRA and HP.[72] Moreover, the overall mean costs per patient were also lower for PRA (€20 544) than for HP (€28 670), with a mean difference of €8126.[73] Based on these data, PRA should be considered, if possible.

In a meta-analysis, emergency laparoscopic surgery for colonic diverticulitis had a lower morbidity rate than open surgery, though the rates of postoperative mortality, severe complications, and reoperation did not differ. However, this meta-analysis was based on both RCTs and retrospective studies. A greater number of high-quality RCTs are necessary to compare laparoscopic surgery and open surgery.[74] Laparoscopic surgery is classified into two types; laparoscopic primary resection and laparoscopic lavage without primary resection. Laparoscopic peritoneal lavage is associated with higher morbidity than laparoscopic primary resection.[75]

Immunosuppressed patients with diverticular disease have an increased risk of developing complicated diverticulitis. The mortality and morbidity rates of immunosuppressed patients were higher than those of immunocompetent patients for emergent surgery (RR: 1.91 and RR: 2.18, respectively), but not for elective surgery (RR: 1.70 and RR: 1.40, respectively).[76] Elective surgery may be planned for immunosuppressed patients with diverticulitis according to a meta-analysis.

3.4 | Recurrence after diverticulitis surgery

A time-to-event analysis for recurrence- and colostomy-free survival was performed using a large retrospective cohort. Of the patients with uncomplicated diverticulitis treated with non-operative methods, 19% underwent elective surgery and 81% were treated medically for recurrent uncomplicated diverticulitis after initial therapy. Patients who underwent elective surgery were associated with lower rates of recurrence than those treated with medical therapy (15% vs 61% at 5 years, OR: 0.17). The rate of colostomy after elective surgery (1.8%) was lower than that after medical therapy (2.3%) at 5 years (OR: 2.3).[77] The recurrence rate of diverticulitis was reported to be 5.8% in a meta-analysis. Six factors related to recurrence after bowel resection with diverticulitis were identified: younger age and irritable bowel syndrome (preoperative); anastomotic level and uncomplicated recurrent diverticulitis (operative); absence of active diverticulitis on pathology and persistence of postoperative pain (postoperative). According to the results of this study, elective surgery prevents diverticulitis recurrence or colostomy risk.[78]

4 | FUTURE PERSPECTIVE AND SUMMARY

In this review, we present key articles on clinical trials and meta-analyses of IBD and diverticulitis from 2020 to 2021. The development of new drugs for IBD is remarkable, and treatment strategies using multiple agents and various techniques are required. It is necessary for surgeons to have a deep understanding of the surgical procedure and perioperative management, as well as the impact of new drugs. In terms of the surgical procedure for CD, it is important to select an optimal procedure that preserves bowel function, minimizes recurrence, and reduces complications. The usefulness of autologous cell transplantation for fistulae on CD has been verified, and it may be clinically applied in the future. It is also important to enhance knowledge on perioperative management associated with IPAA in total proctocolectomy for IBD.

The incidence of diverticulitis is increasing, and more patients are expected to require surgical treatment in the future. According to recent reports, antimicrobial therapy is unnecessary for uncomplicated diverticulitis. Regarding surgical procedures for diverticulitis, both bowel resection and anastomosis are associated with favorable short-term outcomes, higher stoma closure rate, and more reasonable medical costs than HP. The risk factors for the recurrence of diverticulitis are summarized, and these data support the optimal management for postoperative diverticulitis patients. This review consolidates the available knowledge and improves the quality of surgical procedures and perioperative management in treating IBD and diverticulitis.

ACKNOWLEDGEMENTS

We would like to thank Editage (www.editage.com) for English language editing.

REFERENCES

1. Kaplan GG. The global burden of IBD: from 2015 to 2025. Nat Rev Gastroenterol Hepatol. 2015;12(12):720–7.
2. Olaiya B, Renelus BD, Filon M, Saha S. Trends in morbidity and mortality following colectomy among patients with ulcerative colitis in the biologic era (2002–2013): a study using the national inpatient sample. Dig Dis Sci. 2021;66(6):2032–41.
3. Hunt CW, Chaturvedi R, Brown L, et al. Diverticular disease epidemiology: rising rates of diverticular disease mortality across developing nations. Dis Colon Rectum. 2021;64(1):81–90.
4. Ogino T, Mizushima T, Matsuda C, Mori M, Doki Y. Essential updates 2018/2019: colorectal (benign): recent updates (2018–2019) in the surgical treatment of benign colorectal diseases. Ann Gastroenterol Surg. 2020;4(1):30–8.
5. Lorenzo-Pouso AI, Castelo-Baz P, Rodriguez-Zorrilla S, Perez-Sayans M, Vega P. Association between periodontal disease and inflammatory bowel disease: a systematic review and meta-analysis. Acta Odontol Scand. 2021;79(5):344–53.
6. States V, O'Brien S, Rai JP, et al. Pyoderma gangrenosum in inflammatory bowel disease: a systematic review and meta-analysis. Dig Dis Sci. 2020;65(9):2675–85.
7. Alinaghi F, Tekin HG, Burisch J, Wu JJ, Thyssen JP, Egeberg A. Global prevalence and bidirectional association between psoriasis and inflammatory bowel disease-a systematic review and meta-analysis. J Crohns Colitis. 2020;14(3):351–60.
8. Ning L, Liu R, Li S, et al. Increased risk of herpes zoster infection in patients with inflammatory bowel disease: a meta-analysis of cohort studies. Eur J Clin Microbiol Infect Dis. 2020;39(2):219–27.
9. Barberio B, Zamani M, Black CJ, Savarino EV, Ford AC. Prevalence of symptoms of anxiety and depression in patients with inflammatory bowel disease: a systematic review and meta-analysis. Lancet Gastroenterol Hepatol. 2021;6(5):359–70.
10. Gao X, Tang Y, Lei N, et al. Symptoms of anxiety/depression is associated with more aggressive inflammatory bowel disease. Sci Rep. 2021;11(1):1440.
11. Sandborn WJ, Feagan BG, Loftus EV Jr, et al. Efficacy and safety of upadacitinib in a randomized trial of patients with Crohn's disease. Gastroenterology. 2020;158(8):2123–2138 e2128.
12. Feagan BG, Sandborn WJ, Danese S, et al. Ozanimod induction therapy for patients with moderate to severe Crohn's disease: a single-arm, phase 2, prospective observer-blinded endpoint study. Lancet Gastroenterol Hepatol. 2020;5(9):819–28.
13. Sands BE, Feagan BG, Sandborn WJ, et al. Mongersen (GED-0301) for active Crohn's disease: results of a phase 3 study. Am J Gastroenterol. 2020;115(5):738–45.
14. Sandborn WJ, Peyrin-Biroulet L, Zhang J, et al. Efficacy and safety of etrasimod in a phase 2 randomized trial of patients with ulcerative colitis. Gastroenterology. 2020;158(3):550–61.
15. Sandborn WJ, Feagan BG, D'Haens G, et al. Ozanimod as induction and maintenance therapy for ulcerative colitis. N Engl J Med. 2021;385(14):1280–91.
16. Sandborn WJ, Baert F, Danese S, et al. Efficacy and safety of vedolizumab subcutaneous formulation in a randomized trial of patients with ulcerative colitis. Gastroenterology. 2020;158(3):562–572 e512.
17. Atreya R, Peyrin-Biroulet L, Klymenko A, et al. Cobitolimod for moderate-to-severe, left-sided ulcerative colitis (CONDUCT): a phase 2b randomised, double-blind, placebo-controlled, dose-ranging induction trial. Lancet Gastroenterol Hepatol. 2020;5(12):1063–75.
18. Fellermann K, Schiefke I, Racz I, et al. Efficacy and safety of prolonged release budesonide granules in mesalazine-refractory ulcerative colitis: a multi-centre Phase IIa study (TOPICAL-1). United European Gastroenterol J. 2020;8(10):1186–95.
19. Uchino M, Ikeuchi H, Hata K, et al. Does anti-tumor necrosis factor alpha prevent the recurrence of Crohn's disease? Systematic review and meta-analysis. J Gastroenterol Hepatol. 2021;36(4):864–72.
20. Zheng T, Wang X, Chen Z, He A, Zheng Z, Liu G. Efficacy of adjuvant curcumin therapy in ulcerative colitis: a meta-analysis of randomized controlled trials. J Gastroenterol Hepatol. 2020;35(5):722–9.
21. Dulai PS, Raffals LE, Hudesman D, et al. A phase 2B randomised trial of hyperbaric oxygen therapy for ulcerative colitis patients hospitalised for moderate to severe flares. Aliment Pharmacol Ther. 2020;52(6):955–63.
22. Lansdorp CA, Gecse KB, Buskens CJ, et al. Hyperbaric oxygen therapy for the treatment of perianal fistulas in 20 patients with Crohn's disease. Aliment Pharmacol Ther. 2021;53(5):587–97.
23. Singh AK, Jha DK, Jena A, Kumar -MP, Sebastian S, Sharma V. Hyperbaric oxygen therapy in inflammatory bowel disease: a systematic review and meta-analysis. Eur J Gastroenterol Hepatol. 2021Dec 1;33(1S Suppl 1):e564–e573. doi:10.1097/MEG.00000 00000002164. PMID: 33905214
24. Bettenworth D, Bokemeyer A, Kou L, et al. Systematic review with meta-analysis: efficacy of balloon-assisted enteroscopy for dilation of small bowel Crohn's disease strictures. Aliment Pharmacol Ther. 2020;52(7):1104–16.
25. Kelly CR, Yen EF, Grinspan AM, et al. Fecal microbiota transplantation is highly effective in real-world practice: initial results from the FMT National Registry. Gastroenterology. 2021;160(1):183–192 e183.
26. Crothers JW, Chu ND, Nguyen LTT, et al. Daily, oral FMT for long-term maintenance therapy in ulcerative colitis: results of a single-center, prospective, randomized pilot study. BMC Gastroenterol. 2021;21(1):281.

27. Tang LL, Feng WZ, Cheng JJ, Gong YN. Clinical remission of ulcerative colitis after different modes of faecal microbiota transplantation: a meta-analysis. Int J Colorectal Dis. 2020;35(6):1025–34.
28. Haifer C, Saikal A, Paramsothy R, et al. Response to faecal microbiota transplantation in ulcerative colitis is not sustained long term following induction therapy. Gut. 2021;70(11):2210–1.
29. Li SS, Zhu A, Benes V, et al. Durable coexistence of donor and recipient strains after fecal microbiota transplantation. Science. 2016;352(6285):586–9.
30. Paramsothy S, Nielsen S, Kamm MA, et al. Specific bacteria and metabolites associated with response to fecal microbiota transplantation in patients with ulcerative colitis. Gastroenterology. 2019;156(5):1440–1454 e1442.
31. Stevens TW, Haasnoot ML, D'Haens GR, et al. Laparoscopic ileocaecal resection versus infliximab for terminal ileitis in Crohn's disease: retrospective long-term follow-up of the LIR!C trial. Lancet Gastroenterol Hepatol. 2020;5(10):900–7.
32. Ryan EJ, Orsi G, Boland MR, et al. Meta-analysis of early bowel resection versus initial medical therapy in patient's with ileocolonic Crohn's disease. Int J Colorectal Dis. 2020;35(3):501–12.
33. Butt WT, Ryan EJ, Boland MR, et al. Strictureplasty versus bowel resection for the surgical management of fibrostenotic Crohn's disease: a systematic review and meta-analysis. Int J Colorectal Dis. 2020;35(4):705–17.
34. Watanabe K, Sasaki I, Kohyama A, et al. Antimesenteric cutback end-to-end isoperistaltic anastomosis (Sasaki-Watanabe anastomosis) for Crohn's disease: novel surgical technique and early results of surgical anastomotic recurrence. Ann Gastroenterol Surg. 2021;5(4):528–37.
35. Luglio G, Rispo A, Imperatore N, et al. Surgical prevention of anastomotic recurrence by excluding mesentery in Crohn's disease: the SuPREMe-CD study – a randomized clinical trial. Ann Surg. 2020;272(2):210–7.
36. Ng CH, Chin YH, Lin SY, et al. Kono-S anastomosis for Crohn's disease: a systemic review, meta-analysis, and meta-regression. Surg Today. 2021;51(4):493–501.
37. Panes J, Garcia-Olmo D, Van Assche G, et al. Expanded allogeneic adipose-derived mesenchymal stem cells (Cx601) for complex perianal fistulas in Crohn's disease: a phase 3 randomised, double-blind controlled trial. Lancet. 2016;388(10051):1281–90.
38. Dige A, Hougaard HT, Agnholt J, et al. Efficacy of injection of freshly collected autologous adipose tissue into perianal fistulas in patients with Crohn's disease. Gastroenterology. 2019;156(8):2208–2216 e2201.
39. Lightner AL, Dozois EJ, Dietz AB, et al. Matrix-delivered autologous mesenchymal stem cell therapy for refractory rectovaginal Crohn's fistulas. Inflamm Bowel Dis. 2020;26(5):670–7.
40. Zhou C, Li M, Zhang Y, et al. Autologous adipose-derived stem cells for the treatment of Crohn's fistula-in-ano: an open-label, controlled trial. Stem Cell Res Ther. 2020;11(1):124.
41. Maciel Gutierrez VM, Gutierrez Guillen SG, Centeno Flores MW, et al. Safety of allogeneic adipose tissue-derived mesenchymal stem cells for the treatment of complex perianal fistulas not associated with Crohn's disease: a phase I clinical trial. Dis Colon Rectum. 2021;64(3):328–34.
42. Barnhoorn MC, Wasser M, Roelofs H, et al. Long-term evaluation of allogeneic bone marrow-derived mesenchymal stromal cell therapy for Crohn's disease perianal fistulas. J Crohns Colitis. 2020;14(1):64–70.
43. Cao Y, Su Q, Zhang B, Shen F, Li S. Efficacy of stem cells therapy for Crohn's fistula: a meta-analysis and systematic review. Stem Cell Res Ther. 2021;12(1):32.
44. Sachar DB. Management of acute, severe ulcerative colitis. J Dig Dis. 2012;13(2):65–8.
45. Olen O, Erichsen R, Sachs MC, et al. Colorectal cancer in ulcerative colitis: a Scandinavian population-based cohort study. Lancet. 2020;395(10218):123–31.
46. Song EM, Lee HS, Park SH, et al. Clinical characteristics and long-term prognosis of elderly onset ulcerative colitis. J Gastroenterol Hepatol. 2018;33(1):172–9.
47. Komoto S, Higashiyama M, Watanabe C, et al. Clinical differences between elderly-onset ulcerative colitis and non-elderly-onset ulcerative colitis: a nationwide survey data in Japan. J Gastroenterol Hepatol. 2018;33(11):1839–43.
48. Pedersen KE, Jia X, Holubar SD, Steele SR, Lightner AL. Ileal pouch-anal anastomosis in the elderly: a systematic review and meta-analysis. Colorectal Dis. 2021;23(8):2062–74.
49. Dayton MT, Larsen KR. Should older patients undergo ileal pouch-anal anastomosis? Am J Surg. 1996;172(5):pp. 444–447; discussion 447–448.
50. Khan K, Manzoor T, Khan S, Hartley JE. Is diversion free ileal pouch-anal anastomosis a safe procedure? A meta-analysis of 4973 cases. Int J Colorectal Dis. 2021;36(4):657–69.
51. Tamura K, Matsuda K, Yokoyama S, et al. Defunctioning loop ileostomy for rectal anastomoses: predictors of stoma outlet obstruction. Int J Colorectal Dis. 2019;34(6):1141–5.
52. Kitahara T, Sato Y, Oshiro T, Matsunaga R, Nagashima M, Okazumi S. Risk factors for postoperative stoma outlet obstruction in ulcerative colitis. World J Gastrointest Surg. 2020;12(12):507–19.
53. Law CC, Bell C, Koh D, Bao Y, Jairath V, Narula N. Risk of post-operative infectious complications from medical therapies in inflammatory bowel disease. Cochrane Database Syst Rev. 2020;10:CD013256.
54. Guo D, Jiang K, Hong J, Zhang M, Shi Y, Zhou B. Association between vedolizumab and postoperative complications in IBD: a systematic review and meta-analysis. Int J Colorectal Dis. 2021;36(10):2081–92.
55. de Bruyn JR, Bossuyt P, Ferrante M, et al. High-dose vitamin D does not prevent postoperative recurrence of Crohn's disease in a randomized placebo-controlled trial. Clin Gastroenterol Hepatol. 2021;19(8):1573–1582 e1575.
56. Aksan A, Farrag K, Blumenstein I, Schroder O, Dignass AU, Stein J. Chronic intestinal failure and short bowel syndrome in Crohn's disease. World J Gastroenterol. 2021;27(24):3440–65.
57. Jeppesen PB, Gabe SM, Seidner DL, Lee HM, Olivier C. Factors associated with response to teduglutide in patients with short-bowel syndrome and intestinal failure. Gastroenterology. 2018;154(4):874–85.
58. Chandan S, Mohan BP, Kumar A, et al. Safety and efficacy of biological therapy in chronic antibiotic refractory pouchitis: a systematic review with meta-analysis. J Clin Gastroenterol. 2021;55(6):481–91.
59. Hasan B, Yim Y, Ur Rashid M, et al. Hyperbaric oxygen therapy in chronic inflammatory conditions of the pouch. Inflamm Bowel Dis. 2021;27(7):965–70.
60. Jin-Dominguez F, Mansoor E, Panhwar MS, et al. Epidemiology of diverticulitis and prevalence of first-ever colorectal cancer postdiverticulitis in adults in the United States: a population-based national study. Dis Colon Rectum. 2021;64(2):181–9.
61. Aune D, Sen A, Leitzmann MF, Norat T, Tonstad S, Vatten LJ. Body mass index and physical activity and the risk of diverticular disease: a systematic review and meta-analysis of prospective studies. Eur J Nutr. 2017;56(8):2423–38.
62. Tursi A, Violi A, Cambie G, et al. Risk factors for endoscopic severity of diverticular disease of the colon and its outcome: a real-life case-control study. Eur J Gastroenterol Hepatol. 2020;32(9):1123–9.
63. Aune D, Sen A, Norat T, Riboli E. Dietary fibre intake and the risk of diverticular disease: a systematic review and meta-analysis of prospective studies. Eur J Nutr. 2020;59(2):421–32.

64. Hajibandeh S, Hajibandeh S, Smart NJ, Maw A. Meta-analysis of the demographic and prognostic significance of right-sided versus left-sided acute diverticulitis. Colorectal Dis. 2020;22(12):1908–23.
65. Lee KY, Lee J, Park YY, Kim Y, Oh ST. Difference in clinical features between right- and left-sided acute colonic diverticulitis. Sci Rep. 2020;10(1):3754.
66. Jaung R, Nisbet S, Gosselink MP, et al. Antibiotics do not reduce length of hospital stay for uncomplicated diverticulitis in a pragmatic double-blind randomized trial. Clin Gastroenterol Hepatol. 2021;19(3):503–510 e501.
67. van Dijk ST, Chabok A, Dijkgraaf MG, Boermeester MA, Smedh K. Observational versus antibiotic treatment for uncomplicated diverticulitis: an individual-patient data meta-analysis. Br J Surg. 2020;107(8):1062–9.
68. Fowler H, Gachabayov M, Vimalachandran D, Clifford R, Orangio GR, Bergamaschi R. Failure of nonoperative management in patients with acute diverticulitis complicated by abscess: a systematic review. Int J Colorectal Dis. 2021;36(7):1367–83.
69. Lee H, Gachabayov M, Rojas A, Felsenreich DM, Tsarkov P, Bergamaschi R. Systematic review of failure of nonoperative management in complicated sigmoid diverticulitis with abscess. Langenbecks Arch Surg. 2020;405(3):277–81.
70. Patel SV, Hendren S, Zaborowski A, Winter D, for Members of the Evidence Based Reviews in Surgery g. Evidence-based reviews in surgery long-term outcome of surgery versus conservative management for recurrent and ongoing complaints after an episode of diverticulitis: five-year follow-up results of a multicenter randomized controlled trial (DIRECT-Trial). Ann Surg. 2020;272(2):284–7.
71. Gachabayov M, Tuech JJ, Tulina I, Coget J, Bridoux V, Bergamaschi R. Primary anastomosis and nonrestorative resection for perforated diverticulitis with peritonitis: meta-analysis of randomized trials. Colorectal Dis. 2020;22(10):1245–57.
72. Lambrichts DP, Edomskis PP, van der Bogt RD, Kleinrensink GJ, Bemelman WA, Lange JF. Sigmoid resection with primary anastomosis versus the Hartmann's procedure for perforated diverticulitis with purulent or fecal peritonitis: a systematic review and meta-analysis. Int J Colorectal Dis. 2020;35(8):1371–86.
73. Lambrichts DPV, van Dieren S, Bemelman WA, Lange JF. Cost-effectiveness of sigmoid resection with primary anastomosis or end colostomy for perforated diverticulitis: an analysis of the randomized Ladies trial. Br J Surg. 2020;107(12):1686–94.
74. Lin H, Zhuang Z, Huang X, Li Y. The role of emergency laparoscopic surgery for complicated diverticular disease: a systematic review and meta-analysis. Medicine (Baltimore). 2020;99(40):e22421.
75. Azhar N, Johanssen A, Sundstrom T, et al. Laparoscopic lavage vs primary resection for acute perforated diverticulitis: long-term outcomes from the scandinavian diverticulitis (SCANDIV) randomized clinical trial. JAMA Surg. 2021;156(2):121–7.
76. McKechnie T, Lee Y, Kruse C, et al. Operative management of colonic diverticular disease in the setting of immunosuppression: a systematic review and meta-analysis. Am J Surg. 2021;221(1):72–85.
77. Thornblade LW, Simianu VV, Davidson GH, Flum DR. Elective surgery for diverticulitis and the risk of recurrence and ostomy. Ann Surg. 2021;273(6):1157–64.
78. Longchamp G, Abbassi Z, Meyer J, Toso C, Buchs NC, Ris F. Surgical resection does not avoid the risk of diverticulitis recurrence-a systematic review of risk factors. Int J Colorectal Dis. 2021;36(2):227–37.

4

Survey regarding gastrointestinal stoma construction and closure in Japan

Yoshiko Ando[1,2] | Arata Takahashi[3,4,5] | Makoto Fujii[2] | Hiroshi Hasegawa[6] | Toshimoto Kimura[6] | Hiroyuki Yamamoto[4,5] | Tetsuya Tajima[2] | Yukio Nishiguchi[7] | Yoshihiro Kakeji[8] | Hiroaki Miyata[4,5] | Yuko Kitagawa[9]

[1]Department of Nursing, Japanese Red Cross Osaka Hospital, Osaka, Japan

[2]Department of Health Science, Graduate School of Medicine, Osaka University, Osaka, Japan

[3]NCD Data Quality Management Subcommittee, The Japanese Society of Gastroenterological Surgery, Tokyo, Japan

[4]Department of Health Policy and Management, School of Medicine, Keio University, Tokyo, Japan

[5]Department of Healthcare Quality Assessment, Graduate School of Medicine, The University of Tokyo, Tokyo, Japan

[6]Project Management Subcommittee, The Japanese Society of Gastroenterological Surgery, Tokyo, Japan

[7]Department of Surgery, Osaka City Juso Hospital, Osaka, Japan

[8]Database Committee, The Japanese Society of Gastroenterological Surgery, Tokyo, Japan

[9]The Japanese Society of Gastroenterological Surgery, Tokyo, Japan

Correspondence
Yoshiko Ando, Department of Nursing, Japanese Red Cross Osaka Hospital, 5-30 Fudegasaki-cho, Osaka 543-8555, Japan.
Email: y.andou@osaka-med.jrc.or.jp

Abstract

Background and Aim: In Japan, the actual number of stoma constructions and stoma closures is not known. The aim of this study was to conduct a survey to determine the number of gastrointestinal stoma constructions and closures in Japan.

Methods: Enrolled participants comprised patients undergoing selected gastrointestinal surgeries who were recorded in the National Clinical Database. This database uses the "Common Items for Gastrointestinal Surgeons." These procedures were formulated by the Japanese Society of Gastroenterological Surgery during 2013–2018.

Results: According to the National Clinical Database, a total of 154,323 gastrointestinal stomas were constructed between January 1, 2013 and December 31, 2018. By procedure, there were 78,723 cases of stoma construction, 39,653 of abdominoperineal resection, 2470 total pelvic exenteration procedures, and 33,572 Hartmann's procedures. The ratio of stoma closures to stoma constructions increased annually in patients under 70 y of age but not in older patients. Approximately 35% of total colectomies, 60% of proctocolectomies, and 20% of low anterior resections were accompanied by stoma construction. The number of patients with rectal cancer who underwent colostomy increased gradually during the study period and the number who underwent stoma construction increased among older patients.

Conclusion: The number of cases of gastrointestinal stoma construction has increased gradually in Japan, and the proportion of older patients is increasing each year. The purposes and surgical techniques for stoma construction are diverse and are expected to increase in Japan, a super-aged society.

KEYWORDS

colostomy, enterostomy, gastrointestinal stoma closure, gastrointestinal stoma construction, national clinical database, ostomy surgery

1 | INTRODUCTION

Ostomates need to learn new skills after surgery and overcome many challenges so as to return to a normal social life, because defecation management after the construction of a gastrointestinal stoma requires special skills.[1-3] In Japan, it is estimated that there are currently approximately 210,000 people who have received physical disability certificates, which can be applied for after the installation of a permanent stoma.[4] However, the number of temporary stomas and the number of stoma closures cannot be ascertained in the same way, and there are no data available to clearly ascertain the number of new gastrointestinal stomas and the number of people who have them. Additionally, patient background information, such as basic information and surgical information, has not been collected. Thus, it is difficult to grasp the actual situation regarding the number of constructed stomas and stoma closures, together with the patient backgrounds, according to the current official statistics. It is therefore unclear how many ostomates actually exist in Japan at present and the background under which their stoma was constructed. To plan specific support measures for ostomates in Japan, which is a super-aged society unparalleled in the world in terms of its medical care technology and social security system,[5] it is necessary to understand the trends in the construction and closure of gastrointestinal stomas and the current status of the background of gastrointestinal stoma construction.

The National Clinical Database (NCD) of Japan, which began registering data in 2011, is a large nationwide database covering more than 95% of the surgeries performed by general surgeons in Japan. At the end of January in 2021, 5404 facilities have enrolled in the NCD and approximately 1,500,000 cases are registered every year.[6,7] In a validation study using 2016 data conducted by the gastroenterological section of the NCD, the Japanese Society of Gastroenterological Surgery (JSGS), patient demographics, surgical outcomes, and processes were proven to be highly institutionalized.[8,9] Therefore, by extracting cases of gastrointestinal stoma construction and closure from the NCD database, the number of gastrointestinal stomas constructed and their co-procedures, the percentage of stomas constructed among them, and the patient background including age group and preoperative information, can be used to confirm the actual situation of gastrointestinal stoma construction in Japan. At the same time, the number of gastrointestinal stoma closures can serve as a valuable dataset to predict the number of people with temporary stomas. In the present study, we conducted a survey regarding the number of gastrointestinal stoma constructions and closures in Japan.

2 | PARTICIPANTS AND METHODS

The enrolled participants were patients who underwent selected gastrointestinal surgical procedures and who had surgical data recorded in the NCD. The NCD uses the "Common Items for Gastrointestinal Surgeons" as defined in the "Training Curriculum for Board Certified Surgeons in Gastroenterology." These procedures were formulated by the JSGS. The study period covered 2013–2018, and the data were extracted according to the conditions related to the construction of gastrointestinal stoma.

2.1 | Surgical procedure

The total number of cases of gastrointestinal stoma was classified into four categories: abdominoperineal resection (APR), total pelvic exenteration (TPE), Hartmann's procedure, and stoma construction. Stoma construction includes enterostomy and colostomy. To exclude "colostomy" as a route for nutritional injection, cases of concurrent gastric and esophageal surgery were excluded. The total number of stomas was defined as the total number of stomas in the four categories.

For enterostomy and colostomy, those associated with esophageal and gastric surgeries were excluded. In cases of total colectomy, proctocolectomy and ileoanal anastomosis, and low anterior resection (LAR), patients without a record of a concomitant procedure were counted separately from stoma nonconstruction. Stoma closure included enterostoma closure, colostoma closure, and stoma closure.

2.2 | Statistical analysis

Descriptive statistics were conducted for the number of procedures performed, by sex and age group, during 2013–2018 for stoma construction (except for APR, TPE, and Hartmann's procedure), APR, TPE, and Hartmann's procedure. The total number of cases of stoma construction and stoma closure was also analyzed by sex and age group over time. Additionally, the number of patients with and without stoma construction, patients' sex, and patients' age group were counted for the three techniques of total colectomy, proctocolectomy and ileoanal anastomosis, and LAR, and changes over time were examined. In malignant neoplasms of the rectum (International Classification of Diseases, Tenth Revision code: C20), the following characteristics were compared: age at surgery, sex, year of surgery, preoperative chemotherapy within 30 d, preoperative chemotherapy within 90 d, preoperative radiotherapy within 90 d before surgery, American Society of Anesthesiologists physical status (ASA-PS) classification at surgery, Union for International Cancer Control tumor–node–metastasis (UICC TNM) classification, emergency surgery, endoscopic surgery, and characteristics of cancer remnants in the five procedures (LAR with or without diverting stoma, APR, Hartmann's procedure, stoma construction). Additionally, malignant neoplasm and benign tumors were divided into two groups: LAR with or without stoma, age at surgery, sex, year of surgery, presence of diabetes (diet therapy only, oral agents, insulin treatment, no treatment), preoperative presence of dyspnea within 30 d, preoperative ADL within 30 d, chronic obstructive pulmonary disease, preoperative presence of dialysis within 14 d, immediately preoperative highly advanced cancer with multiple metastases, long-term steroid treatment, ASA-PS at surgery, classification at the time of surgery, emergency surgery, presence of endoscopic surgery, preoperative chemotherapy within 30 d and within 90 d, and preoperative radiotherapy within 90 d. For malignant neoplasm, UICC TNM classification and stage were also used as comparison items. All descriptive statistics were performed using IBM SPSS v. 26 (IBM, Armonk NY).

3 | RESULTS

3.1 | Annual changes in stoma construction surgeries by sex and age group

A total of 154,323 gastrointestinal stomas were surgically constructed and reported in the NCD between January 1, 2013 and December 31, 2018. By procedure, there were 78,723 stoma constructions (except for APR, TPE, and Hartmann's procedure), 39,653 APRs, 2470 TPEs, and 33,572 Hartmann's procedures.

During the study period, the number of gastrointestinal stoma construction cases per year increased gradually in both men and women, and the proportion of older patients increased every year. In a comparison of male and female patients, there were 93,271 men and 61,052 women. In patients aged 85 y and older, the number of women was 10,994 and there were 7769 males. The number of stoma construction procedures (except for APR, TPE, Hartmann's procedure) increased among men but remained about the same for women during each year of the study period. The number of APRs performed was about the same each year in both women and men, and the number of Hartmann's procedures increased in both sexes. The number of gastrointestinal stoma constructions has increased gradually in Japan, and the proportion of older patients requiring this procedure increased each year (Table 1, Figure 1).

3.2 | Annual changes in stoma construction and closure by sex and age group

In total, there were 77,910 cases of stoma closure during the study period, with 26,804 cases among women and 51,106 among men. In a comparison by sex, as with colostomy, there were more men than women under 85 y of age and more women than men over 85 y of age. The ratio of stoma closure to stoma construction by age group in each year increased among patients aged 79 y or younger. The ratio of stoma closure to stoma construction in those aged under 60 y increased each year, from 0.64 for women and 0.77 for men in 2013 to 0.80 for women and 1.00 for men in 2018 (Figure 2, Table S1).

3.3 | Number of stoma and nonstoma constructions, according to surgical technique, by sex and age group

The number of total colectomies was 7788 (in 3182 women and 4606 men). Among them, 5090 cases (2073 women, 65.14%; 3017 men, 65.50%) were nonstoma construction and 2698 cases (1109 women, 1589 men) were stoma construction. Surgery with nonstoma construction in both sexes was performed in ~55% of patients under 60 y of age and 70%–75% in those over 70 y of age.

The total number of patients with proctocolectomy and ileoanal anastomosis was 2470 (924 women and 1546 men). Among them, 1018 cases (380 women and 638 men, 41.13% and 41.27%, respectively) were nonstoma construction and 1452 cases (544 women and 908 men) were stoma construction. As with total colectomy, surgery with nonstoma construction in both sexes was performed in ~40% of patients under 60 y of age and in 30%–50% of patients over 60 y of age. Although there was no difference between men and women, there were 1875 patients under the age of 60 y, accounting for 76% of the total.

The total number of LARs was 98 971 (34,555 women and 64,416 men).

Although there was no difference by sex, 23,001 patients were under the age of 60 y, accounting for 76% of the total. Among them, 78,276 cases (women: 28 499 [82.47%], men: 49 777 [77.27%]) were nonstoma construction and 20,695 cases (6056 women, 14,639 men) were stoma construction. In a comparison by sex, the percentage of nonstoma construction was 82.47% in women and 77.27% in men (Figure 3, Table S2).

3.4 | Patient characteristics with stoma and nonstoma construction according to surgical procedures for rectal cancer

Table 2 shows the characteristics of LAR with stoma construction, LAR without stoma construction (nonstoma construction), APR, Hartmann's procedure, and stoma construction without intestinal resection. In total, 21,122 patients had stoma construction and 64,572 had nonstoma construction in LAR. There was no significant difference in the characteristics of patients with and without stomas. The ratio of diverting stoma in LAR to LAR without stoma construction increased each year (Figure 4).

The rate of stage T4b was 2.65% for LAR without diverting stoma and 3.86% for diverting stoma. The APR rate was 9.07%, Hartmann's technique 12.9%, and stoma construction without bowel resection 36.79%. Hartmann's procedure was characterized by a higher percentage of ASA-PS 4 and 5 (5.9%) compared with other procedures, with fewer than 1% for LAR and 1.41% for APR (Table 2).

3.5 | Patient characteristics with malignant and benign tumors in LAR

The characteristics of each malignant neoplasm and benign tumor in LAR are shown in Table 3. There were 93,546 cases of malignant neoplasm, 39 cases of benign tumors, and 5386 cases were unknown. Among malignant neoplasm surgeries, 14.24% of patients in the

TABLE 1 Annual changes in stoma construction by sex and age group

Procedure	Year	Sex	All	Age group (y)							
				< 60	61–64	65–69	70–74	75–79	80–84	85–89	over 90
Total	2013	Female, n	9886	1784	1052	1155	1314	1406	1467	1107	601
		Male, n	14 924	2764	2190	2416	2504	2207	1661	893	289
	2014	Female, n	9828	1735	975	1157	1354	1429	1463	1131	584
		Male, n	15 238	2880	1984	2689	2562	2194	1683	957	289
	2015	Female, n	10 144	1719	913	1352	1388	1442	1567	1153	610
		Male, n	15 720	2872	1964	2845	2618	2376	1759	998	288
	2016	Female, n	10 325	1839	860	1441	1287	1378	1642	1219	659
		Male, n	15 814	2859	1897	3140	2597	2196	1807	996	322
	2017	Female, n	10 576	1776	865	1456	1384	1496	1611	1281	707
		Male, n	15 840	2806	1758	2947	2618	2473	1877	980	381
	2018	Female, n	10 293	1690	813	1398	1406	1467	1577	1260	682
		Male, n	15 735	2728	1657	2881	2771	2480	1842	997	379
Stoma construction (except for APR, TPE, Hartmann's procedure)	2013	Female, n	5277	1051	561	594	675	723	702	603	368
		Male, n	7599	1409	1128	1256	1292	1101	786	449	178
	2014	Female, n	5155	1051	550	590	689	694	667	556	358
		Male, n	7766	1488	1019	1402	1316	1104	811	480	146
	2015	Female, n	5193	998	484	691	692	692	724	571	341
		Male, n	7912	1519	1020	1441	1313	1157	819	477	166
	2016	Female, n	5228	1073	442	719	630	659	759	582	364
		Male, n	7988	1529	962	1570	1339	1080	850	469	189
	2017	Female, n	5350	1014	468	737	673	753	693	628	384
		Male, n	8030	1486	920	1526	1331	1207	883	463	214
	2018	Female, n	5293	1006	448	745	710	707	736	567	374
		Male, n	7932	1425	907	1458	1386	1203	884	475	194

(Continues)

TABLE 1 (Continued)

Procedure	Year	Sex	All	Age group (y)							
				< 60	61–64	65–69	70–74	75–79	80–84	85–89	over 90
Abdominoperineal resection	2013	Female, n	2306	409	279	323	370	338	334	196	57
		Male, n	4363	880	704	739	759	640	441	169	31
	2014	Female, n	2289	415	242	310	363	379	348	181	51
		Male, n	4300	893	624	795	734	585	439	184	46
	2015	Female, n	2346	427	225	367	369	364	348	185	61
		Male, n	4390	848	589	846	777	668	436	193	33
	2016	Female, n	2402	453	230	381	363	340	369	184	82
		Male, n	4381	825	585	954	716	637	440	180	44
	2017	Female, n	2328	432	210	363	344	338	379	192	70
		Male, n	4242	823	519	831	725	657	454	189	44
	2018	Female, n	2198	372	200	334	343	357	319	205	68
		Male, n	4108	757	456	820	762	670	402	194	47
Total pelvic exenteration	2013	Female, n	127	48	22	26	12	12	5	2	0
		Male, n	285	83	67	64	41	22	7	1	0
	2014	Female, n	85	26	10	16	15	11	5	2	0
		Male, n	289	93	47	63	45	33	5	3	0
	2015	Female, n	105	31	15	20	17	11	9	2	0
		Male, n	280	73	60	71	38	29	6	3	0
	2016	Female, n	91	37	11	13	13	9	8	0	0
		Male, n	311	87	52	85	54	26	7	0	0
	2017	Female, n	149	46	24	25	25	20	9	0	0
		Male, n	307	77	62	71	56	32	7	2	0
	2018	Female, n	121	39	17	24	21	9	10	1	0
		Male, n	320	79	41	89	60	36	13	1	1

(Continues)

TABLE 1 (Continued)

Procedure	Year	Sex	All	Age group (y)							
				< 60	61–64	65–69	70–74	75–79	80–84	85–89	over 90
Hartmann's procedure	2013	Female, n	2181	276	191	213	257	335	426	307	176
		Male, n	2685	393	291	358	415	446	428	274	80
	2014	Female, n	2304	245	173	242	288	345	444	392	175
		Male, n	2890	409	295	430	467	474	428	290	97
	2015	Female, n	2510	264	191	275	313	375	487	397	208
		Male, n	3140	432	295	488	491	522	498	325	89
	2016	Female, n	2610	277	177	329	283	370	507	454	213
		Male, n	3145	418	298	533	492	455	512	348	89
	2017	Female, n	2754	285	164	332	342	386	530	462	253
		Male, n	3279	422	260	524	507	579	535	329	123
	2018	Female, n	2687	274	148	296	333	394	513	489	240
		Male, n	3387	472	253	516	565	572	545	327	137

Note: Total is the sum of stoma construction only or bowel resection with stoma construction, abdominoperineal resection, total pelvic exenteration, and Hartmann's procedure.

Abbreviations: APR, abdominoperineal resection; TPE, total pelvic exenteration.

stoma group and 5.34% in the nonstoma group received preoperative chemotherapy 30 d before surgery. The percentage of patients who received preoperative chemotherapy 90 d prior to surgery was 3.58% in the stoma group and 1.89% in the nonstoma group. The preoperative radiation therapy rate was 8.46% in the stoma group and 1.78% in the nonstoma group. Nonlaparoscopic surgery was performed in 33.69% of the stoma group and 45.94% of the nonstoma group. There were no differences in the other patient characteristics (Table 3).

4 | DISCUSSION

In this study we found that the number of cases of stoma construction in Japan has been increasing slowly, and the number of these patients in their 70s and older has been increasing each year. This finding may be due to the fact that some older patients chose to have a stoma construction procedure because of the safety of perioperative management and defecation care[10] or because they have difficulty with stoma closure owing to poor surgical tolerance. This may be true for stoma closure because the ratio of stoma closure to construction has increased in patients under 84 y of age but not in patients over 85 y of age. The high ratio of stoma closure to stoma construction in patients under 59 y of age can also be explained by the fact that surgery for inflammatory bowel disease is often combined with temporary stoma construction,[11] resulting in a high incidence among younger patients.[12]

The total number of stoma construction cases was 24,810 in 2013, 25,066 in 2014, 25,864 in 2015, 26,139 in 2016, 26,416 in 2017, and 26,028 in 2018. However, the number of applications for physical disability certificates owing to rectal/bladder dysfunction with a registered permanent stoma is ~30,000 each year in Japan.[7] Even though the results of this study reflect the sum of temporary and permanent stomas, the total was lower than the number of registrations for physically disability. When we looked at the presence or absence of stoma construction for the three techniques in total colectomy, proctocolectomy, and LAR, the rate of stoma construction was highest for low anterior resection, and stoma construction was performed in ~82% of all cases. Because all of these surgeries are combined with anastomosis of the intestine with preservation of the anus, we considered that this type of stoma construction is positioned as a diverting stoma. In the 1990s and 2000s, it was reported that temporary stoma placement significantly prevented suture failure in low anterior resection.[13-18] Later, in the 2010s, the impact of temporary stoma construction on rates of complication other than suture failure was also examined.[14] Insurance coverage for stents beginning in 2012 has enabled preoperative decompression for colorectal cancer obstruction, decreased the rate of stoma construction before cancer chemotherapy, [19] and has reportedly prevented suture failure in transanal anal drains.[20,21] Whereas the indications for diverting stoma placement are diminishing, there are also reports of

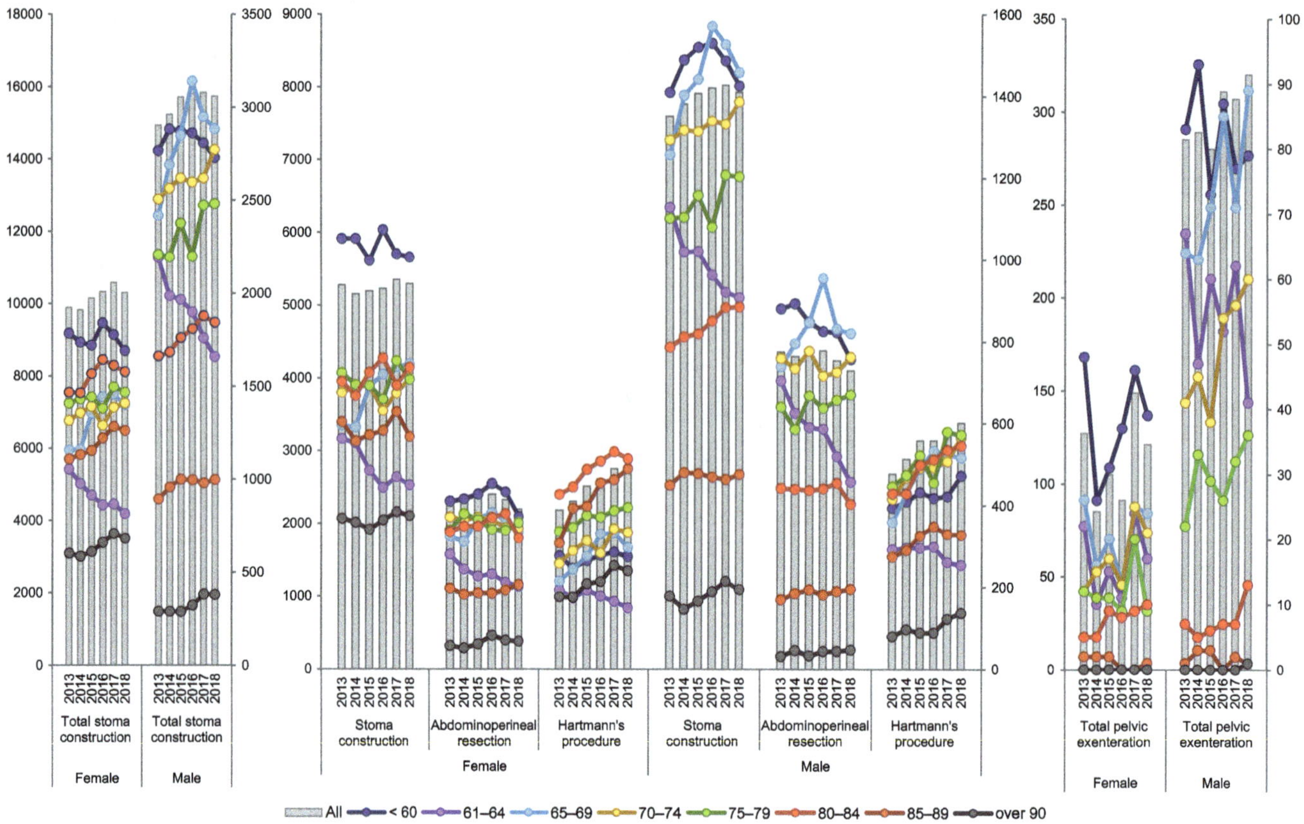

FIGURE 1 Annual changes of surgeries with stoma construction by sex and age group

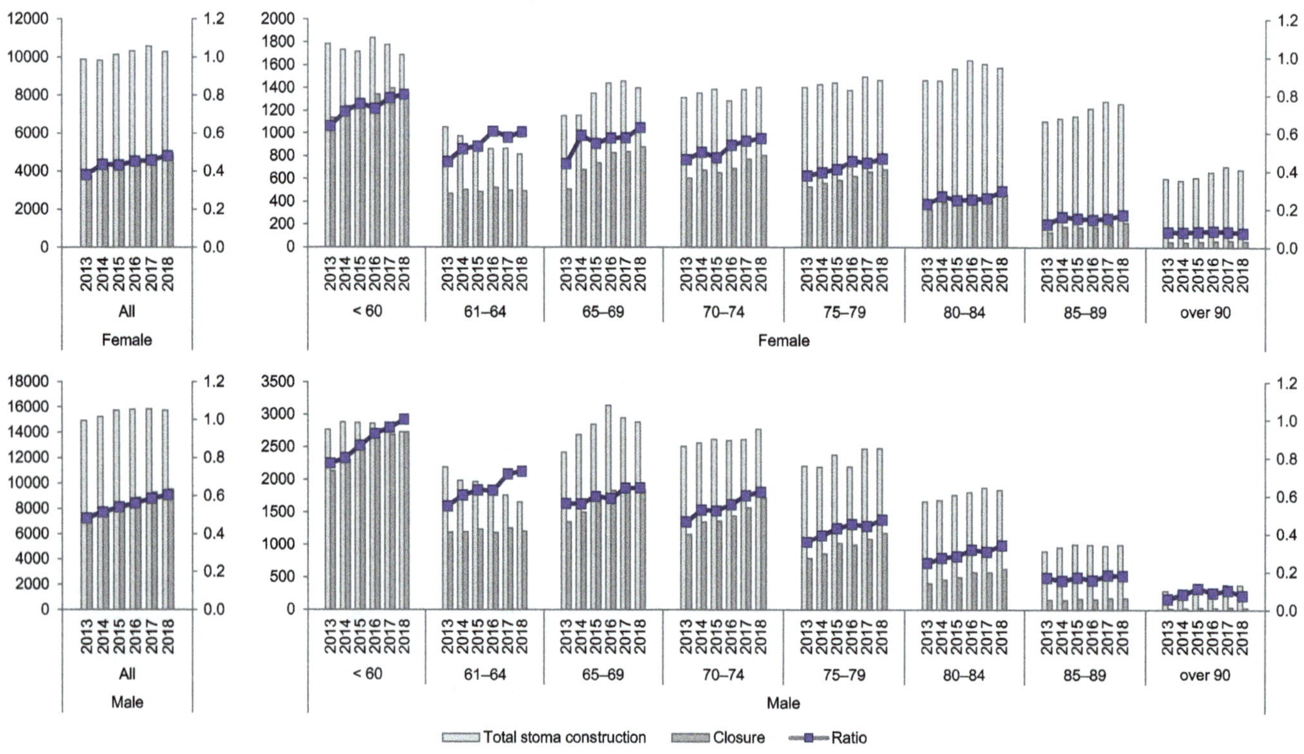

FIGURE 2 Annual changes of stoma construction and closure by sex and age group

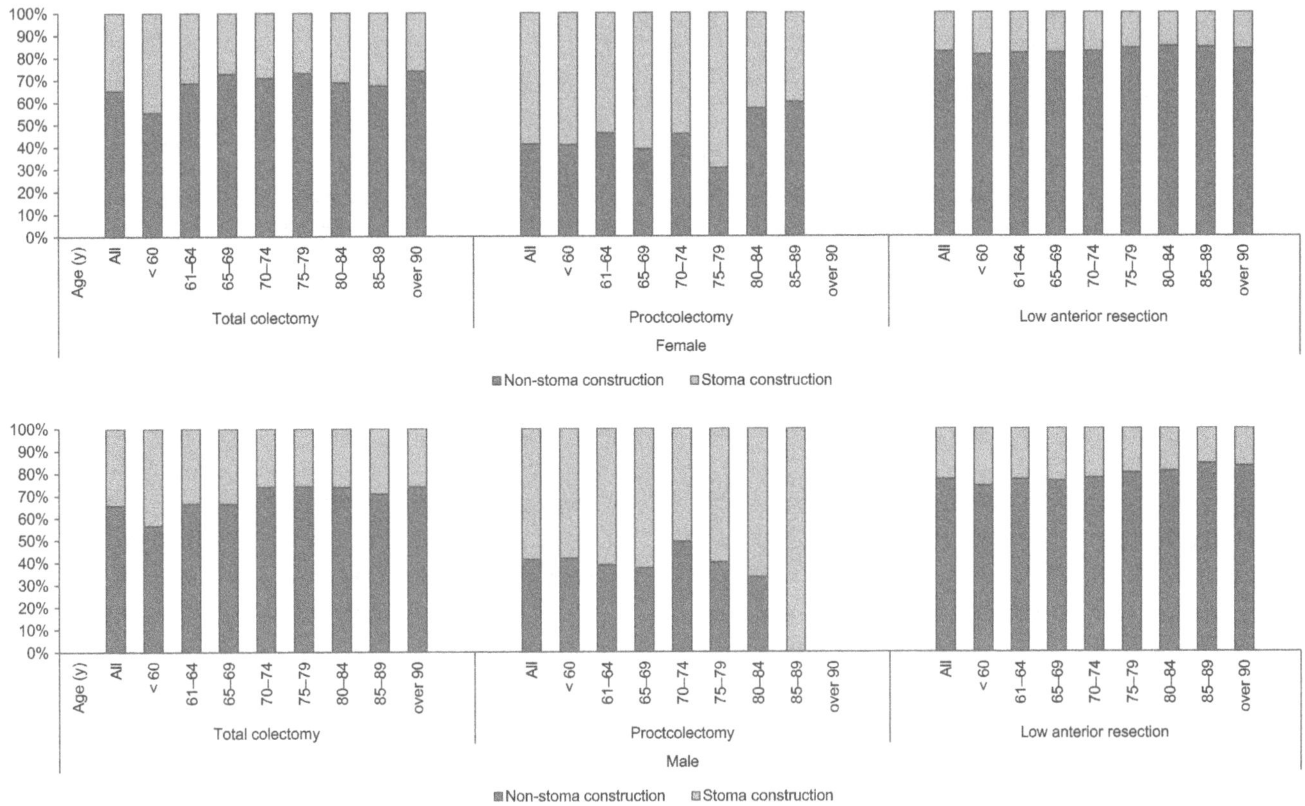

FIGURE 3 Number of stoma construction and no-construction according to the three colorectum operative procedures by sex and age group

risks associated with the use of transanal drains.[18, 22] Additionally, developments such as intraoperative flexible sigmoidoscopy have influenced the widespread use of intraoperative suture confirmation and restorative interventions,[23] and the indications for diverting stoma construction to prevent suture failure and subsequent recurrence in these anus-preserving surgeries are unclear among different institutions and surgeons.[24] Furthermore, these complications and risks are different in robot-assisted surgery.[25,26] Robot-assisted surgery has also been reported to have a higher rate of stoma construction than non-robot-assisted surgery.[25] In Japan, robotic-assisted surgery in the lower rectum has been covered by the national health insurance since 2018. Therefore, future studies should consider robotic-assisted surgery and other types of surgery. Thus, it is expected that the indications for diverting stoma will be transformed with the evolution of surgical instruments, equipment, and techniques.

In rectal cancer, APR, Hartmann's procedure, and stoma construction are characterized by stage progression, as compared with low anterior resection. In particular, Hartmann's procedure has a closure rate of 46%[27] owing to bowel perforation or malignant obstruction as an emergency surgery, suggesting a background of a poor general condition.

Although there are reports that the presence or absence of concomitant stoma construction in LAR is related to age, low albumin, tumor size, distance from the anus, and rectal pressure,[26] the results of the present study showed that the prevalence of preoperative chemotherapy and radiation therapy is a decision-making factor for stoma construction specific to malignant disease.

Surgery for rectal cancer, a typical disease for which a gastrointestinal stoma is placed, can range from APR to LAR to preserve the anus and can require the placement of a permanent stoma, a temporary stoma, or no stoma.[13]

In particular, the rate of stoma construction following curative surgery for rectal cancer is decreasing owing to advances in anus-preserving surgical equipment and techniques.[28] However, the number of stomas is expected to increase in the future, given the increase in the number of patients with rectal cancer and surgeries.[6,] The modest increase in the number of stomas constructed over the 5-year study period may reflect these factors. However, treatment methods progress and change each year. For example, the number of stoma constructions is expected to decrease owing to progress in cancer treatment and the expansion of indications for treatment of gastrointestinal obstruction such as gastrointestinal stenting.[30-32] Stoma construction as a treatment strategy prior to neoadjuvant chemotherapy for advanced colorectal cancer, palliative stoma,[33] and stoma construction as a countermeasure for complications of other diseases and treatments are also increasing,[34] because the period to resection surgery can be longer than that for stenting.[35] Additionally, stoma construction surgeries are

TABLE 2 Patient characteristics for stoma and nonstoma construction according to surgical procedures for rectal cancer (ICD-10 code C20, malignant neoplasms of the rectum)

	Low anterior resection				
	Without diverting stoma	With diverting stoma	Abdominoperineal resection	Hartmann's procedure	Stoma construction without intestinal resection
	n = 64 572	n = 21 122	n = 1412	n = 977	n = 106
Age (y), median (IQR)	68 (61-75)	67 (60-74)	70 (63-77)	74 (66-81)	68 (61-75)
Sex					
Female, n (%)	22 811 (35.33)	6068 (28.73)	405 (28.68)	339 (34.70)	41 (38.68)
Male, n (%)	41 761 (64.67)	15 054 (71.27)	1007 (71.32)	638 (65.30)	65 (61.32)
Year					
2013, n (%)	10 030 (15.53)	2144 (10.15)	229 (16.22)	128 (13.10)	14 (13.21)
2014, n (%)	9748 (15.1)	2692 (12.75)	219 (15.51)	143 (14.64)	21 (19.81)
2015, n (%)	9707 (15.03)	3067 (14.52)	269 (19.05)	171 (17.50)	15 (14.15)
2016, n (%)	12 213 (18.91)	4122 (19.52)	232 (16.43)	170 (17.40)	18 (16.98)
2017, n (%)	11 552 (17.89)	4409 (20.87)	235 (16.64)	176 (18.01)	21 (19.81)
2018, n (%)	11 322 (17.53)	4688 (22.19)	228 (16.15)	189 (19.34)	17 (16.04)
Preoperative chemotherapy-30					
Available, n (%)	1281 (1.98)	806 (3.82)	59 (4.18)	31 (3.17)	4 (3.77)
Not available, n (%)	63 291 (98.02)	20 316 (96.18)	1353 (95.82)	946 (96.83)	102 (96.23)
Preoperative chemotherapy-90					
Available, n (%)	3653 (5.66)	3330 (15.77)	208 (14.73)	62 (6.35)	7 (6.60)
Not available, n (%)	60 919 (94.34)	17 792 (84.23)	1204 (85.27)	915 (93.65)	99 (93.4)
Radiation therapy-90					
Available, n (%)	1292 (2.00)	1950 (9.23)	109 (7.72)	17 (1.74)	3 (2.83)
Not available, n (%)	63 280 (98.00)	19 172 (90.77)	1303 (92.28)	960 (98.26)	103 (97.17)
ASA-PS					
ASA-PS1, n (%)	19 111 (29.6)	4935 (23.36)	331 (23.44)	86 (8.80)	23 (21.70)
ASA-PS2, n (%)	39 261 (60.8)	13 946 (66.03)	889 (62.96)	517 (52.92)	55 (51.89)
ASA-PS3, n (%)	6067 (9.40)	2175 (10.3)	172 (12.18)	316 (32.34)	25 (23.58)
ASA-PS4, n (%)	108 (0.17)	50 (0.24)	18 (1.27)	40 (4.09)	1 (0.94)
ASA-PS5, n (%)	25 (0.04)	16 (0.08)	2 (0.14)	18 (1.84)	2 (1.89)
Tumor stage					
T0 or Tis orT1, n (%)	10 420 (16.14)	3417 (16.18)	71 (5.03)	25 (2.56)	1 (0.94)
T2, n (%)	11 867 (18.38)	4299 (20.35)	239 (16.93)	62 (6.35)	4 (3.77)
T3, (%)	32 488 (50.31)	10 424 (49.35)	816 (57.79)	495 (50.67)	20 (18.87)
T4a, n (%)	7910 (12.25)	2078 (9.84)	146 (10.34)	254 (26.00)	19 (17.92)
T4b, n (%)	1713 (2.65)	816 (3.86)	128 (9.07)	126 (12.9)	39 (36.79)
TX, n (%)	174 (0.27)	88 (0.42)	12 (0.85)	15 (1.54)	23 (21.70)
Node stage					
N0, n (%)	36 826 (57.03)	12 216 (57.84)	677 (47.95)	394 (40.33)	12 (11.32)
N1a or N1b or N1c, n (%)	18 069 (27.98)	5444 (25.77)	412 (29.18)	305 (31.22)	18 (16.98)
N2a or N2b, n (%)	9427 (14.6)	3348 (15.85)	305 (21.6)	207 (21.19)	30 (28.30)
NX, n (%)	250 (0.39)	114 (0.54)	18 (1.27)	71 (7.27)	46 (43.40)

(Continues)

TABLE 2 (Continued)

	Low anterior resection: Without diverting stoma	Low anterior resection: With diverting stoma	Abdominoperineal resection	Hartmann's procedure	Stoma construction without intestinal resection
	n = 64 572	n = 21 122	n = 1412	n = 977	n = 106
Metastasis stage					
M0, n (%)	59 060 (91.46)	19 148 (90.65)	1105 (78.26)	698 (71.44)	52 (49.06)
M1, n (%)	5512 (8.54)	1974 (9.35)	307 (21.74)	279 (28.56)	54 (50.94)
Type of surgery					
Elective surgery, n (%)	64 147 (99.34)	20 799 (98.47)	1345 (95.25)	610 (62.44)	84 (79.25)
Emergency surgery, n (%)	425 (0.66)	323 (1.53)	67 (4.75)	367 (37.56)	22 (20.75)
Approach					
Nonendoscopic surgery, n (%)	29 695 (45.99)	7355 (34.82)	834 (59.07)	756 (77.38)	89 (83.96)
Endoscopic surgery, n (%)	34 877 (54.01)	13 767 (65.18)	578 (40.93)	221 (22.62)	17 (16.04)
Resection margin					
R0, n (%)	60 458 (93.63)	19 745 (93.48)	1250 (88.53)	701 (71.75)	17 (16.04)
R1, n (%)	862 (1.33)	368 (1.74)	65 (4.60)	57 (5.83)	1 (0.94)
R2, n (%)	2846 (4.41)	855 (4.05)	80 (5.67)	178 (18.22)	75 (70.75)
RX, n (%)	406 (0.63)	154 (0.73)	17 (1.20)	41 (4.20)	13 (12.26)

Abbreviations: ASA-PS, American Society of Anesthesiologists physical status; ICD-10, International Classification of Diseases, Tenth Revision; IQR, interquartile range; Preoperative chemotherapy-30, preoperative chemotherapy within 30 d before cancer surgery; Preoperative chemotherapy-90, preoperative chemotherapy within 90 d before cancer surgery; Radiation therapy-90, radiation therapy within 90 d before cancer surgery.

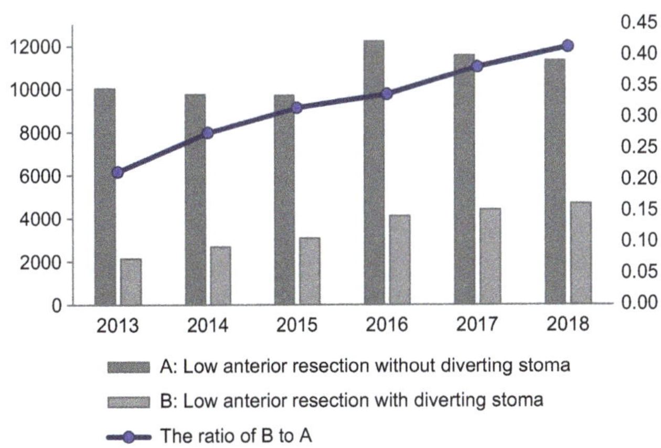

FIGURE 4 Number of low anterior resection with/without diverting stoma

also performed for benign diseases, such as emergency surgery for colonic perforation.[36,37] Thus, it is necessary to consider that the purpose and indications for stoma construction will change and to look at the future trends. In Japan, where the proportion of older people is the highest in the world, the low ratio of stoma closure in the oldest patients in this study and the indications for stoma construction in older people (8) suggest that the number of gastrointestinal ostomates, especially in super-aged populations, will continue to increase in the future.

4.1 | Limitations

In this survey, the background for the construction of a gastrointestinal stoma could not be clarified because it was not linked to the name of the disease in the data source used. Additionally, multiple terms are used to refer to surgical procedures used to create a gastrointestinal stoma, such as "colostomy," which includes enterocutaneous fistula for the purpose of creating an excretion route and enterocutaneous fistula for a route of nutrition injection. Because the purpose of this survey was to determine the route of excretion, we excluded those procedures that were performed in conjunction with esophageal surgery so as to exclude those performed for nutritional infusion.

5 | CONCLUSION

The number of gastrointestinal stomas registered in the NCD during the study period was approximately 25,000 per year, with a moderate increase during 2013–2018. The number of stoma closures was

TABLE 3 Patient characteristics regarding malignant and benign tumors in low anterior resection

	Low anterior resection		Low anterior resection	
	Malignant neoplasm		Benign tumor	
	stoma construction	nonstoma construction	stoma construction	nonstoma construction
	n = 19 181	n = 74 365	n = 13	n = 26
Age (y), mean (SD)	66.18 (11.11)	67.41 (11.33)	62.31 (13.33)	65.81 (10.22)
Sex				
Female, n (%)	5440 (28.36)	26 377 (35.47)	4 (30.77)	11 (42.31)
Male, n (%)	13 741 (71.64)	47 988 (64.53)	9 (69.23)	15 (57.69)
Year				
2013, n (%)	1906 (9.94)	11 491 (15.45)	0 (0)	5 (19.23)
2014, n (%)	2366 (12.34)	11 215 (15.08)	3 (23.08)	3 (11.54)
2015, n (%)	2741 (14.29)	11 143 (14.98)	1 (7.69)	3 (11.54)
2016, n (%)	3745 (19.52)	14 098 (18.96)	5 (38.46)	4 (15.38)
2017, n (%)	4109 (21.42)	13 379 (17.99)	3 (23.08)	7 (26.92)
2018, n (%)	4314 (22.49)	13 039 (17.53)	1 (7.69)	4 (15.38)
Diabetes mellitus				
Insulin therapies, n (%)	15 531 (80.97)	60 875 (81.86)	12 (92.31)	21 (80.77)
No treatment, n (%)	308 (1.61)	1468 (1.97)	0 (0)	0 (0)
Diet therapy, n (%)	2299 (11.99)	8559 (11.51)	1 (7.69)	5 (19.23)
Oral agents, n (%)	735 (3.83)	2362 (3.18)	0 (0)	0 (0)
Dyspnea	308 (1.61)	1101 (1.48)	0 (0)	0 (0)
Not available, n (%)	18 968 (98.89)	73 515 (98.86)	12 (92.31)	26 (100)
During moderate exertion, n (%)	180 (0.94)	763 (1.03)	1 (7.69)	0 (0)
At rest, n (%)	33 (0.17)	87 (0.12)	0 (0)	0 (0)
ADL-30				
Independent, n (%)	18 592 (96.93)	71 754 (96.49)	13 (100)	26 (100)
Partial assistance	479 (2.5)	2247 (3.02)	0 (0)	0 (0)
Total assistance	110 (0.57)	364 (0.49)	0 (0)	0 (0)
ADL-surgery				
Independent, n (%)	18 512 (96.51)	71 500 (96.15)	12 (92.31)	26 (100)
Partial assistance	535 (2.79)	2454 (3.3)	1 (7.69)	0 (0)
Total assistance	134 (0.7)	411 (0.55)	0 (0)	0 (0)
COPD				
Not available, n (%)	18 318 (95.5)	71 922 (96.71)	12 (92.31)	25 (96.15)
Available, n (%)	863 (4.5)	2443 (3.29)	1 (7.69)	1 (3.85)
Dialysis-14				
Not available, n (%)	19 076 (99.45)	73 999 (99.51)	13 (100)	25 (96.15)
Available, n (%)	105 (0.55)	366 (0.49)	0 (0)	1 (3.85)
Multiple metastases				
Not available, n (%)	18 779 (97.9)	72 298 (97.22)	13 (100)	26 (100)
Available, n (%)	402 (2.1)	2067 (2.78)	0 (0)	0 (0)
Steroid therapy				
Not available, n (%)	18 987 (98.99)	73 841 (99.3)	12 (92.31)	24 (92.31)
Discontinuation 30 d before surgery, n (%)	24 (0.13)	80 (0.11)	0 (0)	1 (3.85)

(Continues)

TABLE 3 (Continued)

	Low anterior resection		Low anterior resection	
	Malignant neoplasm		Benign tumor	
	stoma construction	nonstoma construction	stoma construction	nonstoma construction
	n = 19 181	n = 74 365	n = 13	n = 26
Available, n (%)	170 (0.89)	444 (0.6)	1 (7.69)	1 (3.85)
ASA-PS ASA-PS				
ASA-PS1, n (%)	4534 (23.64)	21 691 (29.17)	8 (61.54)	6 (23.08)
ASA-PS2, n (%)	12 596 (65.67)	45 401 (61.05)	3 (23.08)	18 (69.23)
ASA-PS3, n (%)	1988 (10.36)	7106 (9.56)	2 (15.38)	2 (7.69)
ASA-PS4, n (%)	49 (0.26)	137 (0.18)	0 (0)	0 (0)
ASA-PS5, n (%)	14 (0.07)	30 (0.04)	0 (0)	0 (0)
Type of surgery				
Elective surgery, n (%)	18 893 (98.5)	73 824 (99.27)	12 (92.31)	26 (100)
Emergency surgery, n (%)	288 (1.5)	541 (0.73)	1 (7.69)	0 (0)
Approach				
Nonendoscopic surgery, n (%)	6462 (33.69)	34 161 (45.94)	5 (38.46)	10 (38.46)
Endoscopic surgery, n (%)	12 719 (66.31)	40 204 (54.06)	8 (61.54)	16 (61.54)
Preoperative chemotherapy-30				
Available, n (%)	2732 (14.24)	3968 (5.34)	0 (0)	2 (7.69)
Not available, n (%)	16 449 (85.76)	70 397 (94.66)	13 (100)	24 (92.31)
Preoperative chemotherapy-90				
Available, n (%)	686 (3.58)	1408 (1.89)	0 (0)	0 (0)
Not available, n (%)	18 495 (96.42)	72 957 (98.11)	13 (100)	26 (100)
Radiation therapy-90				
Available, n (%)	1623 (8.46)	1324 (1.78)	0 (0)	0 (0)
Not available, n (%)	17 558 (91.54)	73 041 (98.22)	13 (100)	26 (100)
Tumor stage				
T stage, T0, n (%)	127 (0.66)	303 (0.41)		
Tis, n (%)	259 (1.35)	1202 (1.62)		
T1, n (%)	2856 (14.92)	10 064 (13.54)		
T2, n (%)	3974 (20.77)	13 123 (17.66)		
T3, n (%)	9300 (48.6)	37 373 (50.3)		
T4a, n (%)	1908 (9.97)	9685 (13.03)		
T4b, n (%)	632 (3.3)	2321 (3.12)		
TX, n (%)	80 (0.42)	231 (0.31)		
Node stage				
N stage, N0, n (%)	11 247 (58.77)	42 080 (56.63)		
N1a, n (%)	2594 (13.56)	11 557 (15.55)		
N1b, n (%)	2179 (11.39)	9179 (12.35)		
N1c, n (%)	81 (0.42)	298 (0.4)		
N2a, n (%)	1767 (9.23)	6860 (9.23)		
N2b, n (%)	1185 (6.19)	3984 (5.36)		
NX, n (%)	83 (0.43)	344 (0.46)		

(Continues)

TABLE 3 (Continued)

	Low anterior resection		Low anterior resection	
	Malignant neoplasm		Benign tumor	
	stoma construction	nonstoma construction	stoma construction	nonstoma construction
	n = 19 181	n = 74 365	n = 13	n = 26
Metastasis stage				
M stage, M0, n (%)	17 584 (91.89)	67 656 (91.06)		
M1a, n (%)	1221 (6.38)	5036 (6.78)		
M1b, n (%)	308 (1.61)	1512 (2.03)		
M1c, n (%)	23 (0.12)	98 (0.13)		
UICC stage				
Stage, 0, n (%)	252 (1.33)	1178 (1.6)		
Stage, 1, n (%)	5625 (29.72)	18 949 (25.68)		
Stage, 2, n (%)	4896 (25.87)	20 358 (27.59)		
Stage, 3, n (%)	6601 (34.88)	26 652 (36.12)		
Stage, 4, n (%)	1552 (8.2)	6646 (9.01)		

Abbreviations: ADL-30, activities of daily living within 30 d before surgery; ADL-surgery, activities of daily living just before surgery; COPD, chronic obstructive pulmonary disease; Dialysis-14, dialysis within 14 d before surgery; Dyspnea, dyspnea within 30 d before surgery; Multiple metastases, highly advanced cancer with multiple metastases just before surgery; Preoperative chemotherapy-30, preoperative chemotherapy within 30 d before cancer surgery; Preoperative chemotherapy-90, preoperative chemotherapy within 90 d before cancer surgery; Radiation therapy-90, radiation therapy within 90 d before cancer surgery; SA-PS, American Society of Anesthesiologists physical status; Steroid therapy, long-term corticosteroid therapy; UICC, Union for International Cancer Control.

10,000–14,400 per year. The number of stoma closures has also increased. The ratio of concomitant stoma construction surgery was higher in older people, and the ratio of stoma closure was higher in younger patients. The purposes and surgical techniques of stoma construction are diverse and are expected to increase in Japan, which is a super-aged society.

ACKNOWLEDGMENTS

This study was adopted as a new research proposal in the field of gastrointestinal surgery in 2019 by the Japanese Society of Gastroenterological Surgery National Clinical Database (NCD) data utilization study, and was then conducted. We thank all the data managers and hospitals participating in this NCD project for their efforts in entering the data. We thank Analisa Avila, MPH, ELS, of Edanz for editing a draft of this article.

DISCLOSURE

Author contributions: A.T., Y.H. and M.Y. tabulated the data; Y.A. and M.F. drafted the article; Y.N., T.T., H.H., and T.K. proofread the content; and Y.K. and Y.K. gave final approval of the article. All authors have read and approved the final article.

REFERENCES

1. Brown H, Randle J. Living with a stoma: a review of the literature. J Clin Nurs. 2005;14(1):74–81.
2. Richbourg L, Thorpe JM, Rapp CG. Difficulties experienced by the ostomate after hospital discharge. J Wound Ostomy Cont Nurs. 2007;34(1):70–9.
3. Sun V, Grant M, McMullen CK, Altschuler A, Mohler MJ, Hornbrook MC, et al. Surviving colorectal cancer long-term, persistent ostomy-specific concerns and adaptations. J Wound Ostomy Cont Nurs. 2013;40(1):61–72.
4. Data set information: system of social and demographic statistics [Internet]. Japan: Portal Site of Official Statistics of Japan; [June,7,2021]. Available from: https://www.e-stat.go.jp/
5. Department of Economic and Social Affairs, Population Division. World Population Prospects 2019: Volume II: Demographic Profiles. New York: United Nations, 2019.
6. Kakeji Y, Takahashi A, Hasegawa H, Ueno H, Eguchi S, Endo I, et al. Surgical outcomes in gastroenterological surgery in Japan: Report of the National Clinical Database 2011–2018. Ann Gastroent Surg. 2020;4(3):250–74.
7. National Clinical Database [Internet]. Japan: Portal Site of National Clinical Database; [April 25.2021]. Available from: http://www.ncd.or.jp/
8. Kanaji S, Takahashi A, Miyata H, Marubashi S, Kakeji Y, Konno H, et al. Initial verification of data from a clinical database of gastroenterological surgery in Japan. Surg Today. 2019;49(4):328–33.
9. Hasegawa H, Takahashi A, Kanaji S, Kakeji Y, Marubashi S, Konno H, et al. Validation of data quality in a nationwide gastroenterological surgical database: The National Clinical Database site-visit and remote audits, 2016-2018. Ann Gastroenterol Surg. 2021;5(3):296–303.
10. Torer N. Morbidity and mortality of colorectal cancer surgery in octogenarians. Eur Surg. 2016;48(4):215–20.
11. Ryan DP, Doody DP. Restorative proctocolectomy with and without protective ileostomy in a pediatric population. J Pediatr Surg. 2011;46(1):200–3.
12. Estimated age of onset of ulcerative colitis [Internet]. Japan: Japan Intractable Diseases Information Center; [1, July, 2021]. Available from: https://www.nanbyou.or.jp/entry/62
13. Fransvea P, Costa G, D'Agostino L, Sganga G, Serao A. Redo-laparoscopy in the management of complications after laparoscopic colorectal surgery: a systematic review and meta-analysis of surgical outcomes. Tech Coloproctol. 2021;25(4):371–83.

14. Ahmad NZ, Abbas MH, Khan SU, Parvaiz A. A meta-analysis of the role of diverting ileostomy after rectal cancer surgery. Int J Colorectal Dis. 2021;36(3):445–55.
15. Abudeeb H, Hammad A, Ugwu A, Darabnia J, Malcomson L, Maung M, et al. Defunctioning stoma- a prognosticator for leaks in low rectal restorative cancer resection: a retrospective analysis of stoma database. Ann Med Surg. 2012;2017(21):114–7.
16. Huser N, Michalski CW, Erkan M, Schuster T, Rosenberg R, Kleeff J, et al. Systematic review and meta-analysis of the role of defunctioning stoma in low rectal cancer surgery. Ann Surg. 2008;248(1):52–60.
17. Frouws MA, Snijders HS, Malm SH, Liefers GJ, Van de Velde CJH, Neijenhuis PA, et al. Clinical relevance of a grading system for anastomotic leakage after low anterior resection: analysis from a national cohort database. Dis Colon Rectum. 2017;60(7):706–13.
18. Cong ZJ, Fu CG, Wang HT, Liu LJ, Zhang W, Wang H. Influencing factors of symptomatic anastomotic leakage after anterior resection of the rectum for cancer. World J Surg. 2009;33(6):1292–7.
19. Suarez J, Marin G, Vera R, Colibaseanu D, Vila JJ, Ciga MA, et al. Stent placement prior to initiation of chemotherapy in patients with obstructive, nonoperative left sided tumors is associated with fewer stomas. J Surg Oncol. 2017;115(7):856–63.
20. Nishigori H, Ito M, Nishizawa Y. A novel transanal tube designed to prevent anastomotic leakage after rectal cancer surgery: the WING DRAIN. Surg Today. 2017;47(4):513–20.
21. Sterk P, Schubert F, Günter S, Klein P. Anastomotic protection with a transanal tube after rectum resection and total mesorectal excision. Zentralbl Chir. 2001;126(8):601–4.
22. Wang F-G, Yan W-M, Yan M, Song M-M. Outcomes of transanal tube placement in anterior resection: A meta-analysis and systematic review. Int J Surg. 2018;59:1–10.
23. Williams E, Prabhakaran S, Kong JC, Bell S, Warrier SK, Simpson P, et al. Utility of intra-operative flexible sigmoidoscopy to assess colorectal anastomosis: a systematic review and meta-analysis. ANZ J Surg. 2021;91(4):546–52.
24. Saida Yoshihisa, Takahashi Keiichi, Hasegawa Hirotoshi, Yasuno Masamichi, Inomata Masafumi, Yamaguchi Shigeki, Akagi Yoshito, Asano Michio, Iwamoto Shigeyoshi, Kato Takeshi, Kanazawa Akiyoshi, Koyama Motoi, Samura Hironori, Fukunaga Mutsumi, Funahashi Kimihiko, Yamamoto Hirofumi, Enomoto Toshiyuki A Nationwide Survey of Anastomotic Leakage in Rectal Cancer Surgery in Japan (Results of a Questionnaire Survey by the 35th Meeting of the Japan Colorectal Surgical Club). Nippon Daicho Komonbyo Gakkai Zasshi. 2012;65: (7):355. –362. http://dx.doi.org/10.3862/jcoloproctology.65.355
25. Thomas A, Altaf K, Sochorova D, Gur U, Parvaiz A, Ahmed S. Effective implementation and adaptation of structured robotic colorectal programme in a busy tertiary unit. J Robot Surg. 2021;15(5):731–9.
26. Fukui R, Nozawa H, Hirata Y, Kawai K, Hata K, Tanaka T, et al. Low preoperative maximum squeezing pressure evaluated by anorectal manometry is a risk factor for non-reversal of diverting stoma. Langenbecks Arch Surg. 2021;406(1):131–9.
27. Hallam S, Mothe BS, Tirumulaju R. Hartmann's procedure, reversal and rate of stoma-free survival. Ann R Coll Surg Engl. 2018;100(4):301–7.
28. Skelton F, Kunik ME, Regev T, Naik AD. Determining if an older adult can make and execute decisions to live safely at home: a capacity assessment and intervention model. Arch Gerontol Geriatr. 2010;50(3):300–5.
29. Data set information: System of Social and Demographic Statistics [Internet]. Japan: Center for Cancer Control and Information Services, National Cancer Center; [1, July, 2021]. Available from: https://ganjoho.jp/en/public/statistics/short_pred.html
30. Sterpetti AV, Sapienza P, Fiori E, Di Marzo L, Lamazza A. Improved results for left-sided malignant colorectal obstruction with a proper selection for self expandable metal stent placement, surgical resection or diverting stoma. Eur J Surg Oncol. 2020;46(11):2064–7.
31. Arezzo A, Passera R, Lo Secco G, Verra M, Bonino MA, Targarona E, et al. Stent as bridge to surgery for left-sided malignant colonic obstruction reduces adverse events and stoma rate compared with emergency surgery: results of a systematic review and meta-analysis of randomized controlled trials. Gastrointest Endosc. 2017;86(3):416–26.
32. Abelson JS, Yeo HL, Mao J, Milsom JW, Sedrakyan A. Long-term postprocedural outcomes of palliative emergency stenting vs stoma in malignant large-bowel obstruction. JAMA Surg. 2017;152(5):429–35.
33. Sridhar P, Sistla SC, Ali SM, Karthikeyan VS, Badhe AS, Ananthanarayanan PH. Effect of intravenous lignocaine on perioperative stress response and post-surgical ileus in elective open abdominal surgeries: A double-blind randomized controlled trial. ANZ J Surg. 2015;85(6):425–9.
34. Huang XY, Zhong QH, Wang HM, Zhao J, Kuang YY, Guan Q, et al. Diverting colostomy is an effective procedure for ulcerative chronic radiation proctitis patients after pelvic malignancy radiation. BMC Surg. 2020;20(1):9.
35. van Hooft Jeanin E., Tanis Pieter Job, Veld Joyce Valerie, Kumcu Aydan, Amelung Femke Julie, Borstlap Wernard Aat Antoine, Consten Esther Catharina Josephina, Dekker Jan Willem Teunis, van Westreenen Henderik Leendert, Siersema Peter D., ter Borg Frank, Kusters Miranda, Bemelman Wilhelmus Adrianus, de Wilt Johannes Hendrik Willem, Time interval between self-expandable metal stent placement or creation of a decompressing stoma and elective resection of left-sided obstructive colon cancer. Endoscopy. 2021;53: (09):905. –913. http://dx.doi.org/10.1055/a-1308-1487
36. Ansaloni L, Andersson R, Bazzoli F, Catena F, Cennamo V, Di S, et al. Guidelenines in the management of obstructing cancer of the left colon: consensus conference of the world society of emergency surgery (WSES) and peritoneum and surgery (PnS) society. World J Emerg Surg. 2010;5:29.
37. Abdalla S, Brouquet A, Lazure T, Costaglioli B, Penna C, Benoist S. Outcome of emergency surgery for severe neuroleptic-induced colitis: results of a prospective cohort. Colorectal Dis. 2016;18(12):1179–85.

5

Severity of early diagnosed organ/space surgical site infection in elective gastrointestinal and hepatopancreatobiliary surgery

Jun Okui[1,2] | Hideaki Obara[1] | Gaku Shimane[1] | Yasunori Sato[2] | Hirofumi Kawakubo[1] | Minoru Kitago[1] | Koji Okabayashi[1] | Yuko Kitagawa[1]

[1]Department of Surgery, Keio University School of Medicine, Tokyo, Japan

[2]Department of Preventive Medicine and Public Health, Keio University School of Medicine, Tokyo, Japan

Correspondence
Hideaki Obara, Department of Surgery, Keio University School of Medicine, 35 Shinanomachi, Shinjuku-ku, Tokyo, 160-8582, Japan.
Email: obara.z3@keio.jp

Abstract

Background: Organ/space surgical site infection (SSI) is a significant clinical problem. The postdiagnosis course of organ/space SSIs and the impact of its early diagnosis on clinical outcomes are yet to be clarified. Thus, we aimed to investigate the association between the timing of diagnosis and the clinical outcome of organ/space SSI.

Methods: This retrospective, single-center cohort study evaluated patients who underwent elective gastrointestinal or hepatopancreatobiliary surgery between 2016 and 2020. Clinical outcomes were compared between the early group (ie, SSI diagnosed until postoperative day [POD] 4) and normal-late group (ie, SSI diagnosed after POD 5). The primary outcome was the final C-reactive protein (CRP) level within 14 d after organ/space SSI diagnosis.

Results: In total, 110 patients were evaluated. The median time of diagnosis was 7 d postoperatively (interquartile range, 5–9 d postoperatively). Compared with the normal-late group, the early group included a higher proportion of patients with Clavien–Dindo grade ≥IIIb (8/21 vs 11/89, $P = .01$), higher final CRP value within 14 d after SSI diagnosis (mean, 4.49 mg/dL vs 2.27 mg/dL, $P = .01$), longer postoperative length of hospitalization (median, 45.0 d vs 33.0 d; $P = .028$), and worse 1-y overall survival rate (74.8% vs 89.3%, $P = .08$).

Conclusion: Early diagnosed organ/space SSI are originally severe and may therefore be detected earlier. Importantly, early diagnosed organ/space SSI is likely to be severe and refractory.

KEYWORDS
abdominal abscess, anastomotic leak, digestive system surgical procedures, pancreatic fistula, surgical wound infection

1 | INTRODUCTION

Organ/space surgical site infections (SSIs) include various types of pivotal surgical complications, including anastomotic leakage, pancreatic fistula, biliary fistula, or intraabdominal abscess. Organ/space SSI is a significant clinical problem, as it is associated with increased mortality, prolonged hospitalization, increased medical costs,[1] and poor oncological outcomes.[2] Early detection and treatment are speculated to improve the outcomes of organ/space SSI, but diagnosis in the early postoperative period is challenging.[3] A previous study reported that an anastomotic leak in colorectal surgery was diagnosed within a mean of 8.8 d postoperatively.[4]

Delayed diagnosis is mainly attributed to the fact that organ/space SSIs become apparent only after the development of clinical symptoms.[5] Flooden et al suggested that more severe leakages cause symptoms earlier, whereas less severe leakages take longer to develop symptoms.[6] In addition, Morks et al reported that early anastomotic leakage is associated with a higher probability of re-laparotomy than late anastomotic leakage.[7] Many predictive models using postoperative inflammatory markers have been developed for the early detection of organ/space SSIs.[8] However, no study to date has evaluated the postdiagnosis course of organ/space SSIs that could actually be diagnosed early.

Thus, this study aimed to investigate the association between the timing of diagnosis and clinical outcome of organ/space SSI in patients who have undergone either elective gastrointestinal (GI) or hepatopancreatobiliary (HPB) surgery. In particular, we focused on daily changes in C-reactive protein (CRP) levels after diagnosis and subsequent treatment of organ/space SSIs.

2 | METHODS

2.1 | Study design

This retrospective, observational, single-center study was conducted in the Department of Surgery at Keio University Hospital, which is a tertiary care teaching hospital with approximately 1000 beds. The study protocol was approved by the Institutional Review Board of the Keio University School of Medicine (ethics approval number 20120454) and adhered to the Strengthening the Reporting of Observational Studies in Epidemiology guidelines for reporting.[9] The need for informed consent was waived owing to the retrospective nature of the study.

2.2 | Patient selection

The study included patients who underwent elective gastrointestinal and hepatopancreatobiliary surgery with general anesthesia between January 1, 2016, and December 31, 2020. Patients who underwent liver transplant, hernia repair, and abdominal surgery not involving the GI tract or biliary system (eg, adhesive small bowel surgery without intestinal resection, abdominal irrigation for generalized peritonitis, and laparotomy hemostasis) were excluded. Liver transplant was excluded due to the heterogeneous nature of the surgery. In addition, we excluded patients in whom only ileostomy or colostomy was performed because these surgeries have no risk of organ/space SSI. Finally, we also excluded emergency cases because they have a significantly different mechanism of postoperative intraabdominal infection.

Surgical procedures were classified according to the Japan Nosocomial Infections Surveillance (JANIS)[10] surgical classification criteria (Table S1). For patients who underwent simultaneous multiorgan surgeries, only the primary procedure was recorded as the surgical procedure.

2.3 | Definition of organ/space SSI

Anastomotic leakage, pancreatic fistula, biliary fistula, and intraabdominal abscess diagnosed until postoperative day (POD) 30 were considered as organ/space SSIs. Organ/space SSI was diagnosed by fellow and attending surgeons using the Centers for Disease Control and Prevention (CDC) National Healthcare Safety Network (formerly the National Nosocomial Infection Surveillance System) definitions[11] (Table S2). The day when the CDC criteria were met for the first time was designated as the SSI diagnosis date. At Keio University Hospital, all patients with organ/space SSI patients are provided therapeutic intervention of at least antibiotic administration on the day of diagnosis. Therefore, in this study we considered the date of diagnosis as the start date of organ/space SSI treatment.

Pancreatic fistula was evaluated using the CDC definitions for all types of resection organs, instead of the more commonly used International Study Group for Pancreatic Surgery (ISGPS) criteria revised in 2016.[12] This is because our SSI surveillance is based on the national survey. Complications were graded using the Clavien–Dindo classification,[13] and we included only Clavien–Dindo grade ≥II organ/space SSI in the analysis because grade I does not require clinical intervention. Supplementally, grade IIIb requires intervention under general anesthesia, grade IV requires intensive care unit management with life-threatening complications, and grade V indicates the death of a patient.[13] In this study, Clavien–Dindo grade V was defined as death caused by organ/space SSI during the same hospitalization stay. If patients were simultaneously diagnosed with multiple types of organ/space SSIs, the only primary complication was determined as the outcome. In addition, for patients who underwent multiple surgeries during the same hospitalization and developed organ/space SSI, only the surgery that directly caused SSI was counted. Given that the presence or absence of complications is recorded on the surveillance sheet at the time of hospital discharge, patients who developed organ/space SSI after discharge could not be included.

2.4 | Data collection

Patient data from the electronic medical records were reviewed by author J.O. Clinicodemographic data (ie, age, sex, American Society of Anesthesiologists physical status, body mass index, diabetes mellitus, albumin level, and smoking history), intraoperative data (ie, surgical procedures and estimated blood loss), and postoperative data (ie, length of hospitalization and 1-y survival) were collected. Postoperative survival information was collected on August 31, 2021.

2.5 | Primary outcome

Laboratory findings within 14 d after organ/space SSI diagnosis were collected. In particular, we focused on postdiagnosis inflammatory changes (white cell count [WCC] and CRP levels), and thus, we did not collect laboratory data based on the operative day. The final CRP value within 14 d after diagnosis was set as the primary outcome for the following reasons: Nakamura et al investigated the 14-day changes in CRP among patients with persistent inflammatory, immunosuppressed, catabolic syndrome (PIICS)[14] and established that a CRP level of 3.0 mg/dL on day 14 was the optimal cutoff for PIICS diagnosis. Inspired by this research, we investigated the changes in CRP levels over 14 d. Further, since we considered the inflammatory response in the early postdiagnosis period to be highly variable, we focused on the values on day 14 to investigate the final outcome of treatment.

2.6 | Statistical analysis

Univariate analysis was performed to examine the background differences between organ/space SSIs diagnosed until POD 4 (early diagnosis group) and after POD 5 (normal-late diagnosis group). There were several reasons for adopting this division. First, in our previous study the median diagnosis date of organ/space SSI was POD 6 (interquartile range, 4–9 d).[8] Second, postoperative laboratory tests are likely to be performed on odd days in our hospital. Considering the division by odd-numbered days, we thought it was appropriate to set POD 1–4 as the cutoff to define the early diagnosis group.

Continuous variables were presented as the means and standard deviations (SDs) and analyzed using a *t*-test. Meanwhile, categorical variables were presented as frequencies and proportions and analyzed using Fisher's exact test. Length of hospitalization and duration of operation were expressed as median and interquartile range and was analyzed using the Mann–Whitney *U* test. As a supplement, the date of diagnosis by type of organ/space SSI, the date of diagnosis by type of surgical procedure, and final laboratory test date by the date of diagnosis were expressed as median and interquartile range and were analyzed using the Kruskal–Wallis test. Further, organ/space SSI diagnosis date was divided into 2 d and plotted the transition of WCC and CRP for 14 d after the start of organ/space SSI treatment. The reason for dividing by 2 d was that postoperative laboratory tests are likely to be performed on odd days in our hospital. In addition, a local regression line generated using the locally estimated scatterplot smoothing method with 95% confidence interval (CI) was added.[15]

The 1-y overall survival rate was determined by generating Kaplan–Meier survival curves and then comparing these between the two groups using the log-rank test and the Cox proportional hazard model. The hazard ratio (HR) with a 95% CI was estimated. All statistical analyses were performed using R statistical software v. 4.0.3 (R Foundation for Statistical Computing, Vienna, Austria). All *P*-values were two-tailed, and statistical significance was set at $P < .05$.

3 | RESULTS

Among the 3310 patients who underwent elective gastrointestinal and pancreatobiliary surgery, 110 patients (3.3%) developed organ/space SSI (anastomotic leak, n = 38; pancreatic fistula, n = 35; biliary fistula, n = 13; and intraabdominal abscess, n = 24) (Table 1 and S3). In total, 14.2%, 6.5%, and 4.8% developed organ/space SSI after pancreaticoduodenectomy, esophageal surgery, and rectal surgery, respectively (Table 1). The median time between surgery and the diagnosis of organ/space SSI was 7 d (interquartile range, 5–9 d) (Figure 1). The median date of diagnosis by type of organ/space SSI was POD 8.5 for intraabdominal abscess, POD 7 for biliary fistula, POD 6 for anastomotic leakage, and POD 7 for pancreatic fistula (Figure S1). Intraabdominal abscesses tended to be diagnosed late. The median date of diagnosis by type of surgical procedure is shown in Figure S2 and there were no significant differences among procedure types ($P = .83$).

In total, 21 patients (19.1%) and 89 patients (80.9%) were categorized into the early and normal-late diagnosis groups, respectively. The results of univariate analysis are shown in Tables 2 and 3. Preoperative and intraoperative variables did not differ significantly between groups, including surgical procedures and duration of operation. Notably, compared with the normal-late diagnosis group, the early diagnosis group showed a significantly longer median postoperative length of hospitalization (45.0 d vs 33.0 d, respectively; $P = .028$) and had a higher proportion of patients with Clavien–Dindo grade ≥IIIb complications (8/21 vs 11/89, respectively; $P = .01$), and had a higher proportion of patients with relaparotomy (5/21 vs 6/89, $P = .034$).

Postdiagnosis changes in CRP and WCC were followed for 14 d. As shown in Figure S3, the median final laboratory test date was above day 13 in all five groups (POD 1–2, POD 3–4, POD 5–6, POD 7–8, and POD9–). The mean final CRP and WCC values within 14 d tended to increase with an earlier diagnosis date (Figure 2). The final CRP value was significantly higher in the early diagnosis group than in the normal-late group (mean, 4.49 mg/dL vs 2.27 mg/dL; $P = .01$, Table 3). The average CRP and WCC values tended to be higher 14 d after diagnosis in the early diagnosis group (Figure 3).

The 1-y Kaplan–Meier survival curve is shown in Figure 4. Overall, 14 events occurred in our cohort, five events in the early group, and nine events in the normal-late group. The cause of death is shown in Table S5. In both groups, deaths caused by organ/space SSI account for the highest proportion. The overall survival rate was 86.5% (95% CI: 80.1%–93.3%) in the total population, 74.8% (95% CI: 57.8%–96.7%) in the early diagnosis group, and 89.3% (95% CI: 82.9%–96.2%) in the normal-late diagnosis group, with no significant between-group differences ($P = .08$). The HR for survival of the early group compared with the normal-late group was 2.56 (95% CI: 0.86–7.65).

TABLE 1 Organ/space SSI cases stratified by the surgical procedures

Surgical procedures	Keio University Hospital in 2016–2020 (Elective surgery)			JANIS in 2020 (Elective & emergency surgery)*		
	n	Organ/space SSI	Incidence	n	Organ/space SSI	Incidence
ESOP	294	19	6.5%	1563	111	7.1%
GAST-D	319	10	3.1%	7370	254	3.4%
GAST-T	99	1	1.0%	3483	239	6.9%
GAST-O	194	2	1.0%	4932	171	3.5%
SB	226	1	0.4%	7171	220	3.1%
COLO	629	10	1.6%	46 193	1150	2.5%
APPY	35	0	0.0%	13 411	186	1.4%
REC	231	11	4.8%	15 987	883	5.5%
BILI-L	303	14	4.6%	5067	187	3.7%
BILI-PD	190	27	14.2%	3167	562	17.7%
BILI-O	310	13	4.2%	3419	376	11.0%
CHOL	463	2	0.4%	27 340	189	0.7%
SPLE	17	0	0.0%	301	9	3.0%
Total	3310	110	3.3%	68 692	2,392	3.5%

Note:: Data are reported as number of patients (% are calculated on the total patients in the line).

We processed Japan nosocomial infections surveillance (JANIS) data in 2020.

JANIS is the national survey in Japan, in which 2418 hospitals participated. Surgical procedures are classified according to JANIS surgical classification criteria (See Table S1).

Abbreviation: SSI, surgical site infection.

*JANIS does not separate elective and emergency cases for organ/space SSI. We compared the incidence of organ/space SSI including both types of surgery in Table S4.

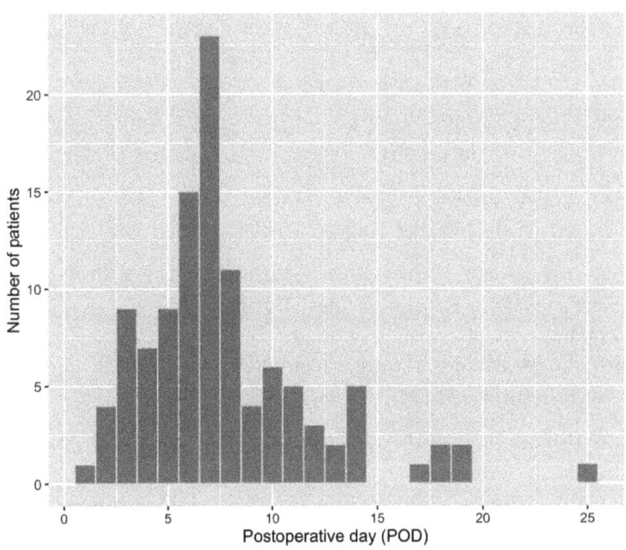

FIGURE 1 Day of organ/space SSI diagnosis. SSI, surgical site infection

4 | DISCUSSION

The postdiagnosis course of organ/space SSIs and the impact of its early diagnosis on clinical outcomes are yet to be clarified. In this study, the median time between surgery and diagnosis was 7 d (interquartile range, 5–9 d). Compared with the normal-late diagnosis group, the early diagnosis group had a longer median postoperative length of hospitalization, a higher proportion of patients with Clavien–Dindo grade ≥IIIb complications, higher final CRP value within 14 d after organ/space SSI diagnosis, and worse overall survival rate. These findings suggest that early diagnosed organ/space SSI cases were originally severe and may, therefore, be detected earlier.

The most important clinical implication of this study is that physicians should be aware that early diagnosed organ/space SSI is likely to be severe and refractory. The early diagnosed group had a worse overall survival rate than did the normal-late group (74.8% vs 89.3%, $P = .08$). Given that these patients showed prominent clinical manifestations from the early postoperative period, organ/space SSI may have been detected early. Notably, considering the expanded use of computed tomography imaging owing to the universal health insurance in Japan, there may have been little delays in the diagnosis. The rigorous assessment of the patients diagnosed in the early postoperative period that they truly have severe disease. These patients should be given antibiotics and undergo swift drainage, regardless of the underlying mechanism. Further, physicians should be cautious against early discharge.

Another clinical implication of this study is that the normal or late-diagnosed organ/space SSI cases are less likely to become severe. The final CRP and WCC values within 14 d postoperatively tended

TABLE 2 Preoperative and intraoperative patient characteristics

	Organ/space SSI diagnosis date		
	POD 1–4 (early diagnosis group)	POD 5– (normal-late diagnosis group)	
n	21	89	P-value
Preoperative information			
Sex = Male	17 (81.0%)	55 (61.8%)	.128
Age	68.2 (9.6)	67.3 (12.3)	.75
Diabetes mellitus	3 (14.3%)	22 (24.7%)	.394
Albumin (g/dL)	3.71 (0.48)	3.90 (0.53)	.155
BMI	22.7 (2.7)	22.4 (3.7)	.79
Past or present smoking habit	13 (61.9%)	40 (44.9%)	.225
ASA-PS			.425
1	4 (19.0%)	30 (33.7%)	
2	15 (71.4%)	52 (58.4%)	
3	2 (9.5%)	7 (7.9%)	
Intraoperative information			
Surgical procedure (%)			.418
ESOP	4 (19.0%)	15 (16.9%)	
GAST-D	2 (9.5%)	8 (9.0%)	
GAST-T	0 (0.0%)	1 (1.1%)	
GAST-O	1 (4.8%)	1 (1.1%)	
SB	1 (4.8%)	0 (0.0%)	
COLO	0 (0.0%)	10 (11.2%)	
REC	2 (9.5%)	9 (10.1%)	
BILI-L	3 (14.3%)	11 (12.4%)	
BILI-PD	7 (33.3%)	20 (22.5%)	
BILI-O	1 (4.8%)	12 (13.5%)	
CHOL	0 (0.0%)	2 (2.2%)	
Laparotomy	13 (61.9%)	48 (53.9%)	.627
Estimated blood loss (mL)	33.1 (18.8)	30.1 (20.5)	.54
Duration of operation (min) (median [IQR])	425 [270-535]	405 [297-512]	.924

Note:: Continuous values represent mean (SD). Categorical values represent n (%).

Continuous variables were analyzed by Welch's *t*-test, and categorical variables were analyzed by Fisher's exact test. Duration of operation was expressed in median and interquartile range, and was analyzed by Mann–Whitney *U* test.

Surgical procedures are classified according to Japan nosocomial infections surveillance (JANIS) surgical classification criteria (See Table S1).

Abbreviations: ASA-PS, American Society of Anesthesiologists physical status; BMI, body mass index; POD, postoperative day; SSI, surgical site infection.

to be lower in those diagnosed later. Our findings suggest that cases diagnosed beyond POD 4 under strict surveillance may not be severe cases. Patients who are diagnosed beyond POD 4 under intensive surveillance may have good outcomes. Several previous studies on colorectal surgery have focused on the timing of diagnosis. Tan et al reported the characteristics of late anastomotic leakage (LAL) diagnosed after POD 30, which included younger patients than the early anastomotic leakage (EAL) group.[16] Flooden et al suggested that early anastomotic leakage and LAL are different entities because of their different anatomical localization of anastomotic leakage points.[6] A previous study also reported that EAL patients are more likely to undergo relaparotomy than LAL patients,[7] and consistent findings were obtained in this study. These findings suggest that organ/space SSI diagnosed in the early stage is severe and refractory. However, these studies were limited to colorectal surgery, and no studies that included all GI and HPB surgeries were conducted.

Many previous studies have reported that postoperative CRP elevation can predict SSI after GI surgery.[17-19] However, although there have been reports that changes in the CRP level can begin as early as the surgery date,[20,21] no study has evaluated the trends in CRP levels by the date of organ/space SSI diagnosis. Previous research suggests a CRP level of 3.0 mg/dL on day 14 is the optimal

TABLE 3 Postoperative outcomes

	Organ/space SSI diagnosis date		
	POD 1–4 (early diagnosis group)	POD 5– (normal-late diagnosis group)	
n	21	89	P-value
Postoperative length of stay (day) (median [IQR])	45.0 [34.0, 73.0]	33.0 [24.0, 52.0]	.028
Postdiagnosis length of stay (day) (median [IQR])	44.0 [30.0, 69.0]	25.0 [14.0, 42.0]	.002
Type of organ/space SSI			.17
Anastomotic leakage	8 (38.1%)	30 (33.7%)	
Pancreatic fistula	8 (38.1%)	27 (30.3%)	
Biliary fistula	4 (19.0%)	9 (10.1%)	
Intraabdominal abscess	1 (4.8%)	23 (25.8%)	
Clavien–Dindo Grade			.006
II	0 (0.0%)	19 (21.3%)	
IIIa	13 (61.9%)	59 (66.3%)	
IIIb	1 (4.8%)	2 (2.2%)	
IVa	2 (9.5%)	1 (1.1%)	
IVb	2 (9.5%)	5 (5.6%)	
V	3 (14.3%)	3 (3.4%)	
Clavien–Dindo Grade IIIb or above	8 (38.1%)	11 (12.4%)	.01
Relaparotomy	5 (23.8%)	6 (6.7%)	.034
Final laboratory test date within 14 d after starting treatment (day)	13.3 (1.6)	12.7 (1.7)	.124
Final WCC (/μL)	7819 (3483)	6909 (2683)	.191
Final CRP (mg/dL)	4.49 (4.62)	2.22 (2.80)	.004

Note:: Continuous values represent mean (SD). Categorical values represent n (%).

Continuous variables were analyzed by Welch's *t*-test, and categorical variables were analyzed by Fisher's exact test. Length of hospitalization was expressed in median and interquartile range, and was analyzed by Mann–Whitney *U* test.

In this study, Clavien–Dindo Grade V was defined as death caused by organ/space SSI during the same hospitalization stay.

Surgical procedures are classified according to Japan nosocomial infections surveillance (JANIS) surgical classification criteria (See Table S1).

Abbreviations: CRP, C-reactive protein; POD, postoperative day; SSI, surgical site infection; WCC, white cell count.

cutoff for PIICS diagnosis, as evaluated by 14-d changes in CRP among patients with PIICS.[14] Similarly, we investigated the changes in CRP levels over 14 d. The results showed higher CRP values prolonged until 14 d in the early diagnosis group than in the normal-late group (mean 4.49 mg/dL vs 2.27 mg/dL; $P = .01$). Collectively, these findings support that prolonged CRP elevation is an important indicator of severity, and thus, it is reasonable to evaluate CRP levels. Additionally, we also investigated the trends in WCC, and the early diagnosed group showed a bimodal curve. The delayed second peak occurred around day 8 after diagnosis, implying severe SSI in the early diagnosis group.

Unlike previous studies that used a combination of primary outcomes, such as in-hospital mortality, cardiovascular complications, incisional SSI, and postoperative remote infections (eg, pneumonia, postoperative urinary tract infections),[22-25] our study focused on organ/space SSI, which is another strength of the present study. When a composite outcome is adopted, it is sometimes difficult to make a clinical interpretation because of the diverse treatment. There are also several options for the management of organ/space SSI; these include antibiotics, bowel rest, percutaneous drainage, and relaparotomy. Further, we focused on organ/space SSIs, due to their severity. Finally, our study has the advantage of accurate observation of organ/space SSI patients owing to its single-center setting.

However, this study also had some limitations. First, we could not investigate whether an earlier diagnosis or intervention resulted in better clinical outcomes. We could only prove the severity of early diagnosed organ/space SSI. Further investigations on the relationship between the timing of diagnosis and outcome are warranted. Prospective studies monitoring the severity of complications and including a control group with delayed treatment are needed; however, such a design is unethical. It would be more appropriate to adjust for potential confounders, such as surgical procedures, Clavien–Dindo grade, and demographic data. However, organ/space

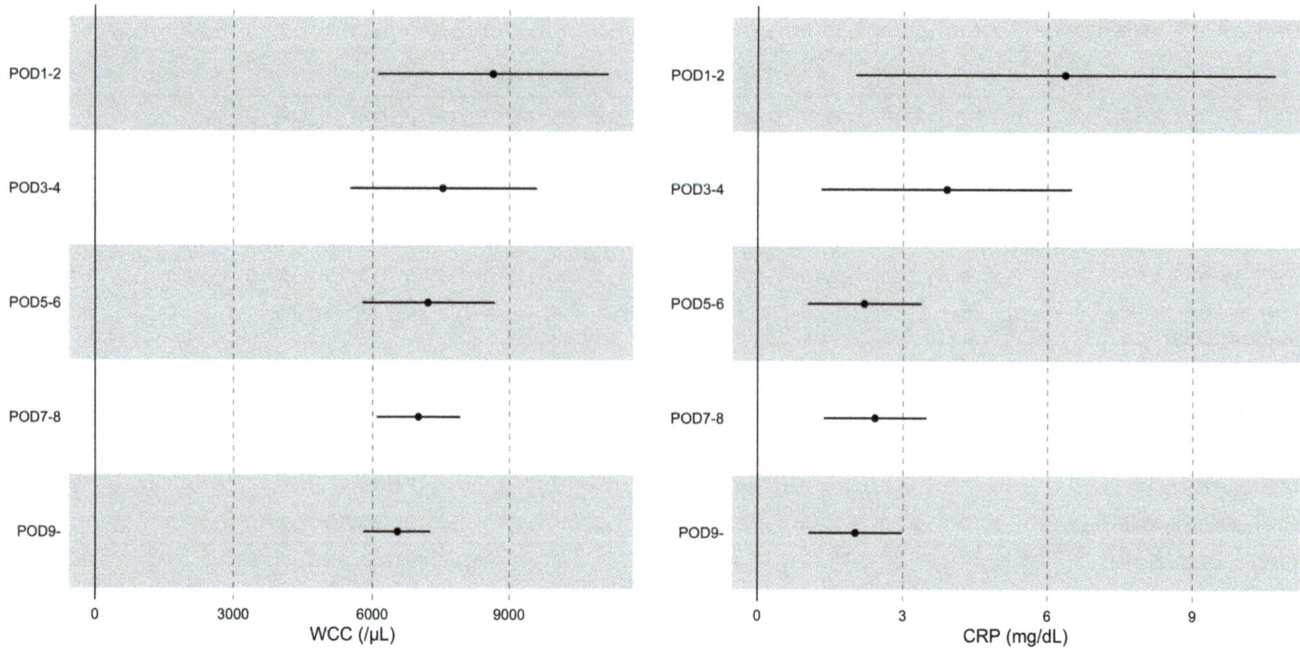

FIGURE 2 Average value of the final WCC and CRP within 14 d after organ/space SSI diagnosis classified by diagnosis date. The period represents the mean value, and the error bar represents the 95% confidence interval. CRP, C-reactive protein; POD, postoperative day; SSI, surgical site infection; WCC, white cell count

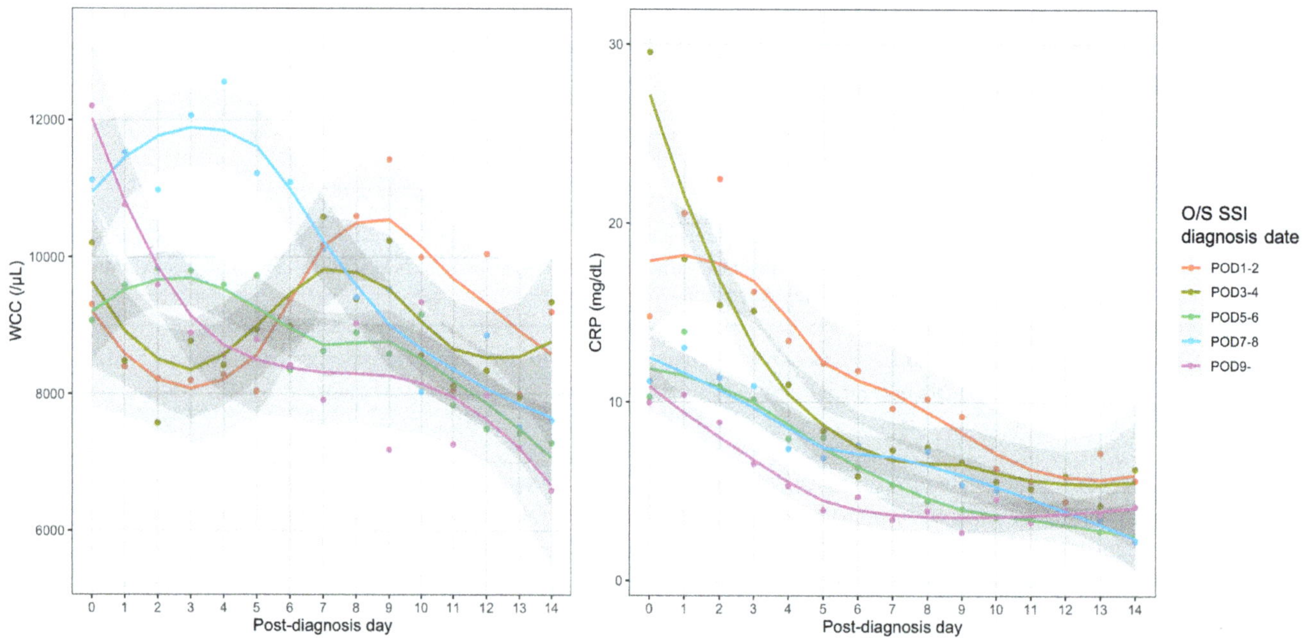

FIGURE 3 Trends in the average values of WCC and CRP within 14 d after organ/space SSI diagnosis classified by diagnosis date. CRP, C-reactive protein; POD, postoperative day; O/S SSI, organ/space surgical site infection; WCC, white cell count

SSI is a rare complication, and thus, this study did not have sufficient power for multivariate analysis.

Second, as described above, this study investigated overall organ/space SSI regardless of the surgical organs; as such, we could not perform a more detailed subgroup analysis according to the type of surgical procedure. For example, the frequency of organ/space SSI varied greatly (14.2% after pancreaticoduodenectomy vs 0.4% after cholecystectomy). The invasiveness of these surgeries varies greatly. Further, because organ/space SSI occurred in only 3.3% of our dataset, the sample size was inadequate to investigate the relationship between the timing of diagnosis and clinical outcomes classified by surgical organs.

Third, given the single-center study setting, we could not externally validate our findings. Treatments for organ/space SSIs differ among facilities, and it directly affects the postdiagnosis inflammatory response. However, it is difficult to collect accurate

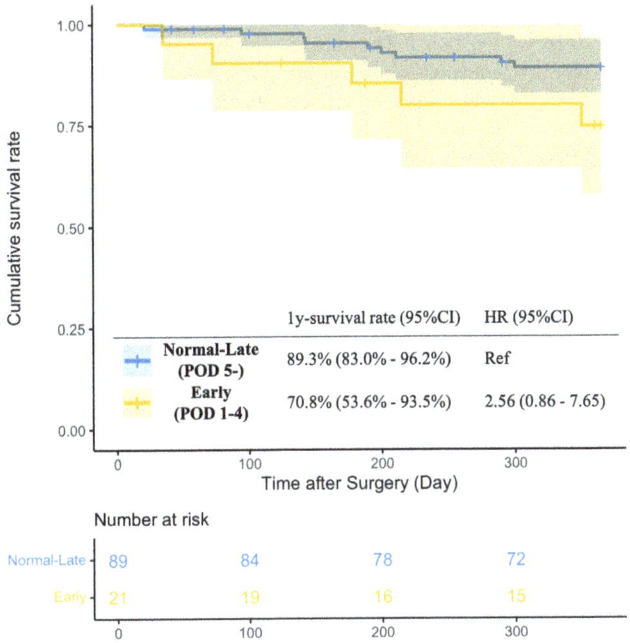

FIGURE 4 Kaplan-Meier curve for 1-y overall survival by timing of organ/space SSI diagnosis. There are 14 events in total (five in the early diagnosis group and nine in the normal-late diagnosis group). The hazard ratio (HR) was estimated using the Cox proportional hazard model. CI, confidence interval; POD, postoperative day; Ref, Reference; SSI, surgical site infection

diagnosis data, including timing, from multiple facilities. Fourth, the diagnosis date may vary depending on the organ/space SSI criteria. For example, pancreatic fistula is commonly evaluated clinically using the ISGPS criteria.[12] However, because our SSI surveillance is based on JANIS, a national survey involving 2418 hospitals, we decided to use the CDC definitions for all types of resection organs.[11] The incidence of organ/space SSI in this study was comparable to that of the national survey in 2020. Unfortunately, JANIS does not separate elective and emergency cases for organ/space SSI; therefore, we compared the incidence of organ/space SSI without excluding emergency cases (Table S4). However, in our previous study based on the same SSI criteria, the median time between surgery and the diagnosis of organ/space SSI was 6 d (interquartile range, 4–9 d),[8] which is not highly different from the 7 d (interquartile range, 5–9 d) in this study. These results show that there is no significant difference between our hospital and other facilities in Japan.

5 | CONCLUSION

Early diagnosed organ/space SSI cases are originally severe and thus may be detected earlier. Physicians should be aware that early diagnosed organ/space SSI is likely to be severe and refractory. For these patients, antibiotics should be selected empirically, drainage should be performed quickly, and clinicians should be cautious about early discharge.

ACKNOWLEDGMENTS

We sincerely appreciate Mr. Koji Yamamoto, Mr. Shigeyuki Munakata, and all the other members of the hospital information system department at Keio University School of Medicine for their tremendous help in data collection.

DISCLOSURE

Author contributions: Okui, Obara, Shimane, Sato, Kawakubo, Kitago, Okabayashi, and Kitagawa contributed to the study conception and design. Okui and Shimane collected the data. Okui and Sato analyzed and interpreted the data. Okui, Obara, Shimane, and Sato drafted the article. Kawakubo, Kitago, Okabayashi, and Kitagawa contributed to the critical revision of the article. All authors have read and approved the final article.

Disclosures outside the scope of this work: Author H.O. received lecture fees from Otsuka Pharmaceutical Factory Inc. Author H.O. was supported by grants from Medtronic Japan Co., Ltd., Japan Blood Products Organization, TAIHO PHARMACEUTICAL CO., LTD, W. L. Gore & Associates, Co., LTD., DAIICHI SANKYO COMPANY, LIMITED, Mitsubishi Tanabe Pharma Corporation, TEIJIN PHARMA LIMITED., KAKEN PHARMACEUTICAL CO., LTD., NOVARTIS PHARMA Co., Ltd., Medtronic Japan Co., Ltd., Japan Blood Products Organization, JMS Co., Ltd., TAIHO PHARMACEUTICAL CO., LTD, MSD KK, KAKEN PHARMACEUTICAL CO., LTD., Mitsubishi Tanabe Pharma Corporation, W. L. Gore & Associates, Co., LTD., NIHON PHARMACEUTICAL CO., LTD., Japan Lifeline Co., Ltd, Medtronic Japan Co., Ltd. JMS Co., Ltd., Japan Blood Products Organization, TAIHO PHARMACEUTICAL CO., LTD. Author Y.K. received lecture fees from CHUGAI PHARMACEUTICAL CO., LTD., TAIHO PHARMACEUTICAL CO., LTD, ASAHI KASEI PHARMA CORPORATION, Otsuka Pharmaceutical Factory Inc, ONO PHARMACEUTICAL CO., LTD., SHIONOGI & CO., LTD., Nippon Covidien Inc, AstraZeneca KK, Ethicon Inc, Bristol-Myers Squibb KK., and Olympus Corporation. Author Y.K. was supported by grants from CHUGAI PHARMACEUTICAL CO., LTD., TAIHO PHARMACEUTICAL CO., LTD, Yakult Honsha Co. Ltd., ASAHI KASEI PHARMA CORPORATION., Ltd., Otsuka Pharmaceutical Co., Ltd., ONO PHARMACEUTICAL CO., LTD., TSUMURA & CO., KAKEN PHARMACEUTICAL CO. LTD., DAINIPPON SUMITOMO PHARMA Co., Ltd., EA Pharma Co., Ltd., Eisai Co., Ltd., Otsuka Pharmaceutical Factory Inc, MEDICON INC., Kyouwa Hakkou Kirin Co., Ltd., Takeda Pharmaceutical Co., Ltd., Toyama Chemical Co., Ltd., Astellas Pharma Inc, TEIJIN PHARMA LIMITED., NIHON PHARMACEUTICAL CO., LTD., and Nippon Covidien Inc Author Y.K. held an endowed chair provided by CHUGAI PHARMACEUTICAL CO., LTD. and TAIHO PHARMACEUTICAL CO., LTD, outside the submitted work. Author Y.K. received other compensation from ONO PHARMACEUTICAL CO., LTD., and Bristol-Myers Squibb KK.

REFERENCES

1. Coello R, Charlett A, Wilson J, Ward V, Pearson A, Borriello P. Adverse impact of surgical site infections in English hospitals. J Hosp Infect. 2005;60(2):93–103.
2. Lawler J, Choynowski M, Bailey K, Bucholc M, Johnston A, Sugrue M. Meta-analysis of the impact of postoperative infective complications on oncological outcomes in colorectal cancer surgery. BJS Open. 2020;4(5):737–47.
3. Doeksen A, Tanis PJ, Vrouenraets BC, van Lanschot JJB, Tets WF. Factors determining delay in relaparotomy for anastomotic leakage after colorectal resection. World J Gastroenterol. 2007;13(27):3721–5.
4. Gessler B, Eriksson O, Angenete E. Diagnosis, treatment, and consequences of anastomotic leakage in colorectal surgery. Int J Colorectal Dis. 2017;32(4):549–56.
5. Sutton CD, Marshall LJ, Williams N, Berry DP, Thomas WM, Kelly MJ. Colo-rectal anastomotic leakage often masquerades as a cardiac complication. Colorectal Dis. 2004;6(1):21–2.
6. Floodeen H, Hallböök O, Rutegård J, Sjödahl R, Matthiessen P. Early and late symptomatic anastomotic leakage following low anterior resection of the rectum for cancer: are they different entities? Colorectal Dis. 2013;15(3):334–40.
7. Morks AN, Ploeg RJ, Sijbrand Hofker H, Wiggers T, Havenga K. Late anastomotic leakage in colorectal surgery: a significant problem. Colorectal Dis. 2013;15(5):e271–5.
8. Okui J, Ueno R, Matsui H, Uegami W, Hayashi H, Miyajima T, et al. Early prediction model of organ/space surgical site infection after elective gastrointestinal or hepatopancreatobiliary cancer surgery. J Infect Chemother. 2020;26(9):916–22.
9. Cuschieri S. The STROBE guidelines. Saudi J Anaesth. 2019;13(Suppl 1):S31–4.
10. Japan Nosocomial Infections Surveillance Ministry of Health, Labour and Welfare [Internet]. [cited 2021 Aug 31]. Available from: https://janis.mhlw.go.jp/english/index.asp
11. Horan TC, Gaynes RP. Surveillance of nosocomial infections. In: MayhallCG, editor. Infect Control Hosp Epidemiol. 3rd ed. Philadelphia: Lippincott Williams & Wilkins, 2004; p. 1659–1702.
12. Bassi C, Marchegiani G, Dervenis C, Sarr M, Abu Hilal M, Adham M, et al. The 2016 update of the International Study Group (ISGPS) definition and grading of postoperative pancreatic fistula: 11 Years After. Surgery. 2017;161(3):584–91.
13. Dindo D, Demartines N, Clavien P-A. Classification of surgical complications: a new proposal with evaluation in a cohort of 6336 patients and results of a survey. Ann Surg. 2004;240(2):205–13.
14. Nakamura K, Ogura K, Nakano H, Naraba H, Takahashi Y, Sonoo T, et al. C-reactive protein clustering to clarify persistent inflammation, immunosuppression and catabolism syndrome. Intensive Care Med. 2020;46(3):437–43.
15. Dayal V. Smoothers and Generalized Additive Models. In: Dayal V, editor. Quantitative Economics with R: A Data Science Approach. Singapore: Springer Singapore; 2020. p. 305–13.
16. Tan WP, Hong EY, Phillips B, Isenberg GA, Goldstein SD. Anastomotic leaks after colorectal anastomosis occurring more than 30 d postoperatively: a single-institution evaluation. Am Surg. 2014;80(9):868–72.
17. Santonocito C, De Loecker I, Donadello K, Moussa MD, Markowicz S, Gullo A, et al. C-reactive protein kinetics after major surgery. Anesth Analg. 2014;119(3):624–9.
18. Dutta S, Fullarton GM, Forshaw MJ, Horgan PG, McMillan DC. Persistent elevation of C-reactive protein following esophagogastric cancer resection as a predictor of postoperative surgical site infectious complications. World J Surg. 2011;35(5):1017–25.
19. Kørner H, Nielsen HJ, Søreide JA, Nedrebø BS, Søreide K, Knapp JC. Diagnostic accuracy of C-reactive protein for intraabdominal infections after colorectal resections. J Gastrointest Surg. 2009;13(9):1599–606.
20. Meyer ZC, Schreinemakers JMJ, Mulder PGH, de Waal RAL, Ermens AAM, van der Laan L. The role of C-reactive protein and the SOFA score as parameter for clinical decision making in surgical patients during the intensive care unit course. PLoS One. 2013;8(2):e55964.
21. Medina Fernández FJ, Muñoz-Casares FC, Arjona-Sánchez A, Casado-Adam A, Gómez-Luque I, Garcilazo Arismendi DJ, et al. Postoperative time course and utility of inflammatory markers in patients with ovarian peritoneal carcinomatosis treated with neoadjuvant chemotherapy, cytoreductive surgery, and HIPEC. Ann Surg Oncol. 2015;22(4):1332–40.
22. Gawande AA, Kwaan MR, Regenbogen SE, Lipsitz SA, Zinner MJ. An Apgar score for surgery. J Am Coll Surg. 2007;204(2):201–8.
23. Le Manach Y, Collins G, Rodseth R, Le Bihan-Benjamin C, Biccard B, Riou B, et al. Preoperative score to predict postoperative mortality (POSPOM): derivation and validation. Anesthesiology. 2016;124(3):570–9.
24. Dalton JE, Kurz A, Turan A, Mascha EJ, Sessler DI, Saager L. Development and validation of a risk quantification index for 30-day postoperative mortality and morbidity in noncardiac surgical patients. Anesthesiology. 2011;114(6):1336–44.
25. Smith RL, Bohl JK, McElearney ST, Friel CM, Barclay MM, Sawyer RG, et al. Wound infection after elective colorectal resection. Ann Surg. 2004;239(5):599–605; discussion 605–7.

6

Robotic pancreaticoduodenectomy for pancreatic head cancer and periampullary lesions

Yi-Ming Shyr | Shin-E Wang | Shih-Chin Chen | Bor-Uei Shyr | Bor-Shiuan Shyr

Division of General Surgery, Department of Surgery, Taipei Veterans General Hospital and School of Medicine, National Yang Ming University, Taipei, Taiwan

Correspondence
Yi-Ming Shyr, Division of General Surgery, Department of Surgery, Taipei Veterans General Hospital, 201, Section 2 Shi-Pai Road, Taipei 112, Taiwan.
Email: ymshyr@gmail.com

Abstract

Pancreaticoduodenectomy, so-called "Whipple operation," is a time-consuming and technically demanding complex operation. Traditionally, this procedure has been performed most usually by open approach, which results in a large and painful wound. With the introduction of laparoscopic and robotic surgery, minimally invasive surgery (MIS) has emerged as a worldwide trend to improve wound cosmesis and to minimize wound pain. Although MIS for pancreaticoduodenectomy has also been attempted at some centers, the role of MIS, either robotic or laparoscopic approach, has not been well-established for complex pancreaticoduodenectomy. Given that laparoscopic pancreaticoduodenectomy has been limited by its technical complexity and the high level of advanced laparoscopic skills required for pancreatic reconstruction, a robotic surgical system is introduced to overcome several limitations related to the laparoscopic approach. Providing high-quality three-dimensional (3-D) vision, high optical magnification, articulation of robotic instruments, greater precision with suture targeting, and elimination of surgeon tremor, robotic surgical systems innovatively perform more delicate and complex procedures involving extensive dissection and suturing techniques such as pancreaticoduodenectomy. Although associated with longer operative time, robotic pancreaticoduodenectomy (RPD) has been claimed to have the benefits of less delayed gastric emptying, less blood loss, shorter length of postoperative stay, and lower wound infection rate, as compared with the traditional open pancreaticoduodenectomy (OPD). Moreover, RPD seems to be not only technically feasible but also justified without compromising the survival outcomes for pancreatic head and ampullary adenocarcinomas. Therefore, RPD could be recommended not only to surgeons but also to patients in terms of surgical feasibility, surgical outcomes, and patient satisfaction.

KEYWORDS

cancer, da Vinci Surgical System, pancreatic head, pancreaticoduodenectomy, periampullary

1 | INTRODUCTION

Pancreaticoduodenectomy, so-called "Whipple operation," is a time-consuming and technically demanding complex operation. Traditionally, this procedure has been performed most usually by open approach, which results in a large and painful wound. With the introduction of laparoscopic and robotic surgery, minimally invasive surgery (MIS) has emerged as a worldwide trend with improving wound cosmesis and mitigating wound pain.[1-5] Although MIS for pancreaticoduodenectomy has also been attempted at some centers, the role of MIS, either by robotic or laparoscopic approach, has not been well-established for the complex pancreaticoduodenectomy. The pancreas team led by Y. M. Shyr and S. E. Wang at Taipei Veterans General Hospital have been endeavoring to develop robotic pancreaticoduodenectomy (RPD) since 2014.[6] With the experience of more than 1580 cases of pancreaticoduodenectomy and over 375 cases of RPD (Figure 1), some remarkable results have been achieved in RPD,[7-9] including: (a) shorter hospital stay after RPD, as early as on post-operative day 6 in five cases of RPD; (b) better cosmesis and smaller wounds, as small as 3 ~ 4 cm by RPD, about 1/10 of the 30 ~ 40 cm wounds by traditional OPD; (c) nearly "no" blood loss in four cases of RPD, with a mean of 120-150 c.c., as compared to 250-500 c.c. blood loss by traditional OPD; (d) short operation time by RPD, as short as 232 minutes. This record of short operation time in RPD was even shorter than the 6-8 hours taken for traditional OPD; (e) successful RPD in a 95-year-old patient, proving RPD is a feasible option in very elderly patients; and (f) low surgical mortality, as low as <3%. Our study showed over 99% of the patients undergoing RPD would like to recommend RPD to those with pancreatic head cancer and periampullary lesions.[2] The pancreatic team, led by Yi-Ming Shyr at Taipei Veterans General Hospital, are highly accredited, having received an Award of Symbol of National Quality, Safety, and Quality (SNQ award) for "Minimally Invasive Robotic Pancreatic Surgery - Small Wound for Major Pancreatic Surgery" in Taiwan in 2019.

2 | MINIMALLY INVASIVE SURGERY IN PANCREATICODUODENECTOMY

Minimally invasive surgery, either laparoscopic or robotic approach, has gained popularity in many surgical fields including pancreatic surgeries.[10-14] Laparoscopic pancreaticoduodenectomy was introduced early in 1994,[15] but its application has been limited by its technical complexity and the high level of surgical

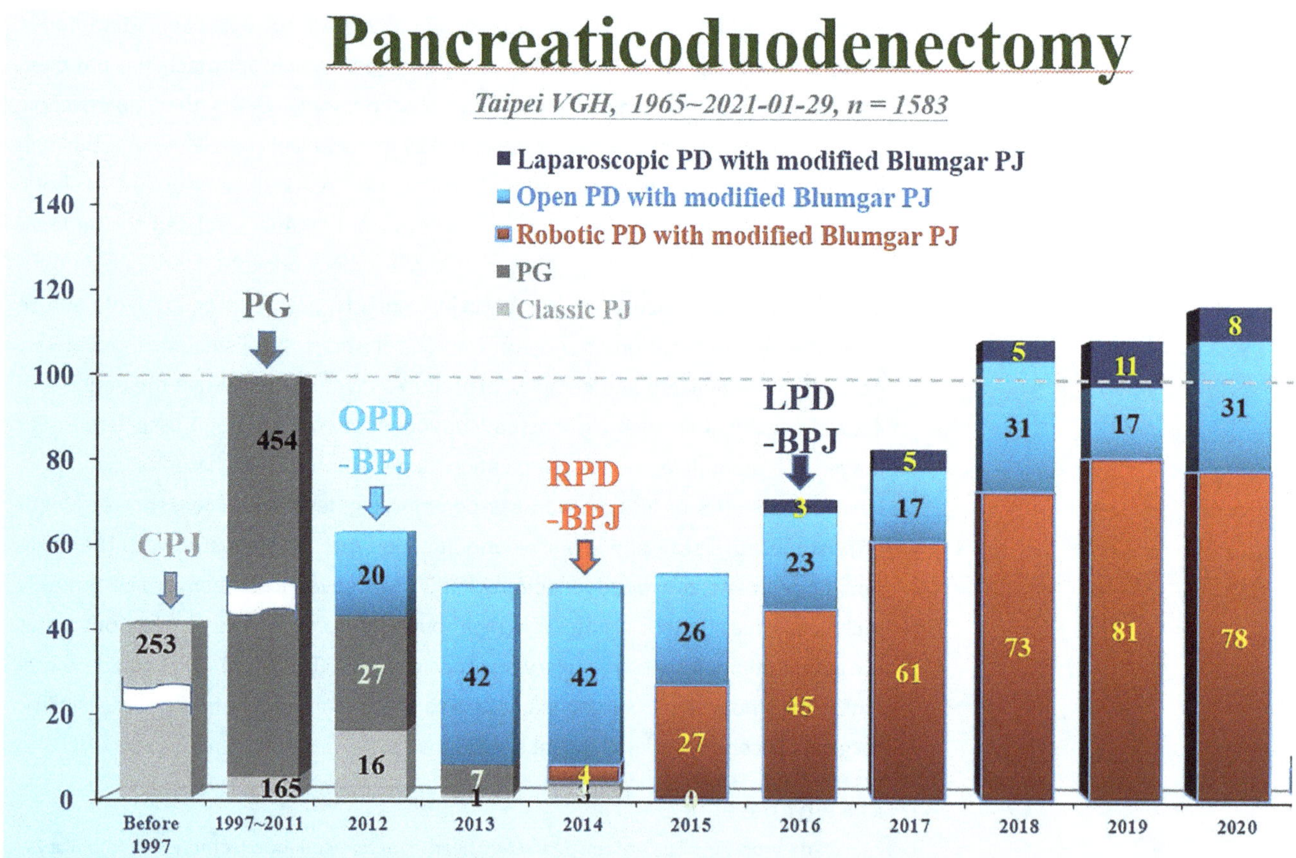

FIGURE 1 Pancreaticoduodenectomy at Taipei Veterans General Hospital. CPJ, classic pancreaticojejunostomy; PG, pancreaticojejunostomy, OPD-BPJ, open pancreaticoduodenectomy with modified Blumgart pancreaticojejunostomy; RPD-BPJ, robotic pancreaticoduodenectomy with modified Blumgart pancreaticojejunostomy; LPD-BPJ, laparoscopic pancreaticoduodenectomy with modified Blumgart pancreaticojejunostomy

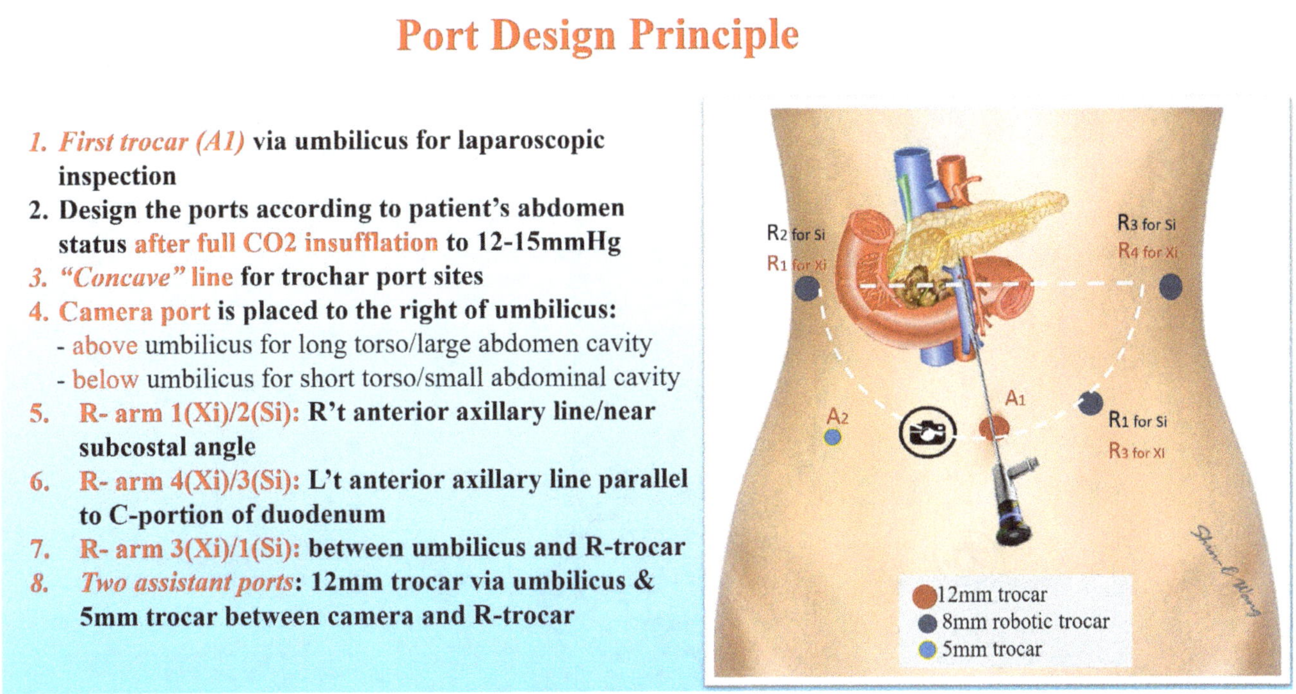

FIGURE 2 Trocar port design principle with six trocar ports including four for robotic and two for assistant instruments

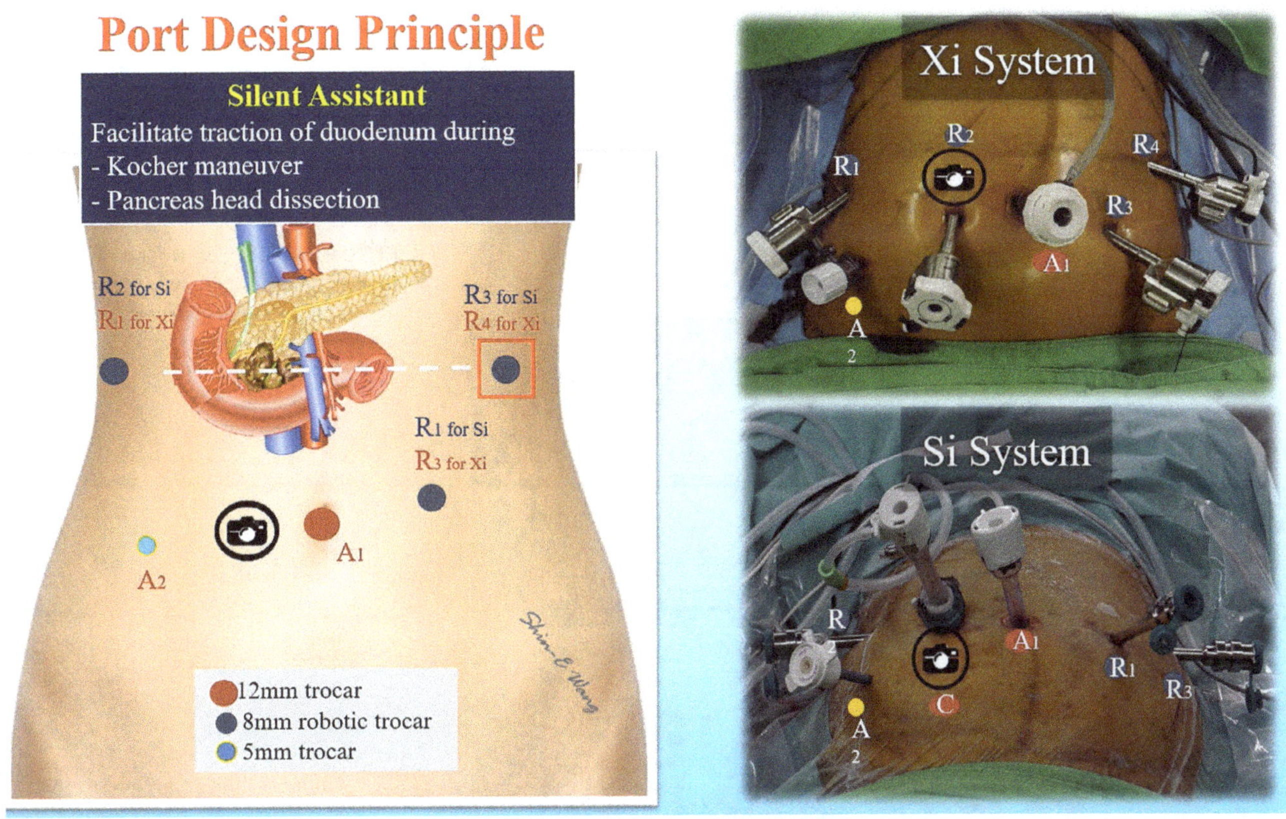

FIGURE 3 Trocar port design for da Vinci Robotic Surgical Systems

skill required. Pancreatic reconstruction requires precise placement of suture needles into a small lumen followed by intracorporeal knot-tying in soft and often friable pancreatic parenchyma. Mastering these complicated operative techniques requires advanced laparoscopic skills and a steep learning curve. With the introduction of da Vinci Robotic Surgical System (Intuitive Surgical,

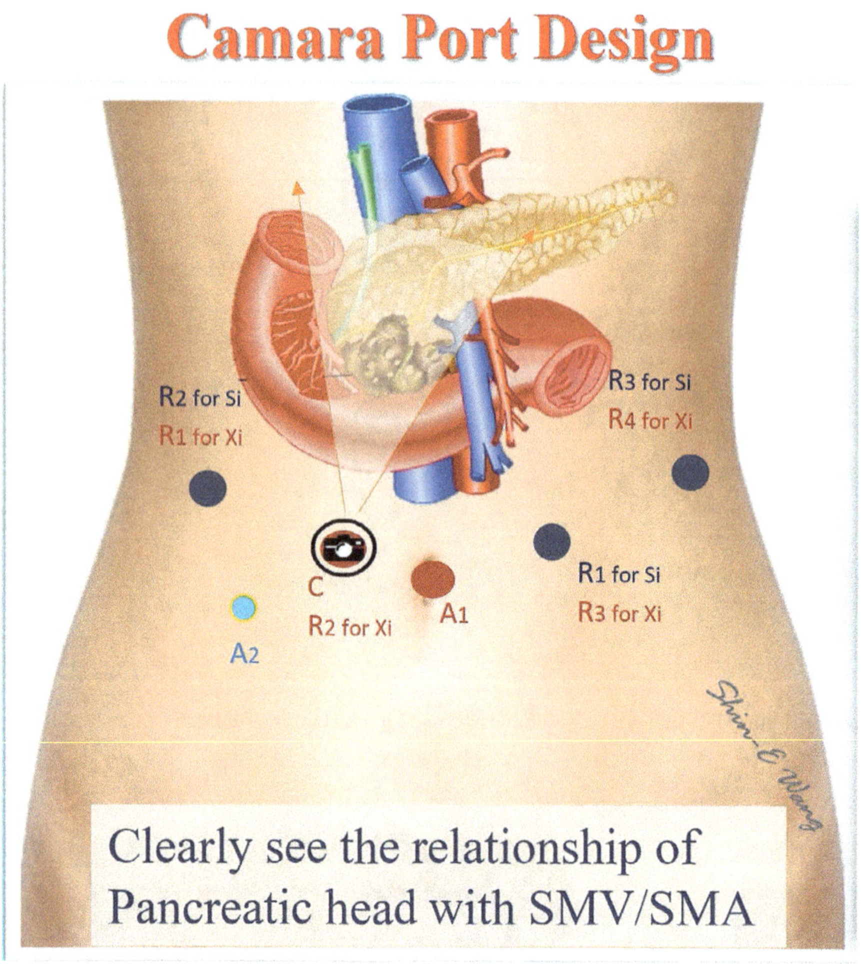

FIGURE 4 The cameral port indicated with "C" is placed about 5 cm to the right of umbilicus. Be this design, the robotic scope can clearly see the relationship of pancreatic head/uncinated process and superior mesenteric vessels during dissection around these vessels

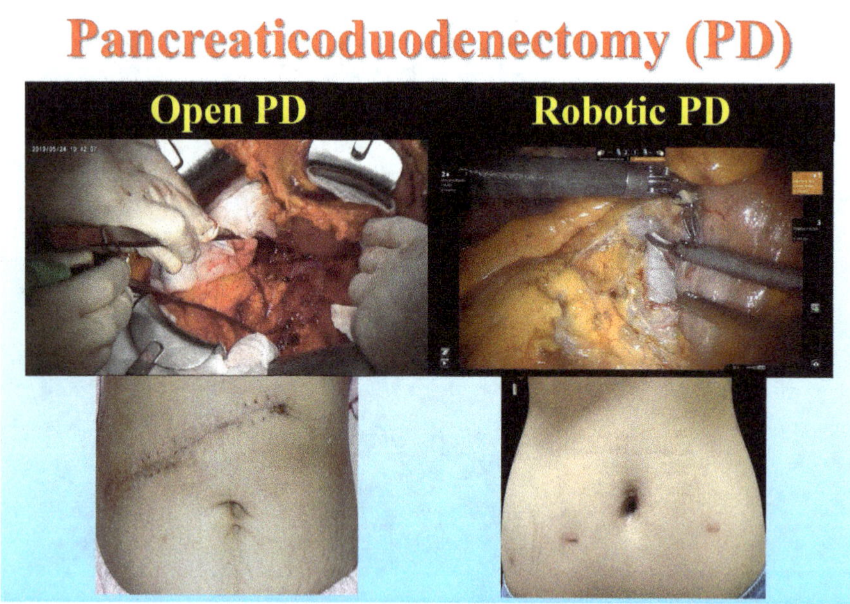

FIGURE 5 Surgical wounds for robotic and traditional open pancreaticoduodenectomy at Taipei Veterans General Hospital

Inc), several limitations related to the laparoscopic approach have been overcome. Providing high-quality three-dimensional (3-D) and optical 10-15 magnification vision, articulated instruments, greater precision with suture targeting, and elimination of surgeon tremor, robotic approach can even enable complex procedures such as Whipple procedure, which involves extensive and complex resection and reconstruction of pancreas, bile duct, and gastrointestinal tract.[12,16,17] However, a major concern about the da Vinci

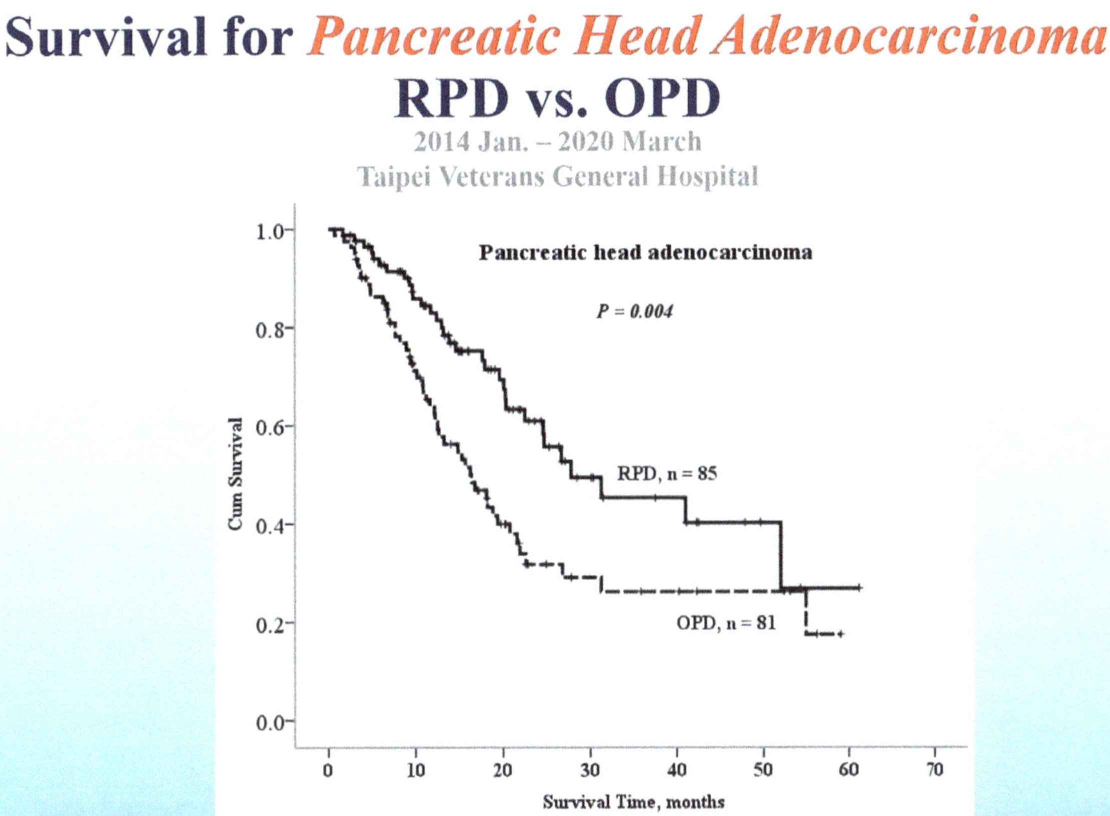

Pancreatic Head Adenocarcinoma	Median (mon.)	Range (mon.)	Mean±SD (mon.)	1-year survival	3-year survival	5-year survival	P value
RPD, n = 85	15.3	1.9 – 61.1	18.9±13.0	82.9%	45.3%	26.8%	0.004
OPD, n = 81	12.3	0.7 – 59.1	16.5±13.9	63.8%	26.2%	17.4%	

FIGURE 6 Survival curves for pancreatic head adenocarcinoma after robotic pancreaticoduodenectomy (RPD) and open pancreaticoduodenectomy (OPD)

Robotic Surgical System is the cost for robotic instruments, one of the reasons that it is not widely accepted as a routine procedure in most centers.[9,10,18–21]

3 | TROCHA PORT DESIGN IN ROBOTIC PANCREATICODUODENECTOMY

da Vinci Robotic Surgical System (Intuitive Surgical, Inc) is used to perform RPD. Six ports including four robotic trocars and two assistant ports are used in both da Vinci Si and Xi Robotic Surgical Systems at Taipei Veterans General Hospital (Figure 2).[5] The trocar designs are similar for da Vinci Si and Xi Surgical Systems (Figure 3). First, a 12-mm trocha as the assistant port is set up via transumbilical incision, and pneumoperitoneum at a pressure level of 12-15 mm Hg is established. Laparoscopic inspection is performed first to check the feasibility and resectability of RPD before docking the robotic system. Three 8-mm robotic ports for working instruments are set up, one along the right anterior axillary line at the same level pancreatic head, another one along the left anterior axillary line at the same level pancreatic head, and the third along the left mid-clavicular line slightly below the umbilicus level. The 8-mm Xi or 12-mm Si camera port is placed at about 3-5 cm to the right of umbilicus. Thus, the robotic camera scope can clearly see the relationship of pancreatic head and superior mesenteric vessels during pancreatic head dissection (Figure 4). A 5-mm trocha as an assistant port is usually placed on the right mid-clavicular line slightly below the camera port.[5,6]

4 | TECHNIQUE OF PANCREATIC RECONSTRUCTION IN ROBOTIC PANCREATICODUODENECTOMY

Pancreatic reconstruction with a modified Blumgart pancreaticojejunostomy (PJ) has been previously described in detail.[1,5,6,22] Briefly, three transpancreatic U-sutures are placed for the horizontal mattress outer sutures on the posterior wall of jejunum, using 3-0 monofilament synthetic absorbable sutures (PDS™). The U-sutures are placed at about 0.8-1 cm from the pancreatic cutting

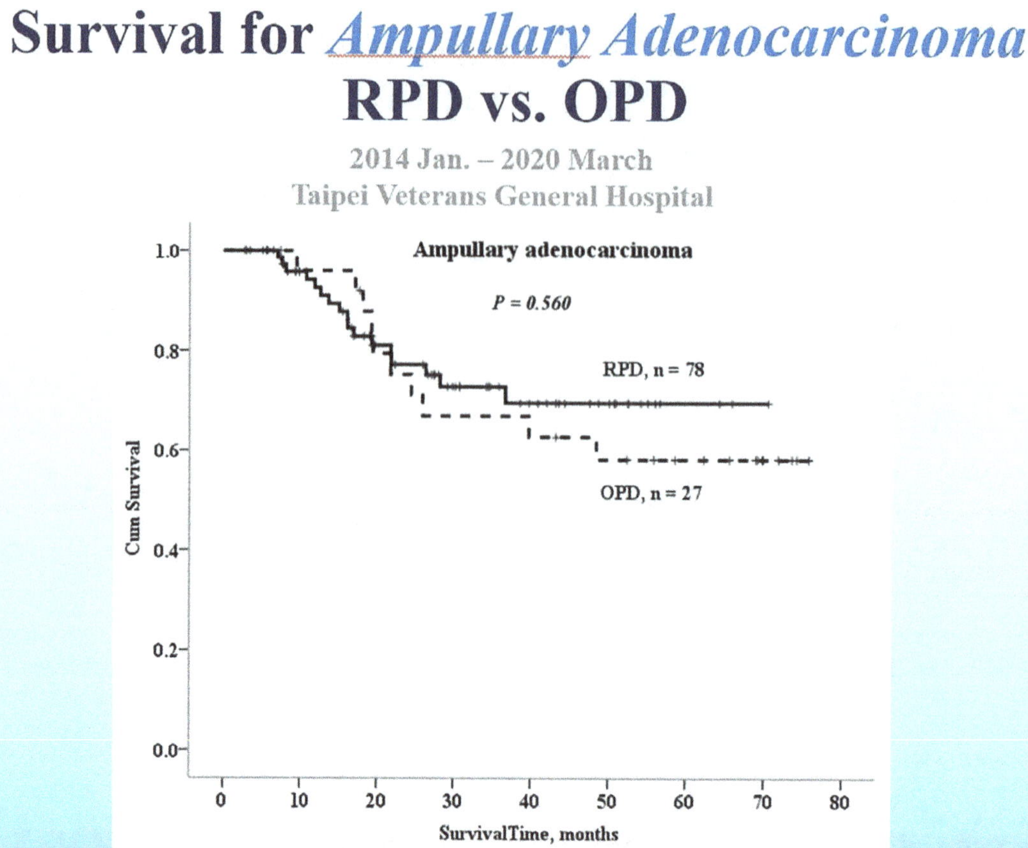

Ampullary Adenocarcinoma	Median (mon.)	Range (mon.)	Mean±SD (mon.)	1-year survival	3-year survival	5-year survival	P value
RPD, n = 78	24.1	3.0 – 70.5	27.0±17.3	92.6%	72.8%	69.5%	0.560
OPD, n = 27	48.4	2.7 – 75.7	43.8±24.9	96.0%	66.9%	58.2%	

FIGURE 7 Survival curves for ampullary adenocarcinoma after robotic pancreaticoduodenectomy (RPD) and open pancreaticoduodenectomy (OPD)

margin. These U-sutures with needles on them are left untied, kept separate, and held with robotic instruments to facilitate inner layer anastomosis. The inner layer duct-to-mucosa anastomosis is performed carefully and precisely by a series of interrupted sutures with 4-0 absorbable synthetic monofilament suture (MonoPlus®), usually six for a normal pancreatic duct and eight or more sutures for a dilated duct. The inner layer sutures are completed one by one by pair-watch technique until the last three sutures. After completing the inner layer duct-to-mucosa anastomosis, the outer layer horizontal mattress sutures on the anterior wall of jejunum are completed, using previously placed U-sutures, which are held and organized by the robotic arm.

5 | MESOPANCREAS DISSECTION

"Mesopancreas dissection," proposed by Inoue et al,[23] is used to describe the extent of lymph node dissection during separation of pancreas head-uncinate process from superior mesenteric vessels. Mesopancreas dissections can be categorized into three levels based on the extent of dissection around and along the superior mesenteric vessels, including level 1 mesopancreas dissection, simply along the right side of superior mesenteric vein (SMV), usually applied for those with benign or low-malignancy potential; level 2 mesopancreas dissection, along the right side of superior mesenteric artery (SMA), and en bloc resection of the corresponding lymph nodes and mesojejunum, but not including the nerve plexus on the SMA, applied for periampullary cancers; level 3 mesopancreas dissection, including en bloc mesopancreas resection with periadventitial tissues including nerve plexus along the right hemi-circumference of SMA from 5 to 11 o'clock, just applied for pancreatic head cancer.[8,23-25]

6 | SURGICAL OUTCOMES AFTER ROBOTIC PANCREATICODUODENECTOMY

It has been claimed that RPD has benefits of less delayed gastric emptying, less blood loss, lower wound infection rate, and shorter postoperative hospital stay, as compared with OPD, according to studies and literature reports.[1,5,7–9,26–29] Our study showed that the biggest complications after RPD are 18.1% occurrence of chyle leakage, followed by 5.7% occurrence of postoperative pancreatic fistula, 4.8% occurrence of intra-abdominal abscess, 3.8% occurrence of delayed gastric emptying, and post pancreatectomy hemorrhage.[2] The wounds after RPD and OPD are shown in Figure 5. We conducted a study of patient satisfaction and quality of life using questionnaires for 105 RPD patients. The results revealed that almost all of the patients responded to this RPD-related survey with "fair" to "excellent" grades for all items, except one (<1%) poor grade for operation service and two (1.9%) "not good" grades for diet tolerance. More than 99% (104/105 = 99.05%) of the patients after RPD were satisfied with the surgical outcomes and would like to recommend RPD to those patients with pancreatic head cancer and periampullary lesions.[2]

7 | SURVIVAL OUTCOMES AFTER ROBOTIC PANCREATICODUODENECTOMY

Survival outcomes after RPD have not been well-studied or reported in the literature.[9] We conducted a retrospective study for survival outcomes of pancreatic head cancer patients undergoing pancreaticoduodenectomy, comparing 85 RPD and 81 OPD patients. This study showed there was a benefit of survival in the RPD group, with 82.9% of 1-year survival, 45.3% of 3-year survival, and 26.8% 5-year survival, as compared with 63.8%, 26.2%, and 17.4%, respectively, in the OPD group, $P = .004$ (Figure 6).[7] For ampullary cancer, there is no survival difference between RPD and OPD groups (Figure 7).[7] At least, RPD is not only technically feasible but also oncologically justifiable without compromising the survival outcomes of pancreatic head and ampullary cancers, although selection bias would be inevitable in this retrospective study.[1,2,9] Prospective randomized control trials or studies of larger sample sizes with long-term follow-up are recommended to reach a reliable conclusion.

ACKNOWLEDGMENTS

This work is funded by grants from the Ministry of Health and Welfare (MOHW107-TDU-B-212-114026A), the Ministry of Science and Technology (MOST 108-2314-B-075 -051 -MY3), and the Taipei Veterans General Hospital (V110C-010 and V110C-011).

REFERENCES

1. Shyr BU, Chen SC, Shyr YM, Wang SE. Surgical, survival, and oncological outcomes after vascular resection in robotic and open pancreaticoduodenectomy. Surg Endosc. 2020;34:377–83.
2. Shyr BU, Shyr BS, Chen SC, Chang IW, Shyr YM, Wang SE. Operative results and patient satisfaction after robotic pancreaticoduodenectomy. Asian J Surg. 2020;43:519–25.
3. Girgis MD, Zenati MS, Steve J, Bartlett DL, Zureikat A, Zeh HJ. Robotic approach mitigates perioperative morbidity in obese patients following pancreaticoduodenectomy. HPB (Oxford). 2017;19:93–8.
4. Kornaropoulos M, Moris D, Beal EW, Makris MC, Mitrousias A, Petrou A, et al. Total robotic pancreaticoduodenectomy: a systematic review of the literature. Surg Endosc. 2017;31:4382–92.
5. Shyr YM, Wang SE, Chen SC, Shyr BU. Robotic pancreaticoduodenectomy in the era of minimally invasive surgery. J Chin Med Assoc. 2020;83:639–43.
6. Shyr BU, Chen SC, Shyr YM, Wang SE. Learning curves for robotic pancreatic surgery-from distal pancreatectomy to pancreaticoduodenectomy. Medicine (Baltimore). 2018;97:e13000.
7. Shyr BU, Shyr BS, Chen SC, Shyr YM, Wang SE. Robotic and open pancreaticoduodenectomy: results from Taipei Veterans General Hospital in Taiwan. Updates in Surgery. 2020. Online ahead of print. https://doi.org/10.1007/s13304-020-00899-z
8. Shyr BU, Shyr BS, Chen SC, Shyr YM, Wang SE. Mesopancreas level 3 dissection in robotic pancreaticoduodenectomy. Surgery. 2021;169:362–8.
9. Wang SE, Shyr BU, Chen SC, Shyr YM. Comparison between robotic and open pancreaticoduodenectomy with modified Blumgart pancreaticojejunostomy: a propensity score-matched study. Surgery. 2018;164:1162–7.
10. Boggi U, Signori S, De Lio N, Perrone VG, Vistoli F, Belluomini M, et al. Feasibility of robotic pancreaticoduodenectomy. Br J Surg. 2013;100:917–25.
11. Napoli N, Kauffmann EF, Menonna F, Perrone VG, Brozzetti S, Boggi U. Indications, technique, and results of robotic pancreatoduodenectomy. Updates Surg. 2016;68:295–305.
12. Napoli N, Kauffmann EF, Palmeri M, Miccoli M, Costa F, Vistoli F, et al. The learning curve in robotic pancreaticoduodenectomy. Dig Surg. 2016;33:299–307.
13. Stafford AT, Walsh RM. Robotic surgery of the pancreas: the current state of the art. J Surg Oncol. 2015;112:289–94.
14. Zureikat AH, Moser AJ, Boone BA, Bartlett DL, Zenati M, Zeh HJ. 250 robotic pancreatic resections: safety and feasibility. Ann Surg. 2013;258(4):554–62; discussion 559–62.
15. Gagner M, Pomp A. Laparoscopic pylorus-preserving pancreatoduodenectomy. Surg Endosc. 1994;8:408–10.
16. Memeo R, Sangiuolo F, de Blasi V, Tzedakis S, Mutter D, Marescaux J, et al. Robotic pancreaticoduodenectomy and distal pancreatectomy: State of the art. J Visc Surg. 2016;153:353–9.
17. Liu R, Zhang T, Zhao ZM, Tan XL, Zhao GD, Zhang X, et al. The surgical outcomes of robot-assisted laparoscopic pancreaticoduodenectomy versus laparoscopic pancreaticoduodenectomy for periampullary neoplasms: a comparative study of a single center. Surg Endosc. 2017;31:2380–6.
18. Guerra F, Checcacci P, Vegni A, di Marino M, Annecchiarico M, Farsi M, et al. Surgical and oncological outcomes of our first 59 cases of robotic pancreaticoduodenectomy. J Visc Surg. 2019;156:185–90.
19. Galvez D, Sorber R, Javed AA, He J. Technical considerations for the fully robotic pancreaticoduodenectomy. J Vis Surg. 2017;3:81.
20. Zeh HJ, Zureikat AH, Secrest A, Dauoudi M, Bartlett D, Moser AJ. Outcomes after robot-assisted pancreaticoduodenectomy for periampullary lesions. Ann Surg Oncol. 2012;19:864–70.
21. Del Chiaro M, Segersvard R. The state of the art of robotic pancreatectomy. Biomed Res Int. 2014;2014:920492. https://doi.org/10.1155/2014/920492
22. Wang SE, Chen SC, Shyr BU, Shyr YM. Comparison of Modified Blumgart pancreaticojejunostomy and pancreaticogastrostomy after pancreaticoduodenectomy. HPB (Oxford). 2016;18:229–35.
23. Inoue Y, Saiura A, Yoshioka R, Ono Y, Takahashi M, Arita J, et al. Pancreatoduodenectomy with systematic mesopancreas dissection using a supracolic anterior artery-first approach. Ann Surg. 2015;262:1092–101.
24. Inoue Y, Saiura A, Tanaka M, Matsumura M, Takeda Y, Mise Y, et al. Technical details of an anterior approach to the superior mesenteric artery during pancreaticoduodenectomy. J Gastrointest Surg. 2016;20:1769–77.
25. Inoue Y, Saiura A, Oba A, Kawakatsu S, Ono Y, Sato T, et al. Optimal extent of superior mesenteric artery dissection during pancreati-

coduodenectomy for pancreatic cancer: balancing surgical and oncological safety. J Gastrointest Surg. 2019;23:1373–83.
26. Yan Q, Xu LB, Ren ZF, Liu C. Robotic versus open pancreaticoduodenectomy: a meta-analysis of short-term outcomes. Surg Endosc. 2020;34:501–9.
27. Podda M, Gerardi C, Di Saverio S, Marino MV, Davies RJ, Pellino G, et al. Robotic-assisted versus open pancreaticoduodenectomy for patients with benign and malignant periampullary disease: a systematic review and meta-analysis of short-term outcomes. Surg Endosc. 2020;34:2390–409.
28. Peng L, Lin S, Li Y, Xiao W. Systematic review and meta-analysis of robotic versus open pancreaticoduodenectomy. Surg Endosc. 2017;31:3085–97.
29. Zureikat AH, Postlewait LM, Liu Y, Gillespie TW, Weber SM, Abbott DE, et al. A Multi-institutional comparison of perioperative outcomes of robotic and open pancreaticoduodenectomy. Ann Surg. 2016;264:640–9.

7

New scoring system for prediction of surgical difficulty during laparoscopic cholecystectomy after percutaneous transhepatic gallbladder drainage

Michinori Matsumoto[1] | Kyohei Abe[1] | Yasuro Futagawa[1] | Kenei Furukawa[2] | Koichiro Haruki[2] | Shinji Onda[2] | Takanori Kurogochi[1] | Nana Takeuchi[1] | Tomoyoshi Okamoto[1] | Toru Ikegami[2]

[1]Department of Surgery, The Jikei University Daisan Hospital, Komae, Japan

[2]Department of Surgery, The Jikei University School of Medicine, Minato-ku, Japan

Correspondence
Michinori Matsumoto, Department of Surgery, The Jikei University Daisan Hospital, 4-11-1 Izumihon-cho, Komae-shi, Tokyo 201-8601, Japan
Email: mmatsumoto4@jikei.ac.jp

Abstract

Background: The surgical difficulty of laparoscopic cholecystectomy (LC) after percutaneous transhepatic gallbladder drainage (PTGBD) remains unknown. This study aimed to establish a scoring system (SS) to predict the necessity of a bailout procedure during LC after PTGBD and to evaluate the relationship between SS and perioperative complications.

Methods: We retrospectively studied 70 patients who underwent LC after PTGBD. Preoperative factors potentially predictive of the need for the bailout procedure were analyzed. The SS included significantly predictive factors, with their cutoff values determined by receiver operating characteristic curves. Patients were assigned a score of 1 when exhibiting only one of these abnormalities. We compared the perioperative factors between three groups with scores of 0, 1, or 2. The SS was applied to another series of 65 patients for validation. We compared the score-2 patient perioperative factors between LC with the bailout procedure and open cholecystectomy from the beginning (OC).

Results: Independent predictors were time until PTGBD after symptom onset and the maximal wall gallbladder thickness (cutoff values: 3 days and 10 mm, respectively). The high-score group was significantly associated with bile duct injury (BDI). The sensitivity and specificity of our SS were 75.0% and 98.1% in validation, respectively. The score-2 OC and laparoscopic subtotal cholecystectomy (LSC) groups had no BDI.

Conclusions: The SS using time until PTGBD after symptom onset and gallbladder wall thickness for predicting the need for the bailout procedure correctly predicted the need. The scores might be associated with the risk of BDI, and LSC or OC might be a better choice for score-2 patients.

KEYWORDS

bile duct injury, laparoscopic cholecystectomy, percutaneous transhepatic gallbladder drainage, receiver operating characteristic, scoring system

1 | INTRODUCTION

Laparoscopic cholecystectomy (LC) has become a standard procedure for benign diseases of the gallbladder (GB) worldwide.[1] Severe inflammation of GB and its surroundings increases both the difficulty of complete LC and the frequency of postoperative complications.[2] Bile duct injury (BDI) is known to occur in a certain proportion of cases, and the prognoses of patients who suffer vasculo-biliary injury (VBI) in particular are poor.[3] Therefore, it is very important to take prudent steps to prevent complications.[4] The Tokyo Guidelines 2018 (TG18) propose management bundles for acute cholecystitis (AC) and cholangitis. When LC for AC is difficult, not only open conversion but also laparoscopic subtotal cholecystectomy (LSC) with the fenestrating or reconstituting and fundus first technique, called the bailout procedure, can be chosen to prevent BDI according to the intraoperative findings.[4]

On the other hand, early surgery for AC cannot be performed for all surgically high-risk patients. Percutaneous transhepatic GB drainage (PTGBD) should be considered the first alternative to cholecystectomy in surgically high-risk patients with AC because several studies have described PTGBD as less invasive and having a lower risk of adverse events than cholecystectomy.[5] However, the degree of surgical difficulty during LC after PTGBD is unknown, and no report has provided scientific evidence of the conditions supporting use of the bailout procedure during LC after PTGBD.

This study aimed to establish a scoring system (SS) to predict the necessity of the bailout procedure during LC after PTGBD and to evaluate the relationship between the SS and perioperative complication.

2 | PATIENTS AND METHODS

The medical records of a series of 178 consecutive patients who had undergone LC or open cholecystectomy after PTGBD for AC between January 2014 and August 2021 in The Jikei University Daisan Hospital and The Jikei University Hospital were retrospectively reviewed. The 178 patients were divided into two groups, one for model development (training cohort) and the other for validation testing (validation cohort). We defined open conversion from LC or LSC with the fenestrating or reconstituting technique as the bailout procedure. In the first 87 patients for the training cohort between 2014 and 2019 in The Jikei University Daisan Hospital, 12 patients who had undergone open cholecystectomy from the beginning (OC) and five patients who had undergone OC with choledochoduodenostomy for cholodocholithiasis were excluded. The remaining 70 patients were divided into 58 patients who had undergone pure LC without the bailout procedure and 12 patients who had undergone LC with the bailout procedure. Independent factors predictive of the necessity of the bailout procedure were examined for the training cohort of the 70 patients. In the validation cohort operated in The Jikei University Daisan Hospital between January 2020 and August 2021 and in The Jikei University Hospital between 2015 and 2020, 12 patients who had undergone OC, five patients who had undergone open cholecystectomy with choledochoduodenostomy for choledocholithiasis, one patient who had undergone open cholecystectomy with choledochojejunostomy for choledocholithiasis, one patient who had undergone LC 7 years after PTGBD, and six patients with unknown data due to PTGBD in other hospitals were excluded. The remaining 65 patients were divided into 53 patients who had undergone pure LC without the bailout procedure and 12 patients who had undergone LC with the bailout procedure. The 65 patients were examined to assess the accuracy of our SS (Figure 1).

Most of PTGBD procedures were performed by physicians in our hospital. The main indication of PTGBD in our hospital was Grade II (moderate) or III (severe) AC according to TG18[5] when the patients could not withstand surgery and were AC refractory to antibiotics. Measurement of the maximum GB wall thickness was performed on the axial or coronal plane of noncontrast or contrast-enhanced computed tomography just before PTGBD because most of the images of abdominal ultrasonography just before or during PTGBD had not been stored.

The following 14 preoperative factors of these patients were analyzed to predict the necessity of the bailout procedure during LC in univariate and multivariate analysis: age, gender, body mass index, procedure (single-port or multi-port LC), American Society of Anesthesiologists physical status classification, age-adjusted Charlson comorbidity index (CCI),[6,7] anticoagulant therapy, past history of upper abdominal surgery, time until PTGBD after symptom onset, time until surgery after PTGBD, maximal GB wall thickness, maximal diameter of impacted stone in the GB, maximal white blood cell (WBC) count in the peripheral blood, and maximal serum value of C-reactive protein. The cutoff score of CCI was determined based on a past report.[8]

The SS was designed by using the significant predictive factors, the cutoff values of which were determined by a receiver operating characteristic (ROC) curve. Patients were assigned to a score of 2 if they had two significant factors predictive of both abnormalities for the respective cutoff values, a score of 1 if they only had one factor predictive of these abnormalities, and a score of 0 if neither abnormality was present. We then compared the 18 perioperative factors, which are the previous 14 preoperative factors and another four perioperative factors (open conversion, subtotal cholecystectomy, BDI, and postoperative complication) among three groups with scores of 0, 1, and 2, respectively. The SS was applied to another series of 65 patients for validation.

Finally, we compared the 21 perioperative factors, which are the previously described 18 perioperative factors and another three operative factors (LSC with fenestrating or reconstituting, operation time, and estimated blood loss during operation) between patients with a score of 2 between 2014 and August 2021 in The Jikei University Daisan Hospital and between 2015 and 2020 in The Jikei University Hospital who underwent LC with the bailout procedure and those who underwent OC.

This retrospective study was approved by the Ethics Committee of The Jikei University School of Medicine (Tokyo, Japan); 27-177 (8062).

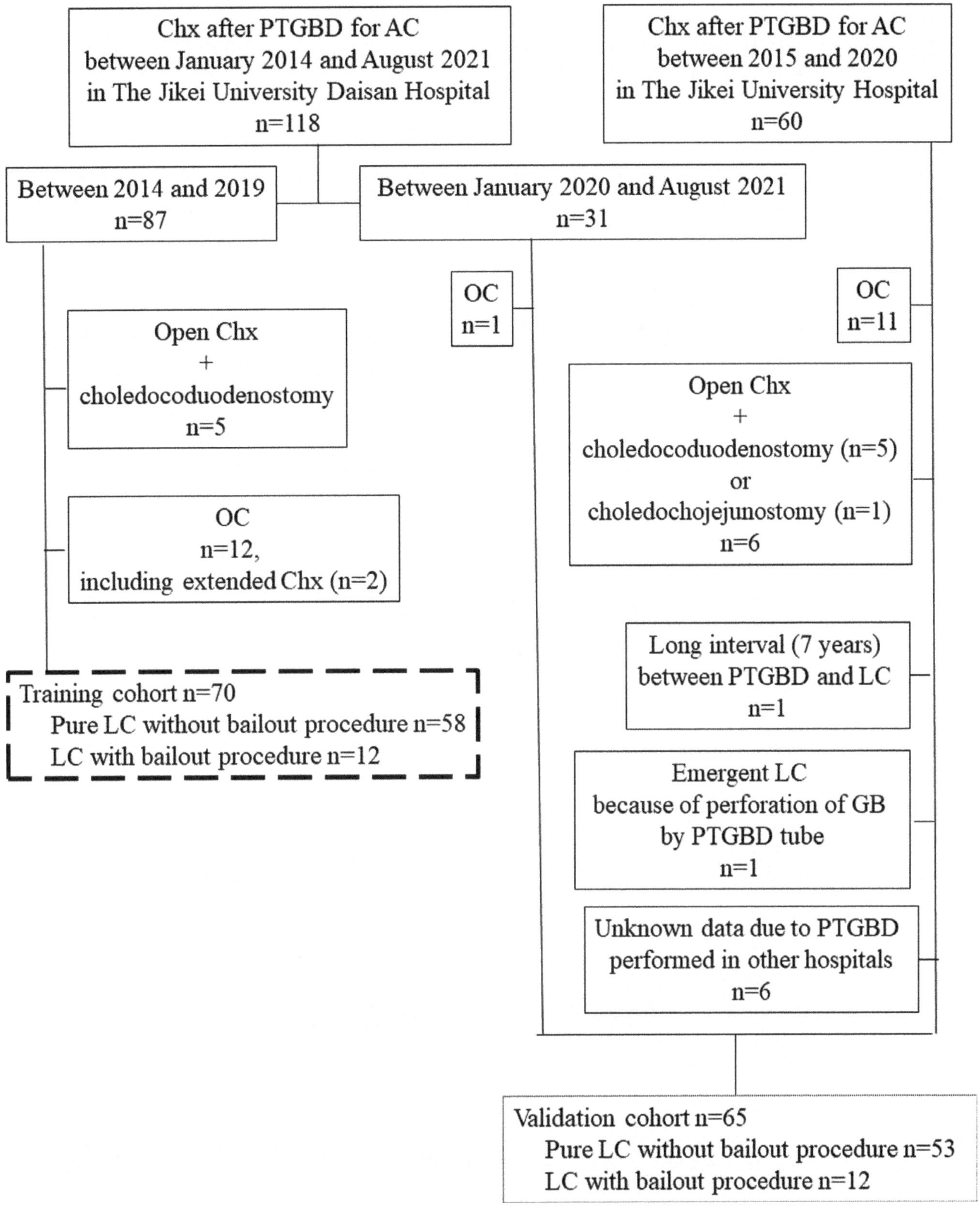

FIGURE 1 Flow diagram describing the patient selection process. AC, acute cholecystitis; PTGBD, percutaneous transhepatic gallbladder drainage; LC, laparoscopic cholecystectomy; Chx, cholecystectomy; OC, open cholecystectomy from the beginning

2.1 | Statistical methods

Continuous data were expressed as the median and range, and compared by the Mann–Whitney *U*-test between two groups and by the Kruskal–Wallis test among three groups. Categorical data were compared by the chi-square test. Univariate factors predictive of the need for the bailout procedure ($P < .05$) were entered into a logistic regression model to identify the independent conversion predictors. Multivariate analysis was performed by a stepwise backward procedure. The accuracy of these independent predictors for the bailout procedure were evaluated by calculating the area under ROC curve (AUROC). The ROC curve was a plot of sensitivity vs 1 − specificity for all possible cutoff values. Cutoff values of these independent predictors were determined by an ROC curve. $P < .05$ was considered to be indicative of statistical significance in all analyses.

3 | RESULTS

3.1 | Characteristics of the clinical patients

The characteristics of the 70 patients are summarized in Table 1. For all cases, there were 51 men and 19 women. The median age was 73 years (range, 28–89 years). All patients who underwent the bailout procedure had open conversion form LC. The conversion rate

TABLE 1 Patient characteristics in the training cohort

	Factor 〔Median (minimum to maximum) or Ratio〕	All cases (n = 70)	Pure LC without bailout procedure (n = 58)	LC with bailout procedure (n = 12)	P-value
Preoperative factor	Age (years old)	73 (28–89)	73.5 (28–89)	68 (43–83)	.809
	Gender (male : female)	51:19	41:17	10:2	.370
	BMI	23.9 (16. 4–32.8)	24.0 (16.6–32.8)	23.6 (16.4–28.4)	.839
	SILS (yes : no)	5:65	4:54	1:11	.860
	ASA-PS (1:2:3)	13:51:6	12:42:4	1:9:2	.380
	CCI (≤5:≤6)	50:20	41:17	9:3	.764
	HT (yes:no)	38:32	30:28	8:4	.344
	DM (yes:no)	19:51	16:42	3:9	.854
	Past history of upper abdominal surgery (yes:no)	3:67	3:55	0:12	.421
	Anticoagulative therapy (yes:no)	17:53	15:43	2:10	.499
	Time until PTGBD after symptom onset (days)	2 (0–16)	2 (0–8)	4 (1–16)	.001
	Time until surgery after PTGBD (days)	64.5 (3–281)	64.5 (3–281)	61 (13–102)	.969
	GB wall thickness (mm)	5 (2–21)	5 (2–15)	11.5 (2–21)	.001
	Maximal diameter of impacted stone (mm)	4 (0–40)	4 (0–40)	7 (3–29)	.093
	Maximal WBC count in the peripheral blood (/μL)	13 ,450 (6800–31,800)	13,000 (6800–27,200)	17,350 (10 800–31,800)	.031
	Maximal serum value of CRP (mg/dL)	19.8 (0.5–40.4)	19.8 (0.5–39.2)	23.3 (14.5–40.4)	.052
Intra- or postoperative factor	Open conversion (yes:no)	12:58	0:58	12:0	<.0001
	LSC with fenestrating or reconstituting (yes:no)	0:70	0:58	0:12	NA
	Subtotal cholecystectomy with fenestrating or reconstituting (yes:no)	5:65	0:58	5:7	<.0001
	BDI during operation (yes:no)	3:0	0:58	3:9	<.0001
	Grade of Clavien–Dindo classification ≤3 (yes:no)	2:68	1:57	1:11	.211

Abbreviations: ASA-PS, the American Society of Anesthesiologists physical status classification; BDI, bile duct injury; BMI, body mass index; CCI, Age-adjusted Charlson comorbidity index; CRP, C-reactive protein; DM, diabetes mellitus; GB, gallbladder; HT, hypertension; LC, laparoscopic cholecystectomy; LSC, laparoscopic subtotal cholecystectomy; NA, not available; PTGBD, percutaneous transhepatic gallbladder drainage; SILS, single-port laparoscopic surgery; WBC, white blood cell.

was 17% (=12/70). The reasons for conversion were as follows: difficulty in dissection at Calot's triangle in five patients, difficulty in dissection for adhesion to the duodenum and/or transverse colon in six patients, and BDI in one patient. Subtotal cholecystectomy was performed for five patients after open conversion; fenestrating in three patients, reconstituting in one patient, and both in one patient. There were three patients with BDI in this training cohort. Of the three cases, one had BDI and another had VBI with injury to the right hepatic artery after open conversion. The other patient had BDI during LC.

3.2 | Univariate and multivariate predictors of the conversion

Significant univariate predictors of the necessity of the bailout procedure during LC after PTGBD were time until PTGBD after symptom onset ($P = .001$), the maximal GB wall thickness ($P = .001$), and the maximal WBC count in the peripheral blood ($P = .031$) (Table 1). Time until PTGBD after symptom onset and the maximal GB wall thickness were independent clinical predictors for the necessity of the bailout procedure during LC after multivariate analysis (odds ratio [OR] = 1.416, 95% confidence interval [CI]: 1.005–1.994, $P = .046$ and OR = 1.423, 95% CI: 1.135–1.784, $P = .002$, respectively) (Table 2).

3.3 | Determination of cutoff values for the independent predictors

The results of the ROC curve of time until PTGBD after symptom onset and the maximal GB wall thickness are shown in Figure 2. The maximal sensitivity and specificity were obtained when the time until PTGBD after symptom onset and the maximal GB wall thickness were 3 d and 10 mm, respectively (AUROC = 0.795, 95% CI: 0.650–0.939, $P = .001$ and AUROC = 0.854, 95% CI: 0.694–1.000. $P < .0001$, respectively) (Figure 2).

3.4 | Univariate analysis of the relationship between patient characteristics and the SS

Two variables were used in the design of the SS. In brief, patients were assigned a score of 2 if they had both a longer time until PTGBD after symptom onset (≥3 days) and a thicker GB wall (≥10 mm), a score of 1 when exhibiting only one of these abnormalities, and a score of 0 if neither abnormality was present (Table 3). This SS design was significantly associated with the open conversion during LC ($P < .0001$) and subtotal cholecystectomy with the fenestrating or reconstituting technique ($P < .0001$) (Table 4). On the other hand, patients with high scores were significantly associated with BDI ($P < .0001$) (Table 4).

3.5 | Validation of the SS for prediction of the bailout procedure

The frequency distribution of the necessity of the bailout procedure during LC according to the time until PTGBD after symptom onset and the maximal GB wall thickness was examined in another series of 65 patients. Table 5 shows the patient characteristics of the 65 patients; of these, 27, 28, and 10 patients had scores of 0, 1, and 2, respectively. Three patients with a score of <2 underwent the bailout procedure during LC. The reasons for conversion were as follows: difficulty in dissection at Calot's triangle in four patients, difficulty in dissection for adhesion to the duodenum and/or transverse colon in two patients, and BDI in one patient. One of the patients who underwent LSC was diagnosed with GB cancer by histopathological examination after surgery. This patient underwent the additional liver bed resection and biliary resection and reconstruction. In univariate analysis, the GB wall in the LC with the bailout procedure group was significantly thicker than the GB wall in the pure LC without the bailout procedure group ($P = .003$). The percentage of patients who required the bailout procedure during LC was 75.0% in patients with a score of 2 ($P < .0001$). The SS was designed using these two variables. By comparing patients with a score of 2 with those with a score of 1 and less, the sensitivity and specificity of our SS for prediction of the bailout procedure were 75.0% (=9/12) and 98.1% (=52/53), respectively (Table 5).

3.6 | Univariate analysis of patient characteristics between patients with a score of 2 from 2014 to August 2021 who underwent LC with the bailout procedure and who underwent OC

Thirteen patients had OC after PTGBD between 2014 and August 2021 in The Jikei University Daisan Hospital and 11 patients had OC after PTGBD between 2015 and 2020 in The Jikei University Hospital. Among the total 24 patients who had OC, nine patients had a score of 2. Table 6 showed that although there was no significant difference between the patients who underwent LC with the bailout procedure and those who underwent OC with a score of 2, none of the patients with a score of 2 who underwent the OC had BDI ($P = .125$). In addition, among patients with a score of 2 who underwent LC with the bailout procedure, only patients who underwent open conversion had BDI while patients who underwent LSC had no BDI.

4 | DISCUSSION

In this study we proposed a new SS to predict the necessity of the bailout procedure during LC after PTGBD, by using significant predictors of time until PTGBD after symptom onset and the maximal GB wall thickness. The SS for the prediction of the

TABLE 2 Logistic regression for independently predicted factors of necessity of the bailout procedure during LC after PTGBD

Predictor	OR	Regression coefficient	95% CI	SE	P-value
Time until PTGBD after symptom onset (days)	1.416	0.348	1.005–1.994	0.175	.046
GB wall thickness (mm)	1.423	0.353	1.135–1.784	0.115	.002

Abbreviations: CI, confidence interval; GB, gallbladder; LC, laparoscopic cholecystectomy; OR, odds ratio; PTGBD, percutaneous transhepatic gallbladder drainage; SE, standard error.

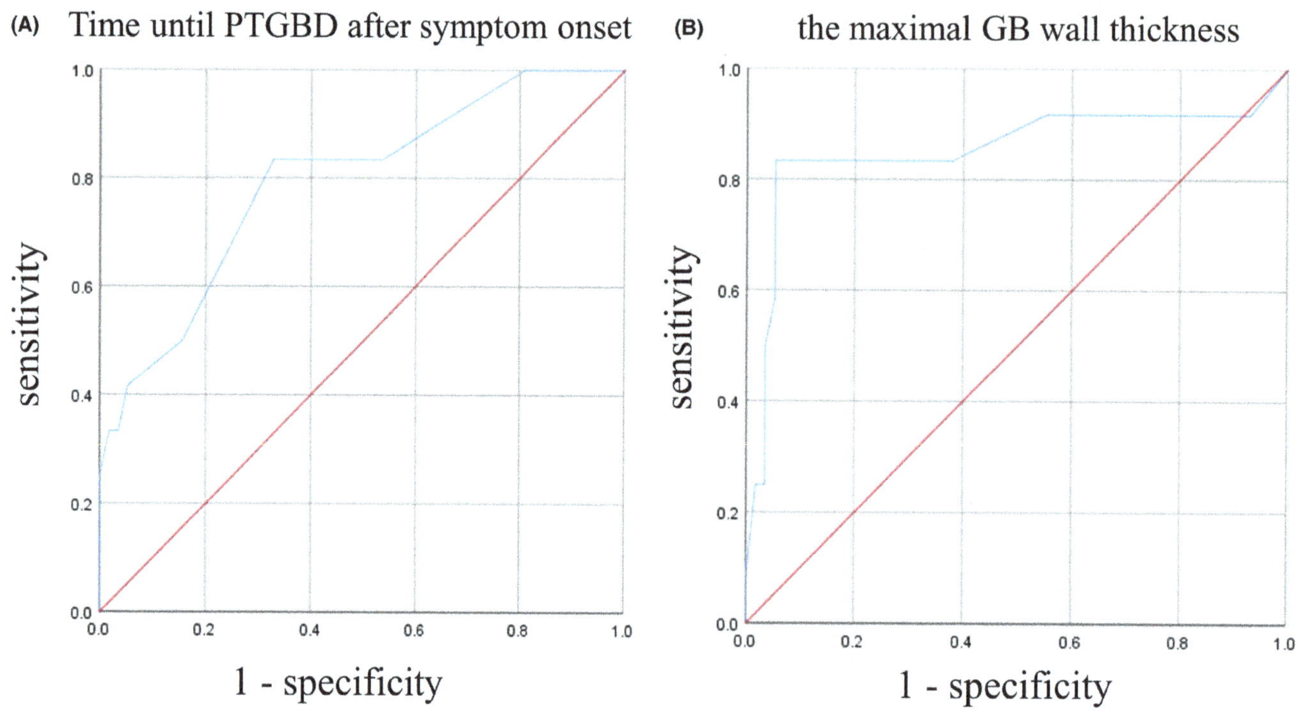

FIGURE 2 Receiver operating characteristic (ROC) curves of the time until PTGBD after symptom onset (A) and the maximal GB wall thickness (B) for predicting the bailout procedure during laparoscopic cholecystectomy. The blue line shows an ROC curve. The red line shows the reference line. (A) Cutoff value, 3 d; sensitivity, 0.833; 1 - specificity, 0.328; AUROC, 0.795; 95% CI, 0.650–0.939; SE, 0.074; $P = .001$. (B) Cutoff value, 10 mm; sensitivity, 0.833; 1 - specificity, 0.053; AUROC, 0.854; 95% CI, 0.694–1.000; SE, 0.082; $P < .0001$. PTGBD, percutaneous transhepatic gallbladder drainage; GB, gallbladder; AUROC, area under receiver operating characteristic curve; CI, confidence index; SE, standard error

TABLE 3 The scoring system for the prediction of the necessity of the bailout procedure during LC

Factors	Point 0	Point 1
Time until PTGBD after symptom onset	<3 days	3 days≤
GB wall thickness	<10 mm	10 mm ≤

Abbreviations: GB, gallbladder; LC, laparoscopic cholecystectomy; PTGBD, percutaneous transhepatic gallbladder drainage.

bailout surgery during LC was significantly associated with a risk of BDI. Despite no significant difference between patients with a score of 2 who underwent LC with the bailout procedure and OC, no patient who underwent the OC had BDI. The use of our novel SS to predict the necessity of the bailout procedure during LC after PTGBD was validated in a separate cohort. By comparing patients with a score of 2 with those with a score of 1 or less, the sensitivity and specificity of our SS for the prediction of the bailout procedure were 75.0% and 98.1%, respectively, and showed acceptable values.

Many previous studies have used factors, such as the open conversion rate, operating time, and incidence of complications as indicators of surgical difficulty.[4] Focusing on the open conversion as an indicator of surgical difficulty, a meta-analysis identified GB wall thickening (>4 to 5 mm) on ultrasound, male sex, advanced age, and obesity as risk factors for open conversion.[9] In this study the maximal GB wall thickness was also found to be an independent predictor of the bailout procedure as open conversion, as in previous reports.[9,10] A thickened GB wall was previously reported to be predictive of a difficult exposure of the anatomy during LC because of increased inflammation, edema, and adhesions.[11,12] Tissue planes

TABLE 4 Patient characteristics in relationship to a scoring system

	Factor [Median (minimum to maximum) or Ratio]	Score 0 (n = 38)	Score 1 (n = 21)	Score 2 (n = 11)	P-value
Preoperative factor	Age (years old)	73 (37–89)	75 (37–83)	65 (28–82)	.264
	Gender (male:female)	26:12	17:4	8:3	.584
	BMI	23.0 (16.6–31.5)	24.8 (19.5–32.8)	24.1 (16.4–28)	.229
	SILS (yes:no)	1:37	2:19	2:9	.186
	ASA-PS (1:2:3)	7:28:3	4:15:2	2:8:1	1.000
	CCI (≤5:≤6)	27:11	14:7	9:2	.664
	HT (yes:no)	18:20	13:8	7:4	.447
	DM (yes:no)	10:28	7:14	2:9	.648
	Past history of upper abdominal surgery (yes:no)	2:36	1:20	0:11	.744
	Anticoagulative therapy (yes:no)	9:29	6:15	2:9	.802
	Time until PTGBD after symptom onset (days)	1 (0–2)	3 (1-8)	4 (3–16)	<.0001
	Time until surgery after PTGBD (days)	69 (3–281)	60 (5–109)	55 (4–102)	.36
	GB wall thickness (mm)	4 (2–9)	5 (2–15)	12 (10–21)	<.0001
	Maximal diameter of impacted stone (mm)	4 (0–60)	4 (0–16)	5 (0–29)	.906
	Maximal WBC count in the peripheral blood (/μL)	13,050 (6800–27,200)	13,600 (7000–22,500)	13,700 (9800–31,800)	.578
	Maximal serum value of CRP (mg/dL)	18.2 (2.7–33.9)	24.2 (6.5–40.4)	19.8 (0.5–36.0)	.322
Intra- or postoperative factor	Open conversion (yes:no)	1:37	2:19	9:2	<.0001
	Subtotal cholecystectomy fenestrating or reconstituting (yes:no)	0:38	1:20	4:7	<.0001
	BDI during operation (yes:no)	0:38	0:21	3:8	<.0001
	Grade of Clavien–Dindo classification ≤3 (yes:no)	0:38	1:20	1:10	.231

Abbreviations: ASA-PS, the American Society of Anesthesiologists physical status classification; BDI, bile duct injury; BMI, body mass index; CCI, Age-adjusted Charlson comorbidity index; CRP, C-reactive protein; DM, diabetes mellitus; GB, gallbladder; HT, hypertension; LSC, laparoscopic subtotal cholecystectomy; PTGBD, percutaneous transhepatic gallbladder drainage; SILS, single-port laparoscopic surgery; WBC, white blood cell.

are less distinct and bleeding is more common due to repetitive inflammation episodes.[13] Therefore, a thickened GB wall might present a more challenging laparoscopic dissection.

On the other hand, although it has been reported that a duration of symptoms of AC >72 hours was an independent predictor of open conversion as a bailout procedure, the time until PTGBD after symptom onset has never been reported.[14] Koo et al reported that it would be easy and safe to dissect the tissue when performing LC within 72 hours of the onset of symptoms of AC because of the phase of edematous cholecystitis.[15,16] Rapid decompression of GB by drainage suppresses progression of inflammation.[17] PTGBD in the phase of edematous cholecystitis seems effective because the inflammation of this phase is reversible.[18,19] Therefore, PTGBD within 3 days of the onset of symptoms might facilitate successful LC after PTGBD.

In this study, although there was no significant difference between patients with a score of 2 who underwent LC with the bailout procedure and those who underwent OC, none of the patients who underwent OC had BDI. In addition, among patients with a score of 2 who underwent LC with the bailout procedure, only patients who underwent open conversion had BDI, while patients who underwent LSC had no BDI. In TG18, LSC is an important procedure that should be considered in order to avoid serious damage to the BDI or blood vessels.[4] However, LSC would require the skill of surgeons and might pose some problems such as postoperative bile leakage, recurrence of GB stone in the remnant GB, or a risk of concomitant GB cancer.[20,21] On the other hand, in a questionnaire survey of experts in Japan, South Korea, and Taiwan, only 17.5% of the respondents said that open conversion made surgery easier[22] and open conversion might not necessarily be safe.[23] The estimated incidence of serious complications, such as BDI or VBI, was reported to be two to five times higher for LC than for open cholecystectomy.[24] In the current study with chronic cholecystitis after PTGBD for AC, two out of four patients with BDI had the accidents after the open conversion. The main reasons for BDI or VBI was misidentification of the anatomy caused by disorientation because of the adhesion from severe

TABLE 5 Patient characteristics in the validation cohort

	Factor [Median (minimum to maximum) or Ratio]	All cases (n = 65)	Pure LC without bailout procedure (n = 53)	LC with bailout procedure (n = 12)	*P*-value
Preoperative factor	Age (years old)	68 (33–91)	68 (33–91)	67 (46–90)	.852
	Gender (male:female)	48:17	38:15	10:2	.408
	BMI	23.0 (7.9–35.0)	23.1 (7.9–35.0)	22.2 (18.4–30.0)	.618
	SILS (yes:no)	0:65	0:53	0:12	NA
	ASA (1:2:3)	12:47:6	10:38:5	2:9:1	.974
	CCI (≤5:≤6)	56:9	45:8	11:1	.540
	HT (yes:no)	28:37	23:30	5:7	.913
	DM (yes:no)	21:44	18:35	3:9	.549
	Past history of upper abdominal surgery (yes:no)	2:63	1:52	1:11	.243
	Anticoagulative therapy (yes:no)	12:53	11:42	1:11	.317
	Time until PTGBD after symptom onset (days)	2 (0–13)	2 (0–11)	3.5 (1–13)	.047
	Time until surgery after PTGBD (days)	57 (1–387)	57 (4–387)	55 (1–345)	.819
	GB wall thickness (mm)	8 (3–16)	7 (3–14)	10.5 (4–16)	.003
	Maximal diameter of impacted stone (mm)	5 (0–48)	5 (0–32)	7.5 (2–48)	.064
	Maximal WBC count in the peripheral blood (/μL)	14 800 (6300–39,300)	14 800 (6300–25,300)	14 550 (8700–39,300)	.833
	Maximal serum value of CRP (mg/dL)	21.86 (1.05–39.24)	23.19 (1.05–39.24)	19.03 (13.25–36.04)	.784
	Score for prediction of the bailout procedure during LC (0:1:2)	27:28:10	24:28:1	3:0:9	<.0001
	Score for prediction of the bailout procedure during LC (0 or 1:2)	55:10	52:1	3:9	<.0001
Intra- or postoperative factor	Open conversion (yes:no)	7:58	0:53	7:5	<.0001
	LSC with fenestrating or reconstituting (yes:no)	4:61	0:53	5:7	<.0001
	Subtotal cholecystectomy with fenestrating or reconstituting (yes:no)	6:59	0:53	7:5	<.0001
	BDI during operation (yes:no)	1:64	0:53	1:11	.034
	Grade of Clavien–Dindo classification ≤3 (yes:no)	5:65	4:49	1:11	.236

Abbreviations:ASA-PS, the American Society of Anesthesiologists physical status classification; BDI, bile duct injury; BMI, body mass index; CCI, Age-adjusted Charlson comorbidity index; CRP, C-reactive protein; DM, diabetes mellitus; GB, gallbladder; HT, hypertension; LC, laparoscopic cholecystectomy; LSC, laparoscopic subtotal cholecystectomy; NA, not available; PTGBD, percutaneous transhepatic gallbladder drainage; SILS, single-port laparoscopic surgery; WBC, white blood cell.

TABLE 6 Patient characteristics with a score of 2

	Factor 〔Median (minimum to maximum) or Ratio〕	OC (n = 9)	LC with bailout procedure (n = 18) LSC (n = 4)	LC with bailout procedure (n = 18) Open conversion (n = 14)	*P*-value
Preoperative factor	Age (years old)	73 (39–91)	66.5 (43–90)		0.705
	Gender (male:female)	7:2	14:4		1.000
	BMI	21.0 (17.1–41.0)	23.8 (16.4–30.0)		0.495
	SILS (yes:no)	0:9	1:17		0.471
	ASA–PS (1:2:3)	1:7:1	1:16:1		0.746
	CCI (≤ 5:6 ≤)	7:2	15:3		0.726
	HT (yes:no)	4:5	12:6		0.268
	DM (yes:no)	2:7	4:14		1.000
	Past history of upper abdominal surgery (yes:no)	2:7	0:18		0.038
	Anticoagulative therapy (yes:no)	3:6	3:15		0.326
	Time until PTGBD after symptom onset (days)	4 (3–17)	5 (3–16)		0.860
	Time until surgery after PTGBD (days)	29 (5–232)	53.5 (5–102)		0.348
	Gallbladder wall thickness (mm)	13 (10–25)	12 (10–21)		0.312
	Maximal diameter of impacted stone (mm)	8 (0–33)	6.5 (2–29)		0.781
	Maximal WBC count in the peripheral blood (/μL)	16 500 (12 200–20,400)	14 700 (8700–39,300)		0.860
	Maximal serum value of CRP (mg/dL)	25.03 (13.30–31.08)	20.65 (13.25–36.04)		0.348
Intra- or postoperative factor	Op time (min)	131 (82–514)	164.5 (80–420)		0.176
	Estimated blood loss during operation (g)	105 (5–510)	100 (5-1,350)		0.668
	Open conversion (yes:no)	0:9	14:4		<0.0001
	LSC with fenestrating or reconstituting (yes:no)	0:9	4:14		0.125
	Subtotal cholecystectomy with fenestrating or reconstituting (yes:no)	3:6	10:8		0.276
	BDI during operation between two groups (yes:no)	0:9	4:14		0.125
	BDI during operation among three groups (yes:no)	0:9	0:4	4:10	0.113
	Grade of Clavien–Dindo classification ≤3 between two groups (yes:no)	0:9	2:16		0.299
	Grade of Clavien–Dindo classification ≤3 among three groups (yes:no)	0:9	0:4	2:12	0.367

Abbreviations: ASA-PS, the American Society of Anesthesiologists physical status classification; BDI, bile duct injury; BMI, body mass index; CCI, Age-adjusted Charlson comorbidity index; CRP, C-reactive protein; DM, diabetes mellitus; GB, gallbladder; HT, hypertension; LC, laparoscopic cholecystectomy; LSC, laparoscopic subtotal cholecystectomy; NA, not available; OC, open cholecystectomy from the beginning; PTGBD, percutaneous transhepatic gallbladder drainage; SILS, single-port laparoscopic surgery; WBC, white blood cell.

inflammation and intraoperative bleeding. Consequently, it might be better to select flexibly LSC or OC according to the skill of the surgeons for patients with a score of 2 after PTGBD because of the higher risks of BDI and needing open conversion.

The current study had several limitations. First, this was a retrospective study. Selection bias for the bailout procedure could arise because the decision to choose the bailout procedure might have varied greatly among surgeons, and the decision depended on the surgeons' skill level. Second, most of the open cholecystectomies or LCs were performed according to the Tokyo Guideline 2013, in which conversion to open cholecystectomy was the only recommendation in patients with AC for which LC was difficult.[25] No patient underwent LSC in the training cohort. According to a systematic review and a meta-analysis, although postoperative bile leakage was more common following LSC than after open conversion, the rates of BDI, postoperative complications, and mortality were all lower.[20,21] In TG18, LSC with fenestrating or reconstituting and the fundus first technique should be chosen to prevent BDI according to the intraoperative findings.[4] In the future, in patients with cholecystitis after PTGBD with a score of 2, outcome of the LSC should be prospectively compared with those of OC.

5 | CONCLUSIONS

We proposed a new SS using the significant factors of time until PTGBD after symptom onset and the maximal GB wall thickness to predict the necessity of the bailout procedure during LC after PTGBD. Our SS for predicting the necessity of a bailout procedure correctly predicted the need and might be associated with a risk of BDI. Therefore, it might be better to select the flexibility of LSC or OC for patients with a score of 2 after PTGBD.

REFERENCES

1. Miyasaka Y, Nakamura M, Wakabayashi G. Pioneers in laparoscopic hepato-biliary-pancreatic surgery. J Hepatobiliary Pancreat Sci. 2018;25(1):109–11.
2. Törnqvist B, Waage A, Zheng Z, Ye W, Nilsson M. Severity of acute cholecystitis and risk of iatrogenic bile duct injury during cholecystectomy, a population-based case-control study. World J Surg. 2016;40(5):1060–7.
3. Törnqvist B, Zheng Z, Ye W, Waage A, Nilsson M. Long-term effects of iatrogenic bile duct injury during cholecystectomy. Clin Gastroenterol Hepatol. 2009;7(9):1013–8; quiz 915.
4. Wakabayashi G, Iwashita Y, Hibi T, Takada T, Strasberg SM, Asbun HJ, et al. Tokyo Guidelines 2018: surgical management of acute cholecystitis: safe steps in laparoscopic cholecystectomy for acute cholecystitis (with videos). J Hepatobiliary Pancreat Sci. 2018;25(1):73–86.
5. Mori Y, Itoi T, Baron TH, Takada T, Strasberg SM, Pitt HA, et al. Tokyo Guidelines 2018: management strategies for gallbladder drainage in patients with acute cholecystitis (with videos). J Hepatobiliary Pancreat Sci. 2018;25(1):87–95.
6. Charlson ME, Pompei P, Ales KL, MacKenzie CR. A new method of classifying prognostic comorbidity in longitudinal studies: development and validation. J Chronic Dis. 1987;40(5):373–83.
7. Charlson M, Szatrowski TP, Peterson J, Gold J. Validation of a combined comorbidity index. J Clin Epidemiol. 1994;47(11):1245–51.
8. Okamoto K, Suzuki K, Takada T, Strasberg SM, Asbun HJ, Endo I, et al. Tokyo Guidelines 2018: flowchart for the management of acute cholecystitis. J Hepatobiliary Pancreat Sci. 2018;25(1):55–72.
9. Philip Rothman J, Burcharth J, Pommergaard HC, Viereck S, Rosenberg J. Preoperative risk factors for conversion of laparoscopic cholecystectomy to open surgery – a systematic review and meta-analysis of observational studies. Digest Surg. 2016;33(5):414–23.
10. Cwik G, Skoczylas T, Wyroślak-Najs J, Wallner G. The value of percutaneous ultrasound in predicting conversion from laparoscopic to open cholecystectomy due to acute cholecystitis. Surg Endosc. 2013;27(7):2561–8.
11. Liu CL, Fan ST, Lai EC, Lo CM, Chu KM. Factors affecting conversion of laparoscopic cholecystectomy to open surgery. Arch Surg (Chicago, Ill: 1960). 1996;131(1):98–101.
12. Wiebke EA, Pruitt AL, Howard TJ, Jacobson LE, Broadie TA, Goulet RJ Jr, et al. Conversion of laparoscopic to open cholecystectomy. An analysis of risk factors. Surg Endosc. 1996;10(7):742–5.
13. Hutchinson CH, Traverso LW, Lee FT. Laparoscopic cholecystectomy. Do preoperative factors predict the need to convert to open? Surg Endosc. 1994;8(8):875–8; discussion 9–80.
14. Asai K, Watanabe M, Kusachi S, Matsukiyo H, Saito T, Kodama H, et al. Risk factors for conversion of laparoscopic cholecystectomy to open surgery associated with the severity characteristics according to the Tokyo guidelines. Surg Today. 2014;44(12):2300–4.
15. Koo KP, Thirlby RC. Laparoscopic cholecystectomy in acute cholecystitis. What is the optimal timing for operation? Arch Surg (Chicago, Ill: 1960). 1996;131(5):540-4; discussion 4-5.
16. Adachi T, Eguchi S, Muto Y. Pathophysiology and pathology of acute cholecystitis: A secondary publication of the Japanese version from 1992. J Hepatobiliary Pancreat Sci. 2021. https://doi.org10.1002/jhbp.912. [Epub ahead of print].
17. Ito K, Fujita N, Noda Y, Kobayashi G, Kimura K, Sugawara T, et al. Percutaneous cholecystostomy versus gallbladder aspiration for acute cholecystitis: a prospective randomized controlled trial. AJR Am J Roentgenol. 2004;183(1):193–6.
18. Teplick SK, Harshfield DL, Brandon JC, Broadwater JR Jr, Cone JB. Percutaneous cholecystostomy in critically ill patients. Gastrointest Radiol. 1991;16(2):154–6.
19. Vogelzang RL, Nemcek AA Jr. Percutaneous cholecystostomy: diagnostic and therapeutic efficacy. Radiology. 1988;168(1):29–34.
20. Elshaer M, Gravante G, Thomas K, Sorge R, Al-Hamali S, Ebdewi H. Subtotal cholecystectomy for "difficult gallbladders": systematic review and meta-analysis. JAMA Surg. 2015;150(2):159–68.
21. Henneman D, da Costa DW, Vrouenraets BC, van Wagensveld BA, Lagarde SM. Laparoscopic partial cholecystectomy for the difficult gallbladder: a systematic review. Surg Endosc. 2013;27(2):351–8.
22. Hibi T, Iwashita Y, Ohyama T, Honda G, Yoshida M, Takada T, et al. The "right" way is not always popular: comparison of surgeons' perceptions during laparoscopic cholecystectomy for acute cholecystitis among experts from Japan, Korea and Taiwan. J Hepatobiliary Pancreat Sci. 2017;24(1):24–32.
23. Lengyel BI, Azagury D, Varban O, Panizales MT, Steinberg J, Brooks DC, et al. Laparoscopic cholecystectomy after a quarter century: why do we still convert? Surg Endosc. 2012;26(2):508–13.
24. Morgenstern L, Wong L, Berci G. Twelve hundred open cholecystectomies before the laparoscopic era. A standard for comparison. Arch Surg (Chicago, Ill: 1960). 1992;127(4):400–3.
25. Yamashita Y, Takada T, Strasberg SM, Pitt HA, Gouma DJ, Garden OJ, et al. TG13 surgical management of acute cholecystitis. J Hepatobiliary Pancreat Sci. 2013;20(1):89–96.

8

Anatomical study of the duodenojejunal uncinate process vein: A key landmark for mesopancreatoduodenal resection during pancreaticoduodenectomy

Masahiko Honjo[1,2] | Taiji Tohyama[1,3] | Kohei Ogawa[1] | Kei Tamura[1] | Katsunori Sakamoto[1] | Akihiro Takai[1] | Jota Watanabe[2] | Hiromi Ohtani[2] | Yasutsugu Takada[1]

[1]Department of Hepato-Biliary-Pancreatic and Breast Surgery, Ehime University Graduate School of Medicine, Shitsukawa, Toon, Japan

[2]Department of Surgery, Ehime Prefectural Central Hospital, Matsuyama, Japan

[3]Department of Surgery, Kurashiki Medical Center, Kurashiki, Japan

Correspondence
Taiji Tohyama, Bakuro-cho, Kurashiki, Okayama, 710-8522, Japan.
Email: taitoh1128@gmail.com

Abstract

Background: The mesopancreas or mesopancreatoduodenum is an important anatomical concept during pancreaticoduodenectomy (PD) in patients with periampullary carcinoma. This study investigated whether the duodenojejunal uncinate process vein (DJUV), which is defined as the vein draining from the upper jejunum to the superior mesenteric vein adjacent to the uncinate process, is a useful anatomical landmark for the caudal border of mesopancreatoduodenum resection during PD.

Methods: This study enrolled 100 adult patients with hepatobiliary pancreatic disease who underwent preoperative multidetector-computed tomography (CT). The anatomy of the key blood vessels involved during PD, and the relationship between these vessels and the DJUV, were analyzed by preoperative CT.

Results: The first jejunal vein was the DJUV in 85 cases, whereas the second jejunal vein was the DJUV in 15 cases. Furthermore, the DJUV was classified into two subtypes depending on its positional relationship with the superior mesenteric artery (SMA). The inferior pancreaticoduodenal artery and vein were located on the cranial side of the DJUV in all cases. The distance between the middle colonic artery, used as a guide for regional lymph nodes, and the point where the DJUV intersected the SMA was within 10 mm in 80% of cases. These results imply that using the DJUV as a landmark for the caudal border of the mesopancreatoduodenum provides a safe approach and enables sufficient dissection of regional lymph nodes and tissues around the SMA.

Conclusion: The DJUV may be a useful anatomical landmark for the caudal border of the mesopancreatoduodenum resection during PD.

KEYWORDS
duodenojejunal uncinate process vein, jejunal vein, mesopancreas, mesopancreatoduodenum, pancreaticoduodenectomy

1 | INTRODUCTION

Multimodal treatment strategies have gradually improved the prognosis of resectable pancreatic cancer, but it remains poor, with a 5-y survival rate of 20%–25% after surgery.[1-4] Pancreaticoduodenectomy (PD) is the only potential curative treatment and is recognized as one of the most influential determinants of survival.[1,5] In 2007, Gockel et al proposed the concept of the mesopancreas, defined as a firm and well-vascularized structure that extends from the posterior face of the head of the pancreas to behind the superior mesenteric vein (SMV) and superior mesenteric artery (SMA).[6] It consists of areolar tissue, adipose tissue, blood vessels, peripheral nerves, and lymph nodes.[6,7] This area is recognized as the primary positive resection margin site and the main site of local recurrence.[8]

The effectiveness of resection of the mesopancreas or pancreato-duodenojejunal mesentery, ie, mesopancreatoduodenum, has been reported.[7,9-11] However, the standard procedure for mesopancreas or mesopancreatoduodenum resection has not been established because the resection boundaries remain unclear.[9,12] Anatomical landmarks that can be identified during surgery include anatomical membranes and blood vessels. The hepatoduodenal ligament, the common hepatic artery, and the root of the SMA and celiac artery are present on the cranial side of the pancreas, and the anterior renal fascia on the inferior vena cava, renal vein, and aorta are present on the dorsal side.[13] Therefore, the boundaries are relatively clear at these sites. However, the caudal borders, particularly the mesenteric dissecting line, are confusing and vary among reports.[10,11,14-16]

The purpose of this study was to investigate whether the pancreato-duodenojejunal mesenteric veins draining into the SMV at the level of the uncinate process, which we named the "duodenojejunal uncinate process vein (DJUV)" could be used as a caudal anatomical landmark for mesopancreas or mesopancreatoduodenum resection during PD. Specifically, we analyzed the anatomy of the key blood vessels involved in PD, and assessed the relationship between these vessels and the DJUV using three-dimensional computed tomography (3D-CT) images based on thin-slice CT examinations.

2 | PATIENTS AND METHODS

2.1 | Patients

All procedures involving human participants followed the ethical standards of the institution and research committee and with the 1964 Declaration of Helsinki and its later amendments or comparable ethical standards. This study was approved by the Ethics Review Boards of Ehime University School of Medicine and Ehime Central Hospital.

In total, 100 patients with hepatobiliary pancreatic disease who underwent preoperative multidetector CT at Ehime University or Ehime Central Hospital between April 2016 and May 2020 were included. The CT data were retrospectively reviewed. We enrolled 68 male and 32 female patients of median age 65 y (range 20–86 y). Their primary conditions were hepatocellular carcinomas (n = 25), metastatic liver tumors (n = 9), liver transplant donor status (n = 11), hilar cholangiocarcinomas (n = 5), distal bile duct carcinomas (n = 16), duodenal papillary tumors (n = 2), a duodenal gastrointestinal stromal tumor (n = 1), gallbladder cancers (n = 2), and pancreatic tumors that did not affect the duodenomesopancreatic region (n = 29; pancreatic body and tail carcinomas [n = 14], intraductal papillary mucinous neoplasms [n = 7], neuroendocrine tumors [n = 5], a serous cystic neoplasm [n = 1], a solid pseudopapillary tumor [n = 1], and a lymphoepithelial cyst [n = 1]). Patients with pancreatic head cancers and large cystic tumors of the pancreas head were excluded, given the hemodynamic changes in the pancreatic head caused by vascular invasion and/or tumor expansion. Also, portal hypertension patients with CT-revealed varices around the lower esophagus or stomach, or with submucosal varices apparent on endoscopic images, were excluded.

2.2 | Definition of DJUV

The following conditions were required for the caudal border of the mesopancreatoduodenum resection for PD. The excisional area included all blood vessels, the nerve plexus, and regional lymph nodes that should be resected. It should be a macroscopically recognizable anatomical structure during surgery. We have recently focused on the jejunal vein in the pancreato-duodenojejunal mesentery that drains from the upper jejunum to the SMV adjacent to the uncinate process via the third and fourth portions of the duodenum. We named this vein the DJUV, and hypothesized that it may be a candidate for the caudal border of the mesopancreatoduodenum during resection.

2.3 | CT protocol and 3D reconstruction

All CT examinations were performed using a 256-slice CT scanner (Brilliance iCT, Philips Healthcare, Andover, MA) running a standardized, multiphasic hepatobiliary-pancreatic protocol. The tube voltage was 120 kVp and the "automated tube current modulation" feature was employed in all cases. The other parameters were as follows: detector collimation, 128 × 0.625 mm; field-of-view (FOV), 350 mm; rotation time, 0.4 sec; and spiral pitch, 0.446. If dynamic CT was planned, precontrast images were obtained first. All patients were given nonionic, iodinated contrast (300–370 mgI/mL) via a 20G intravenous catheter in the antecubital vein; we employed a power injector. The dose of contrast material was determined based on body surface area derived using the DuBois formula: body surface area (m^2) = 0.007184 × height (cm) 0.725 × weight (kg) 0.425. All patients were given 22 gI/m^2 of contrast material over 30 sec. This injection technique was based on a bolus-tracking method. Arterial phase imaging commenced 15 sec later, by which time the trigger threshold of 150 HU in the abdominal aorta had been attained. The portal-venous and delayed phases commenced at 40 and 100 sec after attainment of the trigger threshold, respectively. All series were reconstructed using an iterative reconstruction algorithm (iDose 4; Philips Healthcare).[17]

Synapse Vincent 3D software (Fujifilm, Tokyo, Japan) was used to generate the 3D-CT images. Pancreatic 3D images and arteriographs were obtained during the arterial phase and fused to yield portographs with 0.5-mm-thick slices. All 3D-CT images were reconstructed by a single surgeon. The tributaries of the SMV were numbered in order from the confluence of the splenic vein to distal of the SMV, such as the first and second jejunal veins (J1V and J2V, respectively), and the jejunal artery branches were numbered from the root of the SMA (Figure 1).

2.4 | Anatomical evaluation

The following anatomical findings were analyzed: which jejunal vein corresponded to the DJUV; anatomical variations in the inferior pancreaticoduodenal veins (IPDVs) and inferior pancreaticoduodenal artery (IPDA), and their positional relationships with the DJUV were examined; the distance between the bifurcation of the middle colonic artery (MCA) and the intersection of the DJUV and SMA (the DJUV intersecting point) was measured; and the number of jejunal arteries branching between the root of the SMA and the DJUV intersecting point were counted.

3 | RESULTS

3.1 | Jejunal veins corresponding to the DJUV

Either the J1V or the J2V corresponded to the DJUV in all cases. The J1V was the DJUV (Type 1) in 85 cases, whereas the J2V was the DJUV (Type 2) in 15 cases (Figure 2). The DJUV was divided into two subtypes, depending on its positional relationship with the SMA, ie, running dorsal (subtype a) or ventral (subtype b) to the SMA. There were 70 cases of Type 1a, 15 of Type 1b, 11 of Type 2a, and four of Type 2b. Among the Type 2a and Type 2b cases, the J1V drained into the splenoportal confluence (splenic vein near the confluence of the SMV) in three and two cases, respectively.

3.2 | Anatomical variations in the IPDV

As the IPDVs could not be visualized in one case, 99 cases were analyzed. Three variations were identified: the IPDV drained into the DJUV only, into the SMV only, or into both (Figure 3). Variations were observed in 35, 21, and 14 Type 1a patients; 3, 11, and 0 Type 1b patients; 1, 9, and 1 Type 2a patients; and 0, 3, and 1 Type 2b patients, respectively. In no case did the IPDV join the SMV distal to the DJUV.

3.3 | Anatomical variations in the IPDA

Only one IPDA was confirmed in most cases (Figure 4). The IPDA branched from the J1A in 48 cases, branched directly from the SMA in 39 cases, branched from the J2A in three cases, and branched from the replaced right hepatic artery in two cases. Two IPDAs were observed in the remaining eight cases: one from the J1A and the other from the SMA (n = 5); and both from the J1A (n = 3). The IPDA(s) bifurcated from the more cranial side than the MCA and the DJUV intersecting point in all cases.

3.4 | Distance between the MCA bifurcation and the DJUV intersecting point

According to the General Rules for the Study of Pancreatic Cancer, published by the Japan Pancreas Society, the lymph nodes located between the bifurcation of the MCA and the root of the SMA are regional in cases of cancer of the head of the pancreas (Figure 5).[18] If the distance between the bifurcation of the MCA and the intersection of the DJUV and SMA (DJUV intersecting point) is short; dissecting along the DJUV will reach the SMA at around the bifurcation of the MCA, which is at the distal end of the regional lymph

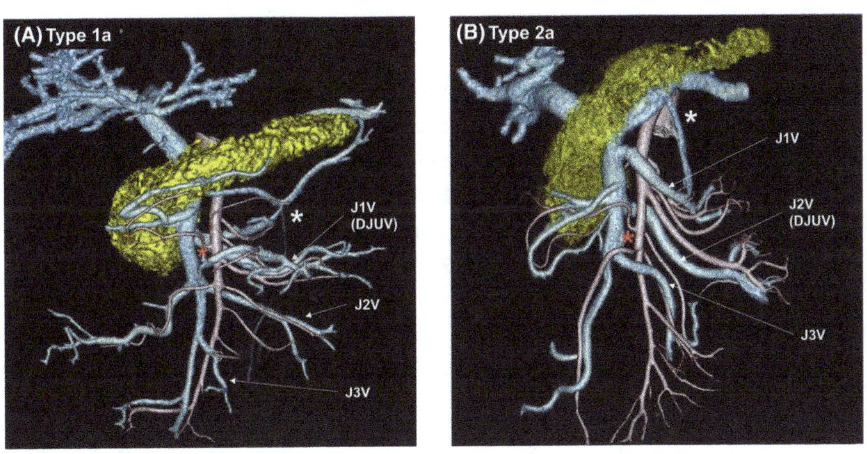

FIGURE 1 Typical DJUV images. (A) Type 1a, in which the J1V corresponds to the DJUV, and runs dorsal to the SMA. (B) Type 2a, in which the J2V corresponds to the DJUV, and runs dorsal to the SMA. DJUV, duodenojejunal uncinate process vein; J1-4A, first to fourth jejunal arteries; J1V-J3V, first to third jejunal veins; white asterisk, inferior mesenteric vein; red asterisk, middle colic artery

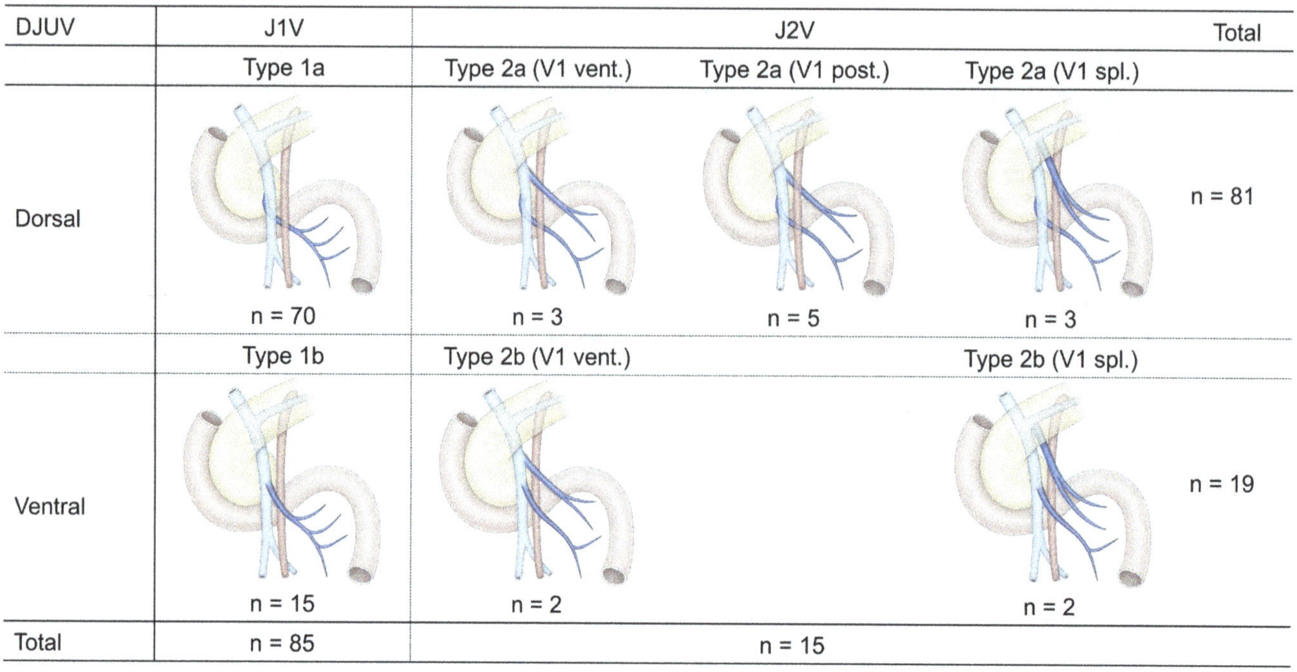

FIGURE 2 Anatomical variations in the DJUV. The J1V was the DJUV (Type 1) in 85 cases, whereas the J2V was the DJUV in 15 cases (Type 2). Next, the DJUV was divided into two subtypes depending on its positional relationship with the SMA, ie, running dorsal (subtype a) or ventral (subtype b) to the SMA. There were 70 cases of Type 1a, 15 cases of Type 1b, 11 cases of Type 2a, and four cases of Type 2b. In Type 2a, the J1V ran along the ventral side of the SMA in three cases, along the dorsal side of the SMA in five cases, and the J1V drained into the splenic vein in three cases. In Type 2b, the J1V ran along the ventral side of the SMA in two cases, and the J1V drained into the splenic vein in two cases. SMA, superior mesenteric artery; DJUV, duodenojejunal uncinate process vein; J1V first jejunal vein; J2V second jejunal vein; V1 vent., the first jejunal vein running ventral to the SMA; V1 dor., the first jejunal vein running dorsally to the SMA; V1 spl., first jejunal vein drained into the splenoportal confluence

nodes. A match was defined as a distance of within 10 mm. When the DJUV was equivalent to the J1V (Type 1), the matching rate was 85.7% for the dorsal type and 73.3% for the ventral type. When the DJUV was equivalent to the J2V (Type 2), the rates were 63.6% and 50%, respectively. The matching rate for all cases was 80%. Of the 20 nonmatching cases, the DJUV crossed the SMA 11 mm or more cephalad to the MCA bifurcation in 10 cases.

3.5 | Number of jejunal arteries branching between the root of the SMA and the DJUV intersecting point

A single jejunal artery (J1A) was identified in nine cases (Table 1). Two arteries (J1A and J2A) were detected in 48 cases, three arteries (J1A, J2A, J3A) in 34 cases, and four arteries (J1A, J2A, J3A, and J4A) in nine cases.

4 | DISCUSSION

In 1982, Heald et al described the concept of the mesorectum, the importance of the surgical principle of the "holy plane," and total mesorectal excision during rectal cancer surgery.[19] In 2007, inspired by the concept of the mesorectum, Gockel et al advocated the concept of the mesopancreas.[6] In Japan, this region is defined as the "pancreatic head nerve plexus II" in the General Rules for the Study of Pancreatic Cancer by the Japan Pancreas Society.[18] Kawabata et al advocated the "mesopancreatoduodenum" as an advance of the mesopancreas concept, which expanded the area for lymphadenectomy to the left side of the SMA.[10,12] Although several surgical procedures have been proposed for mesopancreas or mesopancreatoduodenum resection, the caudal borders, particularly the jejunal mesenteric dissecting line, vary in each report.[10,11,14,16] The present study is the first to determine the anatomical relationships between DJUV and key blood vessels associated with PD, to evaluate mesopancreatoduodenum resection guided by DJUV.

In this study the J1V was regarded as the DJUV (Type 1) in 85% of cases, and the J2V was regarded as the DJUV in 15% of cases. The J1V ran on the dorsal side of the SMA in 70 cases (84%) in which the J1V corresponded to the DUJV, and the J2V ran on the dorsal side of the SMA in 11 cases (73%) in which the J2V corresponded to the DUJV. Previous studies have reported that the J1V runs dorsal to the SMA in 63%–91% of cases.[15,16,20,21] Nagakawa et al reported that the J1V was connected to the uncinate process in 31 of 41 cases (73.8%), and the J2V was connected to the uncinate process in 10 of 41 cases (23.8%) in laparoscopic PD.[22]

Few studies have analyzed the anatomical relationships between the jejunal veins and the IPDA and the IPDV, which are included in

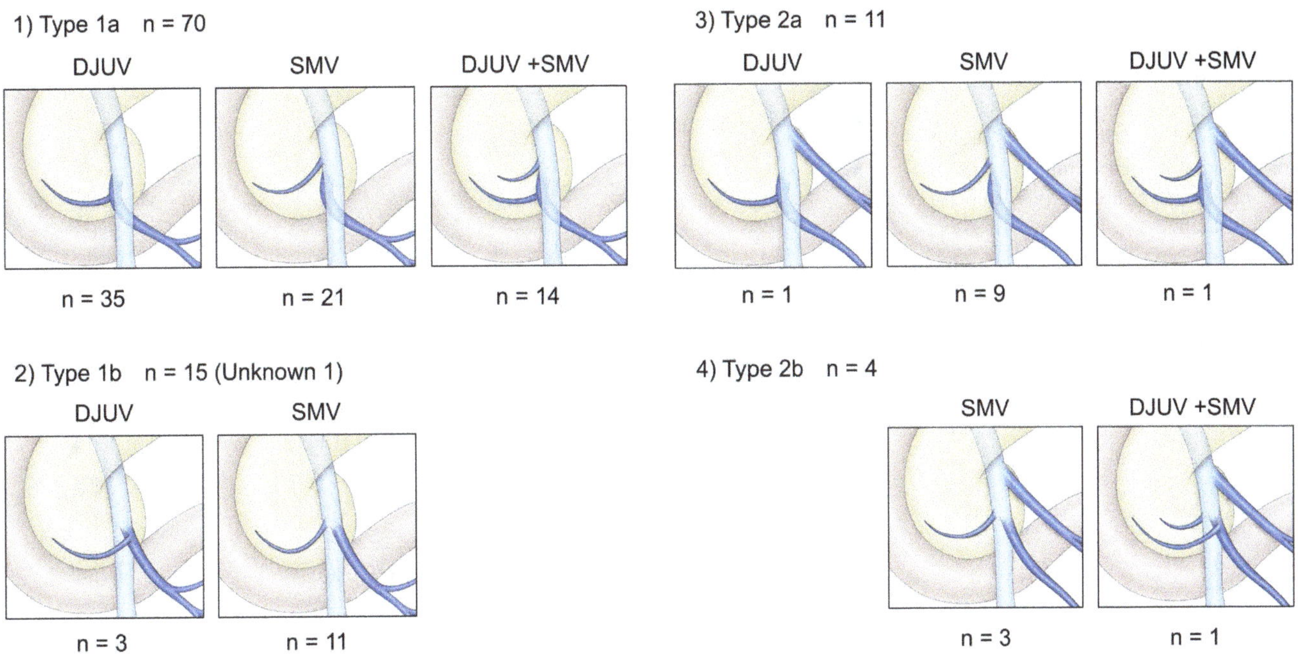

FIGURE 3 Anatomical variations in the IPDV. Three variations were identified: blood return to the DJUV only, blood return to the SMV only, and blood return to both. (1) Type 1a included 35, 21, and 14 cases, respectively. (2) Type 1b included 3, 11, and 0 cases, respectively. (3) Type 2a included 1, 9, and 1 cases, respectively. (4) Type 2b included 0, 3, and 1 cases, respectively. IPDV, inferior pancreaticoduodenal vein; DJUV, duodenojejunal uncinate process vein; SMV, superior mesenteric vein

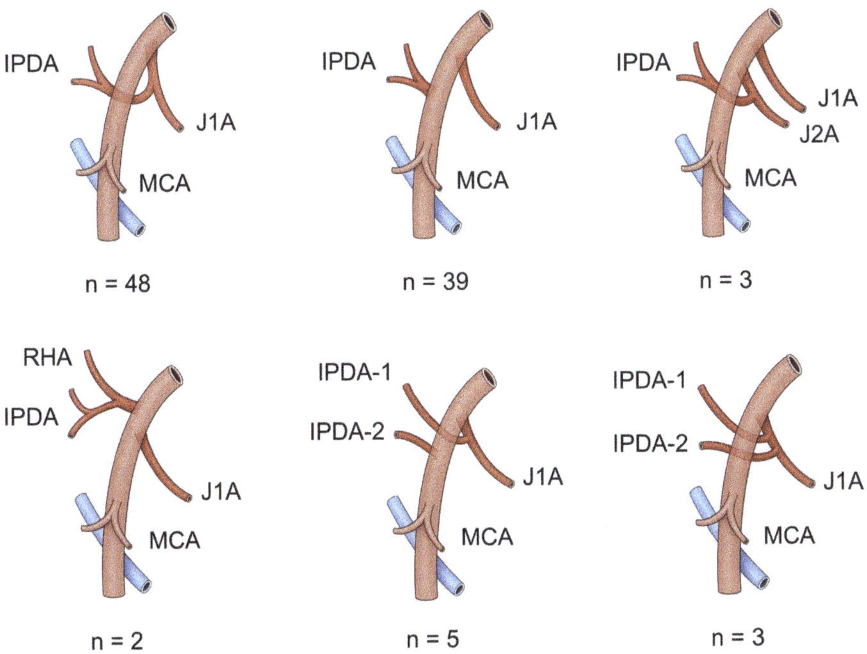

FIGURE 4 Anatomical variations in the IPDA. A single IPDA branched from the J1A in 48 cases, branched directly from the SMA in 39 cases, branched from the J2A in three cases, and branched from a replaced right hepatic artery in two cases. Two IPDAs were observed in the remaining eight cases: one from the J1A and the other from the SMA (n = 5), or both from the J1A (n = 3). IPDA, inferior pancreatoduodenal artery; J1A, first jejunal artery; J2A, second jejunal artery; RHA, right hepatic artery; MCA, middle colic artery; DJUV, duodenojejunal uncinate process vein

the mesopancreatoduodenum.[16] In the present results, three IPDV drainage patterns were observed (Figure 3). In all cases, the IPDVs joined the DJUV or the more cranial side of the SMV. This implies that it is possible to safely dissect between the uncinate process and the SMV by rotating the SMV-DJUV confluence and dissecting along the DJUV, despite the fact that manipulation of this region is associated with a high risk of bleeding in PD patients.[15]

As shown in Figure 4, there were several variations in the branching pattern of the IPDA. The IPDA arose from J1A or J2A in most cases, and all branches were located on the cranial side of the DJUV. This means that all of the IPDA(s) could easily be identified and divided by dissecting the area around the SMA, starting from the intersecting point of the DJUV toward the root of the SMA. Therefore, this approach is thought to be effective in curative resection of the mesopancreatoduodenum, including all the IPDA(s) and nerve plexuses around the IPDA(s).

The positional relationship between the DJUV and the bifurcation of the MCA matched (within 10 mm) in 80% of cases. The

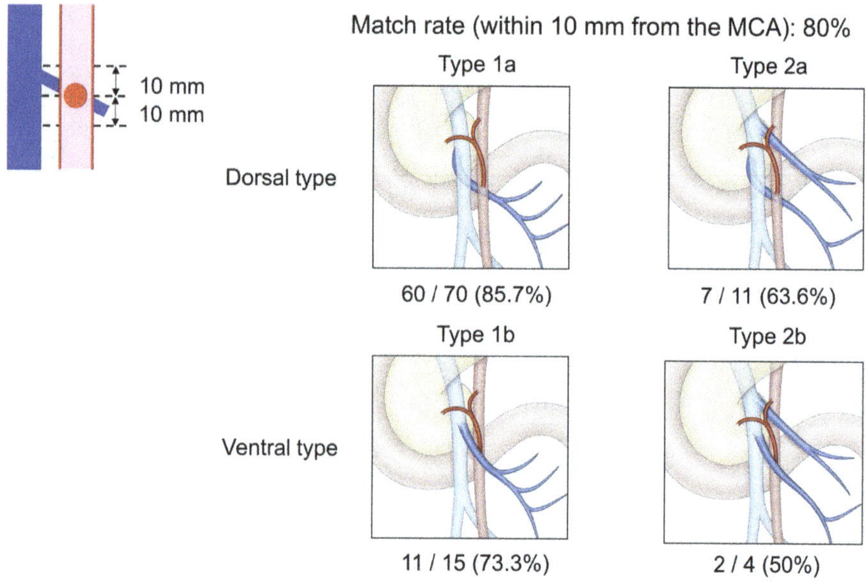

FIGURE 5 Positional relationship of the MCA and the DJUV. Matching was defined as the distance between the bifurcation of the MCA and the intersection of the DJUV and SMA (DJUV crossing point) within 10 mm. Type 1a had a match rate of 85.7%. Type 1b had a match rate of 73.3%. The match rates of Type 2a and Type 2b were lower, at 63.6% and 50%, respectively. The match rate for all cases was 80%. MCA, middle colic artery; DJUV, duodenojejunal uncinate process vein

TABLE 1 Numbers of cases in which jejunal arteries branched between the root of the SMA and the DJUV intersecting point

Jejunal artery branch	Number of cases
J1A	9
J1A + J2A	48
J1A + J2A + J3A	34
J1A + J2A + J3A + J4A	9

matching rate was 85.7% for the most frequent type (Type 1a). These results indicate that dissection along the DJUV will reach close to the vicinity of the root of the MCA in most cases. In Japan, the lymph nodes located between the bifurcation of the MCA and the root of the SMA are considered regional lymph nodes, and lymphadenectomy in this area around the SMA is required during radical PD for cancer of the pancreatic head. The frequency of lymph node metastasis in this area has been reported to be 11%–40%.[23-27] Dissection around the SMA from the intersecting point of the DJUV toward the cranial direction facilitates complete resection of these regional lymph nodes. However, the matching rate was lower in Type 2 cases; such cases require special attention if regional lymphadenectomy is planned.

As shown in Table 1, many jejunal arteries ramify between the root of the SMA and the bifurcation of the MCA, so there is often confusion as to which artery is being dissected when mesenteric resection is performed along the jejunal artery. On the other hand, the DJUV is easy to confirm in the mesentery, so it can be considered a more useful anatomical landmark than the jejunal artery for the standard surgery.

If pancreatic cancer has invaded the confluence of the DJUVs, the confluence must be resected to achieve no residual tumor (ie, R0). However, Kobayashi et al reported that 1 of 32 patients who underwent DJUV sacrifice exhibited severe congestion of the jejunal limb, requiring an emergency jejunal resection.[20] In this study, the

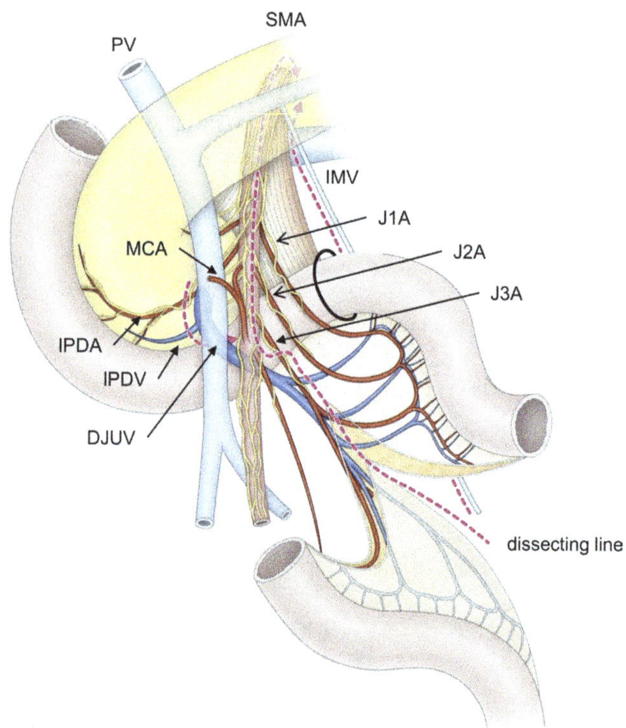

FIGURE 6 Surgical procedures for resecting the mesopancreatoduodenum using the DJUV as a landmark in Type 1a with typical anatomy. Sequentially dissecting the veins from the region of the SMV-DJUV confluence, while inverting the SMV. The DJUV bifurcation was confirmed behind the SMV and serves as a landmark of the endpoint during mesopancreatoduodenum resection. In addition, resecting the caudal border of the mesopancreatoduodenum using the JDUPV as a guide from the left side

DJUV (J1V) had one to five jejunal veins entering the DJUV in most typical Type 1a cases, and the J1V and J2V were nearly confluent in 28 of 70 Type 1a cases (40%) (data not shown).[20] If pancreatic cancer has invaded the DJUV, it is necessary to consider reconstruction based on the anatomical findings, including peripheral arcades. Even in such cases, DJUV-guided mesenteric resection is also effective when considering vascular reconstruction.

Although these anatomical advantages imply the utility of the DJUV as a landmark for mesopancreatoduodenum resection, there are some drawbacks regarding the jejunal arteries. In this study, only the J1A or J1A+J2A originated from the SMA between its root and the DJUV intersecting point in 57% of cases. However, in the other 43% of cases, the J3A or J3A+J4A branched between the two points (Table 1). In such cases, if the duodenojejunal mesentery is transected along the DJUV, multiple jejunal arteries, such as the J3A and J4A, must be transected, which may cause ischemic damage to the elevated jejunum during PD. In clinical practice, circulation from the arterial arcade occasionally compensates for the blood supply, but this is not evaluated preoperatively. Therefore, it may be necessary to shift the cut line of the mesojejunum to the more cranial side in cases in which the jejunal arteries override the DJUV and are distributed along the periphery of the jejunal mesentery (ie, along the J2A) (Figure 6).

This study had some limitations. MD-CT may not reveal all branches of the SMV and SMA, especially the IPDV. Moreover, its retrospective design may be associated with bias. Another is the relatively small sample size. As the vessel anatomy around the head of the pancreas varies widely, further investigation of a larger number of cases is needed to assess the anatomy of the DJUV as a landmark for mesopancreatoduodenum resection. Furthermore, surgical outcomes and patients' prognoses should be evaluated to confirm the validity of the DJUV-guided method.

In conclusion, based on an analysis of the vascular anatomy and positional relationships between the DJUV and key vessels, this study implies the possibility of using the DJUV as a landmark for mesopancreatoduodenum resection. Dissecting along the DJUV as a caudal border may be useful for safe and oncologically curative PD. We believe that this concept contributes to the establishment of a standard PD procedure.

ACKNOWLEDGMENTS

The authors thank Lecturer Megumi Matsuda and Professor Teruhito Kido of the Department of Radiology, Ehime University Graduate School of Medicine, for support and advice on CT imaging methods. We also thank Azusa Okuwa Saikou Inc for preparing the figures.

DISCLOSURE

Author contributions: Tohyama and Honjo contributed to the study conception and design. Tohyama, Honjo, Tamura, Takai, Sakamoto, Ogawa, Watanabe, Ohtani, and Takada participated in data collection or management. Tohyama, Honjo, and Takada contributed to the data analysis and interpretation of the data. Tohyama and Honjo drafted the article. Tohyama, Honjo, and Takada contributed to the article writing and editing. Tohyama and Takada provided critical review. All authors read and approved the final article.

REFERENCES

1. Hartwig W, Hackert T, Hinz U, Gluth A, Bergmann F, Strobel O, et al. Pancreatic cancer surgery in the new millennium: better prediction of outcome. Ann Surg. 2011;254(2):311–9.
2. Cameron JL, He J. Two thousand consecutive pancreaticoduodenectomies. J Am Coll Surg. 2015;220(4):530–6.
3. Conroy T, Hammel P, Hebbar M, Ben Abdelghani M, Wei AC, Raoul JL, et al. FOLFIRINOX or Gemcitabine as Adjuvant Therapy for Pancreatic Cancer. N Engl J Med. 2018;379(25):2395–406.
4. Motoi F, Unno M. Adjuvant and neoadjuvant treatment for pancreatic adenocarcinoma. Jpn J Clin Oncol. 2020;50(5):483–9.
5. Maeda S, Moore AM, Yohanathan L, Hata T, Truty MJ, Smoot RL, et al. Impact of resection margin status on survival in pancreatic cancer patients after neoadjuvant treatment and pancreatoduodenectomy. Surgery. 2020;167(5):803–11.
6. Gockel I, Domeyer M, Wolloscheck T, Konerding MA, Junginger T. Resection of the mesopancreas (RMP): a new surgical classification of a known anatomical space. World J Surg Oncol. 2007;5:44.
7. Quero G, Fiorillo C, Menghi R, Cina C, Galiandro F, Longo F, et al. Total mesopancreas excision for periampullary malignancy: a single-center propensity score-matched comparison of long-term outcomes. Langenbecks Arch Surg. 2020;405(3):303–12.
8. Gaedcke J, Gunawan B, Grade M, Szöke R, Liersch T, Becker H, et al. The mesopancreas is the primary site for R1 resection in pancreatic head cancer: relevance for clinical trials. Langenbecks Arch Surg. 2010;395(4):451–8.
9. Ramia JM, De-la-Plaza R, Manuel-Vazquez A, Lopez-Marcano A, Morales R. Systematic review of the mesopancreas: concept and clinical implications. Clin Transl Oncol. 2018;20(11):1385–91.
10. Kawabata Y, Tanaka T, Nishi T, Monma H, Yano S, Tajima Y. Appraisal of a total meso-pancreatoduodenum excision with pancreaticoduodenectomy for pancreatic head carcinoma. Eur J Surg Oncol. 2012;38(7):574–9.
11. Inoue Y, Saiura A, Yoshioka R, Ono Y, Takahashi M, Arita J, et al. Pancreatoduodenectomy with systematic mesopancreas dissection using a supracolic anterior artery-first approach. Ann Surg. 2015;262(6):1092–101.
12. Nappo G, Perinel J, El Bechwaty M, Adham M. The standardization of pancreatoduodenectomy: where are we? Pancreas. 2016;45(4):493–502.
13. Kitagawa H, Tajima H, Nakagawara H, Makino I, Miyashita T, Terakawa H, et al. A modification of radical antegrade modular pancreatosplenectomy for adenocarcinoma of the left pancreas: significance of en bloc resection including the anterior renal fascia. World J Surg. 2014;38(9):2448–54.
14. Sugiyama M, Suzuki Y, Nakazato T, Yokoyama M, Kogure M, Abe N, et al. Intestinal derotation procedure for facilitating pancreatoduodenectomy. Surgery. 2016;159(5):1325–32.
15. Nakamura M, Nakashima H, Tsutsumi K, Matsumoto H, Muta Y, Ueno D, et al. First jejunal vein oriented mesenteric excision for pancreatoduodenectomy. J Gastroenterol. 2013;48(8):989–95.
16. Ishikawa Y, Ban D, Matsumura S, Mitsunori Y, Ochiai T, Kudo A, et al. Surgical pitfalls of jejunal vein anatomy in pancreaticoduodenectomy. J Hepatobiliary Pancreat Sci. 2017;24(7):394–400.
17. Koiwahara G, Tsuda T, Matsuda M, Hirata M, Tanaka H, Hyodo T, et al. Different enhancement of the hepatic parenchyma in dynamic CT for patients with normal liver and chronic liver diseases and with the dose of contrast medium based on body surface area. Jpn J Radiol. 2015;33(4):194–200.
18. Society JP. Classification of Pancreatic Carcinoma, 4th English Edition edn. Tokyo: Kanehara & Co., Ltd.; 2017.
19. Heald RJ, Husband EM, Ryall RD. The mesorectum in rectal cancer surgery–the clue to pelvic recurrence? Br J Surg. 1982;69(10):613–6.
20. Kobayashi Y, Sakamoto Y, Arita J, Akamatsu N, Kaneko J, Hasegawa K, et al. Vascular anatomy of the jejunal mesentery and complica-

tions associated with division of the first jejunal venous trunk during pancreaticoduodenectomy. J Surg Oncol. 2018;117(6):1297–304.

21. Negoi I, Beuran M, Hostiuc S, Negoi RI, Inoue Y. Surgical anatomy of the superior mesenteric vessels related to colon and pancreatic surgery: a systematic review and meta-analysis. Sci Rep. 2018;8(1):4184.
22. Nagakawa Y, Hosokawa Y, Sahara Y, Takishita C, Hijikata Y, Osakabe H, et al. Approaching the superior mesenteric artery from the right side using the proximal-dorsal jejunal vein preisolation method during laparoscopic pancreaticoduodenectomy. Surg Endosc. 2018;32(9):4044–51.
23. Matsuno S, Egawa S, Fukuyama S, Motoi F, Sunamura M, Isaji S, et al. Pancreatic cancer registry in japan: 20 y of experience. Pancreas. 2004;28(3):219–30.
24. Kanda M, Fujii T, Nagai S, Kodera Y, Kanzaki A, Sahin TT, et al. Pattern of lymph node metastasis spread in pancreatic cancer. Pancreas. 2011;40(6):951–5.
25. Kawabata Y, Tanaka T, Ishikawa N, Hayashi H, Tajima Y. Modified total meso-pancreatoduodenum excision with pancreaticoduodenectomy as a mesopancreatic plane surgery in borderline resectable pancreatic cancer. Eur J Surg Oncol. 2016;42(5):698–705.
26. Qian L, Xie J, Xu Z, Deng X, Chen H, Peng C, et al. The necessity of dissection of no. 14 lymph nodes to patients with pancreatic ductal adenocarcinoma based on the embryonic development of the head of the pancreas. Front Oncol. 2020;10:1343.
27. Imamura T, Yamamoto Y, Sugiura T, Okamura Y, Ito T, Ashida R, et al. Reconsidering the optimal regional lymph node station according to tumor location for pancreatic cancer. Ann Surg Oncol. 2020;28(3):1602–11.

The safety and feasibility of laparoscopic redo surgery for recurrent Crohn's disease: A comparative clinical study of over 100 consecutive patients

Takayuki Ogino[1,2] | Yuki Sekido[1] | Tsuyoshi Hata[1] | Norikatsu Miyoshi[1] | Hidekazu Takahashi[1] | Mamoru Uemura[1] | Hirofumi Yamamoto[1] | Yuichiro Doki[1] | Hidetoshi Eguchi[1] | Tsunekazu Mizushima[1,2]

[1]Department of Gastroenterological Surgery, Osaka University Graduate School of Medicine, Suita, Japan

[2]Department of Therapeutics for Inflammatory Bowel Diseases, Osaka University Graduate School of Medicine, Suita, Japan

Correspondence
Takayuki Ogino, Department of Gastroenterological Surgery, Department of Therapeutics for Inflammatory Bowel Diseases, Osaka University, 2-2-E2 Yamadaoka, Suita, Osaka, 565-0871, Japan.
Email: togino04@gesurg.med.osaka-u.ac.jp

Abstract

Background: Despite advances in medical treatments, most patients with Crohn's disease (CD) will still require surgery, with 20%-50% needing redo surgery within 10 years after the primary procedure. There is no consensus on the application of laparoscopic redo surgery for recurrent CD.

Methods: This study included 107 patients with CD who underwent surgery from 2012 to 2020 at Osaka University Hospital. All procedures were laparoscopic. Patients were grouped based on whether the surgery was redo or primary for evaluation of the safety and feasibility of laparoscopic redo surgery.

Results: The study included 40 patients undergoing redo surgery and 67 having primary surgery. The median age at the time of the procedure was higher for those undergoing redo surgery (43 years vs 34 years, $P < 0.0031$), as were the duration of CD (16.5 years vs 8.3 years, $P < 0.0012$) and number of operating minutes (231.0 min vs 169.0 min, $P < 0.0001$). The remnant bowel length was shorter in the redo surgery group (270.0 cm vs 410.0 cm, $P < 0.0001$). Rates of open conversion were comparable between the two groups (10.0% vs 3.0%, $P = 0.127$), as were postoperative complications (32.5% vs 20.9%, $P = 0.1812$).

Conclusions: These results suggest that laparoscopic redo surgery is safe and feasible, with comparable conversion rates and postoperative complications in experienced institutions.

KEYWORDS
adhesion, Crohn's disease, laparoscopic surgery, redo surgery

1 | INTRODUCTION

Surgery plays a large role in the management of Crohn's disease (CD). With advances involving various biologics and immunomodulators, control of intestinal inflammation and treatment outcomes have been greatly improved.[1] However, 70%-80% of CD patients require surgery during the disease course, and some are at risk for needing redo procedures.[2] Recent studies report overall cumulative rates of redo surgery at 20%-50% within 10 years after the primary surgery.[3,4] Age, preoperative smoking, perianal disease, disease location in the ileocolon, perforating disease, positive microscopic resection margin, and steroid use have been reported as risk factors for redo surgery.[3,4]

No other intestinal disease requires redo surgery as often as CD does. Most CD patients who need redo surgery experience complications such as abscesses, strictures, and intestinal fistulas.[3] They also have an increased risk for postoperative complications, such as intra-abdominal sepsis and anastomotic leakage.[5-7] Results of previous studies indicate that patients with a history of abdominal surgery for CD should be excluded from laparoscopic surgery.[8] Despite the high need for redo surgery, conclusive evaluations of the feasibility and safety of a laparoscopic approach are lacking. Meanwhile, CD surgeons are expected not only to focus on the current surgery but also to consider setting the stage as optimally as possible for a likely redo surgery.

A primary surgery for the non-penetrating type of ileocecal lesion has been widely accepted as a good indication for laparoscopic surgery. Several studies have demonstrated the benefits of laparoscopic surgery for simple CD.[9,10] However, laparoscopic surgery for complex CD is associated with technical difficulties because of features such as widespread inflammation, mesenteric thickness, abscess, and fistula. In particular, redo surgery has often involved dealing with a dense and strong adhesion, making the procedure much more difficult. Thus, few reports are available describing laparoscopic redo surgery for recurrent CD, and of available findings, specific technical issues have been resolved, but the safety, feasibility, and utility have not.

In our experienced institution, we have been aggressively applying laparoscopic surgery in this patient group to minimize abdominal wall destruction and reduce postoperative inflammation. In this study, we assessed the outcomes of laparoscopic redo surgery for recurrent CD compared to outcomes with primary surgery.

2 | METHODS

2.1 | Patients

Since 2012, all procedures in our institution have involved a laparoscopic approach, whether primary or redo surgery. Single incisional laparoscopic surgery (SILS) was selected in principle. Additional ports were used when multiple organ resection was required, and use of more than two additional ports was defined as MULTI. Hand-assisted laparoscopic surgery (HALS) was selected when extensive colectomy was required. HALS was indicated for patients with extensive colonic lesions, whereas SILS was indicated for patients with ileocolic lesions, ileocolic anastomotic lesions, or small intestinal lesions. Open conversion was considered depending on the intraoperative situation. The skin incisions used for each approach are shown in Figure S1.

From January 2012 to December 2020, a total of 131 consecutive patients who underwent surgery for CD intestinal lesions in Osaka University Hospital were included in this study. Patients with surgical indications for perianal diseases or cancer were excluded (Figure 1). The patients were grouped by surgery type (primary or redo), and laparoscopic surgery outcomes were evaluated between the two groups.

Indications for the surgeries were determined in inflammatory bowel disease (IBD) treatment team conferences attended by gastroenterologists, colorectal surgeons, radiologists, nutritionists, and nurses. All surgeries were performed by two qualified and board-certified colorectal surgeons with established endoscopic surgical skills.

2.2 | Surgical technique for redo surgery

All surgery was performed under general anesthesia, with the patient placed in the lithotomy position. An initial laparotomy (3-4 cm) was made in the umbilicus, and adhesions around the previous wound were dissected. For the redo surgeries, most of the surgical sites were located in the ileocolic anastomosis. In these cases, a SILS device with one camera port and two manipulation ports was fitted for performing intra-abdominal procedures, as previously described.[11] After pneumoperitoneum was established, another port was added at the right lower site (planned site of drainage tube) if necessary.

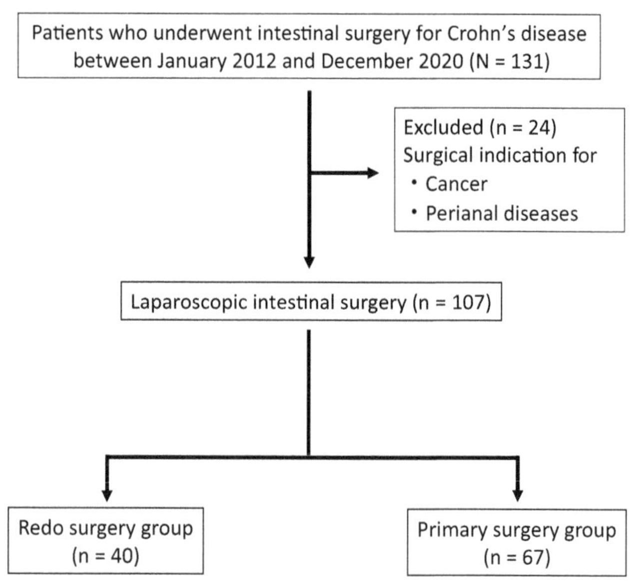

FIGURE 1 Flowchart of patient selection

Laparoscopic redo surgery involved several key features. Sharp and cold dissection was performed for adhesiolysis to minimize the risk of intestinal injury, along with careful manipulation of the intestine and mesentery without grasping inflamed, thickened, and edematous sites. Fistulas between the intestine, abdominal wall, urinary bladder, and inflamed lesion were divided intracorporeally using a stapler if necessary. A cranial approach often allowed easy identification of the retroperitoneal organs. Mobilization of the hepatic flexure and small bowel near the terminal ileum was performed first, and the recurrent area then was approached. After complete mobilization, the affected intestines were exteriorized, and resection and anastomosis were performed extracorporeally. An extension of the skin incision was sometimes needed in cases of bulky mass with inflammation. Careful exploration of the large and small intestines was performed, and the presence or absence of obstruction was confirmed by passage of a balloon inflated to 2 cm from the terminal ileum to the Treitz ligament. After opening of the intestinal lumen at the planned resection line, the inflated balloon was inserted from the site. We folded the intestinal tract like an accordion and forwarded the balloon to the Treitz ligament to assess for the presence or absence of obstruction. For dividing thickened mesentery, we found that ultrasonically activated devices were not sufficient to seal the large blood vessels, so we added transfixion sutures. The affected segment was resected, and a functional end-to-end anastomosis was performed. The stapled lines were oversewn and the defects of the mesentery closed routinely. In cases of a short affected lesion, strictureplasty was performed using the hand-sewn technique. An active drainage tube was routinely placed in Morrison's pouch or Douglas' pouch as previously described.[12]

2.3 | Data collection

Data were retrospectively collected for the comparison between CD patients with redo surgery and those with primary surgery. Patient characteristics included age, sex, body mass index, the American Society of Anesthesiologists physical status (ASA-PS), age at diagnosis, duration of disease, location, prognostic nutrition index, preoperative data, surgical indications, preoperative medication, loss of response, and surgical history. Perioperative data included approach, surgical procedure, operative time, blood loss, length of skin incision, conversion to open surgery, remnant bowel length, postoperative complications, excessive perioperative inflammation, and length of hospital stay.

Loss of response was defined as increased doses of biologics, shortened dosing interval, or changed other biologics within 6 months before surgery. Postoperative complications were defined as complications occurring within 30 days after surgery. Excessive perioperative inflammation was defined as preoperative C-reactive protein (CRP) ≥0.4 mg/dL combined with CRP ≥3.0 mg/dL at postoperative day 7 and/or postoperative peak CRP ≥10 mg/dL.

2.4 | Statistical analysis

All statistical analyses were conducted using GraphPad Prism software, version 5.0 b. The chi-square test and Fisher's exact test were used to compare and analyze categorical variables. All analyses were two-tailed with $P < 0.05$ considered significant.

2.5 | Ethics statement

The protocol for this study was approved by the institutional review board of Osaka University Graduate School of Medicine (#15028). The procedures conformed to the provisions of the Declaration of Helsinki. Written informed consent was obtained from all patients for use of their clinical data.

3 | RESULTS

3.1 | Patient characteristics

In our institution, all intestinal surgeries for CD were started using a laparoscopic approach. A total of 131 consecutive patients underwent intestinal surgery for CD during the study period. We excluded 24 patients with surgical indication for cancer or perianal disease, so that data for 107 patients were analyzed in this study (Figure 1). Of these, 40 (37.4%) had redo surgery and 67 (62.6%) had no history of abdominal surgery for CD.

Patient characteristics are shown in Table 1. The median age at operation was 43 years in the redo group, which was older than patients undergoing primary procedures, who had a median age of 34 years ($P < 0.0031$). The two groups were comparable for sex, body mass index, proportion of ASA-PS, and median age at CD diagnosis. Duration of CD was 16.5 years for those undergoing redo surgery, significantly longer than in the primary group (8.3 years; $P < 0.0012$). The two groups did not differ regarding disease location, perianal disease, preoperative prognostic nutrition index, or CRP values. Preoperative treatments were comparable with regard to anti-tumor necrosis factor-α, anti-interleukin 12/23p40, and corticosteroid therapy. Patients undergoing redo procedures had a numerically higher frequency of immunomodulator use, but not significantly so ($P = 0.052$). Loss of response, rates of emergency operation, and surgical indication were also comparable between the two groups.

For patients having redo procedures, the time since the previous surgery was 9.9 years. In this group, 23 patients (57.5%) had undergone one surgical bowel resection, 14 (35.0%) had a history of two surgeries, and three (7.5%) had undergone more than three surgeries. The approach used for previous surgeries was open in 33 patients (82.5%) and laparoscopic in seven patients (17.5%).

TABLE 1 Patient characteristics

	Redo (n = 40)	Primary (n = 67)	P
Age at operation (y), median ± SD	43.0 ± 11.9	34.0 ± 12.4	0.0031
Sex, n (%)			0.2015
Male	32 (80.0)	46 (68.7)	
Female	8 (20.0)	21 (31.3)	
Body mass index (kg/m^2), median ± SD	18.9 ± 3.1	19.0 ± 3.0	0.9792
ASA-PS, n (%)			0.3947
1	13 (32.5)	25 (37.3)	
2	26 (65.0)	42 (62.7)	
3	1 (2.5)	0 (0.0)	
Age at diagnosis (y), median ± SD	26.5 ± 9.6	25.0 ± 11.6	0.5859
Duration of disease (y), median ± SD	16.5 ± 11.7	8.3 ± 8.0	0.0012
Locations, n (%)			0.6625
Small bowel	18 (45.0)	32 (47.8)	
Colon	3 (7.5)	8 (11.9)	
Ileocolon	19 (47.5)	27 (40.3)	
Perianal diseases	27 (67.5)	41 (61.2)	0.512
Preoperative prognostic nutrition index, median ± SD	42.8 ± 10.8	40.4 ± 8.6	0.1125
Preoperative CRP (mg/dL), median ± SD	0.16 ± 2.21	0.46 ± 3.53	0.2127
Preoperative medication, n (%)[a]			
Anti-tumor necrosis-α	24 (60.0)	38 (56.7)	0.7392
Anti-interleukin 12/23p40	5 (12.5)	8 (11.9)	0.9317
Steroid	2 (5.0)	10 (14.9)	0.1154
Immunomodulator	16 (40.0)	15 (22.4)	0.052
Loss of response	19 (47.5)	30 (44.8)	0.7844
Emergency operation, n (%)	1 (2.5)	7 (10.4)	0.1305
Surgical indication, n (%)			0.091
Fistula/abscess	15 (37.5)	34 (50.7)	
Stenosis	19 (47.5)	32 (47.8)	
Bleeding	1 (2.5)	1 (1.5)	
Ileostomy closure	5 (12.5)	0 (0.0)	
Duration from previous surgery (y), median ± SD	9.9 ± 8.5	-	
Surgical history of bowel resection for CD, n (%)			
1	23 (57.5)	-	
2	14 (35.0)	-	
≥3	3 (7.5)	-	
Approach in previous surgery, n (%)			
Open	33 (82.5)	-	
Laparoscopic	7 (17.5)	-	

[a]Including duplicates.

3.2 | Surgery-related factors

The proportions of the different laparoscopic surgical approaches were comparable between the two groups ($P = 0.5895$). In the redo group, 82.5% had SILS, 5.0% had MULTI, and 12.5% had HALS procedures. In the primary surgery group, 77.6% had SILS, 3.0% had MULTI, and 19.4% had HALS (Table 2). In the redo group, 62.5% had ileocecal resection or ileocolectomy, compared with 53.7% undergoing primary surgery. For some patients in both groups, additional procedures were performed, including partial resection of the small intestine (35.0% of redo and 34.3% of primary surgery patients), right hemicolectomy (2.5% of redo and 3.0% of primary surgery patients), left hemicolectomy (5.0% redo, 4.5% primary), subtotal colectomy (10.0% redo, 14.9% primary), strictureplasty (17.5% redo, 14.9% primary), stoma creation (17.5% redo, 7.5% primary), and stoma closure (10.0% in redo). Operating time was 231.0 ± 93.9 min for the redo group and 169.0 ± 65.1 min for the primary surgery group. As expected, operating time was significantly longer with redo surgeries, given that adhesiolysis was often necessary ($P < 0.0001$). Compared with the primary surgery group, the redo group also had more operative blood loss ($P = 0.0372$), longer skin incisions ($P = 0.0272$), and shorter remnant bowel length ($P < 0.0001$). An incisional extension was performed in 13 patients (32.5%) undergoing redo and 17 (25.4%) having a primary procedure. Of these, open conversion was performed in four patients in the redo group and two in the primary group. The additional length was 2.0 ± 2.8 cm for the redo patients and 1.7 ± 2.0 cm for the primary group. Rates of conversion to open surgery were not significantly different between the two groups ($P = 0.127$). There were four cases of open conversion in the redo group. In the first case, inflammation had spread to the retroperitoneum, and the boundary with the left ureter was unclear. It was difficult to confirm the left ureter in the second case, and there was a severe adhesion between the jejunum and the transverse colon in the third case. The fourth case also involved a strong adhesion between the ileum and the ileo-rectal anastomosis. The primary group included two conversions, one with marked intestinal dilatation and intestinal injury and the other with a widespread enterocutaneous fistula associated with difficult mobilization from the abdominal wall, ileum, and ileal mesentery.

3.3 | Short-term outcomes

Short-term outcomes are shown in Table 3. Postoperative complications were comparable between the two groups (32.5% redo vs 20.9% primary; $P = 0.1812$). Wound infection occurred in eight patients in the redo group and five having primary surgery ($P = 0.0698$). No redo patients had anastomotic leakage, but one primary surgery patient did ($P = 1.000$). Three in each group had small bowel obstruction ($P = 0.6692$), and three redo patients and one primary surgery patient had an intra-abdominal abscess ($P = 0.1460$). One redo patient and three primary surgery patients had gastrointestinal bleeding, and two primary surgery patients had intra-abdominal bleeding

TABLE 2 Operative findings

	Redo (n = 40)	Primary (n = 67)	P
Approach, n (%)			0.5895
SILS	33 (82.5)	52 (77.6)	
MULTI	2 (5.0)	2 (3.0)	
HALS	5 (12.5)	13 (19.4)	
Surgical procedure, n (%)[a]			
Ileocecal resection/ileocolectomy	25 (62.5)	36 (53.7)	
Partial resection of small intestine	14 (35.0)	23 (34.3)	
Right hemicolectomy	1 (2.5)	2 (3.0)	
Left hemicolectomy	2 (5.0)	3 (4.5)	
Subtotal colectomy	4 (10.0)	10 (14.9)	
Strictureplasty	7 (17.5)	10 (14.9)	
Stoma creation	7 (17.5)	5 (7.5)	
Stoma closure	4 (10.0)	0 (0.0)	
Operating time (min), median ± SD	231.0 ± 93.9	169.0 ± 65.1	<0.0001
Blood loss (mL), median ± SD	185.0 ± 188.1	100.0 ± 330.8	0.0372
Skin incision (cm), median ± SD	5.0 ± 2.7	4.0 ± 1.5	0.0272
Conversion to open surgery, n (%)	4 (10.0)	2 (3.0)	0.127
Remnant bowel length (cm), median ± SD	270.0 ± 99.4	410.0 ± 94.6	<0.0001

[a]Including duplicates.

($P = 0.4073$). No redo patients had a catheter infection, but three primary surgery patients did ($P = 0.2911$). The two groups did not differ in postoperative day 7 CRP or postoperative peak CRP. Excessive perioperative inflammation, which is associated with recurrence,[13] also was comparable between the two groups. The groups also did not differ in length of postoperative hospital stay ($P = 0.8653$), and there were no reoperations or postoperative mortalities.

4 | DISCUSSION

Laparoscopic colorectal cancer surgery has become widespread and has been rapidly accepted.[14] In IBD, a laparoscopic approach has already been accepted for simple CD cases, with fewer complications and improved early postoperative outcomes.[9,10] The reported benefits of laparoscopic surgery include reduced postoperative pain, improved respiratory function, less wound infection, less incisional hernia, less small bowel obstruction, earlier resumption of bowel function, shorter hospital stay, and better cosmesis.[9,10,15-17] Especially, reduced rates of small bowel obstruction would indicate lower postoperative adhesion,[18] and suggest attractive advantages in consideration of a later redo surgery (see Supporting Information for case descriptions).

Several studies have described a laparoscopic approach for recurrent CD. Most results indicate a longer operation time, but without significant differences in bleeding, open conversion rates, or complication rates compared with primary surgery.[19-21] Our study also suggests that laparoscopic redo surgery requires a longer operative time, but still with comparable open conversion and postoperative complication rates compared with primary surgery. Studies comparing laparoscopic and open redo surgery have found comparable operation time and complication rates between the two,[17,22,23] but with the advantages of a shorter skin incision, less wound infection, and faster postoperative recovery with laparoscopy.[24] The open conversion rates in these studies were 11% to 31%, and risk factors were dense adhesions, bulky mass, fistula formation, and intraoperative intestinal injury.[21,22,24-27] However, careful interpretations of previous findings are necessary because of patient selection bias for laparoscopic redo surgery in these studies. Our current work represents the first study of consecutive patients all undergoing laparoscopic surgery, regardless of primary or redo surgery, avoiding this selection bias.

Consistent with previous results, we found that laparoscopic redo surgery took longer but did not increase postoperative complications. As noted, laparoscopic redo surgery often entails high technical difficulty because of massive adhesions, the fragility of inflamed lesions, thickened mesentery, inflammatory masses with abscess, and fistulas. In this study, adhesions to the abdominal wall at the previous surgical site could be dissected in all cases. For exteriorizing affected intestines, a midline skin incision was beneficial for evaluation of the entire small intestine and the need for open conversion. Most reasons for open conversion were intraoperative decisions about injury risk to other organs because their orientation could not be established during surgery. To prevent such situations arising during a redo surgery, we recommend two techniques, especially in cases of partial ileal resection or ileocecal resection as a primary surgery. One is mobilization of the right colon to the minimum necessary, and the second is preservation

TABLE 3 Short-term outcomes

	Redo (n = 40)	Primary (n = 67)	P
Complications, n (%)[a]	13 (32.5)	14 (20.9)	0.1812
Wound infection	8 (20.0)	5 (7.5)	0.0698
Anastomotic leakage	0 (0.0)	1 (1.5)	1.000
Small bowel obstruction	3 (7.5)	3 (4.5)	0.6692
Intra-abdominal abscess	3 (7.5)	1 (1.5)	0.146
Bleeding	1 (2.5)	5 (7.5)	0.4073
Catheter infection	0 (0.0)	3 (4.5)	0.2911
Post-operative day 7 CRP (mg/dL), mean ± SD	1.60 ± 4.43	1.61 ± 3.80	0.2527
Postoperative peak CRP (mg/dL), mean ± SD	9.01 ± 5.65	7.06 ± 6.92	0.4654
Excessive perioperative inflammation, n (%)	11 (27.5)	18 (26.9)	0.9431
Reoperation within post-operative day 30	0 (0.0)	0 (0.0)	
Mortality, n (%)	0 (0.0)	0 (0.0)	
Postoperative hospital stay (days), median ± SD	24.0 ± 11.5	25.0 ± 9.3	0.8653

[a]Including duplicates.

of the prepancreatic fascia. These points could lead to significant advantages in a later redo surgery. We also consider SILS a promising technique that could avoid unnecessary intestinal injury, minimize the skin incision, and establish additional ports in the best positions.[28]

The present study has several limitations. Its design was retrospective, and it was conducted in a single institution specializing in IBD and laparoscopic surgery. Most surgeries were performed by two board-certified surgeons, so the findings cannot be generalized to inexperienced centers and surgeons. Perioperative medication and diet, which would affect CD surgery, were selected largely according to clinician discretion and patient condition. This study also identified postoperative hospital stays as long as 20 days or more, whereas most previous results involve hospital stays of less than 1 week, whether for primary or redo surgery.[7,16,20,23,26] Finally, patients were allowed to have an elementary diet after negative CRP in accordance with institutional therapeutic guidelines based on previous results that postoperative inflammation is involved in CD recurrence.[12,25,29]

With the increase in CD patients, laparoscopic redo surgery for recurrent CD will become a common procedure in the near future. Our results suggest that laparoscopic redo surgery is safe and feasible in experienced institutions. Although the quantification of adhesion severity is quite difficult, we have found that the adhesions to the abdominal wall were not very strong in case of previous surgery performed laparoscopically (see Supporting Information for case descriptions). Fewer adhesions would set the stage for easier surgery if a redo is required.

REFERENCES

1. Ogino T, Mizushima T, Matsuda C, Mori M, Doki Y. Essential updates 2018/2019: Colorectal (benign): Recent updates (2018–2019) in the surgical treatment of benign colorectal diseases. Ann Gastroenterol Surg. 2019;4(1):30–8.
2. Bernell O, Lapidus A, Hellers G. Risk factors for surgery and recurrence in 907 patients with primary ileocaecal Crohn's disease. Br J Surg. 2000;87(12):1697–701.
3. de Buck van Overstraeten A, Eshuis EJ, Vermeire S, Van Assche G, Ferrante M, D'Haens GR, et al. Short- and medium-term outcomes following primary ileocaecal resection for Crohn's disease in two specialist centres. Br J Surg. 2017;104(12):1713–22.
4. Shinagawa T, Hata K, Ikeuchi H, Fukushima K, Futami K, Sugita A, et al. Rate of reoperation decreased significantly after year 2002 in patients with Crohn's disease. Clin Gastroenterol Hepatol. 2020;18(4):898–907.
5. Huang W, Tang Y, Nong L, Sun Y. Risk factors for postoperative intra-abdominal septic complications after surgery in Crohn's disease: a meta-analysis of observational studies. J Crohns Colitis. 2015;9:293–301.
6. Brouquet A, Blanc B, Bretagnol F, Valleur P, Bouhnik Y, Panis Y. Surgery for intestinal Crohn's disease recurrence. Surgery. 2010;148:936–46.
7. SICCR Current Status of Crohn's Disease Surgery Collaborative. National variations in perioperative assessment and surgical management of Crohn's disease: a multicentre study. Colorectal Dis. 2020;23:94–104.
8. Wu JS, Birnbaum EH, Kodner IJ, Fry RD, Read TE, Fleshman JW. Laparoscopic-assisted ileocolic resections in patients with Crohn's disease: are abscesses, phlegmons, or recurrent disease contraindications? Surgery. 1997;122:682–8.
9. Maartense S, Dunker MS, Slors JFM, Cuesta MA, Pierik EGJM, Gouma DJ, et al. Laparoscopic-assisted versus open ileocolic resection for Crohn's disease: a randomized trial. Ann Surg. 2006;243:143–9.
10. Milsom JW, Hammerhofer KA, Böhm B, Marcello P, Elson P, Fazio VW. Prospective, randomized trial comparing laparoscopic vs. conventional surgery for refractory ileocolic Crohn's disease. Dis Colon Rectum. 2001;44:1–8.
11. Mizushima T, Nakajima K, Takeyama H, Naito A, Osawa H, Uemura M, et al. Single-incision laparoscopic surgery for stricturing and penetrating Crohn's disease. Surg Today. 2016;46:203–8.
12. Ikeshima R, Mizushima T, Takahashi H, Haraguchi N, Nishimura J, Hata T, et al. The efficacy of active drainage for preventing postoperative organ/space surgical site infections in patients with Crohn's disease. Surg Today. 2018;48:25–32.
13. Ikeda A, Miyoshi N, Fujino S, Iijima H, Takahashi H, Haraguchi N, et al. A Novel predictive nomogram for early endoscopic recurrence after intestinal resection for Crohn's disease. Digestion. 2019;100(4):269–76.
14. Clinical Outcomes of Surgical Therapy Study Group, Nelson H, Sargent DJ, Wieand HS, Fleshman J, Anvari M, et al. A comparison of laparoscopically assisted and open colectomy for colon cancer. N Engl J Med. 2004;350:2050-9.
15. Carmichael H, Peyser D, Vanessa M, Bhasin D, Dean A, Khaitov S, et al. The role of laparoscopic surgery in repeat ileocolic resection for Crohn's disease. Colorectal Dis. 2021;23:2075–84.

16. Chaudhary B, Glancy D, Dixon AR. Laparoscopic surgery for recurrent ileocolic Crohn's disease is as safe and effective as primary resection. Colorectal Dis. 2011;13:1413–6.
17. Aytac E, Stocchi L, Remzi FH, Kiran RP. Is laparoscopic surgery for recurrent Crohn's disease beneficial in patients with previous primary resection through midline laparotomy? A case-matched study. Surg Endosc. 2012;26:3552–6.
18. Krielen P, Stommel MWJ, Pargmae P, Bouvy ND, Bakkum EA, Ellis H, et al. Adhesion-related readmissions after open and laparoscopic surgery: a retrospective cohort study (SCAR update). Lancet. 2020;395(10217):33–41.
19. Celentano V, Sagias F, Flashman KG, Conti J, Khan J. Laparoscopic redo ileocolic resection for Crohn's disease in patients with previous multiple laparotomies. Scand J Surg. 2019;108(1):42–8.
20. Pinto RA, Shawki S, Narita K, Weiss EG, Wexner SD. Laparoscopy for recurrent Crohn's disease: how do the results compare with the results for primary Crohn's disease? Colorectal Dis. 2011;13:302–7.
21. Hasegawa H, Watanabe M, Nishibori H, Okabayashi K, Hibi T, Kitajima M. Laparoscopic surgery for recurrent Crohn's disease. Br J Surg. 2003;90:970–3.
22. Holubar SD, Dozois EJ, Privitera A, Cima RR, Pemberton JH, Young-Fadok T, et al. Laparoscopic surgery for recurrent ileocolic Crohn's disease. Inflamm Bowel Dis. 2010;16:1382–6.
23. Brouquet A, Bretagnol F, Soprani A, Valleur P, Bouhnik Y, Panis Y. A laparoscopic approach to iterative ileocolonic resection for the recurrence of Crohn's disease. Surg Endosc. 2010;24:879–87.
24. Uchikoshi F, Ito T, Nezu R, Tanemura M, Kai Y, Mizushima T, et al. Advantages of laparoscope-assisted surgery for recurrent Crohn's disease. Surg Endosc. 2004;18:1675–9.
25. Moorthy K, Shaul T, Foley RJ. Factors that predict conversion in patients undergoing laparoscopic surgery for Crohn's disease. Am J Surg. 2004;187:47.
26. Goyer P, Alves A, Bretagnol F, Bouhnik Y, Valleur P, Panis Y. Impact of complex Crohn's disease on the outcome of laparoscopic ileocecal resection: a comparative clinical study in 124 patients. Dis Colon Rectum. 2009;52(2):205–10.
27. Bouquot M, Maggiori L, Hain E, Prost a la Denise J, Bouhnik Y, Panis Y. What is the outcome for patients undergoing more than two ileocolonic resections for recurrent Crohn's disease? A comparative study of 569 consecutive procedures. Colorectal Dis. 2019;21:563–9.
28. Maeda K, Nagahara H, Shibutani M, Fukuoka T, Inoue T, Ohira M. A review of reports on single-incision laparoscopic surgery for Crohn's disease. Surg Today. 2019;49(5):361–8.
29. Ohara N, Mizushima T, Iijima H, Takahashi H, Hiyama S, Haraguchi N, et al. Adherence to an elemental diet for preventing postoperative recurrence of Crohn's disease. Surg Today. 2017;47(12):1519–25.

10

Essential updates 2020/2021: Current topics of simulation and navigation in hepatectomy

Yu Saito[1] | Mitsuo Shimada[1] | Yuji Morine[1] | Shinichiro Yamada[1] | Maki Sugimoto[1,2]

[1]Department of Surgery, Tokushima University, Tokushima, Japan

[2]Okinaga Research Institute, Teikyo University, Chiyoda-ku, Japan

Correspondence
Yu Saito, Department of Surgery, Tokushima University, 3-18-15 Kuramoto-cho, Tokushima, 770-8503, Japan.
Email: saito.yu.1001@tokushima-u.ac.jp

Abstract

With the development of three-dimensional (3D) simulation software, preoperative simulation technology is almost completely established. The remaining issue is how to recognize anatomy three-dimensionally. Extended reality is a newly developed technology with several merits for surgical application: no requirement for a sterilized display monitor, better spatial awareness, and the ability to share 3D images among all surgeons. Various technology or devices for intraoperative navigation have also been developed to support the safety and certainty of liver surgery. Consensus recommendations regarding indocyanine green fluorescence were determined in 2021. Extended reality has also been applied to intraoperative navigation, and artificial intelligence (AI) is one of the topics of real-time navigation. AI might overcome the problem of liver deformity with automatic registration. Including the issues described above, this article focuses on recent advances in simulation and navigation in liver surgery from 2020 to 2021.

KEYWORDS
artificial intelligence, extended reality, ICG fluorescence, liver surgery, navigation, simulation

1 | INTRODUCTION

Advances in perioperative care and surgical techniques have significantly improved the outcomes of liver resection during the last three decades. Liver surgery has inherent challenges, including difficult anticipation of complex and variable intrahepatic anatomy and the need for cognitive analysis by the surgeon to integrate preoperative imaging information into the operative field. Therefore, simulation and navigation techniques have been developed in this field.

In preoperative simulation, three-dimensional (3D) simulation technology was developed in Germany in the early 2000s,[1] and immediately thereafter software based on an original algorithm was developed in Japan. The development of intraoperative navigation techniques may also help surgeons to perform liver resections as planned. Intraoperative navigation began with intraoperative ultrasound (US) in 1980[2] and progressed to virtual hepatectomy (Hx),[3-7] real-time virtual sonography,[8-12] and finally indocyanine green (ICG) fluorescence.[13-20] Thus, intraoperative navigation has gradually evolved during the past 40 y.

This biannual review discusses the essential updates to simulation and navigation in Hx that occurred in the 2-y period from 2020 to 2021.

2 | PREOPERATIVE SIMULATION

Preoperative 3D simulation has enabled surgeons to obtain a great deal of information, such as detailed anatomical visualization, the precise volume of each segment and each hepatic venous drainage area, and prediction of postoperative liver failure (POLF). As a result, more aggressive and complicated surgeries can be safely performed. We herein summarize the recent refinements of preoperative simulation in liver surgery from 2020 to 2021 (Table 1).

2.1 | Anatomical visualization: 3D printing liver and extended reality

If a 3D liver model including the tumor, each vessel, and the liver parenchyma is created, it is meaningless to display that model on a 2D monitor or printed paper because of the lack of spatial awareness. Therefore, many reports have described the usefulness of 3D printing of liver models for operative planning or medical education.[21-23] Because 3D printing of the liver results in a model of the patient's own liver, accurate information can be obtained regarding the vessel anatomy, the relationship between the tumor and vessels, and the parenchymal cutting plane. Another advantage of 3D printing is that the operator can freely pick up the patient's own liver. The material used for 3D printing is also being developed in various ways. However, the high cost and complexity of the creation process are undeniable.

Recently, new technologies involving virtual reality (VR), augmented reality (AR), and mixed reality (MR), all of which can be referred to as extended reality (XR), have been developed and applied to various operative simulations. Head mount displays (HMDs) intrinsically provide the user with an egocentric viewpoint and allow the user to work hands-free without a monitor. Especially in VR, the surgeons can be immersed in the patient's own liver. The merits of the application of XR techniques to surgical support include no need for a sterilized display monitor, better spatial awareness, and the ability to share 3D images among all surgeons.[24] XR techniques are applied to preoperative planning or visualization of vessels in liver surgery,[25-27] and XR images are suitable for clinical presentation because of their sharing function. Huettl et al[25] compared 3D printed liver models and VR liver models and concluded that 3D VR liver models enable a better and partially faster anatomical orientation than 3D printed liver models. XR technology is still in its early stages. HMDs should be refined into lighter, simpler, and easier to operate devices.

2.2 | Volumetry: Portal perfusion and venous drainage

Preoperative volumetry is essential to ensuring safe hepatic resection by estimating the volume of both the portal perfusion and venous drainage area. In 2020–2021, Saito et al[28] proposed Hx based on a hybrid concept of the portal perfusion of the anterior segment and venous drainage area of the superior right hepatic vein. The perfusion area of the anterior segment crossed over the superior right

TABLE 1 Preoperative simulation in liver surgery

Author	Year	Category	Article type/Patients' number	Information
Ozer[21]	2021	Anatomical visualization	A case study (n = 5) Questionnaire (n = 22)	3D printing porta-celiac vascular model Surgical plan for resident trainees in Hx
Kuroda[22]	2020	Anatomical visualization	A case study (n = 5) Comparison of surgical outcomes (n = 212)	3D printing liver model Vessel's simulation in donor Hx of LDLT
Larghi[24] Laureiro[23]	2020	Anatomical visualization	A case study (n = 1)	3D printing liver model Surgical plan in hilar cholangiocarcinoma
Huettl[25]	2021	Anatomical visualization	A case study (n = 20) Questionnaire (n = 20)	VR liver Preoperative visualization of vessels in Hx
Boedecker[26]	2021	Anatomical visualization	A case study (n = 1)	VR (immersive into liver) Surgical plan/Clinical presentation in Hx
Pelanis[27]	2020	Anatomical visualization	A case study (n = 1) Questionnaire (n = 28)	MR liver Preoperative visualization of vessels in Hx
Saito[28]	2020	Volumetry	Retrospective single-center study (n = 66)	Hx based on hybrid concept of portal perfusion and venous drainage area
Li[29]	2021	Volumetry	Retrospective single-center study (n = 102)	Simulation of portal or venous associated remnant liver ischemia or congestion
Procopio[30]	2021	Prediction of POLF	Retrospective single-center study (n = 30)	Volumetry using 3D simulation
Araki[32]	2020	Prediction of POLF	Retrospective single-center study (n = 155)	SI in remnant liver with ROB-MRI
Notake[33]	2021	Prediction of POLF	Retrospective single-center study (n = 67)	SI in remnant liver with ROB-MRI

Abbreviations: EOB-MRI, ethoxybenzyl-magnetic; Hx, hepatectomy; LDLT, living-donor liver transplantation; MR, mixed reality; SI, signal intensity; VR, virtual reality.

hepatic vein in one-fourth of the patients in the study. The authors considered that less invasive Hx based on a hybrid concept might be an alternative to right Hx. Li et al[29] preoperatively simulated portal or hepatic vein-associated remnant liver ischemia or congestion, and it led to postoperative complications.

2.3 | Prediction of POLF

Aside from 3D reconstruction or simulation software, also simple liver function simulation is also critical in liver surgery. Preoperative volumetry can estimate the remnant liver volume and predict POLF.[30] Gadolinium ethoxybenzyl diethylenetriamine pentaacetic acid (Gd-EOB-DTPA)-enhanced magnetic resonance imaging (EOB-MRI) can also be used to evaluate liver functional reserve.[31] Functional remnant liver volumetry with signal intensity in EOB-MRI can precisely predict POLF of Hx involving more than one segment.[32] EOB-MRI is also useful for predicting POLF after major Hx for biliary malignancy.[33] In terms of a "one-stop shop" of preoperative simulation, EOB-MRI may be the most useful modality for detecting tumors, simulating vessel anatomy, and estimating remnant functional reserve.

3 | INTRAOPERATIVE NAVIGATION

Navigation in liver surgery began in 1985 when Makuuchi et al[2] performed anatomical resection with dye staining using intraoperative US. Various medical devices have been developed to support the safety and certainty of liver surgery with recent advances in medical engineering technology.

Fluorescent navigation using ICG has been clinically applied in various ways for liver navigation surgery. As described above for preoperative simulation, XR techniques have also been applied to intraoperative support systems. Furthermore, artificial intelligence (AI) technology has been introduced to intraoperative navigation. We herein summarize the recent refinements of intraoperative navigation in liver surgery from 2020 to 2021.

3.1 | ICG staining

Indocyanine green emits a fluorescent wavelength and is clearly visualized when irradiated with near-infrared light (760 nm). In total, 73 articles were found in PubMed in 2020–2021 using the search terms "ICG" and "Liver surgery"; articles describing the intraoperative use of ICG were more limited and can be classified into liver area staining or tumor detection. Recently, ICG has also been widely used in laparoscopic surgery (Table 2).

In 2021, consensus recommendations were established for the use of fluorescence imaging with ICG in hepatobiliary surgery.[34] Seven recommendations were formulated. In area staining, the consensus states that "ICG is helpful in delineating segmental boundaries in both open and minimally invasive liver resection (Recommendation Class IIa/IIb)." In tumor imaging, the consensus states that "ICG is helpful to localize subcapsular tumors within 8 mm of the liver surface or cut surface of the liver parenchyma, and may reduce the risk of positive margins (Recommendation Class IIa/IIb)."

The usefulness of positive and negative staining of each segment has been fully reported. In a retrospective single-center study of 120 cases, Lu et al[35] reported that ICG staining contributed to a shorter operative time and lower amount of intraoperative blood loss and that it helped to achieve a wide surgical margin. Furthermore, ICG staining was performed in special types of Hx, such as laparoscopic donor Hx,[36] robotic Hx,[37] and Hx for hepatolithiasis.[38] Kubo et al[39] used ICG staining for navigation of the venous drainage area of the right hepatic vein. Collaboration with a preoperative 3D simulation modality and intraoperative ICG staining with AR techniques was also introduced in 30 patients undergoing laparoscopic Hx.[40] This new navigation technology contributed to better surgical outcomes; however, its effect on the long-term prognosis remains unclear. In terms of the technical performance of ICG staining, although negative staining is relatively easy, positive staining is sometimes difficult, depending on the location of the tumors, especially in laparoscopic Hx. Xu et al[41] described their failed cases of positive staining, reporting a success rate of around 50%. Performing positive staining requires the surgeon to be proficient in intraoperative laparoscopic US (LUS), comfortable performing US-guided puncture, and skillful in interpreting the preoperative 3D image simulation. The manipulation of LUS is the most demanding part. Therefore, a new kind of LUS probe should be developed for useful positive staining in the future. Because LUS is difficult, Aoki et al[42] performed US-guided preoperative positive percutaneous staining immediately before laparoscopic surgery. This was a very simple technique and may be a reasonable way to resolve the technical difficulty of the procedure.

In tumor detection, ICG is useful to identify not only intrahepatic tumors[43] but also extrahepatic metastatic tumors such as those in the adrenal gland[44] or abdominal wall.[45] Tumor detection with ICG contributes to the safe achievement of surgical margins during liver resection.[46] Purich et al[47] performed a systematic review and meta-analysis of the diagnostic test accuracy of ICG. The sensitivity of intraoperative ICG-related imaging for superficial tumors was high; however, the overall sensitivity was low, at 0.75, suggesting that this technique would have to be used in combination with current identification methods such as intraoperative US. Their study also showed that intraoperative ICG fluorescence imaging was able to detect additional malignant hepatic tumors in 11.6% of patients.

3.2 | XR

In XR techniques, VR is useful for preoperative simulation, allowing the surgeon to become immersed in the patient's own liver with

TABLE 2 ICG navigation in liver surgery

Author	Year	Category	Article type/Patients' number	Information
Wang[34]	2021	Area staining/Tumor detection	Guideline	Recommendation Class; IIa or IIb Evidence level; II-2 or II-3
Lu[35]	2021	Area staining	Retrospective single-center study (n = 120)	Better short-term outcomes and surgical margin
Kim[36]	2021	Area staining	Retrospective single-center study (n = 76)	Laparoscopic donor's Hx Demarcating exact midplane
Marino[37]	2020	Area staining	Retrospective single-center study (n = 40) Positive (n = 20) and Negative (20) staining	Robotic-assisted Hx
He[38]	2020	Area staining	A randomized controlled trial (n = 46)	Hx for hepatolithiasis Better short-term outcomes
Kubo[39]	2020	Area staining	Retrospective single-center study (n = 12)	Determining areas of liver congestion of RHV
Zhang[40]	2020	Area staining	Retrospective single-center study (n = 64)	Collaboration with preoperative 3D simulation and intraoperative ICG
Xu[41]	2020	Area staining	Retrospective single-center study (n = 36)	Technical difficulty in positive staining (Success rate; around 50%)
Aoki[42]	2020	Area staining	A case study (n = 14)	Preoperative positive percutaneous staining before laparoscopic surgery
Lim[43]	2021	Tumor detection	Retrospective single-center study (n = 32)	Detection of intrahepatic tumors
Yamamura[44]	2020	Tumor detection	A case study (n = 1)	Detection of extrahepatic tumors
Hayashi[45]	2021	Tumor detection	A case study (n = 1)	Detection of extrahepatic tumors
Tashiro[46]	2020	Tumor detection	Retrospective single-center study (n = 125)	Better surgical margin
Purich[47]	2020	Prediction of POLF	A systematic review and meta-analysis	overall sensitivity; 0.75 Additional tumor detection; 11.6%

Abbreviation: RHV, right hepatic vein.

TABLE 3 XR navigation in liver surgery

Author	Year	Category	Article type/Patients' number	Information
Golse[48]	2021	AR overlay	A case study (n = 5)	Real-time marker less registration with RGB-D camera
Espinel[49]	2020	AR overlay	A case study (n = 7)	Laparoscope and liver surface as landmark Average registration error <1.0 cm
Prevost[50]	2020	AR overlay	A case study (n = 10)	Laparoscope and 4 points as landmark Mean fiducial registration error 14 mm
Bertrand[51]	2020	AR overlay	A case study (n = 17)	"Hepataug system" Safety and feasibility
Pelanis[52]	2021	AR overlay	A case study (n = 4)	Cone beam CT / Optical tracking system Mean target registration error 3.8 mm
Zhang[53]	2020	AR overlay	Retrospective single-center study (n = 85)	AR contributed to less blood loss and shorter hospital stays
Saito[23]	2020	MR hologram	A case study (n = 2)	Last-minute simulation before Gliisonean pedicle approach
Saito[55]	2021	MR hologram	A case study (n = 2)	Anatomy understanding of intrahepatic anatomy especially in B1 origination
Aoki[56]	2020	MR hologram	A case study (n = 1)	Holography-guided percutaneous puncture in positive staining

Abbreviations: AR, augmented reality; CT, computed tomography; RGB, right green blue.

better spatial awareness. AR or MR techniques should be used with intraoperative navigation tools because surgeons must examine the real operative field in both open and laparoscopic surgery.

In total, 27 articles were found in PubMed in 2020–2021 using the search terms "VR/AR/MR" and "Liver surgery" (Table 3). Most of these reports focused on AR-guided navigation. A preoperatively reconstructed 3D liver model should be overlaid onto the real liver. Unlike for neurosurgery, otolaryngology, and orthopedic surgery, in which rigid structures facilitate a rather unproblematic registration, liver surgery is associated with the problem of deformation of abdominal tissues and organs. This deformation results in a difficult registration procedure, potentially requiring nonrigid registration techniques to achieve sufficient registration accuracy. Therefore, various ways to perform registration of a preoperative 3D liver model have been developed.

Golse et al[48] placed a special camera called the e RGB-D camera in the operation room to perform real-time markerless registration in open liver surgery. In laparoscopic surgery, combination techniques with intraoperative calibration of the laparoscope and various landmarks to define the liver anatomy such as the falciform ligament, edge of the liver, and gall bladder are commonly used.[49-51] Pelanis et al[52] performed intraoperative cone-beam computed tomography (CT) and used an optical tracking system in registration. Target registration error and fiducial registration error were evaluated in those reports[49-52] and ranged from 3.0–14.0 mm. Such an AR overlay navigation system contributed to a reduction in vascular injury and more rapid postoperative recovery.[53] Therefore, more refinements of accurate registration should be implemented in the future.

Mixed reality techniques with 3D computer-generated models called holograms have also been introduced intraoperatively with HMDs. Saito et al used a hologram based on preoperative CT immediately before performing the Glissonean pedicle approach in Hx[54] and a hologram based on intraoperative cholangiography immediately before dissecting the intrahepatic bile duct in biliary surgery.[55] Operators and assistants can share the same hologram from each angle with HMDs and observe the detailed biliary anatomy around the dissected bile duct (Video S1). A system called a "virtual session" was also recently introduced. Conductor (operator), two assistants and a remote participant, who is not in the operating room, can share the hologram in the metaverse. Conductor explains the operative plan to assistants and the remote participant. We plan to apply this system in the field of remote medical care in the near future (Video S2). Strictly speaking, holograms contribute to "last-minute simulation," not navigation. However, the hologram might be a new next-generation operation-support tool in terms of spatial awareness, sharing, and simplicity. Aoki et al[56] also reported holography-guided percutaneous puncture in positive staining with ICG in laparoscopic surgery. As described in the ICG navigation section, positive staining especially in laparoscopic Hx is sometimes difficult, depending on the location of the tumors. This holographic guidance might help the operator to develop a better imagination.

3.3 | AI

Artificial intelligence technology was recently introduced to surgical navigation. AI should provide image recognition, focusing on anatomical structures, image recognition focusing on the surgical procedure itself, and control against incorrect performance of the surgical procedure. AI can already reportedly recognize the surgical process,[57] surgical instruments such as laparoscopic forceps,[58] and anatomical landmarks[59,60] in cholecystectomy or colorectal surgery. AI has also been applied to assessment of surgical skill.[61]

Nazir et al[62] reported a new searching and tagging system that recognizes various anatomical landmarks in laparoscopic liver surgery. Only one article focused on intraoperative navigation with AI in liver surgery from 2020–2021. AI is not yet frequently used in liver surgery, but future technological applications are expected.

To date, AI has only been used for the recognition of anatomical structures based on information of surgical field images. In the future, some suggestions or attention on anatomical structure information that cannot be directly seen in the surgical field are expected. Furthermore, an integrated analysis of real surgical field images and preoperative modalities should be developed for AI navigation surgery.

4 | CONCLUSION

The current status of simulation and navigation in hepatectomy from 2020 to 2021 has been reviewed. Preoperative simulation technology is already almost fully established; the next step is navigation in liver surgery. ICG staining is now widely used for area staining and tumor detection. Some refinements should be developed in terms of positive staining in laparoscopic liver surgery. XR techniques provide amazing new information regarding the liver anatomy, with better spatial awareness; however, the problems of registration and real-time liver deformity remain to be solved. Finally, the development of AI technology is ongoing. The establishment of various simulation and navigation technologies should help surgeons to perform safer liver resection.

REFERENCES

1. Selle D, Preim B, Schenk A, Peitgen HO. Analysis of vasculature for liver surgical planning. IEEE Trans Med Imaging. 2002;21:1344–57.
2. Makuuchi M, Hasegawa H, Yamazaki S. Ultrasonically guided subsegmentectomy. Surg Gynecol Obstet. 1985;161:346–50.
3. Oshiro Y, Yano H, Mitani J, Kim S, Kim J, Fukunaga K, et al. Novel 3-dimensional virtual hepatectomy simulation combined with real-time deformation. World J Gastroenterol. 2015;21(34):9982–92.
4. Oshiro Y, Ohkohchi N. Three-dimensional liver surgery simulation: computer-assisted surgical planning with three-dimensional simulation software and three-dimensional printing. Tissue Eng Part A. 2017;23(11-12):474–80.
5. Mise Y, Tani K, Aoki T, Sakamoto Y, Hasegawa K, Sugawara Y, et al. Virtual liver resection: computer-assisted operation planning using a three-dimensional liver representation. Kokudo N J Hepatobiliary Pancreat Sci. 2013;20(2):157–64.

6. Mise Y, Hasegawa K, Satou S, Shindoh J, Miki K, Akamatsu N, et al. How has virtual hepatectomy changed the practice of liver surgery?: Experience of 1194 virtual hepatectomy before liver resection and living donor liver transplantation. Ann Surg. 2018;268(1):127–33.
7. Aoki T, Murakami M, Koizumi T, Fujimori A, Gareer H, Enami Y, et al. Three-dimensional virtual endoscopy for laparoscopic and thoracoscopic liver resection. J Am Coll Surg. 2015;221(2):e21–6.
8. Sandulescu L, Saftoiu A, Dumitrescu D, Ciurea T. The role of real-time contrast-enhanced and real-time virtual sonography in the assessment of malignant liver lesions. J Gastrointestin Liver Dis. 2009;18(1):103–8.
9. Kasuya K, Sugimoto K, Kyo B, Nagakawa Y, Ikeda T, Mori Y, et al. Ultrasonography-guided hepatic tumor resection using a real-time virtual sonography with indocyanine green navigation (with videos). J Hepatobiliary Pancreat Sci. 2011;18(3):380–5.
10. Satou S, Aoki T, Kaneko J, Sakamoto Y, Hasegawa K, Sugawara Y, et al. Initial experience of intraoperative three-dimensional navigation for liver resection using real-time virtual sonography. Surgery. 2014;155(2):255–62.
11. Takamoto T, Mise Y, Satou S, Kobayashi Y, Miura K, Saiura A, et al. Feasibility of intraoperative navigation for liver resection using real-time virtual sonography with novel automatic registration system. World J Surg. 2018;42(3):841–8.
12. Lv A, Li Y, Qian HG, Qiu H, Hao CY. Precise navigation of the surgical plane with intraoperative real-time virtual sonography and 3D simulation in liver resection. J Gastrointest Surg. 2018;22(10):1814–8.
13. Aoki T, Yasuda D, Shimizu Y, Odaira M, Niiya T, Kusano T, et al. Image-guided liver mapping using fluorescence navigation system with indocyanine green for anatomical hepatic resection. World J Surg. 2008;32(8):1763–7.
14. Aoki T, Murakami M, Koizumi T, Kusano T, Fujimori A, Enami Y, et al. Preoperative tattooing for precise and expedient localization of landmark in laparoscopic liver resection. J Am Coll Surg. 2015;221(5):e97–e101.
15. Ishizawa T, Fukushima N, Shibahara J, Masuda K, Tamura S, Aoki T, et al. Real-time identification of liver cancers by using indocyanine green fluorescent imaging. Cancer. 2009;115:2491–504.
16. Miyata A, Ishizawa T, Tani K, Shimizu A, Kaneko J, Aoki T, et al. Reappraisal of a dye-staining technique for anatomic hepatectomy by the concomitant use of indocyanine green fluorescence imaging. J Am Coll Surg. 2015;221:e27–36.
17. Gotoh K, Yamada T, Ishikawa O, Takahashi H, Eguchi H, Yano M, et al. A novel image-guided surgery of hepatocellular carcinoma by indocyanine green fluorescence imaging navigation. J Surg Oncol. 2009;100:75–9.
18. Kobayashi Y, Kawaguchi Y, Kobayashi K, Mori K, Arita J, Sakamoto Y, et al. Portal vein territory identification using indocyanine green fluorescence imaging: technical details and short-term outcomes. J Surg Oncol. 2017;116:921–31.
19. van der Vorst JR, Schaafsma BE, Hutteman M, Verbeek FP, Liefers GJ, Hartgrink HH, et al. Near-infrared fluorescence-guided resection of colorectal liver metastases. Cancer. 2013;119:3411–8.
20. Nishino H, Hatano E, Seo S, Nitta T, Saito T, Nakamura M, et al. Real-time navigation for liver surgery using projection mapping with indocyanine green fluorescence: development of the novel medical imaging projection system. Ann Surg. 2018;267(6):1134–40.
21. Ozer MA, Uguz A, Unalp OV, Coker A, Govsa F, Guler E, et al. Perceptions of porta-celiac vascular models for hepatic surgery and their use in residency training. Surg Radiol Anat. 2021;43(8):1359–71.
22. Kuroda S, Kihara T, Akita Y, Kobayashi T, Nikawa H, Ohdan H. Simulation and navigation of living donor hepatectomy using a unique three-dimensional printed liver model with soft and transparent parenchyma. Surg Today. 2020;50(3):307–13.
23. Saito Y, Sugimoto M, Imura S, Morine Y, Ikemoto T, Iwahashi S, et al. Intraoperative 3D hologram support with mixed reality techniques in liver surgery. Ann Surg. 2020;271(1):e4–7.
24. Larghi Laureiro Z, Novelli S, Lai Q, Mennini G, D'andrea V, Gaudenzi P, et al. There is a great future in plastics: personalized approach to the management of hilar cholangiocarcinoma using a 3-D-printed liver model. Dig Dis Sci. 2020;65(8):2210–5.
25. Huettl F, Saalfeld P, Hansen C, Preim B, Poplawski A, Kneist W, et al. Virtual reality and 3D printing improve preoperative visualization of 3D liver reconstructions-results from a preclinical comparison of presentation modalities and user's preference. Ann Transl Med. 2021;9(13):1074.
26. Boedecker C, Huettl F, Saalfeld P, Paschold M, Kneist W, Baumgart J, et al. Using virtual 3D-models in surgical planning: workflow of an immersive virtual reality application in liver surgery. Langenbecks Arch Surg. 2021;406(3):911–5.
27. Pelanis E, Kumar RP, Aghayan DL, Palomar R, Fretland ÅA, Brun H, et al. Use of mixed reality for improved spatial understanding of liver anatomy. Minim Invasive Ther Allied Technol. 2020;29(3):154–60.
28. Saito Y, Imura S, Morine Y, Ikemoto T, Yamada S, Shimada M. A hepatectomy based on a hybrid concept of portal perfusion of anterior segment and venous drainage area of superior right hepatic vein. Am Surg. 2020;3134820984872. Online ahead of print.
29. Li XL, Xu B, Zhu XD, Huang C, Shi GM, Shen YH, et al. Simulation of portal/hepatic vein associated remnant liver ischemia/congestion by three-dimensional visualization technology based on preoperative CT scan. Ann Transl Med. 2021;9(9):756.
30. Procopio F, Cimino M, Viganò L, Colombo AE, Franchi E, Costa G, et al. Prediction of remnant liver volume using 3D simulation software in patients undergoing R1vasc parenchyma-sparing hepatectomy for multiple bilobar colorectal liver metastases: reliability, clinical impact, and learning curve. HPB (Oxford). 2021;23(7):1084–94.
31. Yamada S, Shimada M, Morine Y, Imura S, Ikemoto T, Saito Y, et al. A new formula to calculate the resection limit in hepatectomy based on Gd-EOB-DTPA-enhanced magnetic resonance imaging. PLoS One. 2019;14(1):e0210579.
32. Araki K, Harimoto N, Kubo N, Watanabe A, Igarashi T, Tsukagoshi M, et al. Functional remnant liver volumetry using Gd-EOB-DTPA-enhanced magnetic resonance imaging (MRI) predicts post-hepatectomy liver failure in resection of more than one segment. HPB (Oxford). 2020;22(2):318–27.
33. Notake T, Shimizu A, Kubota K, Ikehara T, Hayashi H, Yasukawa K, et al. Hepatocellular uptake index obtained with gadoxetate disodium-enhanced magnetic resonance imaging in the assessment future liver remnant function after major hepatectomy for biliary malignancy. BJS Open. 2021;5(4):zraa048.
34. Wang X, Teh CSC, Ishizawa T, Aoki T, Cavallucci D, Lee SY, et al. Consensus guidelines for the use of fluorescence imaging in hepatobiliary surgery. Ann Surg. 2021;274(1):97–106.
35. Lu H, Gu J, Qian XF, Dai XZ. Indocyanine green fluorescence navigation in laparoscopic hepatectomy: a retrospective single-center study of 120 cases. Surg Today. 2021;51(5):695–702.
36. Kim J, Hong SK, Lim J, Lee JM, Cho JH, Choi Y, et al. Demarcating the exact midplane of the liver using indocyanine green near-infrared fluorescence imaging during laparoscopic donor hepatectomy. Liver Transpl. 2021;27(6):830–9.
37. Marino MV, Podda M, Fernandez CC, Ruiz MG, Fleitas MG. The application of indocyanine green-fluorescence imaging during robotic-assisted liver resection for malignant tumors: a single-arm feasibility cohort study. HPB (Oxford). 2020;22(3):422–31.
38. He K, Hong X, Chi C, Cai C, Wang K, Li P, et al. A new method of near-infrared fluorescence image-guided hepatectomy for patients with hepatolithiasis: a randomized controlled trial. Surg Endosc. 2020;34(11):4975–82.
39. Kubo N, Araki K, Harimoto N, Ishii N, Tsukagoshi M, Igarashi T, et al. Hepatic resection for the right hepatic vein drainage area with indocyanine green fluorescent imaging navigation. J Hepatobiliary Pancreat Sci. 2020;27(7):371–9.

40. Zhang P, Luo H, Zhu W, Yang J, Zeng N, Fan Y, et al. Real-time navigation for laparoscopic hepatectomy using image fusion of preoperative 3D surgical plan and intraoperative indocyanine green fluorescence imaging. Surg Endosc. 2020;34(8):3449–59.
41. Xu Y, Chen M, Meng X, Lu P, Wang X, Zhang W, et al. Laparoscopic anatomical liver resection guided by real-time indocyanine green fluorescence imaging: experience and lessons learned from the initial series in a single center. Surg Endosc. 2020;34(10):4683–91.
42. Aoki T, Koizumi T, Mansour DA, Fujimori A, Kusano T, Matsuda K, et al. Ultrasound-guided preoperative positive percutaneous indocyanine green fluorescence staining for laparoscopic anatomical liver resection. J Am Coll Surg. 2020;230(3):e7–e12.
43. Lim HJ, Chiow AKH, Lee LS, Tan SS, Goh BK, Koh YX, et al. Novel method of intraoperative liver tumour localisation with indocyanine green and near-i nfrared imaging. Singapore Med J. 2021;62(4):182–9.
44. Yamamura K, Beppu T, Sato N, Kinoshita K, Oda E, Yuki H, et al. Complete removal of adrenal metastasis in hepatocellular carcinoma using indocyanine green fluorescent imaging. Anticancer Res. 2020;40(10):5823–8.
45. Hayashi H, Shimizu A, Motoyama H, Kubota K, Notake T, Sugenoya S, et al. Usefulness and limitation of indocyanine green fluorescence for detection of peritoneal recurrence after hepatectomy for hepatocellular carcinoma: a case report. BMC Surg. 2021;21(1):107.
46. Tashiro Y, Aoki T, Hirai T, Koizumi T, Mansou DA, Kusano T, et al. Pathological validity of using near-infrared fluorescence imaging for securing surgical margins during liver resection. Anticancer Res. 2020;40(7):3873–82.
47. Purich K, Dang JT, Poonja A, Sun WYL, Bigam D, Birch D, et al. Intraoperative fluorescence imaging with indocyanine green in hepatic resection for malignancy: a systematic review and meta-analysis of diagnostic test accuracy studies. Surg Endosc. 2020;34(7):2891–903.
48. Golse N, Petit A, Lewin M, Vibert E, Cotin S. Augmented reality during open liver surgery using a markerless non-rigid registration system. J Gastrointest Surg. 2021;25(3):662–71.
49. Espinel Y, Özgür E, Calvet L, Le Roy B, Buc E, Bartoli A. Combining visual cues with interactions for 3D–2D registration in liver laparoscopy. Ann Biomed Eng. 2020;48(6):1712–27.
50. Prevost GA, Eigl B, Paolucci I, Rudolph T, Peterhans M, Weber S, et al. Efficiency, accuracy and clinical applicability of a new image-guided surgery system in 3D laparoscopic liver surgery. J Gastrointest Surg. 2020;24(10):2251–8.
51. Bertrand LR, Abdallah M, Espinel Y, Calvet L, Pereira B, Ozgur E, et al. A case series study of augmented reality in laparoscopic liver resection with a deformable preoperative model. Surg Endosc. 2020;34(12):5642–8.
52. Pelanis E, Teatini A, Eigl B, Regensburger A, Alzaga A, Kumar RP, et al. Evaluation of a novel navigation platform for laparoscopic liver surgery with organ deformation compensation using injected fiducials. Med Image Anal. 2021;69:101946.
53. Zhang W, Zhu W, Yang J, Xiang N, Zeng N, Hu H, et al. Augmented reality navigation for stereoscopic laparoscopic anatomical hepatectomy of primary liver cancer: preliminary experience. J Front Oncol. 2021;25(11):663236.
54. Saito Y, Sugimoto M, Imura S, Morine Y, Ikemoto T, Iwahashi S, et al. Intraoperative 3D hologram support with mixed reality techniques in liver surgery. Ann Surg. 2020;271(1):e4–7.
55. Saito Y, Sugimoto M, Morine Y, Imura S, Ikemoto T, Yamada S, et al. Intraoperative support with three-dimensional holographic cholangiography in hepatobiliary surgery. Langenbecks Arch Surg. 2021. Online ahead of print.
56. Aoki T, Koizumi T, Sugimoto M, Murakami M. Holography-guided percutaneous puncture technique for selective near-infrared fluorescence-guided laparoscopic liver resection using mixed-reality wearable spatial computer. Surg Oncol. 2020;35:476–7.
57. Kitaguchi D, Takeshita N, Matsuzaki H, Oda T, Watanabe M, Mori K, et al. Automated laparoscopic colorectal surgery workflow recognition using artificial intelligence: Experimental research. Int J Surg. 2020;79:88–94.
58. Yamazaki Y, Kanaji S, Matsuda T, Oshikiri T, Nakamura T, Suzuki S, et al. Automated surgical instrument detection from laparoscopic gastrectomy video images using an open source convolutional neural network platform. J Am Coll Surg. 2020;230(5):725–32.e1.
59. Tokuyasu T, Iwashita Y, Matsunobu Y, Kamiyama T, Ishikake M, Sakaguchi S, et al. Development of an artificial intelligence system using deep learning to indicate anatomical landmarks during laparoscopic cholecystectomy. Surg Endosc. 2021;35(4):1651–8.
60. Kitaguchi D, Takeshita N, Matsuzaki H, Hasegawa H, Honda R, Teramura K, et al. Computer-assisted real-time automatic prostate segmentation during TaTME: a single-center feasibility study. Surg Endosc. 2021;35(6):2493–9.
61. Kitaguchi D, Takeshita N, Matsuzaki H, Igaki T, Hasegawa H, Ito M. Development and validation of a 3-dimensional convolutional neural network for automatic surgical skill assessment based on spatio-temporal video analysis. JAMA Netw Open. 2021;4(8):e2120786.
62. Nazir A, Cheema MN, Sheng B, Li P, Li H, Yang P, et al. SPST-CNN: Spatial pyramid based searching and tagging of liver's intraoperative live views via CNN for minimal invasive surgery. J Biomed Inform. 2020;106:103430.

11

Pharmacological treatment to reduce pulmonary morbidity after esophagectomy

Hiroharu Shinozaki[1] | **Tadashi Matsuoka**[1] | **Soji Ozawa**[2]

[1]Department of Surgery, Saiseikai Utsunomiya Hospital, Tochigi, Japan

[2]Department of Gastroenterological Surgery, Tokai University School of Medicine, Kanagawa, Japan

Correspondence
Hiroharu Shinozaki, Department of Surgery, Saiseikai Utsunomiya Hospital, 911-1 Takebayashi, Utsunomiya, Tochigi, 321-0974 Japan.
Email: hiroharu_shinozaki@saimiya.com

Abstract

Esophagectomy for esophageal cancer is one of the most invasive procedures in gastrointestinal surgery. An invasive surgical procedure causes postoperative lung injury through the surgical procedure and one-lung ventilation during anesthesia. Lung injury developed by inflammatory response to surgical insults and oxidative stress is associated with pulmonary morbidity after esophagectomy. Postoperative pulmonary complications negatively affect the long-term outcomes; therefore, an effort to reduce lung injury improves overall survival after esophagectomy. Although significant evidence has not been established, various pharmacological treatments for reducing lung injury, such as administration of a corticosteroid, neutrophil elastase inhibitor, and vitamins are considered to have efficacy for pulmonary morbidity. In this review we survey the following topics: mediators during the perioperative periods of esophagectomy and the efficacy of pharmacological therapies for patients with esophagectomy on pulmonary complications.

KEYWORDS
esophageal cancer, esophagectomy, pharmacological treatment, pulmonary complication

1 | INTRODUCTION

Esophageal cancer is one of the major causes of cancer mortality worldwide, with more than 473,000 new cases and 436,000 deaths annually.[1] Esophagectomy for esophageal cancer plays an important role in the strategy for curative treatment, but is associated with considerable morbidity and mortality.[2-4] Morbidity after esophagectomy is significantly correlated with poor prognosis and especially pulmonary and infectious morbidities affected for long-term outcomes.[5-8] Several studies revealed that postoperative pulmonary complications may be an independent predictor of poor long-term survival in patients undergoing resection of esophageal cancers.[5,6,8] Among recent advances in the perioperative multidisciplinary treatments for the prevention of pulmonary complication,[9,10] we focus on pharmacological treatment and discuss immunological mechanisms related to lung injury caused by esophagectomy in this narrative review.

2 | MEDIATORS DURING THE PERIOPERATIVE PERIODS OF ESOPHAGECTOMY

2.1 | Lung injury during esophagectomy

As one of the most invasive procedures in gastrointestinal surgery, esophagectomy may occasionally cause lung injury postoperatively. Lung injury is associated with tissue injury by the surgical procedure and one-lung ventilation during anesthesia (Figure 1).[11] Surgical insults cause alterations in the hemodynamic, metabolic, and immune responses of patients in the perioperative period, resulting in postoperative complications such as pneumonia.[12] Furthermore, one-lung ventilation during the operation could damage bilateral lungs, that is, the collapsed lung and the other ventilated lung. In the ventilated lung, high lung volume and ventilating pressure, high fraction of inspired oxygen, and capillary shear stress are related to the development of lung injury.[13-15] On the other hand, in the collapsed lung, atelectasis and recruitment, ischemia-reperfusion injury, and manipulation on the lung during the operation are considered to be the main causes of lung injury.[16,17] Not only inflammatory response, but also oxidative stress plays a major role in the development of lung injury following esophagectomy.[11,18-21] In the inflammatory and oxidative stress response, the endothelial glycocalyx is considered to represent a common pathway for the lung injury development during one-lung ventilation, because the endothelial glycocalyx is damaged by most of the recognized lung injurious mechanisms.[22] This response spreads from local to systemic reaction, which is also known as the systemic inflammatory response syndrome (SIRS). SIRS is followed by a compensatory antiinflammatory response syndrome (CARS) as a sequential reaction, which potentially predisposes the host to septic complications.[23]

2.2 | Cytokine cascades and pulmonary inflammation

Various cytokine cascades, which consist of a complex biochemical network, are activated in acute response to surgical insults and work with diverse effects after invasive surgery. The invasive procedures such as esophagectomy sometimes cause an exaggerated production of proinflammatory cytokines, which can lead to systemic hemodynamic instability or metabolic derangements.[12] In particular, tumor necrosis factor-α (TNF-α) and interleukin 1β (IL-1β) are promoted by macrophages and monocytes at the primary local operative site, and play a key role during the acute phase response to surgical insults.[24] Stimulated by TNF-α and IL-1β, this acute phase response is followed by the production and release of interleukin (IL)-6.[25] Several previous studies reported that surgical insults produce inflammatory mediators such as IL-6, IL-8, high-mobility group box chromosomal protein-1 (HMGB-1), or neutrophil elastase in esophagectomy and the elevation of these mediators was associated with pulmonary inflammation.[26-28]

2.3 | Microcirculatory dysfunction and local inflammation

Higher invasive surgery generally tends to have more intraoperative blood loss and microcirculatory disturbances due to hypoperfusion, which is thought to involve endogenous TNF-α release.[12,29] These inflammatory responses are also associated with an increase in microvascular hyperpermeability, which can lead to postoperative complications such as lung injury and cardiovascular dysfunction.[29] Moreover, microcirculatory disturbances following high invasive surgery are also related to alterations in intestinal permeability, which

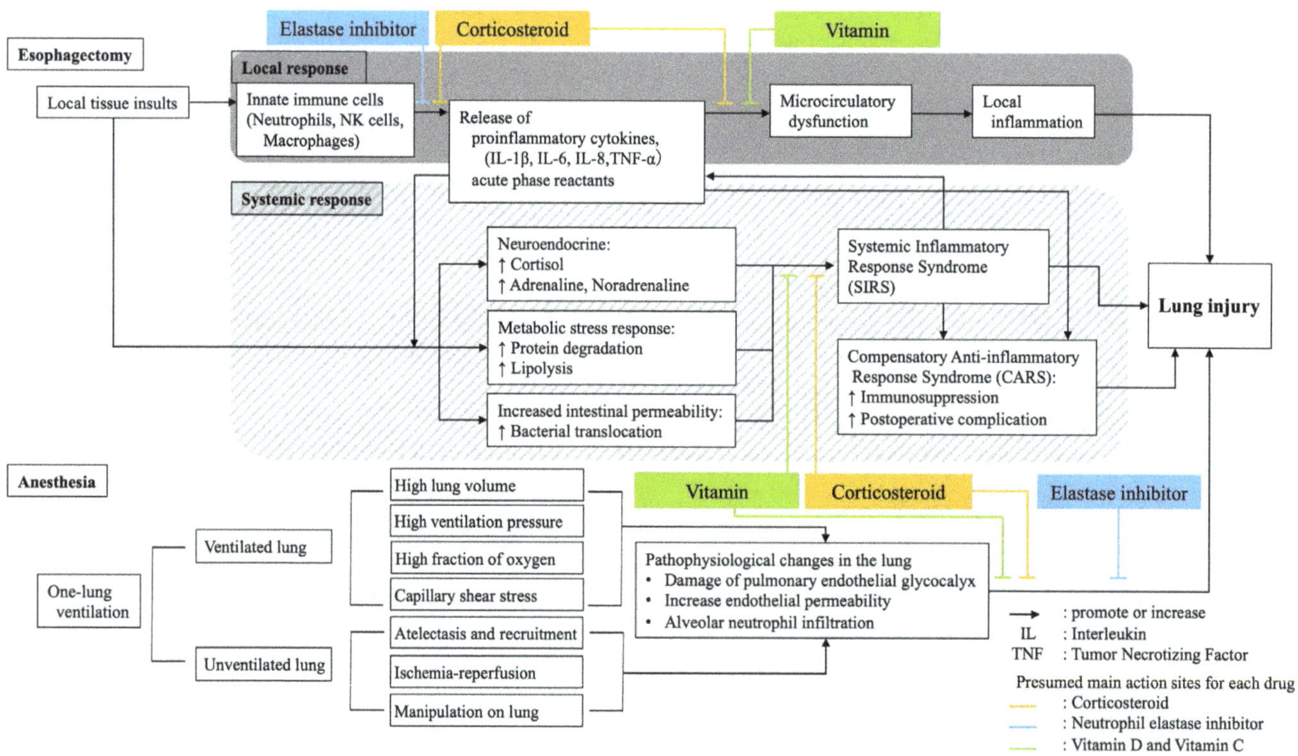

FIGURE 1 Schema of lung injury during esophagectomy. Colored lines indicate the presumed main action sites of each drug

can lead to postoperative bacterial translocation and can exacerbate surgically induced SIRS and postoperative lung injury following esophagectomy.[11,30,31]

2.4 | Metabolic alterations

Invasive surgery such as esophagectomy reduces metabolism for ~24 h postoperatively and subsequently causes a catabolic phase.[32] In the catabolic phase, an increase in endogenous steroid hormone as a counter-response, induced by TNF-α and IL-1β, causes inhibition of protein synthesis, increased muscular protein degradation, and mobilization of fats by lipolysis.[33-35] In postoperative metabolic alterations, which occurs frequently in invasive surgery, it is vital to attenuate the catabolic response and support an anabolic phase effectively, which follows a catabolic phase and yields protein synthesis.[36] Early enteral nutrition reduces the catabolic response to surgical stress and supports an anabolic phase effectively, which can improve surgical outcomes, including pulmonary complications.[36,37]

2.5 | Innate immune alterations

Although IL-6 functions as a proinflammatory cytokine in the early postoperative period, it can also exert antiinflammatory effects by attenuating TNF-α and IL-1 activity[38] and inducing macrophages to release prostaglandin E2 and IL-10,[39,40] which are central reactions in the CARS in esophagectomy.[41-44] Invasive surgery such as esophagectomy also produces alterations in innate immune homeostasis, in which, total systemic CD4+ and CD8+ T-lymphocyte counts are reduced markedly.[44-46] These immunosuppressed states in the CARS predispose the host to sepsis and are also associated with mortality and significant morbidity, such as postoperative pulmonary complications.[47-51] Moreover, these states have been associated with an increased rate of tumor progression and metastasis formation in patients with malignant diseases.

2.6 | Minimally invasive esophagectomy and inflammatory response

Recently, minimally invasive esophagectomy (MIE) such as thoracoscopic, mediastinoscopic, or robot-assisted esophagectomy is performed more frequently for esophageal cancer treatment. MIE reduces surgical insults, which are related to the reduction of mortality and morbidities.[52,53] In addition, it is reported that minimally invasive surgery including thoracoscopic and laparoscopic surgery can significantly reduce the rate of tumor progression when compared with open surgery, attenuating suppression of natural killer and lymphokine-activated killer cell cytotoxicity, which lead to prevention of the accelerated tumor growth.[54,55]

TABLE 1 Incidence of postoperative pulmonary complications after esophagectomy with or without steroids

			Patient number		Administration of the drug			Pulmonary complications				
Author	Study design	Year	MP group	Control	Dose	Timing	Duration	MP group (%)	Control (%)	Risk ratio	95% CI	P value
Yano et al[59]	RCT	2005	20	20	500 mg	Preoperative	120 min	6 (20)	3 (15)	2.00	(0.58-6.91)	.450
Takeda et al[65]	RCT	2003	7	10	10 mg/kg	Before anesthesia	NA	0 (0)	0 (0)	NA	NA	NA
Sato et al[48]	RCT	2002	33	33	10 mg/kg	Preoperative	30 min	3 (13)	10 (30)	0.30	(0.09-0.99)	.061
Takemura et al[60]	RCT	1999	9	9	250 mg	Preoperative	30 min	1 (11)	0 (0)	3.00	(0.14-65.16)	1.000
Matsutani et al[61]	RCT	1998	14	19	10 mg/kg	Before anesthesia	NA	0 (0)	2 (11)	0.27	(0.01-5.15)	.496
Takeda et al[62]	RCT	1997	15	15	30 mg/kg	Before anesthesia	NA	0 (0)	5 (33)	0.09	(0.01-1.51)	.042
Sayama et al[63]	RCT	1994	8	9	250 mg	Preoperative	120-180 min	1 (13)	1 (11)	1.13	(0.08-15.19)	1.000
Engelman et al[64]	Meta-analysis	210	175	171						0.41	(0.24-0.71)	
Weiji et al[58]	Meta-analysis	2014	281	286						0.69	(0.26-1.79)	

Abbreviations: MP, methylprednisolone; NA, not available; RCT, randomized control trial.

3 | PHARMACOLOGICAL TREATMENTS

In order to attenuate these acute responses, various treatments based on the pharmacological effect were developed and performed. Here we discuss and review some of the pharmacological treatments to reduce pulmonary complications in esophagectomy for esophageal cancer.

3.1 | Corticosteroid

Corticosteroid suppresses the production of cytokines such as IL-6 and TNF-α in monocytes and macrophages. In esophagectomy, these cytokines are associated with tissue injury from the surgical procedure and one-lung ventilation further develops postoperative lung injury. Therefore, the presence of a corticosteroid is considered to reduce lung injury by reducing these inflammatory and oxidative responses.[56] It was reported that corticosteroids had no effect on serum cytokines already released.[57] Therefore, a corticosteroid was mainly administrated preoperatively or at the induction of anesthesia, which was reported to reduce postoperative IL-6 levels and the incidence of peripheral leukocytopenia caused by surgical stress.[58]

Based on these theoretical mechanisms, the perioperative corticosteroid for patients with transthoracic esophagectomy was conventionally administered to improve mortality and pulmonary complications in Asia, especially in Japan. To evaluate the efficacy of perioperative corticosteroid, several studies were performed (Table 1).[48,59-65] Sato et al pointed out the effect of the preoperative methylprednisolone on the reduction of pulmonary complications.[48] On the other hand, Takeda et al reported no significant differences in the incidence of pulmonary complications.[65] As the sample size in each study was relatively small and, due to the lack of consensus, the efficacy of perioperative corticosteroid remains controversial. Engelman et al performed a meta-analysis from eight randomized control studies (RCTs) and reported that preoperative methylprednisolone usage significantly decreased the incidence of pulmonary complications without an increase of the incidence of other complications such as anastomotic leakage and infections.[64] On the other hand, Weijs et al performed a meta-analysis from seven RCTs and reported that there was no significant effect of perioperative methylprednisolone usage on the incidence of pulmonary complications or other complications such as anastomotic leakage and infections.[58] Based on these nonconclusive results, the Japanese esophageal cancer practice guidelines weakly recommend the clinical use of perioperative corticosteroid administration.[66,67] In addition, patients in these meta-analyses were all treated by transthoracic esophagectomy, and not MIE. To date, the efficacy of MIE has been reported and has become increasingly popular.[3,68-72] MIE is considered to reduce the invasiveness of the operation and decrease postoperative pulmonary complications.[68-70] Several studies evaluating the efficacy of MIE reported a significant reduction in the incidence of pulmonary complications compared to that of open esophagectomy.[71,72] Based on these reports, the efficacy of the perioperative corticosteroid for patients with MIE may be limited due to the relatively less incidence of pulmonary complication in MIE. To clarify the relationships between the use of the perioperative corticosteroid and MIE, further randomized controlled trials are needed.

3.2 | Neutrophil elastase inhibitor

Sivelestat sodium hydrate, a synthetic neutrophil elastase inhibitor, can competitively inhibit neutrophil elastase activity enhanced by IL-8 during surgical stress. This synthetic neutrophil elastase inhibitor is thought to be related to the increase in lung vascular permeability.[73-75] In addition, sivelestat sodium hydrate suppresses proinflammatory cytokines, including IL-1β and IL-6, similar to the mechanisms of corticosteroids.[28]

These antiinflammatory mechanisms are considered to improve postoperative lung injury in esophagectomy. Sivelestat sodium hydrate may be considered for clinical use to attenuate lung injury after esophagectomy,[26] but its use is not approved by insurance in Japan. Although several studies have shown the therapeutic effect of a neutrophil elastase inhibitor, its efficacy in a clinical setting remains controversial (Table 2).[27,28,76-81] Kuwahara et al reported that perioperative administration of neutrophil elastase inhibitor at the beginning of surgery did not shorten the duration of mechanical ventilation after thoracoscopic esophagectomy (median [h] interquartile range [IQR], 24.5 [24.3-28.7] vs 24.5 [23.9-49.1], $P = .796$).[27] On the other hand, Makino et al evaluated the efficacy of neutrophil elastase inhibitor in an RCT and reported that perioperative neutrophil elastase inhibitor at the beginning of surgery maintained postoperative pulmonary function following video-assisted esophagectomy and shortened the duration of mechanical ventilation (median [h] [IQR], 89.5 [57.3-121.7] vs 204 [77.4-330.6], $P = .046$).[76] Suda et al also reported that perioperative administration of neutrophil elastase inhibitor, which is intravenously administered immediately after surgery, shortened the duration of mechanical ventilation after transthoracic esophagectomy (median [day] [IQR], 1.5 [1-1.5] vs 2 [1.5-2], $P = .008$).[28] Due to the limited sample size and conflicting conclusion from these studies, Wang et al performed a systematic review and meta-analysis to evaluate the benefit and safety of neutrophil elastase inhibitor administration. This meta-analysis, including data from nine studies, revealed that neutrophil elastase inhibitor administration significantly decreased the duration of mechanical ventilation and the incidence of acute lung injury.[82] The administration of the neutrophil elastase inhibitor did not decrease the incidence of pneumonia, intensive care unit stay, or postoperative hospital stay. However, this meta-analysis included trials of non-RCTs and had dissimilar procedures, such as minimally invasive or traditional surgery, which could affect patient outcomes. In addition, the combined effect of corticosteroids and neutrophil elastase inhibitors was not evaluated. Therefore, multi-institutional RCTs with a large sample size are needed to validate the efficacy of perioperative neutrophil elastase inhibitor administration for esophagectomy.

TABLE 2 Incidence of postoperative pulmonary complications after esophagectomy with or without neutrophil elastase inhibitor

Author	Study design	Year	Surgical approach	Adjunct therapy	Patients number: EI Group	Patients number: Control	Administration of the drug: Dose	Administration of the drug: Timing	Administration of the drug: Duration	Pulmonary complications: EI Group	Pulmonary complications: Control	Risk ratio	95%CI	P value
[a]Kawahara et al[27]	RCT	2010	MIE	MP	10	10	300 mg/d	Beginning of surgery	72 h	2 (20%)	2 (20%)	1.00	(0.17–5.77)	1.000
[a]Makino et al[76]	RCT	2011	MIE	None	16	15	4.8 mg/kg/d	Beginning of surgery	7 d	4 (25%)	3 (20%)	1.25	(0.33–4.68)	1.000
[a]Ono et al[77]	Non–RCT	2007	Thoracotomy	None	7	10	4.8 mg/kg/d	ICU admission	6 d	0 (0%)	7 (70%)	0.09	(0.01–1.35)	0.004
[a]Mimatsu et al [78]	Non-RCT	2011	Thoracotomy	NA	22	20	4.8 mg/kg/d	ICU admission	5 d	NA	NA	1.21	(0.31–4.77)	NA
[a]Iwahashi et al[79]	Non-RCT	2011	Thoracotomy	MP	15/15	15	4.8 mg/kg/d	Closure of the chest	2 d/5 d	0 (0%)	1 (1%)	0.33	(0.01–7.58)	0.333
[a]Nishiyama et al[80]	Non-RCT	2012	Thoracotomy	None	26	27	4.8 mg/kg/d	Beginning of surgery	3 d	3 (10%)	4 (16%)	0.78	(0.19–3.15)	1.000
[a]Nagai et al[81]	Non-RCT	2013	Thoracotomy	MP	42	35	4.8 mg/kg/d	Beginning of surgery	3 d	5 (12%)	4 (11%)	1.04	(0.30–3.59)	1.000
[a]Wang,et al[82]	Meta-analysis	2015			153	147						0.84	(0.47–1.50)	
[b]Suda et al[28]	RCT	2007	Thoracotomy	None	18	25	4.8 mg/kg/d	Immediately after surgery	6 d	0 (0%)	1 (0%)	0.47	(0.02–11.01)	1.000
[b]Makino et al[76]	RCT	2011	MIE	None	16	15	4.8 mg/kg/d	Beginning of surgery	7 d	2 (13%)	8 (53%)	0.23	(0.06–0.93)	0.023
[b]Wang,et al[82]	Meta-analysis	2015			34	40						0.27	(0.08–0.93)	

Abbreviations: EI, neutrophil elastase inhibitor; MIE, minimally invasive esophagectomy; MP, methylprednisolone; NA, not available; RCT, randomized control trial.

[a]Pneumonia was evaluated as a pulmonary complication.

[b]Acute lung injury was evaluated as a pulmonary complication.

3.3 | Vitamins

Some vitamins have cell-protective effects. Vitamin D, which is a regulator of nitric oxide synthesis in endothelial cells, enhances the activity of antioxidative enzymes attenuating reactive oxygen species (ROS), and inhibits production of proinflammatory mediators such as TNF-α and IL-6 by suppressing nuclear factor kappa B (NF-κB) signaling. These protective effects of vitamin D are considered to protect the pulmonary endothelium[83] and are considered to reduce postoperative lung injury. Vitamin C also attenuates inflammatory cytokines such as TNF-α and IL-6. Vitamin C also reduces oxidative stress by scavenging free radicals, preventing further damage to the alveolar capillaries. Vitamin C inhibits the activation of neutrophil, resulting in the increase of alveolar fluid clearance and preventing lung vascular endothelial injury.[84] Studies have shown that these effects are synergically enhanced by the presence of corticosteroids.[84,85]

A couple of studies evaluated the efficacy of several vitamin therapies, including trials using vitamins D and C (Table 3). Parekh et al conducted a randomized, placebo-controlled trial to evaluate the efficacy of vitamin D for patients with open esophagectomy or MIE.[86] In this study, a single oral preoperative vitamin D administration did not improve postoperative lung function. On the other hand, recent studies reported that vitamin C was applied to various conditions such as septic shock and acute respiratory distress syndrome (ARDS).[84,85,87] We have reported the therapeutic effect of the combination therapy of vitamin C and corticosteroid on postoperative lung function after esophagectomy.[88] However, this study was a single-center retrospective study and a before-after study with a small sample size. Therefore, additional large-scale prospective studies are required.

3.4 | Others

Drugs that suppress the production of inflammatory mediators, such as cytokines or antioxidant agents that have cell-protective effects have the possibility of reducing pulmonary morbidity by attenuating lung injury during invasive surgery, theoretically. However, few drugs other than steroids, vitamin C, vitamin D, and neutrophil elastase inhibitor have been reported to be clinically effective. In this context, gas inhalation therapy might have the potential to reduce pulmonary morbidity after esophagectomy. β-agonist inhalation effectively treats ARDS through decreasing inflammatory cell infiltration and cytokine release, augmenting alveolar fluid clearance, and improving alveolar capillary barrier function.[89] However, Perkins et al reported that there is no significant difference in the incidence of ARDS in postoperative patients with esophagectomy between β-agonists, salmeterol, and placebo (odds ratio [OR], 1.25; 95% confidence interval [CI], 0.71-2.22).[90] Inhaled nitric oxide, a well-known inhalant for the treatment of lung injury, was considered to decrease pulmonary artery pressure and improve oxygenation, but has not shown efficacy for ARDS.

TABLE 3 Incidence of postoperative pulmonary complications after esophagectomy with or without vitamins

Drug					Patients number		Administration of the drug			Pulmonary complications					
Author	Study design	Year	Surgical approach	Adjunct therapy	Vit. Group	Control	Dose	Timing	frequency	Vit. Group	Control	Risk ratio	95% CI	P value	P/F ratio improvement
Vit. D															
Parekh et al[86]	RCT	2018	Thoracotomy	None	33	35	7.5 mg	Preopeartive	Single dose	17 (52%)	17 (49%)	1.06	(0.66-1.71)	1.000	No
Vit. C															
Matsuoka et al[88]	Non-RCT	2019	Thoracoscopy	MP	6	11	1.5 g	Beginning of surgery	Every 6 h for 4 d	2 (33%)	5 (45%)	0.73	(0.20-2.70)	1.000	Yes

Abbreviations: MP, methylprednisolone; RCT, randomized control trial; Vit., vitamin.

The specific therapeutic effects of nitric oxide inhalation for postoperative lung injury in esophagectomy remains unclear, as no study targeted the population of patients with esophagectomy.[91] These inhalation therapies need further investigation to be considered one of the mainstream treatment options.

4 | CONCLUSION

Lung injury following esophagectomy is associated with an invasive surgical procedure and one-lung ventilation during anesthesia. Surgical insults cause alterations in hemodynamic, metabolic, and immune responses, and one-lung ventilation damages bilateral lungs by inflammatory and oxidative stress responses. Local response to tissue insults spreads to a systemic response through inflammatory mediators resulting in lung injury. Some of the pharmacological treatments for preventing lung injury have the potential to improve pulmonary morbidity after esophagectomy. However, further prospective studies with large samples are needed to confirm the efficacy of those therapies to establish better perioperative management for esophagectomy.

ACKNOWLEDGMENTS

The authors thank Ms. Izu Inada (Department of Gastroenterological Surgery, Tokai University School of Medicine) for assisting us in preparing this article.

DISCLOSURE

Author Contribution: Hiroharu Shinozaki and Soji Ozawa devised the main conceptual ideas for this article. Hiroharu Shinozaki and Tadashi Matsuoka selected and reviewed references and wrote the initial draft of the manuscript. All authors critically reviewed the manuscript.

REFERENCES

1. Kamangar F, Nasrollahzadeh D, Safiri S, Sepanlou SG, Fitzmaurice C, Ikuta KS, et al. The global, regional, and national burden of oesophageal cancer and its attributable risk factors in 195 countries and territories, 1990–2017: a systematic analysis for the Global Burden of Disease Study 2017. Lancet Gastroenterol Hepatol. 2020;5:582–97.
2. Takeuchi H, Miyata H, Gotoh M, et al. A risk model for esophagectomy using data of 5354 patients included in a Japanese nationwide web-based database. Ann Surg. 2014;260:259–66.
3. Yoshida N, Yamamoto H, Baba H, et al. Can minimally invasive esophagectomy replace open esophagectomy for esophageal cancer? Latest analysis of 24,233 esophagectomies from the japanese national clinical database. Ann Surg. 2020;272:118–24.
4. Ozawa S, Koyanagi K, Ninomiya Y, Yatabe K, Higuchi T. Postoperative complications of minimally invasive esophagectomy for esophageal cancer. Ann Gastroenterol Surg. 2020;4:126–34.
5. Kataoka K, Takeuchi H, Mizusawa J, Igaki H, Ozawa S, Abe T, et al. Prognostic Impact of Postoperative Morbidity After Esophagectomy for Esophageal Cancer: Exploratory Analysis of JCOG9907. Ann Surg. 2017;265:1152–7.
6. Saeki H, Tsutsumi S, Tajiri H, Yukaya T, Tsutsumi R, Nishimura S, et al. Prognostic significance of postoperative complications after curative resection for patients with esophageal squamous cell carcinoma. Ann Surg. 2017;265:527–33.
7. Yamashita K, Makino T, Miyata H, Miyazaki Y, Takahashi T, Kurokawa Y, et al. Postoperative infectious complications are associated with adverse oncologic outcomes in esophageal cancer patients undergoing preoperative chemotherapy. Ann Surg Oncol. 2016;23:2106–14.
8. Baba Y, Yoshida N, Shigaki H, Iwatsuki M, Miyamoto Y, Sakamoto Y, et al. Prognostic impact of postoperative complications in 502 patients with surgically resected esophageal squamous cell carcinoma. Ann Surg. 2016;264:305–11.
9. Watanabe M, Okamura A, Toihata T, Yamashita K, Yuda M, Hayami M, et al. Recent progress in perioperative management of patients undergoing esophagectomy for esophageal cancer. Esophagus. 2018;15:160–4.
10. Yoshida N, Harada K, Iwatsuki M, Baba Y, Baba H. Precautions for avoiding pulmonary morbidity after esophagectomy. Ann Gastroenterol Surg. 2020;4:480–4.
11. Boshier P, Marczin N, Hanna G. Pathophysiology of acute lung injury following esophagectomy. Dis Esophagus. 2015;28:797–804.
12. Choileain NN, Redmond HP. Cell response to surgery. Arch Surg. 2006;141:1132–40.
13. Chu EK, Whitehead T, Slutsky AS. Effects of cyclic opening and closing at low-and high-volume ventilation on bronchoalveolar lavage cytokines. Crit Care Med. 2004;32:168–74.
14. Rozé H, Lafargue M, Batoz H, Picat MQ, Perez P, Ouattara A, et al. Pressure-controlled ventilation and intrabronchial pressure during one-lung ventilation. Br J Anaesth. 2010;105:377–81.
15. Lohser J, Slinger P. Lung injury after one-lung ventilation: a review of the pathophysiologic mechanisms affecting the ventilated and the collapsed lung. Anesth Analg. 2015;121:302–18.
16. Douzinas EE, Kollias S, Tiniakos D, Evangelou E, Papalois A, Rapidis AD, et al. Hypoxemic reperfusion after 120 mins of intestinal ischemia attenuates the histopathologic and inflammatory response. Crit Care Med. 2004;32:2279–83.
17. Silva PL, Moraes L, Santos RS, Samary C, Ramos MBA, Santos CL, et al. Recruitment maneuvers modulate epithelial and endothelial cell response according to acute lung injury etiology. Crit Care Med. 2013;41:e256–e265.
18. Ferrari RS, Andrade CF. Oxidative stress and lung ischemia-reperfusion injury. Oxid Med Cell Longev. 2015;2015:1–14.
19. Baudouin S. Lung injury after thoracotomy. Br J Anaesth. 2003;91:132–42.
20. Yamada T, Hisanaga M, Nakajima Y, Kanehiro H, Watanabe A, Ohyama T, et al. Serum interleukin-6, interleukin-8, hepatocyte growth factor, and nitric oxide changes during thoracic surgery. World J Surg. 1998;22:783–90.
21. Misthos P, Katsaragakis S, Milingos N, Kakaris S, Sepsas E, Athanassiadi K, et al. Postresectional pulmonary oxidative stress in lung cancer patients. The role of one-lung ventilation. Eur J Cardiothorac Surg. 2005;27:379–83.
22. Chappell D, Jacob M, Hofmann-Kiefer K, Bruegger D, Rehm M, Conzen P, et al. Hydrocortisone preserves the vascular barrier by protecting the endothelial glycocalyx. Anesthesiology. 2007;107:776–84.
23. Bone RC. Immunologic dissonance: a continuing evolution in our understanding of the systemic inflammatory response syndrome

(SIRS) and the multiple organ dysfunction syndrome (MODS). Ann Intern Med. 1996;125:680-7.
24. Baumann H, Gauldie J. The acute phase response. Immunol Today. 1994;15:74-80.
25. Baigrie R, Lamont P, Kwiatkowski D, Dallman M, Morris P. Systemic cytokine response after major surgery. Br J Surg. 1992;79:757-60.
26. Akamoto S, Okano K, Sano T, Yachida S, Izuishi K, Usuki H, et al. Neutrophil elastase inhibitor (sivelestat) preserves antitumor immunity and reduces the inflammatory mediators associated with major surgery. Surg Today. 2007;37:359-65.
27. Kawahara Y, Ninomiya I, Fujimura T, Funaki H, Nakagawara H, Takamura H, et al. Prospective randomized controlled study on the effects of perioperative administration of a neutrophil elastase inhibitor to patients undergoing video-assisted thoracoscopic surgery for thoracic esophageal cancer. Dis Esophagus. 2010;23:329-39.
28. Suda K, Kitagawa Y, Ozawa S, Miyasho T, Okamoto M, Saikawa Y, et al. Neutrophil elastase inhibitor improves postoperative clinical courses after thoracic esophagectomy. Dis Esophagus. 2007;20:478-86.
29. Yamauchi J-I, Vollmar B, Wolf B, Menger MD. Role of TNF-α in local surgical trauma-induced microvascular dysfunction. Dig Surg. 1999;16:400-6.
30. Roumen RM, van der Vliet JA, Wevers RA, Goris RJA. Intestinal permeability is increased after major vascular surgery. J Vasc Surg. 1993;17:734-7.
31. Rush B Jr. Irreversibility in hemorrhagic shock is caused by sepsis. Am Surg. 1989;55:204-8.
32. Woolf PD. Hormonal responses to trauma. Crit Care Med. 1992;20:216-26.
33. Hill A, Hill G. Metabolic response to severe injury. Br J Surg. 1998;85:884-90.
34. Singer M, De Santis V, Vitale D, Jeffcoate W. Multiorgan failure is an adaptive, endocrine-mediated, metabolic response to overwhelming systemic inflammation. Lancet. 2004;364:545-8.
35. Zamir O, Hasselgren P-O, Higashiguchi T, Frederick JA, Fischer JE. Tumour necrosis factor (TNF) and interleukin-1 (IL-1) induce muscle proteolysis through different mechanisms. Mediators Inflamm. 1992;1:247-50.
36. Wray CJ, Mammen JM, Hasselgren P-O. Catabolic response to stress and potential benefits of nutrition support. Nutrition. 2002;18:971-7.
37. Peng J, Cai J, Niu Z-X, Chen L-Q. Early enteral nutrition compared with parenteral nutrition for esophageal cancer patients after esophagectomy: a meta-analysis. Dis Esophagus. 2016;29:333-41.
38. Tilg H, Trehu E, Atkins MB, Dinarello CA, Mier JW. Interleukin-6 (IL-6) as an anti-inflammatory cytokine: induction of circulating IL-1 receptor antagonist and soluble tumor necrosis factor receptor p55. Blood. 1994;83:113-8.
39. Sheeran P, Hall G. Cytokines in anaesthesia. Br J Anaesth. 1997;78:201-19.
40. Ayala A, Lehman DL, Herdon CD, Chaudry IH. Mechanism of enhanced susceptibility to sepsis following hemorrhage: interleukin-10 suppression of T-cell response is mediated by eicosanoid-induced interleukin-4 release. Langenbecks Arch Surg. 1994;129:1172-8.
41. Mokart D, Capo C, Blache J, Delpero JR, Houvenaeghel G, Martin C, et al. Early postoperative compensatory anti-inflammatory response syndrome is associated with septic complications after major surgical trauma in patients with cancer. Br J Surg. 2002;89:1450-6.
42. Ogata M, Okamoto K, Kohriyama K, Kawasaki T, Itoh H, Shigematsu A. Role of interleukin-10 on hyporesponsiveness of endotoxin during surgery. Crit Care Med. 2000;28:3166-70.
43. Biffl WL, Moore EE, Moore FA, Peterson VM. Interleukin-6 in the injured patient: marker of injury or mediator of inflammation? Ann Surg. 1996;224:647-64.
44. Yamaguchi Y, Hihara J, Hironaka K, Ohshita A, Okita R, Okawaki M, et al. Postoperative immunosuppression cascade and immunotherapy using lymphokine-activated killer cells for patients with esophageal cancer: Possible application for compensatory anti-inflammatory response syndrome. Oncol Rep. 2006;15:895-901.
45. Yadavalli GK, Auletta JJ, Gould MP, Salata RA, Lee JH, Heinzel FP. Deactivation of the innate cellular immune response following endotoxic and surgical injury. Exp Mol Pathol. 2001;71:209-21.
46. Dietz A, Heimlich F, Daniel V, Polarz H, Weidauer H, Maier H. Immunomodulating effects of surgical intervention in tumors of the head and neck. Otolaryngol Head Neck Surg. 2000;123:132-9.
47. Okamura A, Takeuchi H, Matsuda S, Ogura M, Miyasho T, Nakamura R, et al. Factors affecting cytokine change after esophagectomy for esophageal cancer. Ann Surg Oncol. 2015;22:3130-5.
48. Sato N, Koeda K, Ikeda K, Kimura Y, Aoki K, Iwaya T, et al. Randomized study of the benefits of preoperative corticosteroid administration on the postoperative morbidity and cytokine response in patients undergoing surgery for esophageal cancer. Ann Surg. 2002;236:184-90.
49. Frick VO, Justinger C, Rubie C, Graeber S, Schilling MK, Lindemann W. Thoracotomy procedures effect cytokine levels after thoracoabdominal esophagectomy. Oncol Rep. 2012;27:258-64.
50. Angele MK, Faist E. Clinical review: Immunodepression in the surgical patient and increased susceptibility to infection. Crit Care. 2002;6:298.
51. Neidhardt R, Keel M, Steckholzer U, Safret A, Ungethuem U, Trentz O, et al. Relationship of Interleukin-10 plasma levels to severity of injury and clinical outcome in injured patients. J Trauma Acute Care Surg. 1997;42:863-71.
52. Brune IB, Wilke W, Hensler T, Holzmann B, Siewert JR. Downregulation of T helper type 1 immune response and altered pro-inflammatory and anti-inflammatory T cell cytokine balance following conventional but not laparoscopic surgery. Am J Surg. 1999;177:55-60.
53. Takeuchi H, Miyata H, Ozawa S, Udagawa H, Osugi H, Matsubara H, et al. Comparison of short-term outcomes between open and minimally invasive esophagectomy for esophageal cancer using a nationwide database in Japan. Ann Surg Oncol. 2017;24:1821-7.
54. Allendorf JD, Bessler M, Kayton ML, Oesterling SD, Treat MR, Nowygrod R, et al. Increased tumor establishment and growth after laparotomy vs laparoscopy in a murine model. Arch Surg. 1995;130:649-53.
55. Wildbrett P, Oh A, Carter JJ, Schuster H, Bessler M, Jaboci CA, et al. Increased rates of pulmonary metastases following sham laparotomy compared to CO2 pneumoperitoneum and the inhibition of metastases utilizing perioperative immunomodulation and a tumor vaccine. Surg Endosc. 2002;16:1162-9.
56. Gao Q, Mok HP, Wang WP, Xiao F, Chen LQ. Effect of perioperative glucocorticoid administration on postoperative complications following esophagectomy: a meta-analysis. Oncol Lett. 2014;7:349-56.
57. Riad M, Mogos M, Thangathurai D, Lumb PD. Steroids. Curr Opin Crit Care. 2002;8:281-4.
58. Weijs TJ, Dieleman JM, Ruurda JP, Kroese AC, Knape HJ, van Hillegersberg R. The effect of perioperative administration of glucocorticoids on pulmonary complications after transthoracic oesophagectomy: a systematic review and meta-analysis. Eur J Anaesthesiol. 2014;31:685-94.
59. Yano M, Taniguchi M, Tsujinaka T, Fujiwara Y, Yasuda T, Shiozaki H, et al. Is preoperative methylprednisolone beneficial for patients undergoing esophagectomy? Hepatogastroenterology. 2005;52:481-5.
60. Takemura S, Miya K, Takao H, Umemoto T, Saji S. Influence of corticosteroid preoperative administration for surgical stress of the oesophageal cancer patients during peri-and postoperative periods. Jpn J Gastroenterol Surg. 1999;32:1113-41.

61. Matsutani T, Onda M, Sasajima K, Miyashita M. Glucocorticoid attenuates a decrease of antithrombin III following major surgery. J Surg Res. 1998;79:158–63.
62. Takeda S, Ogawa R, Nakanishi K, Kim C, Miyashita M, Sasajima K, et al. The effect of preoperative high dose methylprednisolone in attenuating the metabolic response after oesophageal resection. Eur J Surg. 1997;163:511–7.
63. Sayama J, Shineha R, Yokota K-I, Hirayama K, Higuchi N, Ohe H, et al. Control of the excessive reaction after surgery for esophageal carcinoma with preoperative administration of the corticosteroids. Jpn J Gastroenterol Surg. 1994;27:841–8.
64. Engelman E, Maeyens C. Effect of preoperative single-dose corticosteroid administration on postoperative morbidity following esophagectomy. J Gastrointest Surg. 2010;14:788–804.
65. Takeda S, Takeda S, Kim C, Ikezaki H, Nakanishi K, Sakamoto A, et al. Preoperative administration of methylprednisolone attenuates cytokine-induced respiratory failure after esophageal resection. J Nippon Med Sch. 2003;70:16–20.
66. Kitagawa Y, Uno T, Oyama T, Kato K, Kato H, Kawakubo H, et al. Esophageal cancer practice guidelines 2017 edited by the Japan Esophageal Society: part 1. Esophagus. 2019;16:1–24.
67. Kitagawa Y, Uno T, Oyama T, et al. Esophageal cancer practice guidelines 2017 edited by the Japan esophageal society: part 2. Esophagus. 2019;16:25–43.
68. Naffouje SA, Salloum RH, Khalaf Z, Salti GI. Outcomes of open versus minimally invasive ivor-lewis esophagectomy for cancer: a propensity-score matched analysis of NSQIP database. Ann Surg Oncol. 2019;26:2001–10.
69. Yerokun BA, Sun Z, Yang CJ, Gulack BC, Speicher PJ, Adam MA, et al. Minimally invasive versus open esophagectomy for esophageal cancer: a population-based analysis. Ann Thorac Surg. 2016;102:416–23.
70. Sihag S, Kosinski AS, Gaissert HA, Wright CD, Schipper PH. Minimally invasive versus open esophagectomy for esophageal cancer: a comparison of early surgical outcomes from the society of thoracic surgeons national database. Ann Thorac Surg. 2016;101(4):1281–9; discussion 8–9.
71. Sakamoto T, Fujiogi M, Matsui H, Fushimi K, Yasunaga H. Comparing perioperative mortality and morbidity of minimally invasive esophagectomy versus open esophagectomy for esophageal cancer: a nationwide retrospective analysis. Ann Surg. 2019.
72. Kubo N, Ohira M, Yamashita Y, et al. The impact of combined thoracoscopic and laparoscopic surgery on pulmonary complications after radical esophagectomy in patients with resectable esophageal cancer. Anticancer Res. 2014;34:2399–404.
73. Duswald KH, Jochum M, Schramm W, Fritz H. Released granulocytic elastase: an indicator of pathobiochemical alterations in septicemia after abdominal surgery. Surgery. 1985;98:892–9.
74. Matsuzaki K, Hiramatsu Y, Homma S, Sato S, Shigeta O, Sakakibara Y. Sivelestat reduces inflammatory mediators and preserves neutrophil deformability during simulated extracorporeal circulation. Ann Thorac Surg. 2005;80:611–7.
75. Tamakuma S, Ogawa M, Aikawa N, Kubota T, Hirasawa H, Ishizaka A, et al. Relationship between neutrophil elastase and acute lung injury in humans. Pulm Pharmacol Ther. 2004;17:271–9.
76. Makino H, Kunisaki C, Kosaka T, Akiyama H, Morita S, Endo I. Perioperative use of a neutrophil elastase inhibitor in video-assisted thoracoscopic oesophagectomy for cancer. Br J Surg. 2011;98:975–82.
77. Ono S, Tsujimoto H, Hiraki S-I, Takahata R, Kimura A, Kinoshita M, et al. Effects of neutrophil elastase inhibitor on progression of acute lung injury following esophagectomy. World J Surg. 2007;31:1996–2001.
78. Mimatsu K, Oida T, Kawasaki A, Kano H, Kuboi Y, Amano S. Influence of neutrophil elastase inhibitor on the postoperative course in patients with esophageal cancer after transthoracic esophagectomy. Hepatogastroenterology. 2011;58:1583–7.
79. Iwahashi M, Nakamori M, Nakamura M, Ojima T, Naka T, Yamaue H. Optimal period for the prophylactic administration of neutrophil elastase inhibitor for patients with esophageal cancer undergoing esophagectomy. World J Surg. 2011;35:1573–9.
80. Nishiyama J, Matsuda M, Ando S, Hirasawa M, Suzuki T, Makuuchi H. The effects of the early administration of sivelestat sodium, a selective neutrophil elastase inhibitor, on the postoperative course after radical surgery for esophageal cancer. Surg Today. 2012;42:659–65.
81. Nagai Y, Watanabe M, Baba Y, Iwatsuki M, Hirashima K, Karashima R, et al. Preventive effect of sivelestat on postoperative respiratory disorders after thoracic esophagectomy. Surg Today. 2013;43:361–6.
82. Wang ZQ, Chen LQ, Yuan Y, Wang WP, Niu ZX, Yang YS, et al. Effects of neutrophil elastase inhibitor in patients undergoing esophagectomy: a systematic review and meta-analysis. World J Gastroenterol. 2015;21:3720–30.
83. Chen SF. 1 alpha, 25-Dihydroxyvitamin D3 decreased ICAM-1 and ELAM-1 expressions on pulmonary microvascular endothelial cells and neutrophil motivation. J Steroid Biochem Mol Biol. 1995;52:67–70.
84. Marik PE. Hydrocortisone, ascorbic acid and thiamine (HAT Therapy) for the treatment of sepsis. Focus on ascorbic acid. Nutrients. 2018;10:1762.
85. Marik PE, Khangoora V, Rivera R, Hooper MH, Catravas J. Hydrocortisone, vitamin C, and thiamine for the treatment of severe sepsis and septic shock: a retrospective before-after study. Chest. 2017;151:1229–38.
86. Parekh D, Dancer RCA, Scott A, D'Souza VK, Howells PA, Mahida RY, et al. Vitamin D to prevent lung injury following esophagectomy-a randomized placebo-controlled trial. Crit Care Med. 2018;46:e1128–e1135.
87. Marik PE, Long A. ARDS complicating pustular psoriasis: treatment with low-dose corticosteroids, vitamin C and thiamine. BMJ Case Rep. 2018;2018:bcr2017223475.
88. Matsuoka T, Shinozaki H, Ozawa S, Izawa Y, Koyanagi K, Kawarai Lefor A, et al. Administration of corticosteroids, ascorbic acid, and thiamine improves oxygenation after thoracoscopic esophagectomy. Ann Thorac Cardiovasc Surg. 2020;26:133–9.
89. Perkins GD, McAuley DF, Richter A, Thickett DR, Gao F. Bench-to-bedside review: beta2-Agonists and the acute respiratory distress syndrome. Crit Care. 2004;8:25–32.
90. Perkins GD, Gates S, Park D, Gao F, Knox C, Holloway B, et al. The beta agonist lung injury trial prevention. A randomized controlled trial. Am J Respir Crit Care Med. 2014;189:674–83.
91. Adhikari NK, Dellinger RP, Lundin S, Payen D, Vallet B, Gerlach H, et al. Inhaled nitric oxide does not reduce mortality in patients with acute respiratory distress syndrome regardless of severity: systematic review and meta-analysis. Crit Care Med. 2014;42:404–12.

12

Usefulness of bacterial culture of drainage fluid for predicting surgical site infection after crohn's disease surgery

Momoko Ichihara[1] | Takayuki Ogino[1,2] | Makoto Fujii[3] | Naotsugu Haraguchi[1] | Hidekazu Takahashi[1] | Norikatsu Miyoshi[1] | Mamoru Uemura[1] | Yuichiro Doki[1] | Hidetoshi Eguchi[1] | Tsunekazu Mizushima[1,2]

[1]Department of Gastroenterological Surgery, Osaka University Graduate School of Medicine, Osaka, Japan

[2]Department of Therapeutics for Inflammatory Bowel Diseases, Osaka University Graduate School of Medicine, Osaka, Japan

[3]Division of Health Science, Osaka University Graduate School of Medicine, Osaka, Japan

Correspondence
Takayuki Ogino, Osaka University, 2-2-E2 Yamadaoka, Suita, Osaka, 565-0871, Japan.
Email: togino04@gesurg.med.osaka-u.ac.jp

Abstract

Aim: Early detection of surgical site infection (SSI) allows for appropriate management after Crohn's disease (CD) surgery. The aim of this study was to evaluate the usefulness of bacterial culture of postoperative drainage fluid after CD surgery.

Methods: This study included 110 patients with CD who underwent surgery with bowel resection between January 2010 and March 2020 at Osaka University Hospital. Patients with only perianal surgery or incomplete records were excluded. Risk factors for SSI were evaluated in the context of clinical findings, including bacterial culture of postoperative drainage fluid, and bacterial species related to SSI were also examined.

Results: Of 110 patients, 18 (16.4%) developed SSI. Organ/space SSI developed in six, and a positive bacterial culture of drainage fluid (D-Posi) was found in five (83.3%). Of 104 patients without organ/space SSI, 31 (29.8%) were D-Posi ($P = .027$). Similarly, 68.8% with incisional SSI were D-Posi, whereas 26.6% without incisional SSI were D-Posi ($P = .0021$). Multivariate analysis revealed that D-Posi was an independent risk factor in both organ/space and incisional SSI. Bacterial examination showed that *Pseudomonas aeruginosa* and *Enterococcus faecalis* were significantly detected in patients with SSI.

Conclusion: This study suggests the usefulness of postoperative drainage fluid bacterial culture for early diagnosis of SSI after CD surgery.

KEYWORDS
bacterial culture, CD, drainage fluid, SSI

1 | INTRODUCTION

Crohn's disease (CD) involves chronic intestinal inflammation and differences in gut bacterial species compared with healthy controls.[1,2] Despite improvements in medical treatments, 70%–90% of patients will undergo surgery in their lifetime.[3] More than half of them will require surgical intervention within 15 y of previous operations because of recurrence or new lesions occurrence.[4-6] Postoperative complications may not only delay resumption of medication but also trigger recurrence and complicate subsequent surgeries because of adhesions.[7,8] If complications are detected in the early phase, exacerbations could be avoided and prognosis improved.[7,8] For these reasons, accurate predictors of complications are needed.

Surgical site infection (SSI) is one of the postoperative complications, and the rate of SSI after CD surgery is higher than after colorectal cancer surgery.[4,9-11] Several SSI risk factors have been identified in patients with CD, including anemia, a longer duration of surgery, and higher intraoperative lactate level.[4,11] Although these are indirect risk factors for SSI, a direct factor is bacterial contamination of the surgical site.[12] Few reports, however, have described the association between positive bacterial culture of lavage or drainage fluid and SSI in gastrointestinal surgery.[12-14] To our knowledge, no studies have evaluated the role of positive bacterial culture of drainage fluid (D-Posi) after CD surgery.

We hypothesized that D-Posi could predict SSI in the early phase after CD surgery. The aims of this study were to evaluate the clinical impact of D-Posi in detecting SSI and the characteristics of detected bacterial species after CD surgery.

2 | METHODS

2.1 | Patients

A total of 245 consecutive patients who underwent CD surgery between January 2010 and March 2020 at Osaka University Hospital were included in this study. We excluded 125 patients who underwent perianal surgery only and 10 patients with incomplete records (Figure 1). Informed consent was obtained from all patients before the surgery. The study protocol was approved by the Institutional Review Board of Osaka University Hospital (# 15028).

2.2 | Perioperative management and surgical procedure

Prophylactic antibiotics with second-generation cephalosporin (cefmetazole) were intravenously administered within 30 min before skin incision, repeatedly at 3-h intervals during surgery, and postoperatively twice a day until postoperative day (POD) 2. Drainage tubes were placed in a Morrison's pouch or Douglas' pouch. Before March 2012, we performed closed passive drainage using surgeon's choice of a SILASCON duple drain (Kaneka Medical Products, Japan) or closed active drainage using a BLAKE silicone drain (Ethicon, Cincinnati, OH). After April 2012, closed active drainage was used in all cases.

A wound protector was used during surgery, and intraperitoneal lavage was performed before wound closure. All surgical staff changed gloves after bowel anastomosis. The peritoneum was closed by a running suture with 3-0 Vicryl (Ethicon). The muscular fascia was closed by a knotted suture with 1-PDS PLUS (Ethicon). The wound was washed with 200 mL of saline before closure of the skin by a buried suture with 4-0 PDS plus (Ethicon). Board-certified surgeons performed all surgeries.

2.3 | Outcome measurement and definition of SSI

For evaluating candidate risk factors for SSI, we collected medical records data on patient characteristics including age, sex, body mass index (BMI), American Society of Anesthesiologists score, duration of disease, behavior (nonstricturing and nonpenetrating, stricturing, or penetrating), preoperative laboratory data, antitumor necrosis factor alpha (TNF)-α use, steroid use, and frequency of surgery. We also collected data on surgical variables, including type of surgery (open or laparoscopic), surgical site (small bowel, colon, ileocolon, or

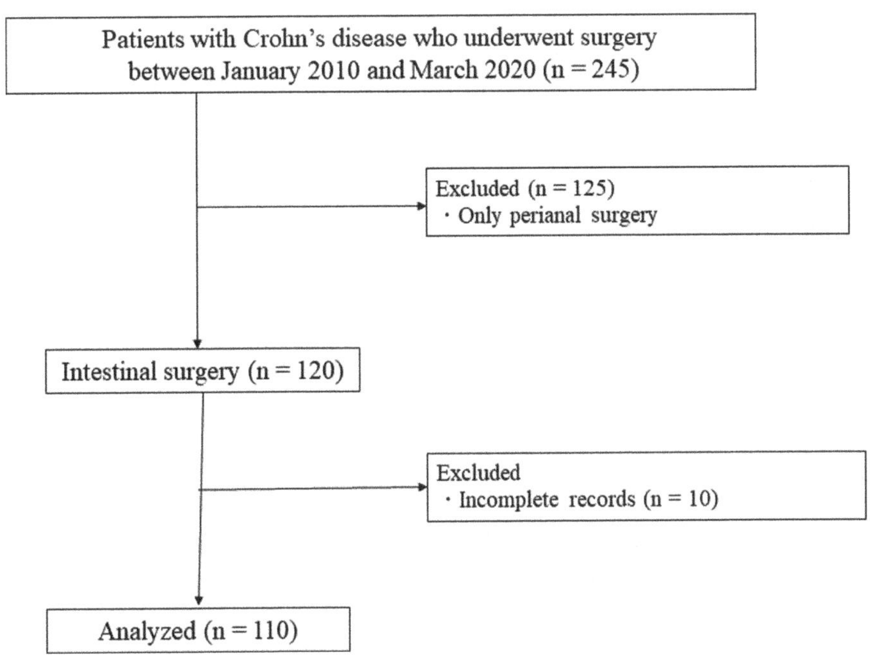

FIGURE 1 Flow chart of participant inclusion in the study

rectum), with or without abdominoperineal resection (APR), ostomy creation, surgical wound classification, duration of surgery, intraoperative bleeding, transfusion, and D-Posi. The surgical staff examined the wounds daily, and bacterial culture of drainage fluid was performed on POD 1 and 4 in all cases. The definition of D-Posi was detection of bacteria in the drainage fluid at POD 1 or 4.

Surgical site infection was defined according to the US Centers for Disease Control and Prevention classifications,[4,15] as an infection that occurred at the surgical site within 30 d after surgery with at least one of the following observations: purulent discharge from the incision or from the drain placed into the organ/space; bacteria isolated by culturing fluid or tissue from the incision or the organ/space; an open wound with signs and symptoms of infection; and/or an abscess or other evidence of infection found on examination of the incision or the organ/space.[11,16]

2.4 | Detection method of bacterial species

Bacterial culture of drainage fluid was performed on the same day a sample was submitted. The sample was smeared for detecting the type by gram staining, and then coated on both Agar's and Ringer's medium. Results of the gram staining were available the same day. The bacterial species were examined with matrix-assisted laser desorption/ionization-time-of-flight mass spectrometry using colonies on Agar medium. On the day following sample submission, D-Posi status and bacterial species were identified. The antibiotic sensitivity was identified at 2 d after sample submission. If the amount of bacteria was limited, this step sometimes took a few more days and up to 1–2 wk for very low counts associated with using Ringer's medium.

2.5 | Statistical analysis

All statistical analyses were performed using JMP 15 (SAS Institute, Cary, NC).

The reference values were determined according to the median values about age, duration of disease, C-reactive protein, duration of surgery, and intraoperative bleeding, and also according to the standard values of white blood cell (WBC), hemoglobin, platelet and albumin, and BMI. Patients' backgrounds, surgical variables, and postoperative results were compared using the Chi-squared or Fisher's exact test for categorical variables, as appropriate. Odds ratios (ORs) were used to evaluate the relationship between SSI and different factors. Variables from comparisons yielding $P < .1$ in the univariate analysis were entered into a multivariate analysis. For multivariate analysis, we used a logistic regression model to investigate the factors associated with SSI incidence. The predictive accuracy and area under the curve (AUC) were calculated. Receiver operating characteristic analyses were performed to compare the performance of variables as SSI risk predictors. Risk factors, excluding D-Posi, with a univariate $P < .1$, were defined as "Others" and "Others" together with D-Posi was defined as "Combination." Diagnostic accuracy was judged using the diagnostic OR (DOR), which is not affected by disease frequency and incidence of complications. Statistical significance was defined as $P < .05$. The ratios were calculated as follows:

$$\text{Positive likelihood ratio (LR}(+)) = \text{sensitivity}/(1-\text{specificity});$$

$$\text{Negative likelihood ratio (LR}(-)) = (1-\text{sensitivity})/\text{specificity};$$

$$\text{DOR} = \text{positive LR}/\text{negative LR}.$$

3 | RESULTS

3.1 | Patient characteristics

Data for 110 patients were analyzed and the characteristics of the 84 men and 26 women are shown in Table 1. The median age at surgery was 39.5 y, and 36 patients (32.7%) were D-Posi. The APR accounted for 10 patients (9.1%). The median duration of surgery was 203.5 min, and the median intraoperative bleeding was 145 mL. Seven patients (6.4%) received a blood transfusion. A total of 17 patients (15.5%) received preoperative antibiotics for high inflammatory response with penetrating disease.

3.2 | Postoperative complications

Postoperative complications were diagnosed in 28 patients (25.5%), including overall SSI in 18 (16.4%), incisional SSI in 16 (14.5%), and organ/space SSI in six (5.5%) (12 had incisional SSI only, two had organ/space SSI only, and four had both types of SSI). Gastrointestinal bleeding occurred in five patients (4.5%), intra-abdominal bleeding in one (0.9%), subcutaneous bleeding in one (0.9%), ileus in five (4.5%), catheter infection in four (3.6%), and femoral nerve palsy in one (0.9%). Severe complications (Clavien–Dindo grade ≥ III) were observed in seven patients (6.4%). There were no perioperative deaths.

3.3 | SSI risk factors

For analyses, 18 patients were in the overall SSI group and compared with the other 92 patients in the nonoverall SSI group. Univariate analysis of risk factors associated with overall SSI identified preoperative WBC ≥9400/μL, open surgery, APR, a longer duration of surgery, a high degree of intraoperative bleeding, and D-Posi (Table 2). Risk factors for incisional SSI were WBC ≥9400/μL, APR, a longer duration of surgery, and D-Posi; the only risk factor associated with organ/space SSI was D-Posi. Of the patients with incisional SSI, 68.8% (11/16) were D-Posi, whereas 26.6% (25/ 94) without incisional SSI were D-Posi ($P = .0021$). Similarly, 83.3% (5/6) with organ/space SSI were D-Posi, and 29.8% (31/104) without organ/space were D-Posi ($P = .027$) (Table 3). In multivariate analyses, only

TABLE 1 Patient characteristics (N = 110)

	N*
Preoperative	Median (range)
Age, y	39.5 (14–72)
Male/female	84/26
BMI, kg/m^2	19.0 (14.0–28.4)
ASA score ≥2, n (%)	71 (64.5%)
Duration of disease, y	10 (0–41)
Behavior	
Nonstricturing & nonpenetrating	7 (6.4%)
Stricturing	41 (37.2%)
Penetrating	62 (56.4%)
Preoperative WBC, per μL	5260 (1990–16 890)
Preoperative Hb, g/dL	12.0 (7.3–16.1)
Preoperative platelet ×10^4, per μL	28.8 (6.8–57.8)
Preoperative albumin, g/dL	3.5 (1.5–4.9)
Preoperative CRP, mg/dL	0.20 (0–22.4)
Preoperative use of anti-TNF-α antibody	78 (70.9%)
Preoperative use of steroid	11 (10%)
Frequency of surgery (primary/redo)	66/44
Surgical	
Open/laparoscopic	13/97
Surgical site	
Small bowel/colon/ileocolon/rectum	21/14/65/10
APR, n (%)	10 (9.1%)
Ostomy creation	18
Wound class (II/III/IV)	95/8/7
Duration of surgery, min	203.5 (105–748)
Intraoperative bleeding, mL	145 (0–8050)
Transfusion, n (%)	7 (6.4%)
D-Posi, n (%)	36 (32.7%)

Abbreviations: APR, abdominoperineal resection; ASA, American Society of Anesthesiologists; BMI, body mass index; CRP, C-reactive protein; D-Posi, bacterial culture positive of postoperative drainage fluid; Hb, hemoglobin; WBC, white blood cell count.

*Median (range) unless otherwise specified.

D-Posi emerged as an independent risk factor of overall, incisional, and organ/space SSI. In addition, high BMI was also an independent risk factor for incisional SSI (Table 4).

Abdominoperineal resection has been reported as a risk factor for incisional and organ/space SSI, leading to assess also the clinical impact of D-Posi with exclusion of APR.[11] Of 100 patients with APR excluded, overall SSI developed in 14 patients: 10 with incisional SSI only, two with organ/space only, and two with both. Eleven (78.6%) with overall SSI were D-Posi, whereas 20 (23.3%) without overall SSI were D-Posi ($P = .0004$). We found that 75% with incisional SSI were D-Posi and 22.0% without incisional SSI were D-Posi ($P = .002$). Similarly, 75% with organ/space SSI were D-Posi, and 29.2% without organ/space SSI were D-Posi ($P = .091$). Multivariate analysis identified D-Posi as an independent risk factor in overall SSI and incisional SSI also among the patients with APR excluded.

3.4 | Treatment details for the case of D-Posi

Of 110 patients, 36 were D-Posi, 19 (52.8%) of whom received only prophylactic antibiotics. Four (11.1%) had longer administration of cefmetazole for a few days. Nine (25.0%) were switched to other antibiotics with broad-spectrum activity, based on the detected bacterial species. Four (11.1%) were switched to other antibiotics and had percutaneous drainages. Among the patients with D-Posi, confirming their status took a median of 2 d in 13 patients with SSI and 5 d in 23 patients with non-SSI. Identifying antibiotic sensitivity took a median of 4 (2–17) d. The period for detecting D-Posi was significantly shorter in the SSI group compared to the non-SSI group ($P = .007$), possibly because of different bacterial loads.

3.5 | Comparison of predictive and diagnostic accuracy

Next, we evaluated the predictive and diagnostic ability of D-Posi. In overall SSI, the AUC for D-Posi was 0.736, and the DOR was 7.81, and the AUC was higher than the "Others" group (AUC = 0.733). Values for the "Combination" were the highest, with an AUC of 0.819 and DOR of 21.3 (Figure 2A and Table 5). In organ/space SSI, the AUC for D-Posi was 0.768, and the DOR was 11.8 (Figure 2C and Table 5), while D-Posi was not a strong predictor for incisional SSI compared to "Others" and "Combination," with an AUC of 0.711 and DOR of 6.07 (Figure 2B and Table 5). The negative predictive value was above 90% in all groups.

3.6 | Characteristics of detected bacteria

We investigated which bacteria were associated with SSI risk. In univariate analysis, *Pseudomonas aeruginosa* and *Enterococcus faecalis* were significantly associated with overall SSI ($P = .0024$ and .017, respectively). *Pseudomonas aeruginosa* was frequently detected in patients with incisional and organ/space SSI *Klebsiella pneumoniae* and *E. faecalis* were often frequently detected in patients with organ/space SSI (Table S1). The comparison of detected bacteria between SSI and D-Posi were also performed. Of 16 patients with incisional SSI, seven (43.8%) had the same organism detected from both samples. Among six patients with organ/space SSI, four (66.6%) had the same organism in both samples (Table S2). Of 18 patients with SSI, six organisms were subjected to an antibiotic sensitivity test of both samples. Most of the antibiotic sensitivity results were the same in both samples, and the examined organisms were resistant to the prophylactic antibiotic cefmetazole (Table S3).

TABLE 2 Univariate analysis of risk factors associated with overall surgical site infection (SSI)

	Overall SSI group, n (%) (n = 18)	Nonoverall SSI group, n (%) (n = 92)	OR	95% CI	P
Preoperative backgrounds					
Age ≥40 y	10 (55.6%)	45 (48.9%)	1.31	0.47-3.60	.607
Male	15 (83.3%)	69 (75.0%)	1.67	0.44-6.28	.450
BMI ≥22 kg/m^2	7 (38.9%)	21 (22.8%)	2.15	0.74-6.24	.159
ASA score ≥2	12 (66.7%)	59 (64.1%)	1.12	0.38-3.26	.837
Duration of disease ≥10 y	9 (50.0%)	47 (51.6%)	0.94	0.34-2.57	.898
Behavior					
Penetrating/nonpenetrating	8/10	54/38	0.56	0.20-1.56	.269
Preoperative WBC ≥9.4 × 10^3/μL	5 (27.8%)	9 (9.8%)	3.55	1.03-12.3	.045[a]
Preoperative Hb <12 g/dL	12 (66.7%)	43 (46.7%)	2.28	0.79-6.59	.129
Preoperative platelet ≥32 × 10^4/μL	9 (50.0%)	31 (33.7%)	1.97	0.71-5.46	.193
Preoperative albumin <3.5 g/dL	9 (52.9%)	38 (41.8%)	1.57	0.55-4.44	.396
Preoperative CRP ≥0.2 mg/dL	11 (61.1%)	43 (46.7%)	1.79	0.64-5.03	.269
Preoperative use of anti-TNF-α antibody	13 (72.2%)	65 (70.7%)	1.08	0.35-3.33	.893
Preoperative use of steroid	2 (11.1%)	9 (9.8%)	1.15	0.22-5.84	.864
Frequency of surgery; redo	9 (50.0%)	35 (38.0%)	1.63	0.59-4.50	.347
Surgical backgrounds					
Open/Laparoscopic	5/13	8/84	4.04	1.14-14.2	.030[a]
Surgical site					
Small bowel	3	18	0.25	0.04-1.45	.123
Colon	2	12	0.25	0.04-1.77	.166
Ileocolon	9	56	0.24	0.06-1.03	.054
Rectum	4	6	Reference = 1		
APR	4 (22.2%)	6 (6.52%)	4.10	1.02-16.4	.046[a]
Ostomy creation	5 (27.8%)	13 (14.1%)	2.34	0.71-7.66	.161
Wound class ≥III	3 (16.7%)	12 (13.0%)	1.33	0.34-5.30	.683
Duration of surgery ≥204 min	14 (77.8%)	41 (44.6%)	4.35	1.33-14.2	.015[a]
Intraoperative bleeding ≥145 mL	13 (72.2%)	42 (45.7%)	3.10	1.02-9.39	.046[a]
Transfusion	2 (11.1%)	5 (5.4%)	2.18	0.39-12.2	.377
D-Posi	13 (72.2%)	23 (25.0%)	7.80	2.51-24.2	.0004[a]

Abbreviations: 95% CI, 95% confidence interval; APR, abdominoperineal resection; ASA, American Society of Anesthesiologists; BMI, body mass index; CRP, C-reactive protein; D-Posi, bacterial culture–positive postoperative drainage fluid; Hb, hemoglobin; OR, odds ratio; WBC, white blood cell count.

[a]$P < .05$

Of 110 patients, only four patients underwent bacterial culture of intraoperative samples (*Proteus vulgaris* detected in one case, *Bacteroides fragilis* in one, *K. pneumoniae* and *Escherichia coli* in one, and none detected in the fourth case). Of these four patients, two were D-Posi, but the detected bacteria were different from the intraoperative samples, and none of the four patients developed SSI.

4 | DISCUSSION

In patients with CD, it is important to detect SSI in the early phase and prevent worsening, because infectious complications could increase the recurrence risk.[7,8,17,18] Thus, accurate predictors of SSI are needed in this patient population. Several studies have

TABLE 3 Univariate analysis of risk factors associated with incisional surgical site infection (SSI) and organ space SSI

	Incisional SSI				Organ/space SSI			
	Incisional SSI, n (%) (n = 16)	Nonincisional SSI, n (%) (n = 94)	OR (95% CI)	P	Organ/space SSI, n (%) (n = 6)	Nonorgan/space SSI, n (%) (n = 104)	OR (95% CI)	P
Preoperative backgrounds								
Age ≥40 y	10 (62.5%)	45 (47.9%)	1.8 (0.61–5.40)	.284	1 (16.7%)	54 (51.9%)	0.19 (0.02–1.64)	.130
Male	14 (87.5%)	70 (74.5%)	2.4 (0.51–11.34)	.269	4 (66.7%)	80 (76.9%)	0.60 (0.10–3.48)	.569
BMI ≥22 kg/m^2	7 (43.8%)	21 (22.3%)	2.7 (0.90–8.13)	.077	1 (16.7%)	27 (26.0%)	0.57 (0.06–5.10)	.616
ASA score ≥2	10 (62.5%)	61 (64.9%)	0.90 (0.30–2.70)	.853	4 (66.7%)	67 (64.4%)	1.1 (0.19–6.32)	.911
Duration of disease ≥10 y	8 (50.0%)	48 (51.6%)	0.94 (0.32–2.71)	.905	4 (66.7%)	52 (50.5%)	2.0 (0.34–11.18)	.448
Behavior								
Penetrating/ nonpenetrating	6/10	56/38	0.41 (0.14–1.21)	.11	4/2	58/48	1.59 (0.28–9.05)	.604
Preoperative WBC ≥9.4 × 10^3/μL	5 (31.3%)	9 (9.6%)	4.3 (1.22–15.15)	.024[a]	1 (16.7%)	13 (12.5%)	1.4 (0.15–12.95)	.767
Preoperative Hb <12 g/dL	10 (62.5%)	45 (47.9%)	1.8 (0.61–5.40)	.284	4 (66.7%)	51 (49.0%)	2.1 (0.36–11.85)	0.410
Preoperative platelet ≥32 × 10^4/μL	9 (56.3%)	31 (33.0%)	2.6 (0.89–7.67)	.081	2 (33.3%)	38 (36.5%)	0.87 (0.15–4.97)	.874
Preoperative albumin <3.5 g/dL	7 (46.7%)	40 (43.0%)	1.2 (0.39–3.46)	.791	3 (50.0%)	44 (43.1%)	1.3 (0.25–6.85)	.742
Preoperative CRP ≥0.2 mg/dL	11 (68.8%)	43 (45.7%)	2.6 (0.84–8.10)	.097	2 (33.3%)	52 (50.0%)	0.50 (0.09–2.85)	.435
Preoperative use of anti-TNF-α antibody	11 (68.8%)	67 (71.3%)	0.89 (0.28–2.79)	.837	6 (100%)	72 (69.2%)	NA	NA
Preoperative use of steroid	2 (12.5%)	9 (9.6%)	1.35 (0.26–6.91)	.719	1 (16.7%)	10 (9.6%)	1.90 (0.20–17.73)	.581
Frequency of surgery; redo	8 (50.0%)	36 (38.3%)	1.61 (0.56–4.67)	.380	3 (50.0%)	41 (39.4%)	1.54 (0.30–7.98)	.609

TABLE 3 (Continued)

	Incisional SSI				Organ/space SSI			
	Incisional SSI, n (%) (n = 16)	Nonincisional SSI, n (%) (n = 94)	OR (95% CI)	*P*	Organ/space SSI, n (%) (n = 6)	Nonorgan/space SSI, n (%) (n = 104)	OR (95% CI)	*P*
Surgical backgrounds								
Open/laparoscopic	4/12	9/85	3.1 (0.84–11.83)	.090	2/4	11/93	4.2 (0.69–25.8)	.118
Surgical site								
Small bowel/	2	19	0.16 (0.02–1.09)	.061	2	19	0.42(0.05–3.53)	.425
Colon or ileocolon/	10	69	0.22 (0.05–0.91)	.036[a]	2	77	0.10(0.01–0.84)	.034[a]
rectum	4	6	Reference=1		2	8	Reference=1	
APR	4 (25.0%)	6 (6.4%)	4.9 (1.20–19.86)	.027[a]	2 (33.3%)	8 (7.7%)	6.0 (0.95–37.94)	.057
Ostomy creation	4 (25.0%)	14 (25.9%)	1.9 (0.53–6.76)	.319	2 (33.3%)	16 (15.4%)	2.8 (0.46–16.29)	.265
Wound class ≥III	2 (12.5%)	13 (13.8%)	0.89 (0.18–4.38)	.886	1 (16.7%)	14 (13.5%)	1.29 (0.140–11.83)	.824
Duration of surgery ≥204 min	12 (75.0%)	43 (45.7%)	3.6 (1.07–11.84)	.039[a]	5 (83.3%)	50 (48.1%)	5.4 (0.61–47.83)	.130
Intraoperative bleeding ≥145 mL	11 (68.8%)	44 (46.8%)	2.5 (0.81–7.76)	.113	5 (83.3%)	50 (48.1%)	5.4 (0.61–47.83)	.130
Transfusion	2 (12.5%)	5 (5.3%)	2.5 (0.45–14.4)	.292	0 (0%)	7 (6.7%)	NA	NA
D-Posi	11 (68.8%)	25 (26.6%)	6.1 (1.92–19.21)	.0021[a]	5 (83.3%)	31 (29.8%)	11.8 (1.32–105.0)	.027[a]

Abbreviations: 95% CI, 95% confidence interval; APR, abdominoperineal resection; ASA, American Society of Anesthesiologists; BMI, body mass index; CRP, C-reactive protein; D-Posi, bacterial culture–positive postoperative drainage fluid; Hb, hemoglobin; NA, not applicable; OR, odds ratio; WBC, white blood cell count.

[a]$P < .05$.

TABLE 4 Multivariate analysis of risk factors associated with surgical site infection (SSI)

	OR	95% CI	P
Overall SSI			
Preoperative WBC ≥9.4 × 10³/μL	1.83	0.40-8.44	.439
Open	1.59	0.37-6.92	.534
APR	1.82	0.32-10.3	.495
Duration of surgery ≥204 min	2.49	0.55-11.3	.237
Intraoperative bleeding ≥145 mL	1.30	0.31-5.48	.722
D-Posi	6.00	1.79-19.9	.0036[a]
Incisional SSI			
BMI ≥22 kg/m²	4.77	1.17-19.5	.030[a]
Preoperative WBC ≥9.4 × 10³/μL	1.60	0.28-9.07	.598
Preoperative platelet ≥32 × 10⁴/μL	2.90	0.71-11.9	.139
Preoperative CRP ≥0.2 mg/dL	1.52	0.32-7.23	.598
Open	2.04	0.38-11.1	.408
APR	2.91	0.43-19.9	.276
Duration of surgery ≥204 min	1.78	0.39-8.13	.451
D-Posi	5.59	1.42-22.0	.014[a]
Organ/space SSI			
APR	4.63	0.65-33.0	.126
D-Posi	10.6	1.26-96.1	.037[a]

Abbreviations: 95% CI, 95% confidence interval; APR, abdominoperineal resection; D-Posi, bacterial culture-positive postoperative drainage fluid; OR, odds ratio; WBC, whiteblood cell count.

[a]$P < .05$.

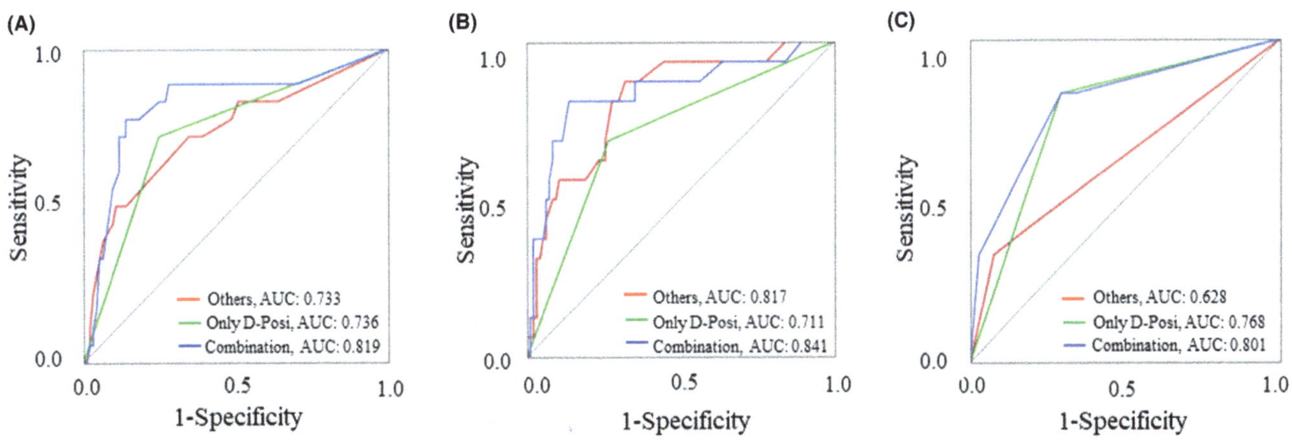

FIGURE 2 Receiver operating characteristic curve analysis based on risk factors other than D-Posi, D-Posi, or a combination of both for surgical site infection (SSI). (A) Overall SSI. (B) Incisional SSI. (C) Organ/space SSI. AUC, area under the curve. D-Posi, positive bacterial culture of drainage fluid

suggested that D-Posi could have predictive associations with predicting SSI.[12,14] Sugiura et al reported that bacterial culture-positive peritoneal lavage fluid correlated with SSI and pancreatic fistula after pancreaticoduodenectomy.[12] Migita et al showed that D-Posi was an independent risk factor among clinical and surgical variables for intra-abdominal abscess after gastrectomy.[14] Routine use of prophylactic drainage has been reported not to decrease postoperative complications in colorectal surgeries, including ileocecal resection or right hemicolectomy.[19,20] However, undrained fluid could cause intra-abdominal abscess because of bacterial leakage from the mesentery in patients with CD.[21] Compared with patients with cancer, patients with CD also have a higher risk of infection because of low nutrition, the use of immunosuppressive drugs, and the presence of fistulas and abscess. Therefore, we routinely placed prophylactic drainage for our patients with CD. This study is the first to investigate the impact of D-Posi and detected bacteria in these patients. The results identified D-Posi as an independent predictor of SSI, with an AUC >0.8 in the early phase.

TABLE 5 Diagnostic accuracies for predicting surgical site infection (SSI)

	Sensitivity (%)	Specificity (%)	PPV (%)	NPV (%)	LR (+)	LR (-)	DOR
Overall SSI							
Others	50.0	89.1	47.4	90.1	4.60	0.56	8.20
D-Posi	72.2	75.0	36.1	93.2	2.89	0.37	7.81
Combination	77.8	85.9	51.9	95.2	5.50	0.26	21.3
Incisional SSI							
Others	87.5	68.1	31.8	97.0	2.74	0.18	14.9
D-Posi	68.8	73.4	30.6	93.2	2.59	0.43	6.07
Combination	81.3	86.2	50.0	96.4	5.88	0.22	27.0
Organ/space SSI							
Others	33.3	92.3	20.0	96.0	4.33	0.72	6.00
D-Posi	83.3	70.2	13.9	98.6	2.80	0.24	11.8
Combination	83.3	70.2	13.9	98.6	2.80	0.24	11.8

Abbreviations: DOR, diagnostic odds ratio; D-Posi, bacterial culture–positive postoperative drainage fluid; LR (−), negative likelihood ratio; LR (+), positive likelihood ratio; NPV, negative predictive value; PPV, positive predictive value.

[a]$P < .05$.

Organ/space SSI usually becomes evident around POD 7 or later.[22,23] To prevent worsening, early administration of antibiotics is recommended for suspected cases after gastrointestinal surgery.[24,25] Percutaneous drainage also can preclude the need for surgical intervention for intra-abdominal abscess.[26] In our study, six patients had organ/space SSI, and all were diagnosed at POD 8 (POD 5–15) because computed tomography diagnosis of organ/space SSI was mainly performed following symptom progression. The negative predictive value of diagnosing SSI was >95% with the use of D-Posi, suggesting its potential to allow prediction of SSI on POD 4. Of six patients with organ/space SSI, four with D-Posi were switched to other antibiotics with broad-spectrum activity on POD 4.5 (POD 2–7), and one patient continued receiving antibiotics from 14 d before surgery until POD 11 because of high inflammation with penetrating disease. Identifying the D-Posi status might allow us perform empirical treatment in the early phase before the definitive diagnosis.

Several studies have demonstrated that patients with CD have gut bacterial alterations characterized by reduced bacterial diversity, depletion of Firmicutes or Bacteroides, and enrichment of Proteobacteria.[1,2,27-29] However, the causative bacteria of SSI in patients with CD have not been reported. A previous study showed that *E. faecalis*, *S. aureus*, and *P. aeruginosa* were often isolated from SSI following lower intestinal tract surgery.[30] Our data also showed that *E. faecalis* and *P. aeruginosa* were significantly detected in CD patients with organ/space SSI. Because *P.aeruginosa* affected immunosuppressed patients, careful management would be essential for CD patients under treatment.[31,32] The current findings suggest that organisms at the site of SSI were resistant to the prophylactic antibiotic cefmetazole and that most of the antibiotic sensitivity results were the same between drainage fluid and of SSI bacterial culture. This suggested that sensitivity results in drainage fluid could guide the choice of an antibiotic.

The present study had several limitations. First, these results were based on a single-center retrospective cohort study, including some selection bias that could not be avoided. Second, the impact of preoperative medicines, such as biologics except anti-TNF-α therapy, immune suppressants, and 5-aminosalicylic acid were not evaluated in this study. A larger study that includes these factors is needed.

In conclusion, this study confirmed the clinical usefulness of D-Posi for SSI and demonstrated the association of bacteria species with CD surgery. Bacterial culture of drainage fluid represents an easy, noninvasive, and inexpensive tool to perform appropriate management of SSI.

ACKNOWLEDGMENT

The authors thank the staff at Osaka University Hospital.

DISCLOSURES

The study protocol was approved by the Institutional Review Board of Osaka University Hospital (# 15028).

Informed consent was obtained from all patients before the surgery.

This research was not preregistered in an independent, institutional registry (N/A).

This research was not an animal study (N/A).

The authors T.O. and T.M. were supported by the KINSHUKAI GROUP.

Author T.M. was partly supported by a research grant from the Osaka Medical Research Foundation for Intractable Disease, JSP KAKENHI (20K17615), Danone Institute of Japan Foundation (DIJF R01-24), and Astellas Pharma Global Development (Grant No. IDRS2017A0000577).

AUTHOR CONTRIBUTIONS

Study concept and design: M.I., T.O., and T.M. Acquisition of data: M.I., T.O., and T.M. Statistical analysis and interpretation of data: M.I., T.O., and M.F. Drafting of the article: M.I. and T.O. Critical revision of the article for important intellectual content: all authors. Supervision: Y.D. and H.E.

REFERENCES

1. Machiels K, Pozuelo Del Río M, Martinez-De la Torre A, Xie Z, Pascal Andreu V, Sabino J, et al. Early postoperative endoscopic recurrence in Crohn's disease is characterised by distinct microbiota recolonisation. J Crohns Colitis. 2020;14(11):1535–46.
2. Wright EK, Kamm MA, Wagner J, Teo SM, Cruz P, Hamilton AL, et al. Microbial factors associated with postoperative Crohn's disease recurrence. J Crohns Colitis. 2017;11(2):191–203.
3. Byrne J, Stephens R, Isaacson A, Yu H, Burke C. Image-guided percutaneous drainage for treatment of post-surgical anastomotic leak in patients with Crohn's disease. J Crohns Colitis. 2016;10(1):38–42.
4. Liu S, Miao J, Wang G, Wang M, Wu X, Guo K, et al. Risk factors for postoperative surgical site infections in patients with Crohn's disease receiving definitive bowel resection. Sci Rep. 2017;7(1):9828.
5. Olaisen M, Flatberg A, Granlund AVB, Røyset ES, Martinsen TC, Sandvik AK, et al. Bacterial mucosa-associated microbiome in inflamed and proximal noninflamed ileum of patients with Crohn's disease. Inflamm Bowel Dis. 2021;27(1):12–24.
6. Ogino T, Mizushima T, Matsuda C, Mori M, Doki Y. Essential updates 2018/2019: Colorectal (benign): Recent updates (2018–2019) in the surgical treatment of benign colorectal diseases. Ann Gastroenterol Surg. 2020;4(1):30–8.
7. Riss S, Schuster I, Papay P, Mittlböck M, Stift A. Repeat intestinal resections increase the risk of recurrence of Crohn's disease. Dis Colon Rectum. 2013;56:881–7.
8. Guo Z, Cao L, Guo F, Gong J, Li Y, Gu L, et al. The presence of postoperative infectious complications is associated with the risk of early postoperative clinical recurrence of Crohn's disease. World J Surg. 2017;41(9):2371–7.
9. Bhakta A, Tafen M, Glotzer O, Ata A, Chismark AD, Valerian BT, et al. Increased incidence of surgical site infection in IBD patients. Dis Colon Rectum. 2016;59(4):316–22.
10. Uchino M, Ikeuchi H, Tsuchida T, Nakajima K, Tomita N, Takesue Y. Surgical site infection following surgery for inflammatory bowel disease in patients with clean-contaminated wounds. World J Surg. 2009;33(5):1042–8.
11. Uchino M, Ikeuchi H, Bando T, Chohno T, Sasaki H, Horio Y, et al. Efficacy of preoperative oral antibiotic prophylaxis for the prevention of surgical site infections in patients with Crohn disease: a randomized controlled trial. Ann Surg. 2019;269(3):420–6.
12. Sugiura T, Mizuno T, Okamura Y, Ito T, Yamamoto Y, Kawamura I, et al. Impact of bacterial contamination of the abdominal cavity during pancreaticoduodenectomy on surgical-site infection. Br J Surg. 2015;102(12):1561–6.
13. Minervini S, Bentley S, Youngs D, Alexander-Williams J, Burdon DW, Keighley MR. Prophylactic saline peritoneal lavage in elective colorectal operations. Dis Colon Rectum. 1980;23(6):392–4.
14. Migita K, Takayama T, Matsumoto S, Wakatsuki K, Tanaka T, Ito M, et al. Impact of bacterial culture positivity of the drainage fluid during the early postoperative period on the development of intra-abdominal abscesses after gastrectomy. Surg Today. 2014;44(11):2138–45.
15. Allegranzi B, Zayed B, Bischoff P, Kubilay NZ, de Jonge S, de Vries F, et al. New WHO recommendations on intraoperative and postoperative measures for surgical site infection prevention: an evidence-based global perspective. Lancet Infect Dis. 2016;16(12):e288–303.
16. Garner JS, Jarvis WR, Emori TG, Horan TC, Hughes JM. CDC definitions for nosocomial infections, 1988. Am J Infect Control. 1988;16(3):128–40.
17. Mizushima T, Nakajima K, Takeyama H, Naito A, Osawa H, Uemura M, et al. Single-incision laparoscopic surgery for stricturing and penetrating Crohn's disease. Surg Today. 2016;46(2):203–8.
18. Ikeshima R, Mizushima T, Takahashi H, Haraguchi N, Nishimura J, Hata T, et al. The efficacy of active drainage for preventing postoperative organ/space surgical site infections in patients with Crohn's disease. Surg Today. 2018;48(1):25–32.
19. Zhang HY, Zhao CL, Xie J, Ye YW, Sun JF, Ding ZH, et al. To drain or not to drain in colorectal anastomosis: a meta-analysis. Int J Colorectal Dis. 2016;31(5):951–60.
20. Yeh CY, Changchien CR, Wang JY, Chen JS, Chen HH, Chiang JM, et al. Pelvic drainage and other risk factors for leakage after elective anterior resection in rectal cancer patients: a prospective study of 978 patients. Ann Surg. 2005;241(1):9–13.
21. Ha CWY, Martin A, Sepich-Poore GD, Shi B, Wang Y, Gouin K, et al. Translocation of viable gut microbiota to mesenteric adipose drives formation of creeping fat in humans. Cell. 2020;183(3):666–83.e17.
22. Tanaka K, Kumamoto T, Nojiri K, Takeda K, Endo I. The effectiveness and appropriate management of abdominal drains in patients undergoing elective liver resection: a retrospective analysis and prospective case series. Surg Today. 2013;43(4):372–80.
23. Torzilli G, Olivari N, Del Fabbro D, Gambetti A, Leoni P, Gendarini A, et al. Bilirubin level fluctuation in drain discharge after hepatectomies justifies long-term drain maintenance. Hepatogastroenterology. 2005;52(64):1206–10.
24. Kamiya S, Hiki N, Kumagai K, Honda M, Nunobe S, Ohashi M, et al. Two-point measurement of amylase in drainage fluid predicts severe postoperative pancreatic fistula after gastric cancer surgery. Gastric Cancer. 2018;21(5):871–8.
25. Fritz S, Hartwig W, Lehmann R, Will-Schweiger K, Kommerell M, Hackert T, et al. Prophylactic antibiotic treatment is superior to therapy on-demand in experimental necrotising pancreatitis. Crit Care. 2008;12(6):R141.
26. Clancy C, Boland T, Deasy J, McNamara D, Burke JP. A meta-analysis of percutaneous drainage versus surgery as the initial treatment of Crohn's disease-related intra-abdominal abscess. J Crohns Colitis. 2016;10(2):202–8.
27. Liguori G, Lamas B, Richard ML, Brandi G, da Costa G, Hoffmann TW, et al. Fungal dysbiosis in mucosa-associated microbiota of Crohn's disease patients. J Crohns Colitis. 2016;10(3):296–305.
28. Manichanh C, Borruel N, Casellas F, Guarner F. The gut microbiota in IBD. Nat Rev Gastroenterol Hepatol. 2012;9(10):599–608.
29. Khor B, Gardet A, Xavier RJ. Genetics and pathogenesis of inflammatory bowel disease. Nature. 2011;474(7351):307–17.
30. Takesue Y, Kusachi S, Mikamo H, Sato J, Watanabe A, Kiyota H, et al. Antimicrobial susceptibility of pathogens isolated from surgical site infections in Japan: Comparison of data from nationwide surveillance studies conducted in 2010 and 2014–2015. J Infect Chemother. 2017;23(6):339–48.
31. Sadikot RT, Blackwell TS, Christman JW, Prince AS. Pathogen-host interactions in Pseudomonas aeruginosa pneumonia. Am J Respir Crit Care Med. 2005;171(11):1209–23.
32. Matsunaga T, Miyata H, Sugimura K, Asukai K, Yanagimoto Y, Takahashi Y, et al. Clinical usefulness of a perioperative bacteriological culture to treat patients with postoperative pneumonia after esophagectomy. Ann Gastroenterol Surg. 2018;3(1):57–64.

13

Adapted systemic inflammation score as a novel prognostic marker for esophageal squamous cell carcinoma patients

Daichi Nomoto[1] | Yoshifumi Baba[1,2] | Takahiko Akiyama[1] | Kazuo Okadome[1] | Masaaki Iwatsuki[1] | Shiro Iwagami[1] | Yuji Miyamoto[1] | Naoya Yoshida[1] | Masayuki Watanabe[3] | Hideo Baba[1,4]

[1]Department of Gastroenterological Surgery, Graduate School of Medical Sciences, Kumamoto University, Kumamoto, Japan

[2]Department of Next-Generation Surgical Therapy Development, Graduate School of Medical Sciences, Kumamoto University, Kumamoto, Japan

[3]Department of Gastroenterological Surgery, Cancer Institute Hospital, Japanese Foundation for Cancer Research, Tokyo, Japan

[4]Center for Metabolic Regulation of Healthy Aging, Kumamoto University, Kumamoto, Japan

Correspondence
Hideo Baba, Department of Gastroenterological Surgery, Graduate School of Medical Sciences, Kumamoto University, 1-1-1 Honjo, Chuo-ku, Kumamoto, 860-8556 Japan.
Email: hdobaba@kumamoto-u.ac.jp

Abstract

Background: The adapted systemic inflammation score (aSIS), calculated from serum albumin and the lymphocyte-to-monocyte ratio, has been reported to be a novel prognostic marker for some types of cancers. However, the prognostic impact of aSIS in patients with esophageal squamous cell carcinoma (ESCC) remains controversial. This study aimed to examine the prognostic effects of aSIS in a large cohort of 509 ESCC patients.

Methods: Preoperative aSIS was retrospectively calculated for 509 ESCC patients who underwent curative resection. Time-dependent receiver operating characteristics (t-ROC) curves were used for comparing the prognostic impact.

Results: Patients with high aSIS showed significantly poorer overall survival (OS) than patients with low aSIS (log rank $P < .001$). The multivariate analysis revealed that aSIS was an independent prognostic factor for overall survival (multivariate hazard ratio 1.76; 95% confidence interval 1.13–2.75; $P = .013$). The t-ROC analysis showed that aSIS was more sensitive than other nutritional prognostic factors (controlling for nutritional status, systemic inflammation score, and the neutrophil-to-lymphocyte ratio).

Conclusion: Preoperative aSIS may be a useful prognostic biomarker in ESCC patients who underwent curative resection.

KEYWORDS
adapted systemic inflammation score, esophageal squamous cell carcinoma, prognosis

1 | INTRODUCTION

Esophageal cancer is the sixth leading cause of cancer death and the seventh most common cancer worldwide.[1] Despite the development of multidisciplinary treatment strategies, including surgery, chemotherapy, radiotherapy, and chemoradiotherapy, the prognosis of patients with esophageal cancer, including those who underwent complete resection, remains poor. Thus, better prognostic biomarkers are needed for making appropriate treatment decisions for esophageal cancer patients.

The systemic inflammation score (SIS) was developed as a new scoring system based on serum albumin (Alb) and the lymphocyte-to-monocyte ratio (LMR). SIS has been reported as a powerful prognostic marker for clear-cell renal cell carcinoma and colorectal cancer.[2,3] The cutoff value of LMR in SIS was the median value for patients with renal cell carcinoma. Therefore, Lin et al developed a modified SIS (mSIS) with optimized LMR cutoff values for gastric cancer patients using the software X-tile (Yale University, New Haven, CT).[4] The mSIS has been shown to be superior to SIS as a predictive indicator for gastric cancer.[5] Several studies have examined the prognostic role of SIS and mSIS in esophageal squamous cell carcinoma (ESCC).[6-8] However, previous data on SIS, mSIS, and clinical outcomes for ESCC have been inconclusive because previous studies were limited by small sample sizes (n < 443). Considering the importance of a potential prognostic marker for ESCC, the assessment of SIS and clinical outcome using a large number of ESCC cases is needed.

In this study we reoptimized the LMR cutoff values as 3.3 using the software X-tile according to esophageal cancer patients' cohort, and defined adapted SIS (aSIS). The prognostic effects of aSIS were examined in a large cohort of 509 ESCC patients. Our non-biased database enabled us to examine whether the influence of aSIS on clinical outcome was modified by numerous other variables. Furthermore, the predictive value of aSIS was compared with that of other known nutritional prognostic factors (Controlling Nutritional Status [CONUT] and Neutrophil-to-Lymphocyte ratio [NLR]).

2 | MATERIALS AND METHODS

2.1 | Patients

Between April 2005 and December 2017, 751 consecutive patients with esophageal cancer who underwent curative resection at Kumamoto University Hospital were enrolled. Of these patients, patients who underwent salvage esophagectomy (53), pharyngolaryngoesophagectomy (27), transhiatal esophagectomy (11), and non-curative surgery (R1 or R2 resection) (53) and with other histological types (93) and who lack peripheral monocyte data (5) were excluded from the study. Thus, a total of 509 patients with esophageal cancer who underwent subtotal esophagectomy were eventually included in the study. We classified the clinical tumor stage according to the Union for International Cancer Control (UICC) TNM classification of malignant tumors, seventh edition.[9] Patients were followed up as outpatients every 1–3 mo after discharge until death or December 2019, whichever came first. Overall survival (OS) was defined as the period from the date of surgery to the date of death. Cancer-specific survival (CSS) was defined as the period from the date of surgery to the date of death owing to esophageal cancer. Patients' clinicopathological characteristics were obtained retrospectively from the medical records. These characteristics included age, sex, body mass index (BMI), comorbidity, preoperative therapy, clinical tumor stage, OS, and CSS. Written informed consent was obtained from each patient, and the study was approved by the Institutional Review Board of Kumamoto University (#1909). The term "prognostic marker" was used throughout this article according to the Reporting Recommendations for Tumor Marker Prognostic Studies (REMARK) guidelines.[10]

2.2 | The aSIS and other scoring systems

Serum samples were obtained and analyzed within 7 d before esophagectomy. The aSIS was calculated from serum albumin and peripheral LMR (Figure 1). The LMR cutoff value was calculated using the software X-tile,[4] which determined the LMR cutoff value as 3.3 (Figure S1).

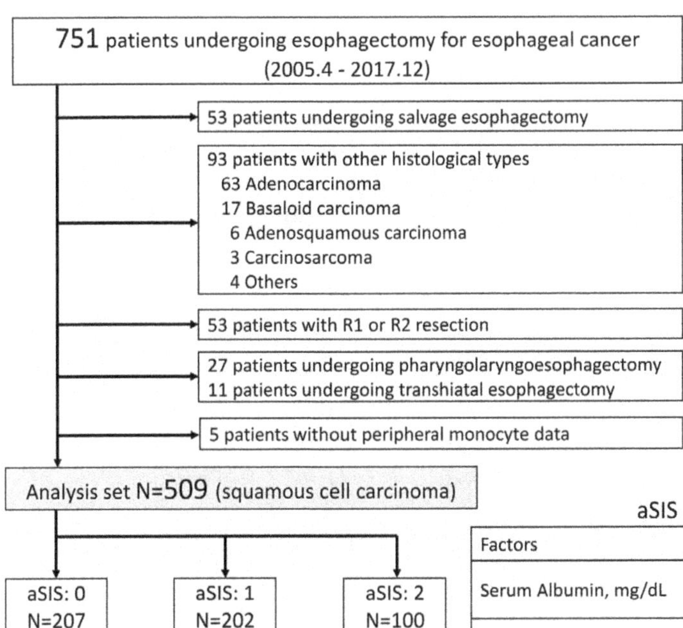

aSIS

Factors	Score	
Serum Albumin, mg/dL	≥ 4	0
	< 4	1
Lymphocyte:monocyte ratio	≥ 3.3	0
	< 3.3	1

FIGURE 1 Flow chart of the analyzed cases and the definition of adapted systemic inflammation score

NLR and CONUT scores were calculated as described previously.[11-13]

2.3 | Statistical analyses

All statistical analyses were performed using JMP v. 10 (SAS Institute, Cary, NC) and EZR (Saitama Medical Center, Jichi Medical University, Japan). Categorical variables were presented as numbers or percentages, and the groups were compared using the chi-squared test or Fisher's exact test. Continuous variables are presented as mean values and standard deviations, and the mean values were compared using Student's *t*-test. For survival analysis, the Kaplan–Meier method was used for evaluating the survival time distribution, and the log-rank test was performed for comparisons. The multivariate Cox proportional hazards model was constructed for computing hazard ratios (HRs) and 95% confidence intervals (CIs) according to aSIS containing clinicopathological factors potentially related to the clinical outcome. Time-dependent receiver operating characteristic curves (ROCs) for the prognostic values of NLR, CONUT, SIS, and aSIS were estimated using the R package "timeROC" (https://cran.r-project.org/web/packages/timeROC/index.html). Variables with $P < .05$ in the univariate analysis were subjected to the multivariate model using a stepwise backward elimination procedure with a threshold $P < .05$. Statistical significance was set at $P < .05$.

TABLE 1 Patient characteristics

Variables	Total N	aSIS 0	aSIS 1	aSIS 2	*P* value
All cases	509	207	202	100	
Mean age ±SD	66.3 ± 8.0	64.6 ± 8.0	67.8 ± 7.8	67.2 ± 8.3	< .01
Sex, male	446 (88%)	178 (86%)	176 (87%)	92 (92%)	.31
Performance status					
0	443 (87%)	190 (92%)	175 (87%)	78 (78%)	< .01
1	57 (11%)	17 (8%)	21 (10%)	19 (19%)	
2	9 (2%)	0 (0%)	6 (3%)	3 (3%)	
Body Mass Index					
<18.5	61 (12%)	16 (8%)	26 (13%)	19 (19%)	< .01
18.5 ≤, <25	368 (72%)	146 (70%)	151 (75%)	71 (71%)	
25≤	80 (16%)	45 (22%)	25 (12%)	10 (10%)	
Alcohol use, Yes	483 (95%)	197 (95%)	192 (95%)	94 (94%)	.91
Tobacco use, Yes	436 (86%)	168 (82%)	176 (87%)	92 (92%)	.026
Comorbidity, Present	392 (77%)	145 (70%)	166 (82%)	81 (81%)	< .01
Preoperative treatment					
Present	195 (38%)	44 (21%)	91 (45%)	60 (60%)	< .01
Absent	314 (62%)	163 (79%)	111 (55%)	40 (40%)	
Tumor location					
Ce	2 (1%)	1 (1%)	1 (1%)	0 (0%)	.71
Ut	72 (14%)	31 (15%)	32 (16%)	9 (9%)	
Mt	279 (55%)	112 (54%)	113 (56%)	54 (54%)	
Lt	143 (28%)	58 (28%)	51 (25%)	34 (34%)	
Ae	13 (2%)	5 (2%)	5 (2%)	3 (3%)	
Clinical stage					
I	252 (50%)	140 (68%)	89 (44%)	23 (23%)	< .01
II	89 (17%)	30 (14%)	39 (19%)	20 (20%)	
III	143 (28%)	26 (13%)	68 (34%)	49 (49%)	
IV	25 (5%)	11 (5%)	6 (3%)	8 (8%)	
Postoperative treatment					
Present	96 (19%)	50 (24%)	30 (15%)	16 (16%)	.053
Absent	413 (81%)	157 (76%)	172 (85%)	84 (84%)	

Abbreviations: aSIS, adapted systemic inflammation score; SD; standard deviation.

3 | RESULTS

3.1 | mSIS and clinicopathological characteristics

Of the 509 ESCC patients, 446 (88%) were men and 63 (12%) were women. The mean age was 66.3 y (range, 41–89 y). Patients were segregated into three groups based on the aSIS: 207 patients (40%) in the aSIS = 0 group, 202 (40%) in the aSIS = 1 group, and 100 (20%) in the aSIS = 2 group (Figure 1). The relationships between aSIS and clinicopathological factors are presented in Table 1. Older age, poorer performance status (PS), lower BMI, and higher clinical stage were significantly associated with higher aSIS (each $P < .05$).

3.2 | Correlations between the aSIS and short-term outcomes of surgery

The short-term outcomes after surgery according to the aSIS are presented in Table 2. High aSIS was significantly associated with a higher incidence of pulmonary morbidity ($P < .01$). Other complications and complication severity were not associated with aSIS. We checked the correlation between aSIS and patients' characteristics affecting pulmonary morbidity such as a respiratory function or surgical procedure. Regarding a respiratory function, we analyzed percent vital capacity (%VC) and forced expiratory volume in 1 sec as a percentage of forced vital capacity (FEV1.0%). %VC decreased significantly as aSIS increased (Figure S2; $P < .001$). On the other hand, there was no significant correlation between FEV1.0% and aSIS (Figure S2; $P = .698$). Regarding a surgical procedure, we checked minimally invasive esophagectomy (MIE) and open esophagectomy (OE). There were more patients with aSIS:2 and fewer patients with aSIS:0 in the OE group than in the MIE group (Figure S2; $P = .011$).

3.3 | Adapted systemic inflammation score and patient survival

The impact of aSIS on clinical outcomes was assessed in ESCC patients. There were 168 deaths among the 509 patients, including 96 esophageal cancer-specific deaths. The median follow-up time for censored patients was 4.0 y. The Kaplan-Meier analysis showed that there was a significant difference in the OS and CSS among the three groups (both log rank $P < .01$). The 3-y OS rates in groups 0, 1, and 2 were 84.1%, 74.6%, and 57.3%, respectively (Figure 2). The 3-y CSS rates in groups 0, 1, and 2 were 87.5%, 81.3%, and 72.0%, respectively (Figure 2).

In the univariate analysis, a high aSIS score was associated with poor OS (HR 2.50, 95% CI 1.65–3.79, $P < .01$) (Table 3). For patient factors, advanced age (HR 1.56, 95% CI 1.14–2.17, $P < .01$), lower BMI (HR 1.81, 95% CI 1.16–2.71, $P < .01$), and poor PS (HR 2.09, 95% CI 1.41–3.01, $P < .01$) were significantly associated with poor OS. For tumor factors, clinical stage (HR 2.19, 95% CI 1.60–2.97, $P < .01$) was significantly associated with poor OS. In the multivariate analysis, aSIS was an independent prognostic factor for the OS (multivariate HR 1.81, 95% CI 1.16–2.81, $P < .01$). The other independent prognostic factors were advanced age, low BMI, poor PS, and postoperative complications.

3.4 | Survival analysis of interactions between aSIS and other factors

We next determined whether the influence of aSIS on the OS was affected by any clinicopathological factors. The effect of aSIS was not significantly modified by comorbidity, BMI, Brinkman Index, sex, or age ($P > .11$ for all interactions) (Figure 3A). Interestingly, a potential modifying effect of preoperative treatment on the relationship between the aSIS and OS was observed (P for interaction = .055).

TABLE 2 Short-term outcome of surgery

Variables	Total N	aSIS 0	aSIS 1	aSIS 2	P value
All cases (Subtotal esophagectomy)	509	207	202	100	
Operating time (min) ±SD	562 ± 121	579 ± 129	552 ± 115	548 ± 114	.033
Blood loss (g) ±SD	475 ± 556	467 ± 684	437 ± 382	568 ± 555	.15
Postoperative morbidity, CDc ≥II	193 (38%)	81 (39%)	67 (33%)	45 (45%)	.12
Postoperative morbidity, CDc ≥IV	33 (6%)	12 (6%)	11 (5%)	10 (10%)	.31
Surgical site infection	125 (25%)	56 (27%)	48 (24%)	21 (21%)	.48
Pulmonary morbidity	87 (17%)	31 (15%)	28 (14%)	28 (28%)	< .01
Cardiovascular morbidity	29 (6%)	12 (6%)	11 (5%)	6 (6%)	.98
Anastomotic leakage	64 (13%)	31 (15%)	18 (9%)	15 (15%)	.12
Reoperation	35 (7%)	14 (7%)	16 (8%)	5 (5%)	.63

Abbreviations: aSIS, adapted systemic inflammation score; CDc, Clavien-Dindo classification; SD, standard deviation.

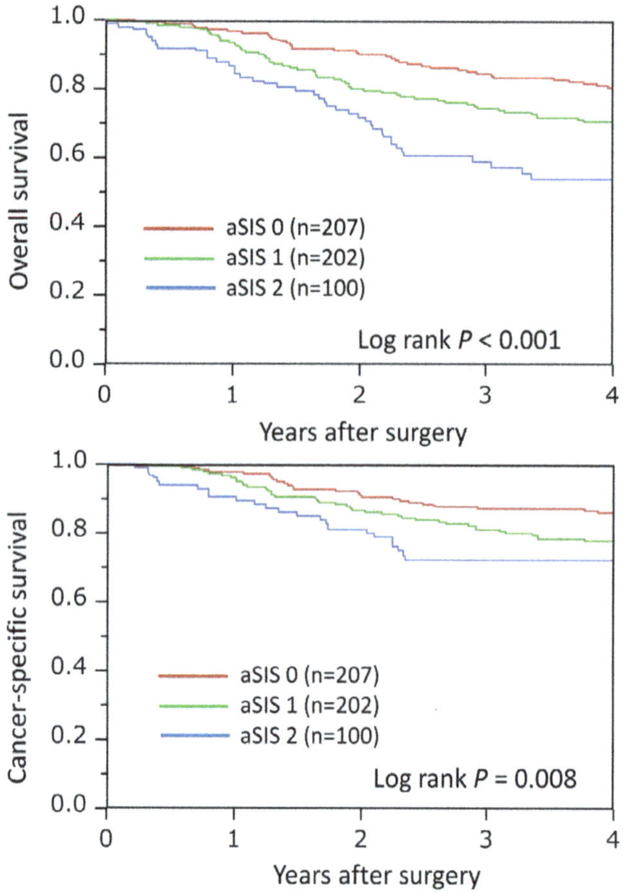

Number at risk

	0	1	2	3	4
aSIS 0	207	199	182	158	122
aSIS 1	202	186	154	123	98
aSIS 2	100	82	66	39	30

FIGURE 2 Kaplan–Meier curves for the overall survival (OS) and cancer-specific survival in esophageal squamous cell carcinoma patients according to adapted systemic inflammation score stratification

Among patients who did not receive preoperative treatment, the high mSIS had a significantly shorter OS (log rank $P < .001$). In contrast, among patients who received preoperative treatment, there was no significant difference in the OS for the high aSIS and low aSIS (log rank $P = .676$) (Figure 3B). Similarly, a potential modifying effect of cStage on the relationship between the mSIS and OS was also observed (P for interaction = .030). Among patients with cStage I, II, the high mSIS had a significantly shorter OS (log rank $P < .001$) (Figure S3).

Furthermore, we divided the patients into those who received preoperative treatment and those who did not, and further analyzed the patients' characteristics and prognostic factors.

In patients without preoperative treatment, the relationships between aSIS and clinicopathological factors are presented in Table S1. Older age, poorer PS, lower BMI, and higher clinical stage were significantly associated with higher aSIS (each $P < .05$). High aSIS was significantly associated with a higher incidence of pulmonary morbidity ($P < .01$). In the multivariate Cox regression analysis for OS, aSIS was an independent prognostic factor for the OS (multivariate HR 2.27, 95% CI 1.18–4.19, $P = .02$; Table S3). These results for patients who did not receive preoperative treatment were in good agreement with the analysis results of all 509 patients.

On the other hand, in patients with preoperative treatment, the relationships between aSIS and clinicopathological factors are presented in Table S2. Older age, and smoker were significantly associated with higher aSIS (each $P < .05$). Unlike patients without preoperative treatment, high aSIS was not significantly associated with a higher incidence of pulmonary morbidity ($P = .62$). Furthermore, in the univariate and multivariate Cox regression analysis for OS, aSIS was not an independent prognostic factor for the OS (univariate HR 1.23, 95% CI 0.68–2.26, $P = .50$; Table S4).

3.5 | Comparison of aSIS with other prognostic scoring systems

Time-dependent area under the curve (AUC)-of-ROC curves of aSIS and other prognostic scoring systems (CONUT, SIS, and NLR) was constructed for the prediction of OS (Figure 4). When the predictive performance for the OS was compared after 1-5 y of follow-up, the AUC values of the aSIS were similar to those of the SIS and CONUT, and were significantly higher than those of the NLR.

4 | DISCUSSION

In this study we examined the prognostic effects of aSIS in a large cohort of 509 patients with ESCC. We found that high aSIS was associated with poor prognosis, suggesting that aSIS status could be used as a marker to identify patients who are likely to have unfavorable clinical outcomes. Additionally, the t-ROC analysis showed that aSIS was more sensitive than other nutritional prognostic factors (CONUT, NLR, and SIS). Given that better prognostic biomarkers are needed for making appropriate treatment decisions for patients with esophageal cancer, our observations are likely to have clinical implications.

Systemic inflammation plays an important role in the tumor microenvironment. Several investigations have revealed that inflammation in the tumor microenvironment promotes tumor proliferation, angiogenesis, metastasis, inhibition of tumor immunity, and resistance to anticancer treatment.[14] Several studies have also shown the predictive value of nutrition and systemic inflammation markers (eg, CONUT and NLR) in patients who underwent curative resection for various cancers. CONUT was calculated from the serum Alb level, total cholesterol concentration, and total lymphocyte count. NLR was calculated from the neutrophil-to-lymphocyte ratio.

SIS is a new scoring system based on serum Alb and LMR. Chang et al first reported that SIS predicts the postoperative prognosis of

TABLE 3 Cox regression analysis for overall survival

Variables	Univariate analysis HR (95% CI)	P value	Multivariate analysis HR (95% CI)	P value
Age (≥ 65 vs <65)	1.56 (1.14-2.17)	< .01	1.46 (1.03-2.07)	.032
Sex (male vs female)	1.18 (0.74-1.98)	.52		
Brinkman Index (≥800 vs <800)	1.05 (0.77-1.42)	.77		
Body Mass Index				
(≥25 vs <25)	0.72 (0.44-1.12)	.15		
(<18.5 vs ≥18.5)	1.81 (1.16-2.71)	< .01	1.67 (1.06-2.53)	.028
Performance Status (1, 2 vs 0)	2.09 (1.41-3.01)	< .01	1.54 (1.01-2.27)	.043
Comorbidity (+ vs -)	1.52 (1.04-2.29)	.028	1.16 (0.77-1.78)	.48
cStage (III, IV vs I, II)	2.19 (1.60-2.97)	< .01	1.38 (0.90-2.12)	.14
Preoperative treatment (+ vs -)	2.18 (1.59-2.97)	< .01	1.50 (0.98-2.27)	.060
Preoperative aSIS				
(1 vs 0)	1.76 (1.23-2.54)	< .01	1.36 (0.93-2.01)	.11
(2 vs 0)	2.50 (1.65-3.79)	< .01	1.81 (1.16-2.81)	< .01
Postoperative complications				
CDc ≥IIIb (+ vs -)	1.72 (1.11-2.56)	.016	1.74 (1.12-2.63)	.016

Abbreviations: CDc, Clavien-Dindo classification; CI, confidence interval; HR, hazard ratio.

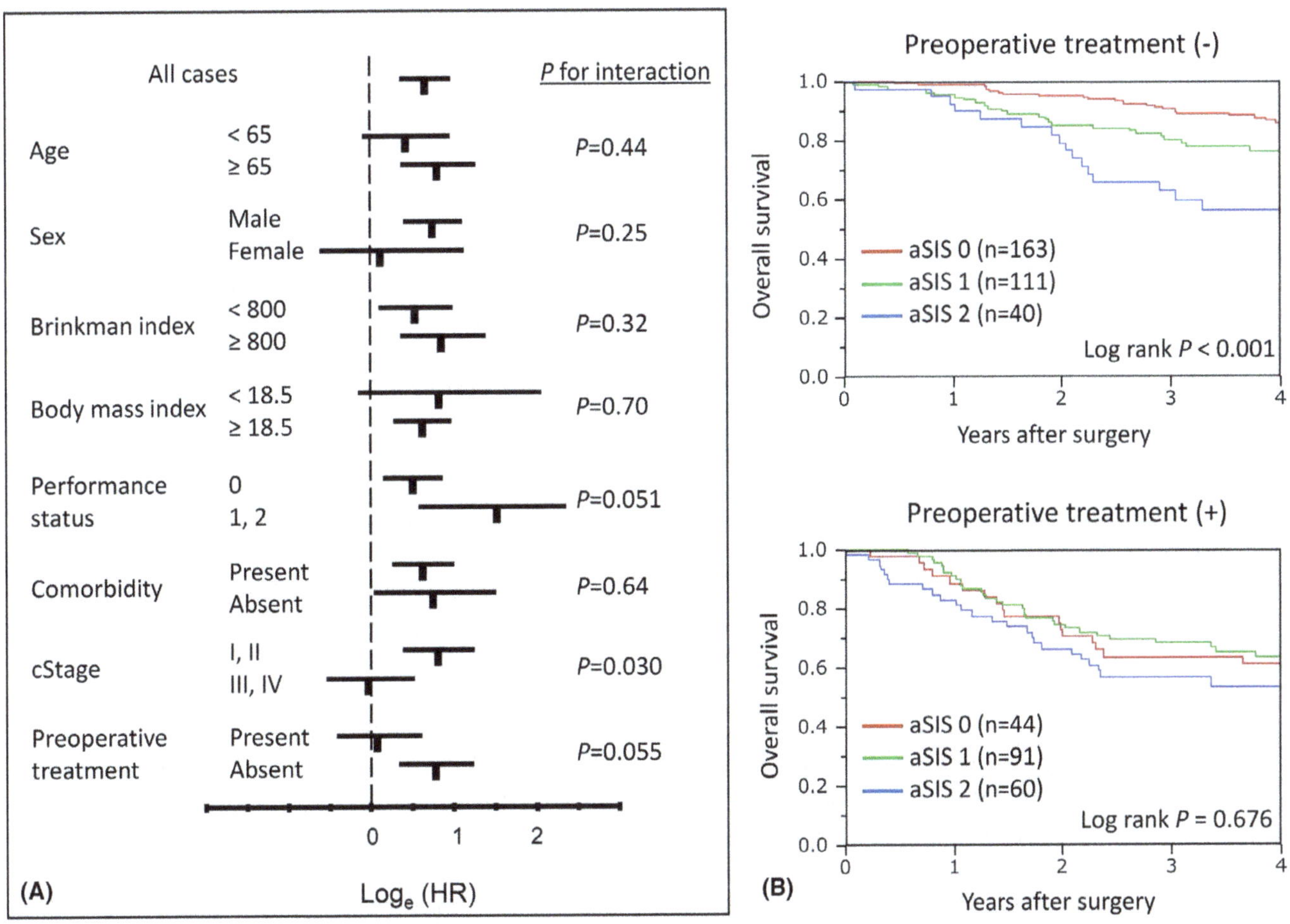

FIGURE 3 A: Relationship between the adapted systemic inflammation score (aSIS) and OS. Log$_e$(HRs) plots of the OS rate in aSIS 0 (low) and aSIS 1, 2 (high) groups are shown. B: Kaplan-Meier curves for OS in patients with esophageal squamous cell carcinoma, according to the aSIS stratification. The upper panel includes patients who did not receive any preoperative treatment. The lower panel includes patients who received preoperative treatment. aSIS, modified systemic inflammation score; OS, overall survival; HRs, hazards ratio

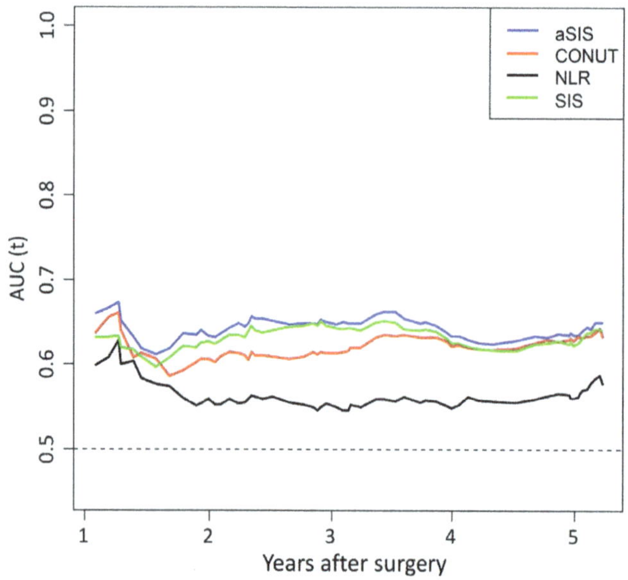

FIGURE 4 The time-dependent AUC-of-ROC curves of aSIS and other prognostic scoring systems (CONUT, SIS, NLR) for the prediction of OS. AUC-of-ROC, area under the curve of the receiver operating characteristics; CONUT, controlling nutritional status; SIS, systemic inflammation score; aSIS, adapted systemic inflammation score; NLR, neutrophil-to-lymphocyte ratio

patients with clear-cell renal cell carcinoma, and the cutoff value of LMR was 4.44 based on the median value of LMR.[2] Higher SIS was associated with poorer OS in colorectal cancer[3,15] and gastric cancer.[16,17] However, Lin et al showed that SIS was not an independent prognostic factor for gastric cancer patients based on a multivariate analysis.[5] They determined a new cutoff value of LMR at 3.4 using the software X-tile[4] and constructed the mSIS. The mSIS was the only significant independent biomarker, and a higher mSIS score was associated with 5-y OS.

Two previous studies on ESCC showed that a high SIS was significantly associated with poorer OS.[6,7] There was only one study focusing on the prognostic role of mSIS in ESCC patients.[8] Kanda et al analyzed patients with esophageal cancer using Lin's cutoff value of 3.4, without using the software X-tile, and reported that a higher mSIS was associated with poorer disease-free survival in 443 ESCC patients.[8] However, all of these studies were limited by small sample sizes (n < 450). In contrast to previous studies, our study evaluated preoperative aSIS in a much larger cohort of over 500 ESCC patients. Furthermore, the LMR cutoff value was optimized at 3.3 for ESCC patients using the software X-tile. In our study aSIS was a significant independent prognostic biomarker and the higher aSIS was associated with poorer OS and CSS. Importantly, aSIS was more sensitive than other nutritional prognostic factors, namely, CONUT, NLR, and SIS. The reason why aSIS was more sensitive than SIS might be the difference in the LMR cutoff value (the LMR cutoff values in aSIS and SIS were 3.3 and 4.44, respectively). In ESCC patients, The LMR cutoff value 4.44 was strict and many patients were assigned to SIS:2 (SIS 2:32%, aSIS 2:20%), and it might not be possible to stratify patients with poor SIS. The reason why aSIS was more sensitive than CONUT and NLR might be the difference in each prognostic factor's components. Especially, it might be affected by the fact that only aSIS includes monocytes, not CONUT and NLR. Peripheral monocyte count appeared to be useful prognostic marker in a large cohort of patients with ESCC.[18] However, the precise molecular mechanism by which monocytes might predict clinical survival is not understood. One hypothesized pathogenic mechanism is that monocytes are recruited by some cytokines and chemokines around the tumor and differentiate into tumor-associated macrophages (TAMs), which facilitate multiple tumorigenic mechanisms. Type 2 macrophages, in particular, have a tumorigenic effect that includes tumor initiation, invasion, angiogenesis, and metastasis.[19] We have previously reported that the presence of a high-density of TAMs was associated with significantly worse OS in patients with resected ESCC.[20] Therefore, an elevated absolute monocyte count may indicate the presence of TAMs.

The biological mechanism underlying the relationship between the systemic impact of aSIS and prognosis is still unknown. One mechanism may involve the relationship between systemic inflammation and tumor immunity (tumor infiltrating lymphocytes [TILs]). We have previously revealed the correlation between TIL status and total lymphocyte count in peripheral blood. TILs might promote antitumor immunity and might be associated with improved outcomes in ESCC patients.[21] Further experimental studies are necessary for investigating these mechanisms in ESCC.

Interestingly, we found that the prognostic effect of the aSIS differed according to the neoadjuvant treatment status. Low aSIS was associated with high OS among patients who did not undergo neoadjuvant treatment. In contrast, in patients who underwent neoadjuvant treatment, there was no association between the aSIS and OS. The most probable reason could be that many patients with neoadjuvant treatment have advanced-stage ESCC and poor prognosis (Table S2). On the other hand, 50% of patients without neoadjuvant treatment were cStage I (Table S1). Second, in the clinical setting for esophageal cancer treatment, preoperative therapy might negatively affect the patients' systemic nutritional and immunological status. In fact, comparing preneoadjuvant treatment and preoperative blood sampling values, Alb levels and lymphocyte count decreased significantly (Alb 4.0 ± 0.4 vs 3.7 ± 0.4, $P < .01$; lymphocytes 1766 ± 597 vs 1486 ± 584, $P < .01$), and monocyte count tended to decrease (434 ± 174 vs 413 ± 160, $P = .14$). Approximately 67% of the patients with aSIS of 0 before neoadjuvant treatment showed elevated preoperative aSIS. This could affect their clinical outcome via the local tumor immune response.[22]

This study has several limitations. First, this was a retrospective study. Second, the patients were included from just our institution. The significance of aSIS needs to be validated using other cohorts.

In conclusion, our large cohort study with more than 500 cases revealed that the preoperative aSIS was associated with the clinical outcome in ESCC patients who underwent curative resection. Furthermore, aSIS was more sensitive than other nutritional prognostic factors. Considering the relationship between nutritional status and local tumor immunity, our findings may have considerable clinical implications. Future studies are needed for confirming our findings as well as for elucidating the exact mechanisms by which the nutritional status affects local tumor immunity.

ACKNOWLEDGMENT

We thank Editage (www.editage.com) for English language editing.

REFERENCES

1. Bray F, Ferlay J, Soerjomataram I, Siegel RL, Torre LA, Jemal A. Global cancer statistics 2018: GLOBOCAN estimates of incidence and mortality worldwide for 36 cancers in 185 countries. CA Cancer J Clin. 2018;68(6):394–424.
2. Chang Y, An H, Xu L, Zhu Y, Yang Y, Lin Z, et al. Systemic inflammation score predicts postoperative prognosis of patients with clear-cell renal cell carcinoma. Br J Cancer. 2015;113(4):626–33.
3. Suzuki Y, Okabayashi K, Hasegawa H, Tsuruta M, Shigeta K, Kondo T, et al. Comparison of preoperative inflammation-based prognostic scores in patients with colorectal cancer. Ann Surg. 2018;267(3):527–31.
4. Camp RL, Dolled-Filhart M, Rimm DL. X-tile: a new bio-informatics tool for biomarker assessment and outcome-based cut-point optimization. Clin Cancer Res. 2004;10(21):7252–9.
5. Lin J-X, Lin J-P, Xie J-W, Wang J-B, Lu J, Chen Q-Y, et al. Prognostic importance of the preoperative modified systemic inflammation score for patients with gastric cancer. Gastric Cancer. 2019;22(2):403–12.
6. Han L, Song Q, Jia Y, Chen X, Wang C, Chen P, et al. The clinical significance of systemic inflammation score in esophageal squamous cell carcinoma. Tumour Biol. 2016;37(3):3081–90.
7. Fu X, Li T, Dai Y, Li J. Preoperative systemic inflammation score (SIS) is superior to neutrophil to lymphocyte ratio (NLR) as a predicting indicator in patients with esophageal squamous cell carcinoma. BMC Cancer. 2019;19(1):721.
8. Kanda M, Koike M, Tanaka C, Kobayashi D, Hattori N, Hayashi M, et al. Modified systemic inflammation score is useful for risk stratification after radical resection of squamous cell carcinoma of the esophagus. Ann Surg Oncol. 2019;26(13):4773–81.
9. Sobin LH, Gospodarowicz MK, Wittekind C. TNM Classification of Malignant Tumours, 8th edn. Oxford: Wiley-Blackwell; 2010.
10. McShane LM, Altman DG, Sauerbrei W, Taube SE, Gion M, Clark GM. Reporting recommendations for tumor marker prognostic studies (REMARK). J Natl Cancer Inst. 2005;97(16):1180–4.
11. Sharaiha RZ, Halazun KJ, Mirza F, Port JL, Lee PC, Neugut AI, et al. Elevated preoperative neutrophil:lymphocyte ratio as a predictor of postoperative disease recurrence in esophageal cancer. Ann Surg Oncol. 2011;18(12):3362–9.
12. Yodying H, Matsuda A, Miyashita M, Matsumoto S, Sakurazawa N, Yamada M, et al. Prognostic significance of neutrophil-to-lymphocyte ratio and platelet-to-lymphocyte ratio in oncologic outcomes of esophageal cancer: a systematic review and meta-analysis. Ann Surg Oncol. 2016;23(2):646–54.
13. De Ulíbarri JI, González-Madroño A, de Villar NG, et al. CONUT: a tool for controlling nutritional status. First validation in a hospital population. Nutr Hosp. 2005;20(1):38–45.
14. Mantovani A, Allavena P, Sica A, Balkwill F. Cancer-related inflammation. Nature. 2008;454(7203):436–44.
15. Feng Y, Liu L, Zhu Y. Systemic inflammation score in locally advanced rectal cancer patients following total mesorectal excision. Onco Targets Ther. 2019;12:6617–22.
16. Sato B, Kanda M, Tanaka C, Kobayashi D, Iwata N, Hattori N, et al. Significance of preoperative systemic inflammation score in short-term and long-term outcomes of patients with pathological T2–4 gastric cancer after radical gastrectomy. World J Surg. 2018;42(10):3277–85.
17. Ma M, Weng M, Chen F, Hu Y, Lai J, Wang Y, et al. Systemic inflammation score is a prognostic marker after curative resection in gastric cancer. ANZ J Surg. 2019;89(4):377–82.
18. Han L, Jia Y, Song Q, Wang N, Wang J, Bai B, et al. Prognostic significance of preoperative absolute peripheral monocyte count in esophageal squamous cell carcinoma. Dis Esophagus. 2016;29(7):740–6.
19. Quail DF, Joyce JA. Microenvironmental regulation of tumor progression and metastasis. Nat Med. 2013;19(11):1423–37.
20. Yagi T, Baba Y, Okadome K, Kiyozumi Y, Hiyoshi Y, Ishimoto T, et al. Tumour-associated macrophages are associated with poor prognosis and programmed death ligand 1 expression in oesophageal cancer. Eur J Cancer. 2019;111:38–49.
21. Yagi T, Baba Y, Ishimoto T, Iwatsuki M, Miyamoto Y, Yoshida N, et al. PD-L1 expression, tumor-infiltrating lymphocytes, and clinical outcome in patients with surgically resected esophageal cancer. Ann Surg. 2019;269(3):471–8.
22. Okadome K, Baba Y, Yagi T, Kiyozumi Y, Ishimoto T, Iwatsuki M, et al. Prognostic nutritional index, tumor-infiltrating lymphocytes, and prognosis in patients with esophageal cancer. Ann Surg. 2020;271(4):693–700.

14

Is proximal gastrectomy indicated for locally advanced cancer in the upper third of the stomach?

Motonari Ri[1] | Koshi Kumagai[1] | Ken Namikawa[2] | Shinichiro Atsumi[1] | Masaru Hayami[1] | Rie Makuuchi[1] | Satoshi Ida[1] | Manabu Ohashi[1] | Takeshi Sano[1] | Souya Nunobe[1]

[1]Department of Gastroenterological Surgery, Cancer Institute Hospital, Japanese Foundation for Cancer Research, Tokyo, Japan

[2]Department of Gastroenterology, Cancer Institute Hospital, Japanese Foundation for Cancer Research, Tokyo, Japan

Correspondence
Souya Nunobe, Department of Gastroenterological Surgery, Cancer Institute Hospital, Japanese Foundation for Cancer Research, 3-8-31 Ariake, Koto-ku, Tokyo, 135-8550, Japan.
Email: souya.nunobe@jfcr.or.jp

Abstract

Aim: To treat upper third gastric cancer, proximal gastrectomy (PG), a function-preserving procedure, is recommended for early lesions when at least half the distal stomach can be preserved, while total gastrectomy (TG) is standard for locally advanced lesions. Oncological feasibility, when applying PG for such lesions, remains unknown.

Methods: We reviewed patients undergoing TG for clinical (c) T2–T4 upper third gastric cancer between 2006 and 2015. Preoperative tumor locations were further classified into the cardia, fornix, and gastric body based on endoscopic findings. The metastatic rate and therapeutic value index for lymph node (LN) dissection were determined, and characteristics of patients with distal LN (No. 4d, 5, and 6) metastasis (DLNM) were reviewed. In addition, patients with pathological tumor invasion to the middle third (M) region were investigated.

Results: We studied 167 patients. There were 8 (4.8%) with DLNM and 41 (24.6%) with pathological tumor invasion to the M region. As to regional stations, therapeutic indices for LN dissection at stations No. 4d, 5, 6, and 12a were zero or extremely low. No DLNM was detected in cT2 lesions or cT3/T4 lesions located within the cardia and/or the fornix. In addition, none of the lesions located within the cardia and/or the fornix by preoperative endoscopy extended to the M region in the pathological specimen.

Conclusions: For upper third gastric cancer, PG without No. 12a dissection might be acceptable for cT2–T4 lesions located within the cardia and/or the fornix when considering the risk of DLNM and cancer-positivity in the distal stump.

KEYWORDS

distal margin, locally advanced gastric cancer, lymph node metastasis, proximal gastrectomy, therapeutic index, upper third gastric cancer

1 | INTRODUCTION

Worldwide, gastric cancer is among the most life-threatening malignant neoplasms.[1,2] The incidence of gastric cancer in the upper third of the stomach has recently been rising in both Western and Asian countries.[3-5] As a therapeutic strategy for upper third gastric cancer indicated for surgical treatment, proximal gastrectomy (PG), a function-preserving procedure, is advocated for lesions diagnosed at an early stage when more than half of the distal stomach can be preserved.[6] In contrast, total gastrectomy (TG) is now the standard procedure for locally advanced lesions in the upper third of the stomach.[6]

Comparing TG and PG for early gastric cancer, PG is considered to be more advantageous in mitigating body weight loss, maintaining nutritional status, and not causing deterioration of quality of life postoperatively.[7-9] Therefore, provided that oncological safety is assured, PG may also be the preferred surgical treatment for locally advanced gastric cancer in the upper third region. As to esophagogastric junctional (EGJ) cancer, PG can be selected even for an advanced tumor if the primary lesion is less than 4 cm in size, based on the oncological safety of lymph node (LN) metastasis, as stated in the Japanese gastric cancer treatment guidelines.[6]

However, there are oncological concerns when applying PG for advanced upper third gastric malignancies other than EGJ tumors. That is, an optimal extent of LN dissection in performing PG for advanced cancer has not yet been established, with only a few reports focusing on this issue,[10,11] nor has the relationship between actual locations of primary lesions and LN metastasis been investigated in sufficient detail. Moreover, it is essential to ensure an adequate distal tumor margin and sufficient volume of the remnant stomach after gastric dissection.

Here we evaluated pathological metastasis involving the aforementioned regional LNs and the distal tumor margin in patients undergoing TG for clinically advanced gastric cancer in the upper third of the stomach. The present results are anticipated to contribute to determining the criteria for applying PG to advanced lesions.

2 | METHODS

2.1 | Patients

From January 2006 to December 2015, patients who underwent TG for cT2–4 gastric cancer, preoperatively diagnosed as being located within the upper third region of the stomach without or with esophageal invasion, at the Department of Gastroenterological Surgery, Cancer Institute Hospital, Tokyo, Japan, were registered in this study. Although D2 LN dissection was usually performed during TG for advanced lesions, a few patients underwent TG with D1/D1+ LN dissection at the discretion of the main surgeon, based on patient background factors such as age, performance status, comorbidities, and so on. The exclusion criteria were as follows: (a) EGJ cancer with its center located within 2 cm of the EGJ, as defined by the Japanese gastric cancer treatment guidelines,[12] (b) macroscopic type 4 (diffuse infiltrative) lesion, (c) remnant gastric cancer, (d) simultaneous multiple gastric cancers, (e) the presence of other primary malignant disease, (f) history of preoperative chemotherapy, and (g) R1/R2 resection. This study was approved by the Institutional Review Board of the Cancer Institute Hospital (No. 2017-1187).

2.2 | Assessment of clinical staging

For clinical T factor diagnosis, findings obtained by endoscopy and the features noted on computed tomography (CT) by an experienced radiologist were reviewed, and the depth of tumor invasion of the wall was finally determined at the gastric cancer team conference including surgeons, endoscopists, and chemotherapists. Regional LNs with a long-axis diameter of 10 mm or more on CT were diagnosed as metastatic nodes and their station numbers were also examined. Clinical stages were determined according to the 14th edition of the Japanese Classification of Gastric Carcinoma.[13]

2.3 | Pathological metastasis and therapeutic value index for LNs at each station

As to the regional LNs to be dissected, the rate of LN metastasis and the therapeutic value index for dissection of LNs at each station were examined, including LNs not defined as meeting the extent of lymphadenectomy in PG for early cancer. The rate of metastasis was calculated by dividing the number of patients with metastasis at the nodal station by the number of patients in whom that station was retrieved. Moreover, the therapeutic values of each dissected LN were determined using the therapeutic value index proposed by Sasako et al.[14] This index was obtained by multiplying the rate of nodal metastasis by the 5-y overall survival (OS) for each nodal station. The 5-y OS in patients with LN metastasis was calculated for each station, irrespective of nodal metastasis at other stations. In addition, clinical details of patients with distal LN metastasis (DLNM), that is, metastasis to LNs at stations No. 4d, 5, and/or 6, which could not be removed during PG, were investigated.

2.4 | Evaluation of tumor location based on preoperative endoscopy and pathological specimen

We assessed tumor location preoperatively based on the endoscopic findings. In particular, the locations of the distal tumor border were further divided into three regions, ie, the cardia, the fornix, and the gastric body (Figure 1). The location of the cardia was defined as being within 2 cm of the EGJ in the stomach. Representative endoscopic photographs of tumors included in this study are presented in Figure 2. In addition, tumor locations were also determined postoperatively using the pathological specimen, and divided into the upper third or middle third (M) regions of the stomach.

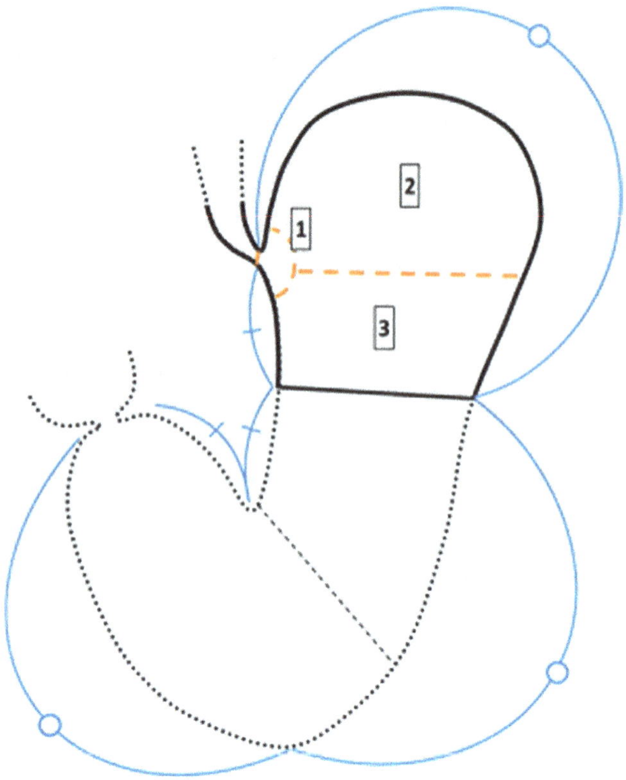

FIGURE 1 Classification of tumor location in the upper third of the stomach based on endoscopic findings. Locations of the distal tumor border in gastric cancers of the upper third were divided into three regions based on the endoscopic findings: (1) the cardia, (2) the fornix, (3) the gastric body

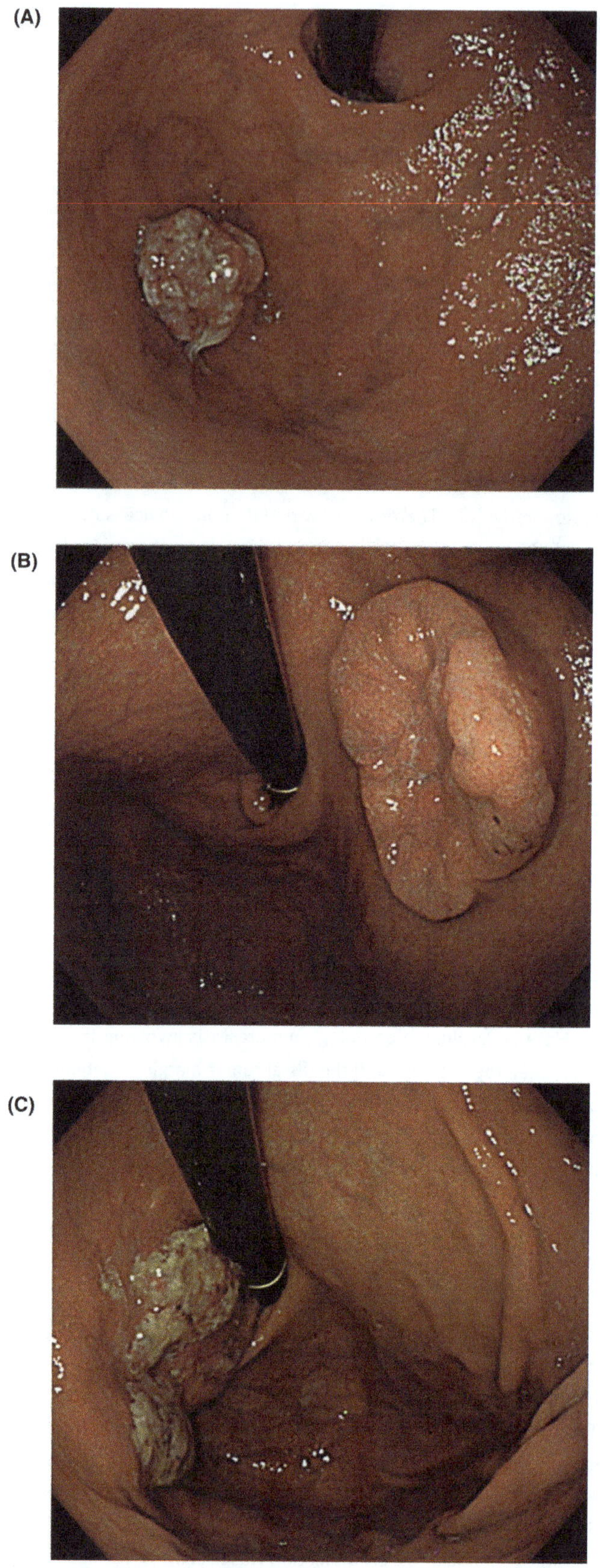

FIGURE 2 Representative endoscopic photographs showing tumor locations. (A) Located within the fornix. (B) Located within the gastric body. (C) Located in both the gastric body and the cardia

3 | STATISTICAL ANALYSIS

The patient background characteristics, surgical details, and pathological findings were collected from our database and information contained in electronic medical records. The relationships between clinical characteristics and pathological findings, including LN metastasis and tumor location, were investigated. All continuous variables are expressed as median values. Statistical analyses were conducted using the Mann–Whitney *U*-test and the chi-squared test. A *P*-value less than .05 was considered to indicate a statistically significant difference. All statistical analyses were performed with JMP Pro 13 (SAS Institute Japan, Japan) for windows.

4 | RESULTS

4.1 | Clinicopathological characteristics

Patient clinical characteristics are shown in Table 1. In total, 167 patients were included in this study. As to the location of the distal tumor border according to preoperative endoscopy, 12 patients (7.2%) had lesions limited to the cardia or the fornix. Although 23

TABLE 1 Characteristics of the patients

	All (n = 167)
Sex, n (%)	
Male	116 (69.5)
Female	51 (30.5)
Age, years [IQR]	67 [59-73]
Tumor location, n (%)	
U	151 (90.4)
UE	16 (9.6)
Location of distal tumor border by endoscopy, n (%)	
Cardia or fornix	12 (7.2)
Gastric body	155 (92.8)
Tumor circumference, n (%)	
Less	46 (27.5)
Gre	22 (13.2)
Ant	24 (14.4)
Post	71 (42.5)
Circ	4 (2.4)
Clinical macroscopic type, n (%)	
0	35 (21.0)
1	14 (8.4)
2	39 (23.4)
3	76 (45.5)
5	3 (1.8)
Preoperative tumor size, mm [IQR]	40 [30-55]
Clinical T factor, n (%)	
T2	65 (38.9)
T3	41 (24.6)
T4	61 (36.5)
Clinical N factor, n (%)	
N0	144 (86.2)
N+	23 (13.8)
Region of clinical lymph node metastasis	
Left area of cardia (No. 2)	1 (4.2)
Lesser curvature (No. 1 and 3)	21 (87.5)
Supra-pancreas (No. 7, 8a, 9 and 11p)	2 (8.3)
Splenic hilum (No. 10)	0 (0)
Distal area (No. 4d, 5 and 6)	0 (0)
Surgical approach, n (%)	
Open	163 (97.6)
Laparoscopic	4 (2.4)
Type of lymph node dissection, n (%)	
D2 or more	156 (93.4)
D1 or D1+	11 (6.6)

Abbreviation: IQR, interquartile range.

patients (13.8%) were clinically diagnosed as having LN metastasis, none of them had swollen LNs at stations No. 4d, 5, and/or 6. As to pathological findings (Table 2), there were 8 patients (4.8%) with DLNM, and 41 (24.6%) showing tumor invasion to the M region in the pathological specimen.

4.2 | Rate of LN metastasis and therapeutic value index of LN dissection for each station

Table 3 shows the LN metastasis rate, 5-y OS, and the therapeutic value index for dissection of each LN station. In patients with cT2 lesions, the metastatic rate and the therapeutic index of LN were both zero at stations No. 4d, 5, and 6. On the other hand, the LN metastasis rate was zero only at station No. 6 of the three stations examined patients with cT3/T4 tumors. Among the regional stations examined, however, the therapeutic indices of LN dissection at stations No. 4d and 5 were extremely low, at 1.0 and 1.4, respectively. The therapeutic index for dissection of LNs at station No. 12a was also zero in all patients.

TABLE 2 Pathological findings

	All (n = 167)
Pathological tumor size, mm [IQR]	50 [38-75]
Histology, n (%)	
Differentiated	72 (43.1)
Undifferentiated	92 (55.1)
Others	3 (1.8)
Pathological T factor, n (%)	
T1	16 (9.6)
T2	29 (17.4)
T3	55 (32.9)
T4	67 (40.1)
Pathological N factor, n (%)	
N0	78 (46.7)
N1	34 (20.4)
N2	26 (15.6)
N3	29 (17.4)
Pathological stage, n (%)	
I	39 (23.4)
II	63 (37.7)
III	61 (36.5)
IV	4 (2.4)
DLNM, n (%)	
Yes	8 (4.8)
No	159 (95.2)
Pathological tumor invasion to the M region, n (%)	
Yes	41 (24.6)
No	126 (75.4)

Abbreviations: DLNM, distal lymph node (stations No. 4d, 5, and 6) metastasis; IQR, interquartile range; M region, middle third of the stomach.

TABLE 3 Metastatic ratio and therapeutic value index for dissection of LNs at each station

Station of LN	No. of metastatic LNs/retrieved LNs	Metastatic ratio (%)	5-y overall survival (%)	Therapeutic index
(a) cT2 lesions				
1	9/65	13.8	44.4	6.2
2	5/58	8.6	80.0	6.9
3	19/65	29.2	78.9	23.1
4sa	3/58	5.2	66.7	3.4
4sb	3/61	4.9	33.3	1.6
4d	0/65	0.0	0.0	0.0
5	0/47	0.0	0.0	0.0
6	0/65	0.0	0.0	0.0
7	3/64	4.7	33.3	1.6
8a	1/65	1.5	0.0	0.0
9	2/62	3.2	50.0	1.6
10	2/19	10.5	50.0	5.3
11p	5/65	7.7	40.0	3.1
11d	2/26	7.7	0.0	0.0
12a	0/25	0.0	0.0	0.0
(b) cT3-4 lesions				
1	25/101	24.8	40.0	9.9
2	20/96	20.8	45.0	9.4
3	46/102	45.1	54.3	24.5
4sa	10/87	11.5	30.0	3.4
4sb	6/97	6.2	16.7	1.0
4d	6/102	5.9	16.7	1.0
5	1/73	1.4	100.0	1.4
6	1/101	1.0	0.0	0.0
7	23/102	22.5	56.5	12.7
8a	3/102	2.9	33.3	1.0
9	8/97	8.2	50.0	4.1
10	10/70	14.3	20.0	2.9
11p	16/95	16.8	31.3	5.3
11d	6/60	10.0	16.7	1.7
12a	0/50	0.0	0.0	0.0

4.3 | Patients with DLNM

Table 4 shows the clinicopathological and demographic characteristics of eight patients with DLNM. All primary lesions extended to the gastric body, and all had a depth of cT3 or cT4. All but one of the seven patients were diagnosed at far advanced stages of disease, pStage III or IV, with extensive LN metastasis.

4.4 | Patients with pathological tumor invasion to M region

Table 5 compares the clinicopathological factors between patients with and without pathological tumor invasion to the M region. The proportions of females and patients with cT4 lesions were significantly higher among those with than those without pathological invasion to the M region. Preoperative and pathological tumor sizes were significantly greater in patients with than in those without pathological invasion to the M region. In addition, none of the tumors limited to the cardia and/or the fornix based on preoperative endoscopy extended to the M region in the pathological specimen.

5 | DISCUSSION

We evaluated the pathological status of regional LNs, the therapeutic index for each nodal station, and the pathological tumor location in patients undergoing TG for cT2–4 upper third gastric cancer, to

TABLE 4 Characteristics of patients with DLNM

No.	Gender	Age, years	Distal border of tumor	Clinical macroscopic type	Preoperative tumor size, mm	cT factor	Histology	pT factor	pN factor	pStage
1	Female	67	Gastric body	Type 3	100	cT4a	Undiff.	pT4a	pN3b	IIIC
2	Female	61	Gastric body	Type 3	55	cT3	Undiff.	pT4a	pN3a	IVA
3	Male	71	Gastric body	Type 3	60	cT4a	Undiff.	pT4a	pN3b	IIIC
4	Male	79	Gastric body	Type 3	60	cT4b	Undiff.	pT4b	pN3b	IVA
5	Male	59	Gastric body	Type 3	40	cT3	Diff.	pT4a	pN3a	IIIC
6	Male	81	Gastric body	Type 3	60	cT4a	Diff.	pT4a	pN3a	IIIC
7	Male	73	Gastric body	Type 1	35	cT3	Diff.	pT1b	pN1	IB
8	Female	48	Gastric body	Type 3	50	cT4a	Undiff.	pT4a	pN3a	IIIC

Abbreviations: DLNM, distal lymph node (stations No. 4d, 5, and 6) metastasis; Undiff., undifferentiated type.

explore the possibility of applying PG for these lesions. The following findings were obtained in the present study. Among the regional LNs examined, the therapeutic indices for dissection of LNs at stations No. 4, 5, 6, and 12a were zero or extremely low. Moreover, no DLNM was detected in cT2 lesions or cT3/T4 lesions located within the cardia/fornix. In addition, the lesions located within the cardia/fornix by preoperative endoscopy did not extend to the M region in the pathological specimen. Therefore, PG without No. 12a dissection might be indicated for lesions within the cardia/fornix, considering the oncological aspects of DLNM and the risk of cancer-positivity in the distal margin.

Several studies have focused on the frequency of DLNM in locally advanced cancers in the upper third of the stomach, and all obtained similar results.[10,11,14] In particular, Yura et al suggested that the frequency of DLNM in pT2/T3 lesions in the upper region was extremely low, and that no therapeutic effect was obtained by dissecting these LNs.[11] However, patients were not studied according to clinical T factors, but instead only according to pathological T factors in all of the previous investigations. Given that surgical treatment is determined based on the preoperative diagnosis including the clinical T factor and that clinicopathological discrepancies among T categories are possible, the results obtained from the present study, which included taking clinical T factors into account, appear to be reliable.

Moreover, tumor locations were further divided into three regions based on preoperative endoscopic findings, revealing that DLNM is unlikely to develop in locally advanced lesions, even with serosal invasion, when they are located above the gastric body. Although greater tumor diameter is considered to carry a risk of deeper wall invasion,[15-17] PG might be acceptable for such lesions because a sufficient distal margin can be maintained. In addition, given that all patients with DLNM were pathologically diagnosed as having far advanced disease stages, ie, pStage IIIC or IV, except in one case, surgical treatment alone would not have achieved satisfactory long-term survival. Thus, patients with DLNM require perioperative multidisciplinary treatments.

As specified in the current guidelines,[6] lymph node dissection with D1 or D1 plus can be applied in PG for early lesions, while the optimal extent of lymphadenectomy in PG for advanced stage cancer remains unknown. Although LNs at the distal stations cannot be removed because blood flow to the remnant stomach must be preserved, it is possible to dissect LNs at stations No. 10, 11d, and 12a, which are not included among the LNs defined as being suitable for PG with D1 or D1 plus. Based on several reports indicating that No. 12a LN dissection has no therapeutic effect, which is consistent with the results of the present study,[10,11,14] it may be reasonable to omit lymphadenectomy of station No. 12a when performing PG for advanced lesions. On the other hand, the frequency of No. 10 LN metastasis in proximal advanced gastric cancer is not low, reportedly being 10.7%–16.5%,[18-20] which is similar to the result obtained in this study. Splenectomy for No. 10 LN dissection should be determined according to the results of a randomized controlled trial.[21]

Insufficient volume of the remnant stomach after PG is reportedly associated with deterioration of postoperative quality of life and skeletal muscle loss.[22,23] In practice, the aim is generally to preserve more than 2/3 of the preoperative gastric volume in performing PG for early lesions.[7,24] Even when applying PG to advanced tumors, it is apparently essential that at least half of the distal stomach, as recommended in the guidelines, be preserved.[6] Large tumors and pathologically advanced T stage are reportedly risk factors for

TABLE 5 Comparison between patients with and without pathological tumor invasion to the M region

	No pathological invasion to M region	Pathological invasion to M region	
	(n = 126)	(n = 41)	P value
Sex, n (%)			
Male	93 (73.8)	23 (56.1)	.032
Female	33 (26.2)	18 (43.9)	
Age, years [IQR]	67 [60-73]	63 [54-75]	.142
Tumor location, n (%)			
U	116 (92.1)	35 (85.4)	.205
UE	10 (7.9)	6 (14.6)	
Location of distal tumor border by endoscopy, n (%)			
Cardia or fornix	12 (9.5)	0 (0)	.040
Gastric body	114 (90.5)	41 (100)	
Clinical macroscopic type, n (%)			
0	25 (19.8)	10 (24.4)	.444
1	13 (10.3)	1 (2.4)	
2	29 (23.0)	10 (24.4)	
3	56 (44.4)	20 (48.8)	
5	3 (2.4)	0 (0)	
Preoperative tumor size, mm [IQR]	40 [30-50]	50 [40-60]	<.001
Clinical T factor, n (%)			
T2	56 (44.4)	9 (22.0)	<.001
T3	34 (27.0)	7 (17.1)	
T4	26 (28.6)	25 (61.0)	
Histology, n (%)			
Differentiated	57 (45.2)	15 (36.6)	.605
Undifferentiated	67 (53.2)	25 (61.0)	
Others	2 (1.6)	1 (2.4)	
Pathological tumor size, mm [IQR]	48 [35-62]	80 [52-95]	<.001
Pathological T factor, n (%)			
T1	15 (11.9)	1 (2.4)	.030
T2	24 (19.1)	5 (12.2)	
T3	44 (34.9)	11 (26.8)	
T4	43 (34.1)	24 (58.5)	
Pathological stage, n (%)			
I	34 (27.0)	5 (12.2)	.124
II	48 (38.1)	15 (36.6)	
III	42 (33.3)	19 (46.3)	
IV	2 (1.6)	2 (4.9)	

Abbreviations: IQR, interquartile range; M region, middle third of the stomach.

a positive resection margin in gastric cancer surgery, similar to the characteristics of patients with pathological tumor invasion to the M region in this study.[25-27] However, this study suggested that more than half of the stomach might be preserved even with locally advanced gastric cancer, provided that the lesion is located within the cardia and/or the fornix.

This study has several limitations. First, this was a retrospective study with a small sample size conducted at a single institution. Moreover, we were not able to perform a multivariate analysis because there were too few patients with DLNM in this cohort. The most recent cases could not be included in the present study due to this being a 5-y survival analysis. Second, the therapeutic effect of dissecting LNs at station No. 11d remains unclear due to the insufficient number of cases. In addition, whether dissection of No. 3b LNs has any clinical benefit could not be evaluated because not all of the No. 3 LNs were recorded separately, ie, as No. 3a or 3b LNs, in our database. This is because the nodes at station No. 3 were divided into 3a and 3b LNs according to the revision of the 14th edition of the Japanese Classification of Gastric Carcinoma in 2010.[13] When performing PG for locally advanced lesions, complete dissection of LNs at station No. 3 including the No. 3b might be essential, along with not leaving a significant volume of the remnant stomach due to the necessity of securing an appropriate margin. The optimal extent of LN dissection at station No. 3 is a topic for future study. Third, functions of the remnant stomach such as peristalsis and retention after PG for locally advanced cancer were not evaluated. A multicenter study with a large sample size is required to clarify these issues and overcome the limitations of this study.

In conclusion, for locally advanced gastric cancer in the upper third of the stomach, PG without No. 12a dissection might be acceptable for lesions located within the cardia and/or the fornix, given that neither DLNM nor a distal cancer-positive margin was detected in these cases.

DISCLOSURE

The protocol for this research project was approved by the Institutional Review Board of the Cancer Institute Hospital and conforms to the provisions of the Declaration of Helsinki. Approval No. 2017-1187. Informed consent was obtained from all of the subjects.

REFERENCES

1. Ferlay J, Soerjomataram I, Dikshit R, Eser S, Mathers C, Rebelo M, et al. Cancer incidence and mortality worldwide: sources, methods and major patterns in GLOBOCAN 2012. Int J Cancer. 2015;136(5):E359–86.
2. Torre LA, Bray F, Siegel RL, Ferlay J, Lortet-Tieulent J, Jemal A. Global cancer statistics, 2012. CA Cancer J Clin. 2015;65(2):87–108.
3. Wu H, Rusiecki JA, Zhu K, Potter J, Devesa SS. Stomach carcinoma incidence patterns in the United States by histologic type and anatomic site. Cancer Epidemiol Biomarkers Prev. 2009;18(7):1945–52.
4. Ahn HS, Lee HJ, Yoo MW, Jeong S-H, Park D-J, Kim H-H, et al. Changes in clinicopathological features and survival after gastrectomy for gastric cancer over a 20-year period. Br J Surg. 2011;98(2):255–60.
5. Deans C, Yeo MSW, Soe MY, Shabbir A, Ti TK, So JBY. Cancer of the gastric cardia is rising in incidence in an Asian population and is associated with adverse outcome. World J Surg. 2011;35(3):617–24.
6. Japanese Gastric Cancer Association. Japanese gastric cancer treatment guidelines 2018 (5th edition). Gastric Cancer. 2021;24:1–21.
7. Hayami M, Hiki N, Nunobe S, Mine S, Ohashi M, Kumagai K, et al. Clinical outcomes and evaluation of laparoscopic proximal gastrectomy with double-flap technique for early gastric cancer in the upper third of the stomach. Ann Surg Oncol. 2017;24(6):1635–42.
8. Tanioka T, Waratchanont R, Fukuyo R, Saito T, Umebayashi Y, Kanemoto E, et al. Surgical and nutritional outcomes of laparoscopic proximal gastrectomy versus total gastrectomy: a meta-analysis. Surg Endosc. 2020;34(3):1061–9. https://doi.org/10.1007/s00464-019-07352-2
9. Takiguchi N, Takahashi M, Ikeda M, Inagawa S, Ueda S, Nobuoka T, et al. Long-term quality-of-life comparison of total gastrectomy and proximal gastrectomy by postgastrectomy syndrome assessment scale (PGSAS-45): a nationwide multi-institutional study. Gastric Cancer. 2015;18(2):407–16.
10. Haruta S, Shinohara H, Hosogi H, Ohkura YU, Kobayashi N, Mizuno A, et al. Proximal gastrectomy with exclusion of no. 3b lesser curvature lymph node dissection could be indicated for patients with advanced upper-third gastric cancer. Gastric Cancer. 2017;20(3):528-35.
11. Yura M, Yoshikawa T, Otsuki S, Yamagata Y, Morita S, Katai H, et al. Oncological safety of proximal gastrectomy for T2/T3 proximal gastric cancer. Gastric Cancer. 2019;22(5):1029–35.
12. Japanese Gastric Cancer A. Japanese gastric cancer treatment guidelines 2014 (ver. 4). Gastric Cancer. 2017;20(1):1–19.
13. Japanese Gastric Cancer Association. Japanese classification of gastric carcinoma: 3rd English edition. Gastric Cancer. 2011;14(2):101–12.
14. Sasako M, McCulloch P, Kinoshita T, Maruyama K. New method to evaluate the therapeutic value of lymph node dissection for gastric cancer. Br J Surg. 1995;82(3):346–51.
15. Wang X, Wan F, Pan J, Yu GZ, Chen Y, Wang JJ. Tumor size: a non-neglectable independent prognostic factor for gastric cancer. J Surg Oncol. 2008;97(3):236–40.
16. Wang HM, Huang CM, Zheng CH, Li P, Xie J-W, Wang J-B, et al. Tumor size as a prognostic factor in patients with advanced gastric cancer in the lower third of the stomach. World J Gastroenterol. 2012;18(38):5470–5.
17. Guo P, Li Y, Zhu Z, Sun Z, Chong LU, Wang Z, et al. Prognostic value of tumor size in gastric cancer: an analysis of 2,379 patients. Tumour Biol. 2013;34(2):1027–35.
18. Shin SH, Jung H, Choi SH, An JY, Choi MG, Noh JH, et al. Clinical significance of splenic hilar lymph node metastasis in proximal gastric cancer. Ann Surg Oncol. 2009;16(5):1304–9.
19. Sasada S, Ninomiya M, Nishizaki M, Harano M, Ojima Y, Matsukawa H, et al. Frequency of lymph node metastasis to the splenic hilus and effect of splenectomy in proximal gastric cancer. Anticancer Res. 2009;29(8):3347–51.
20. Kosuga T, Ichikawa D, Okamoto K, Komatsu S, Shiozaki A, Fujiwara H, et al. Survival benefits from splenic hilar lymph node dissection by splenectomy in gastric cancer patients: relative comparison of the benefits in subgroups of patients. Gastric Cancer. 2011;14(2):172–7.
21. Sano T, Sasako M, Mizusawa J, Yamamoto S, Katai H, Yoshikawa T, et al. Randomized controlled trial to evaluate splenectomy in total gastrectomy for proximal gastric carcinoma. Ann Surg. 2017;265(2):277–83.
22. Inada T, Yoshida M, Ikeda M, Yumiba T, Matsumoto H, Takagane A, et al. Evaluation of QOL after proximal gastrectomy using a newly developed assessment scale (PGSAS-45). World J Surg. 2014;38(12):3152–62.
23. Ri M, Nunobe S, Makuuchi R, Ida S, Kumagai K, Ohashi M, et al. Key factors for maintaining postoperative skeletal muscle mass after laparoscopic proximal gastrectomy with double-flap technique reconstruction for early gastric cancer. J Gastrointest Surg. 2021;25(6):1569–72.
24. Hosoda K, Washio M, Mieno H, Moriya H, Ema A, Ushiku H, et al. Comparison of double-flap and OrVil techniques of laparoscopy-assisted proximal gastrectomy in preventing gastroesophageal reflux: a retrospective cohort study. Langenbecks Arch Surg. 2019;404(1):81–91.
25. Lee JH, Ahn SH, Park DJ, Kim HH, Lee HJ, Yang HK. Clinical impact of tumor infiltration at the transected surgical margin during gastric cancer surgery. J Surg Oncol. 2012;106(6):772–6.
26. Bissolati M, Desio M, Rosa F, Rausei S, Marrelli D, Baiocchi GL, et al. Risk factor analysis for involvement of resection margins in gastric and esophagogastric junction cancer: an Italian multicenter study. Gastric Cancer. 2017;20(1):70–82.

15

Prognostic value of carbohydrate antigen 19-9 and the surgical margin in extrahepatic cholangiocarcinoma

Ryusei Yamamoto | Teiichi Sugiura | Ryo Ashida | Katsuhisa Ohgi | Mihoko Yamada | Shimpei Otsuka | Katsuhiko Uesaka

Division of Hepato-Biliary-Pancreatic Surgery, Shizuoka Cancer Center, Shizuoka, Japan

Correspondence
Teiichi Sugiura, Division of Hepato-Biliary-Pancreatic Surgery, Shizuoka Cancer Center, 1007 Shimo-Nagakubo, Sunto-Nagaizumi, Shizuoka 411-8777, Japan.
Email: t.sugiura@scchr.jp

Abstract

Aim: The prognostic value of the perioperative carbohydrate antigen 19-9 (CA19-9) value and the prognostic relationship between the CA19-9 value and the surgical margin in extrahepatic cholangiocarcinoma (EHCC) have not been fully discussed.

Methods: A total of 390 patients who underwent curative resection for EHCC between 2002 and 2018 were retrospectively analyzed. According to the perioperative CA19-9 value, patients were divided into three groups: preoperative normal (Normal, n = 178), preoperative high and postoperative normal (Normalization, n = 155), and preoperative high and postoperative high (Nonnormalization, n = 57). Survival was analyzed according to the perioperative CA19-9 value and surgical margin.

Results: The optimal cutoff value of CA19-9 was 37 U/mL. Overall survival (OS) was significantly stratified according to the perioperative CA19-9 value. The 5-y OS rates in the Normal, Normalization, and Nonnormalization groups were 53%, 38%, and 23%, respectively ($P < .001$). Although the locoregional recurrence rate was comparable among the groups, the Normal group exhibited distant recurrence less frequently in comparison to the other groups. In the Normal group, the margin status had a significant impact on the OS (surgical resection with a negative margin [R0], 59% vs a microscopically positive margin [R1], 7% at 5-y, $P < .001$). In contrast, in the Normalization and Nonnormalization groups, the OS rate of the R0 and R1 resection groups did not differ to a statistically significant extent.

Conclusion: The perioperative CA19-9 value was related to the prognosis of resectable EHCC. A preoperative CA19-9 value of ≥37 U/mL reflected systemic disease. R0 resection did not affect the survival in this patient group.

KEYWORDS
carbohydrate antigen 19-9, extrahepatic cholangiocarcinoma, surgical margin

1 | INTRODUCTION

Surgical resection with a negative margin (R0) has been regarded as the key to achieving long-term survival with extrahepatic cholangiocarcinoma (EHCC).[1,2] However, the prognostic impact of R0 resection is sometimes limited in advanced EHCC, such as in cases with lymph node metastasis or abnormally high carbohydrate antigen 19-9 (CA19-9) values.[3–5]

Given the anatomical complexity of the biliary system, locally advanced EHCC often requires extended surgery to achieve R0 resection, including trisectionectomy,[6] combined vascular resection and reconstruction (VR),[7,8] and hepatopancreatoduodenectomy (HPD).[9–11] However, these extensive surgeries are associated with high morbidity and mortality rates.[10–13] Thus, high-risk surgeries should be performed for patients who are expected to benefit from R0 resection. However, the significance of R0 resection has not been fully discussed. Although it is difficult to predict the presence of lymph node metastasis in the preoperative setting,[14] the CA19-9 value can be evaluated easily. Therefore, if the CA19-9 value could be used to predict the prognosis of EHCC, it might help avoid overly invasive surgery.

Abnormally high CA19-9 values have been reported to be a prognostic factor in resectable EHCC, and to imply the systemic disease status.[15–18] Recently, the perioperative change of CA19-9 has been regarded as an important marker in biliary tract cancer; however, its prognostic value in EHCC has not been sufficiently assessed.[5,19–21] The prognostic relationship between CA19-9 and the surgical margin remains unclear. A few studies have briefly reported an association between the perioperative CA19-9 value and the surgical margin in biliary tract cancer[5,19,21]; however, no studies have investigated this association in detail in a population limited to patients with EHCC.

The present study thoroughly investigated survival according to the perioperative CA19-9 value in patients who underwent resection of EHCC with curative intent. Furthermore, the prognostic value of R0 resection was assessed in groups of patients stratified according to the perioperative CA19-9 value, in order to reveal the significance of radical resection.

2 | METHODS

This was a retrospective review of a prospectively maintained EHCC database. Patients who underwent resection for pathologically confirmed EHCC at Shizuoka Cancer Center between September 2002 and December 2018 were reviewed. To avoid the influence of jaundice on CA19-9, patients in whom the total bilirubin value was >2.0 mg/dL at the time of CA19-9 measurement were excluded.[5] Patients who exhibited CA19-9 values of <2 U/mL were excluded because they were judged to be nonsecretors of CA19-9 (lack of Lewis antigen glycosyl transferase).[19,22] Patients whose perioperative CA19-9 values were not measured were also excluded. Biliary drainage was routinely performed for patients with jaundice, mainly via an endoscopic approach. Portal vein embolization was performed when the future liver remnant was judged to be insufficient.[23] Neoadjuvant treatment was not performed. Adjuvant treatment was only performed in exceptional cases. Patients who participated in the BCAT trial[24] received adjuvant gemcitabine chemotherapy, and those who participated in the ASCOT trial[25] received adjuvant S-1 chemotherapy. Some patients who exhibited a microscopically positive margin (R1) at the hepatic bile duct received 5-FU or S-1 chemotherapy and radiotherapy; the decision on the administration of adjuvant chemoradiotherapy was left to the patient, after providing them with sufficient information to give their informed consent.[26] This study was approved by our Institutional Ethics Committee (approval number J2020-87-2020-1-3).

2.1 | Evaluation of CA19-9

The preoperative CA19-9 value was usually measured within 2 weeks before the day of surgery, after the resolution of jaundice and cholangitis. The postoperative CA19-9 value was usually measured at 2 weeks after the day of discharge. The institutional cutoff value of CA19-9 was 37 U/mL, according to the standard reference value.[27] In the present study, the cutoff values of CA19-9 were determined by a minimum *P*-value analysis,[28] which was performed to identify the preoperative and postoperative CA19-9 values that were associated with the best overall survival (OS).

Eligible patients were divided to three groups according to their perioperative CA19-9 value: preoperative normal (Normal group), preoperative high and postoperative normal (Normalization group), and preoperative high and postoperative high (Nonnormalization group).

2.2 | Surgery and pathology

The standard surgical procedure in the author's institution was hepatectomy with extrahepatic bile duct resection for perihilar cholangiocarcinoma and pancreatoduodenectomy for distal cholangiocarcinoma.[29] The regional lymph nodes were dissected in all patients. Paraaortic lymph node sampling was performed, but surgical resection was typically performed if the intraoperative frozen section diagnosis yielded a positive result. When necessary, HPD and/or VR were aggressively performed to achieve R0 resection. Postoperative complications were graded according to the Clavien–Dindo classification.[30]

Pathological examinations were performed in accordance with the International Union Against Cancer (UICC) TNM classification 7th edition.[31] In the present study, carcinoma in situ at the ductal margin was defined as R0, because it did not affect OS.[1]

2.3 | Postoperative follow-up

The median follow-up period of the censored patients was 47 mo in the present study. The site of recurrence was confirmed based on radiologic or histologic evidence. Locoregional recurrence was specifically defined as a local ill-defined mass at the site of choledochojejunostomy, the hepatic artery, or the portal vein, accompanied by positive positron emission tomography findings, increased tumor marker levels, and an increase in size over time on serial imaging performed to detect disease progression.[26]

2.4 | Statistical analyses

Continuous data were described as the median and interquartile range and were compared using the Mann–Whitney *U*-test. Categorical variables were compared using Fisher's exact test. The cutoff values of continuous variables according to OS were determined based on a minimum *P*-value analysis.[28] Survival curves were generated using the Kaplan–Meier method, and differences were compared by a log-rank test. A Cox proportional hazards model, with stepwise backward-forward selection, was used for a multivariate analysis. Two-sided $P < .05$ were considered statistically significant. All statistical analyses were performed using the R software program (v. 4.0.3; The R Foundation for Statistical Computing, Vienna, Austria).

3 | RESULTS

In all, 491 consecutive patients underwent resection for EHCC with curative intent, including 272 patients with perihilar cholangiocarcinoma and 219 patients with distal cholangiocarcinoma. A total of 101 patients were excluded for the following reasons (some overlapped): preoperative CA19-9 value not recorded (n = 4); total bilirubin ≥2.0 mg/dL at the measurement of the CA19-9 value (n = 68); CA19-9 < 2 U/mL (n = 19); and postoperative CA19-9 value not recorded (n = 20). After applying the exclusion criteria, 390 patients were included in the present study.

In the minimum *P*-value analysis, the optimal cutoff value of preoperative and postoperative CA19-9 was determined to be 37 U/mL; this was the same as the standard cutoff value (Figure 1). The patients were grouped according to their perioperative CA19-9 values as follows: Normal group, n = 178 (46%); Normalized group, n = 155 (40%); and Nonnormalized group, n = 57 (15%).

Table 1 shows the patient characteristics according to the perioperative CA19-9 values. The median preoperative CA19-9 values of the Normal, Normalization, and Nonnormalization groups were 16, 104, and 311 U/mL, respectively, and each difference was statistically significant. The median postoperative CA19-9 values of the Normal, Normalization, and Nonnormalization groups were 10, 13, and 75 U/mL, respectively, and each difference was statistically significant. Distal cholangiocarcinoma was more frequently observed in the Normal group in comparison to the other groups. The R0 resection rates of the Normal, Normalization, and Nonnormalization groups were 90%, 87%, and 79%, respectively. R1 at the ductal margin was observed in 4%, 7%, and 9% of cases, respectively. R1 at the radial margin was observed in 6%, 8%, and 12% of cases, respectively. Two patients in the Normalization group had R1 at both the ductal and radial margins.

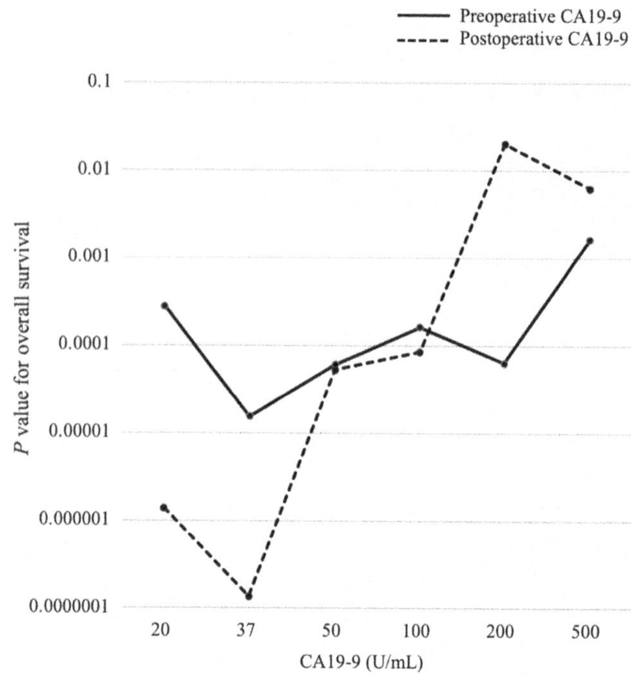

FIGURE 1 The optimal cutoff value of preoperative and postoperative CA19-9 for overall survival was determined to be 37 U/mL. CA19-9, carbohydrate antigen 19-9

Figure 2 shows the OS according to the perioperative CA19-9 values. Survival was clearly stratified according to the perioperative CA 19-9 values. The 5-y OS rates in the Normal, Normalization, and Nonnormalization groups were 53%, 38%, and 23%, respectively, and each difference was statistically significant ($P < .001$). The same tendency was also observed when patients with distant metastasis were excluded from the analysis (Figure S1). Moreover, a similar tendency was observed when patients were divided into perihilar cholangiocarcinoma (Figure S2) and distal cholangiocarcinoma (Figure S3) groups.

Table 2 shows the sites of recurrence according to the perioperative CA19-9 values. The locoregional recurrence rate did not differ significantly among the groups (Normal group, 15%; Normalization group, 13%; Nonnormalization group, 11%). The frequency of distant recurrence in the Normal group was significantly lower in comparison to the other groups (Normal group, 38%; Normalization group, 54%; Nonnormalization group, 65%). The same tendency was also observed when patients with distant metastasis were excluded (Table S1).

Figure 3 shows the OS according to the surgical margin status in each of the groups. In the Normal group, OS was significantly better in patients who received R0 resection than in those who received R1 resection (59% vs 7% at 5-y, $P <.001$). In the Normalization and Nonnormalization groups, the OS of the patients who received R0 resection was not significantly different from that in patients who received R1 resection. The same tendency was also observed when patients with distant metastasis were excluded (Figure S1). Moreover, a similar tendency was observed when patients were divided into perihilar cholangiocarcinoma (Figure S2) and distal cholangiocarcinoma (Figure S3) groups.

TABLE 1 Clinicopathologic characteristics according to the perioperative CA19-9 value

	(A) Normal	(B) Normalization	(C) Nonnormalization	P[d]		
	(n = 178)	(n = 155)	(n = 57)	A vs B	A vs C	B vs C
Age (y)[a]	70 (66–75)	71 (65–75)	72 (65–77)	.958[e]	.702[e]	.686[e]
Sex ratio, M:F	128:50	111:40	46:11	1	.226	.218
Preoperative CA19-9 (U/mL)[a]	16 (9–22)	104 (61–266)	311 (103–1211)	<.001[e]	<.001[e]	<.001[e]
Postoperative CA19-9 (U/mL)[a]	10 (6–17)	13 (8–21)	75 (46–125)	.024[e]	<.001[e]	<.001[e]
Preoperative CEA (ng/mL)[a]	2.0 (1.4–3.0)	2.4 (1.6–3.8)	3.7 (2.4–6.2)	.003[e]	<.001[e]	<.001[e]
Postoperative CEA (ng/mL)[a]	1.9 (1.4–2.6)	1.9 (1.4–2.8)	3.1 (2.2–4.2)	.772[e]	<.001[e]	<.001[e]
Location				<.001	<.001	.227
Perihilar	91 (51)	108 (70)	45 (79)			
Distal	87 (49)	47 (30)	12 (21)			
Biliary drainage	130 (73)	113 (73)	39 (68)	1	.502	.606
Albumin (g/dL)[a]	4.3 (4.0–4.3)	4.0 (3.7–4.2)	3.8 (3.6–4.1)	.117[e]	.007[e]	.109[e]
Total bilirubin (mg/dL)[a]	0.7 (0.5–1.0)	0.9 (0.7–1.3)	0.8 (0.6–1.2)	<.001[e]	.080[e]	.330[e]
C-reactive protein (mg/dL)[a]	0.20 (0.08–0.52)	0.52 (0.16–1.41)	0.52 (0.18–1.04)	<.001[e]	.004[e]	.638[e]
Operative procedure				<.001	<.001	.107
Hepatectomy	66 (37)	94 (61)	34 (60)			
Pancreatoduodenectomy	70 (39)	37 (24)	8 (14)			
Hepatopancreatoduodenectomy	42 (24)	24 (15)	15 (26)			
Vascular resection	34 (19)	51 (33)	18 (32)	.005	.066	1
Blood transfusion	38 (21)	41 (27)	17 (30)	.303	.210	.608
Complication, grade ≥3[b]	106 (60)	80 (52)	28 (49)	.152	.171	.759
Hospital stay (day)[a]	26 (19–39)	25 (18–38)	25 (17–43)	.621[e]	.906[e]	.738[e]
Histology, G2/G3	111 (62)	105 (68)	37 (65)	.357	.755	.743
T classification, T3/T4[c]	87 (49)	96 (62)	34 (60)	.020	.173	.754
Lymph node metastasis	58 (33)	73 (47)	32 (56)	.072	.002	.279
Distant metastasis	5 (3)	10 (7)	3 (5)	.121	.406	1
Surgical margin				.563	.057	.253
R0	161 (90)	135 (87)	45 (79)			
R1 at ductal margin	7 (4)	10 (7)	5 (9)			
R1 at radial margin	10 (6)	12 (8)	7 (12)			
Adjuvant treatment	18 (10)	20 (13)	7 (12)	.491	.627	1

Note: Values in parentheses are percentages unless otherwise indicated.

Abbreviations: CA19-9, carbohydrate antigen; CEA, carcinoembryonic antigen.

[a]Values are median (interquartile range).

[b]According to the Clavien–Dindo classification.

[c]According to the UICC 7th edition.

[d]Fisher's exact test.

[e]Mann–Whitney *U*-test.

The multivariate analysis revealed that both the preoperative CA19-9 value ($P = .018$) and the postoperative CA19-9 value ($P < .001$) were independently associated with OS (Table 3).

4 | DISCUSSION

The present study showed the utility of the perioperative CA19-9 value and the prognostic relationship between the perioperative CA19-9 value and the surgical margin in a relatively large cohort of patients with resectable EHCC. The optimal cutoff value was determined to be 37 U/mL. Patients in whom the preoperative CA19-9 value was <37 U/mL showed a good prognosis, and greatly benefited from R0 resection. The preoperative CA19-9 value of ≥37 U/mL reflected the presence of systemic disease. R0 resection did not affect survival in this patient group.

Hepato-biliary-pancreatic surgeons have made efforts to achieve complete eradication of EHCC through extended hepatectomy, VR,

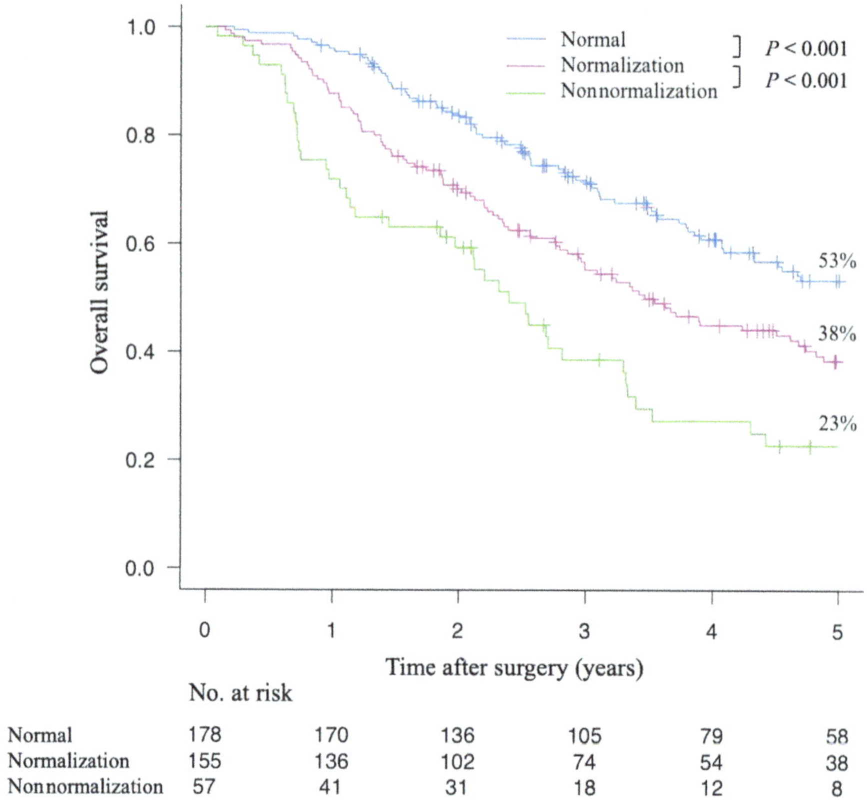

FIGURE 2 Overall survival according to the perioperative carbohydrate antigen 19-9 value

TABLE 2 Site of recurrence according to the perioperative CA19-9 value

	(A) Normal	(B) Normalization	(C) Nonnormalization	P		
	(n = 178)	(n = 155)	(n = 57)	A vs B	A vs C	B vs C
Locoregional recurrence	27 (15)	20 (13)	6 (11)	.637	.512	.814
Distant recurrence	67 (38)	84 (54)	37 (65)	.003	<.001	.210
Liver	32 (18)	42 (27)	8 (14)	.049	.550	.067
Retroperitoneal lymph node	20 (11)	16 (10)	14 (25)	.860	.017	.013
Peritoneal	13 (7)	24 (16)	14 (25)	.023	.001	.157
Lung	10 (6)	16 (10)	5 (9)	.151	.368	1
Others	6 (3)	14 (9)	6 (11)	.037	.076	.792

Note: Values in parentheses are percentages.

and HPD, approaches that require highly sophisticated surgical skills and perioperative management approaches.[6-11,29] In the present study, VR and HPD were performed for 103 patients (26%) and 81 patients (21%), respectively. However, some patients did not benefit from R0 resection, despite receiving aggressive surgery, and showed high morbidity and mortality. A few studies reported the prognostic relationship between CA19-9 and R0 resection in biliary tract cancer among patients with normalized and nonnormalized CA19-9 values.[5,19,21] However, the significance of R0 resection in patients with normal CA19-9 values has not been reported. The present study showed that patients with preoperative CA19-9 values of <37 U/mL—but not those with values of ≥37 U/mL—benefited from R0 resection.

It is known that CA19-9 influences the prognosis of biliary tract cancer; the standard cutoff value is 37 U/mL.[5,19,20,27] However, the optimal cutoff value of CA19-9 for EHCC remains controversial. Wang et al[18] reported a cutoff value of 150 U/mL, but their sample size was very limited. Although Lee et al[21] reported a cutoff value of 300 U/mL, preoperative CA19-9 >300 U/mL did not remain a significant factor in their multivariate analysis. Based on the statistical analysis of the present study, the cutoff value of 37 U/mL was found to be appropriate. Moreover, the multivariate analysis revealed that preoperative and postoperative CA19-9 values of ≥37 U/mL were both independent prognostic factors. Therefore, the standard cutoff value of 37 U/mL was found to be the optimal cutoff value for CA19-9.

Recently, the usefulness of the perioperative change in CA19-9 in patients with resectable biliary tract cancer has received attention.[5,19-21] It is obvious that the Nonnormalization group would show a dismal prognosis. Yamashita et al[19] reported that patients with normalized CA19-9 showed equivalent survival to those with normal CA19-9. However, two-thirds of their cohort was composed of

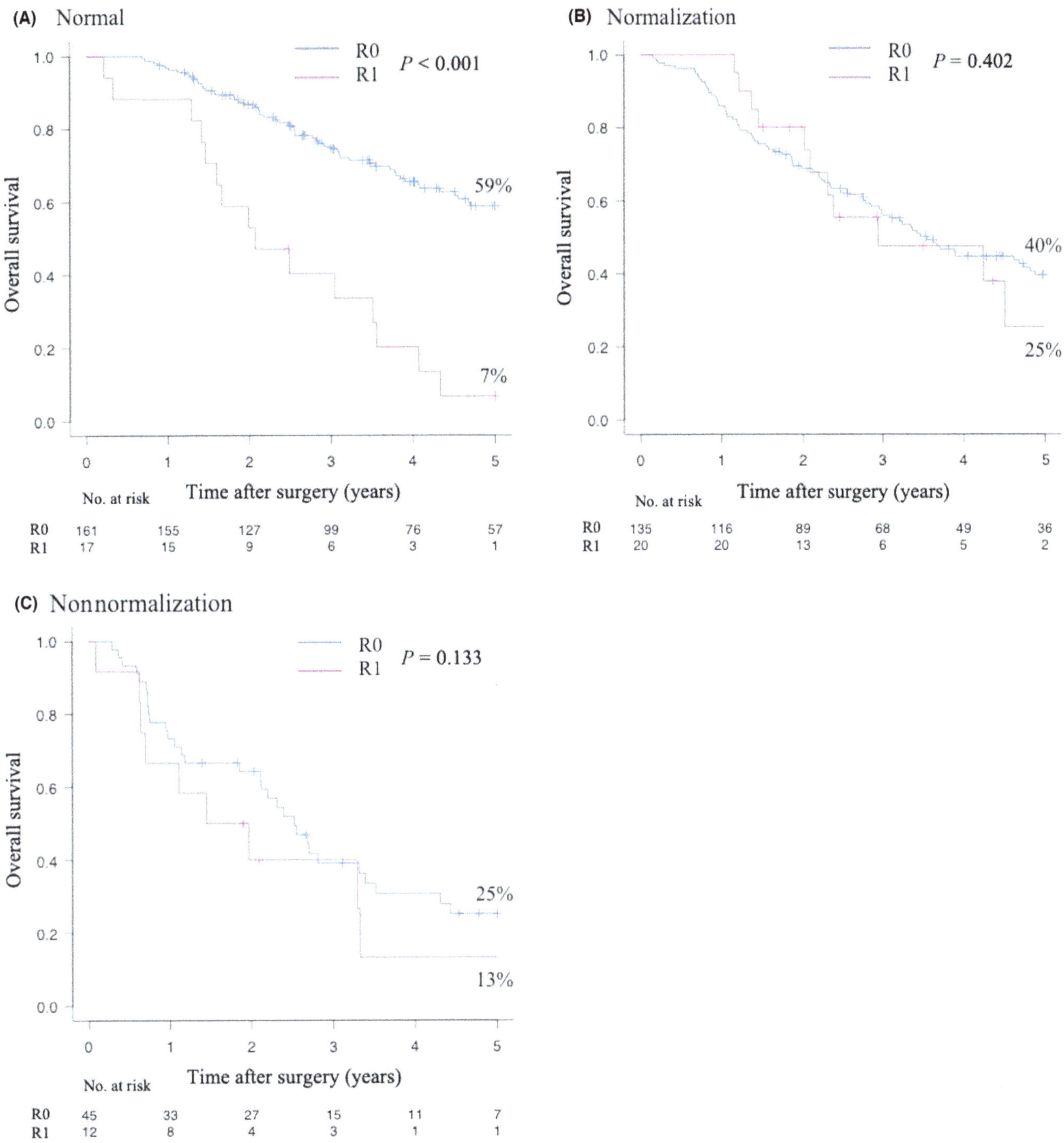

FIGURE 3 Overall survival according to surgical margin in each group. A: Normal group. B: Normalization group. C: Nonnormalization group

patients with intrahepatic cholangiocarcinoma; thus, it may be difficult to directly apply their results to resectable EHCC. Lee et al[21] reported that among a cohort of patients with resected perihilar cholangiocarcinoma, patients with normal CA19-9 values and those with normalized CA19-9 showed similar OS; however, their surgical outcomes seemed to be poor, as the R0 resection rate in patients with normal CA19-9 values was 62%, while the 5-y OS rate was only 29%. If the R0 resection rate could be further improved, a prognostic difference might have been observed between patients with normal and normalized CA19-9 values. In the present study, OS in the Normalization group was significantly poorer in comparison to the Normal group, which was similar to the results reported by Kim et al[20] The locoregional recurrence rate did not differ among the groups. However, in the Normal group distant recurrence was observed less frequently in comparison to the other groups, while the distant recurrence rate did not differ between the Normalization and Nonnormalization groups. Namely, a high preoperative CA19-9 value reflects systemic disease in patients with EHCC. In these patients, a satisfactory prognosis could not be achieved by

TABLE 3 Univariate and multivariate analyses of factors associated with overall survival

Variables	n	OS (%) 3-y	OS (%) 5-y	P^b	Multivariate HR (95% CI)	P^c
Age (y)						
<75	270	62.6	44.9	.052		
≥75	120	55.4	38.5			
Gender						
Female	105	67.9	56.2	.012		
Male	285	57.4	37.8			
Preoperative CA19-9 (U/mL)						
<37	178	71.8	53.3	<.001	1.00 (reference)	.015
≥37	212	50.9	34.3		1.42 (1.07-1.89)	
Postoperative CA19-9 (U/mL)						
<37	322	64.3	47.1	<.001	1.00 (reference)	<.001
≥37	68	41.5	23.5		1.84 (1.34-2.52)	
Preoperative CEA (ng/mL)						
<3.0	250	66.6	48.0	<.001		
≥3.0	140	49.1	33.8			
Postoperative CEA (ng/mL)						
<3.0	287	64.4	45.3	<.001		
≥3.0	47.0	47.0	35.4			
Location						
Perihilar	244	57.1	39.9	.040		
Distal	146	66.1	48.5			
Albumin (g/dL)						
<4.0	186	51.1	33.3	<.001	1.50 (1.15-1.97)	.003
≥4.0	204	68.5	50.1		1.00 (reference)	
Hepatopancreatoduodenectomy						
Absent	308	61.3	42.8	.677		
Present	82	56.5	43.1			
Vascular resection						
Absent	287	66.8	49.4	<.001	1.00 (reference)	<.001
Present	103	41.7	23.8		1.83 (1.37-2.45)	
Blood transfusion						
Absent	294	60.2	41.9	.842		
Present	96	60.6	45.8			
Histologic grade						
G1	137	71.9	54.4	<.001	1.00 (reference)	<.001
G2/G3	253	54.1	36.6		1.76 (1.31-2.36)	
T classification[a]						
T1/T2	173	68.3	51.0	.002		
T3/T4	217	54.1	36.7			
Lymph node metastasis						
Absent	227	70.2	54.7	<.001	1.00 (reference)	<.001
Present	163	46.1	25.5		1.67 (1.26-2.20)	
Distant metastasis						
Absent	372	61.6	44.1	.020		

(Continues)

TABLE 3 (Continued)

Variables	n	OS (%) 3-y	5-y	P^b	Multivariate HR (95% CI)	P^c
Present	18	30.8	15.4			
Surgical margin						
R0	341	62.7	46.5	<.001	1.00 (reference)	<.001
R1	49	43.2	15.1		1.89 (1.31–2.74)	
Adjuvant treatment						
Absent	345	59.4	43.2	.913	1.00 (reference)	.029
Present	45	67.9	38.3		0.61 (0.39–0.95)	

Abbreviations: CA19-9, carbohydrate antigen; CEA, carcinoembryonic antigen; CI, confidence interval; HR, hazard ratio; OS, overall survival.
[a]According to the UICC 7th edition.
[b]Log-rank test.
[c]Cox hazard test.

radical resection alone. These results suggest that R0 resection was meaningful in the Normal group but not in the Normalization or Nonnormalization groups.

The present authors would not discourage hepato-biliary-pancreatic surgeons from aiming for R0 resection in cases in which the CA19-9 value is ≥37 U/mL; however, in these cases excessive surgery, such as HPD with VR, should be considered after extremely careful patient selection. Conversely, in patients with CA19-9 values of <37 U/ml, such procedures should be performed because R0 resection offers the best chance of achieving long-term survival.

The present study was associated with some limitations, including its retrospective nature and single-center setting. The results of this study cannot be applied to patients with jaundice or CA19-9 values of <2 U/mL. The period from surgery to postoperative CA19-9 measurement differed according to the individual length of postoperative hospital stay, which seemed to affect the postoperative CA19-9 value. However, this period could not affect the postoperative CA19-9 value because the half-life of CA19-9 is only 0.5 d.[32] Furthermore, the number of subjects was not sufficient to draw broad interpretations. Thus, a multi-institutional study with a large cohort should be conducted to validate the findings of the present study.

In conclusion, the perioperative CA19-9 value was related to the prognosis of resectable EHCC. The preoperative CA19-9 value of ≥37 U/mL reflected a systemic disease status. R0 resection did not affect survival in this patient group.

REFERENCES

1. Igami T, Nagino M, Oda K, Nishio H, Ebata T, Yokoyama Y, et al. Clinicopathologic study of cholangiocarcinoma with superficial spread. Ann Surg. 2009;249(2):296–302.
2. Ribero D, Amisano M, Lo Tesoriere R, Rosso S, Ferrero A, Capussotti L. Additional resection of an intraoperative margin-positive proximal bile duct improves survival in patients with hilar cholangiocarcinoma. Ann Surg. 2011;254(5):776–81.
3. Komaya K, Ebata T, Shirai K, Ohira S, Morofuji N, Akutagawa A, et al. Recurrence after resection with curative intent for distal cholangiocarcinoma. Br J Surg. 2017;104(4):426–33.
4. Komaya K, Ebata T, Yokoyama Y, Igami T, Sugawara G, Mizuno T, et al. Recurrence after curative-intent resection of perihilar cholangiocarcinoma: analysis of a large cohort with a close postoperative follow-up approach. Surgery. 2018;163(4):732–8.
5. Kato Y, Takahashi S, Gotohda N, Konishi M. Prognostic impact of the initial postoperative CA19-9 level in patients with extrahepatic bile duct cancer. J Gastrointest Surg. 2016;20(8):1435–43.
6. Natsume S, Ebata T, Yokoyama Y, Igami T, Sugawara G, Shimoyama Y, et al. Clinical significance of left trisectionectomy for perihilar cholangiocarcinoma: an appraisal and comparison with left hepatectomy. Ann Surg. 2012;255(4):754–62.
7. Maeta T, Ebata T, Hayashi E, Kawahara T, Mizuno S, Matsumoto N, et al. Pancreatoduodenectomy with portal vein resection for distal cholangiocarcinoma. Br J Surg. 2017;104(11):1549–57.
8. Mizuno T, Ebata T, Yokoyama Y, Igami T, Yamaguchi J, Onoe S, et al. Combined vascular resection for locally advanced perihilar cholangiocarcinoma. Ann Surg. 2020. https://doi.org/10.1097/SLA.0000000000004322
9. Ebata T, Yokoyama Y, Igami T, Sugawara G, Takahashi YU, Nimura Y, et al. Hepatopancreatoduodenectomy for cholangiocarcinoma: a single-center review of 85 consecutive patients. Ann Surg. 2012;256(2):297–305.
10. Welch JC, Gleeson EM, Karachristos A, Pitt HA. Hepatopancreatoduodenectomy in North America: are the outcomes acceptable? HPB. 2020;22(3):360–7.
11. D'Souza MA, Valdimarsson VT, Campagnaro T, Cauchy F, Chatzizacharias NA, D'Hondt M, et al. Hepatopancreatoduodenectomy -a controversial treatment for bile duct and gallbladder cancer from a European perspective. HPB. 2020;22(9):1339–48.
12. Otsubo T, Kobayashi S, Sano K, Misawa T, Ota T, Katagiri S, et al. Safety-related outcomes of the Japanese Society of Hepato-Biliary-Pancreatic Surgery board certification system for expert surgeons. J Hepatobiliary Pancreat Sci. 2017;24(5):252–61.
13. Endo I, Hirahara N, Miyata H, Yamamoto H, Matsuyama R, Kumamoto T, et al. Mortality, morbidity and failure to rescue in hepatopancreatoduodenectomy: an analysis of 422 patients registered in the National Clinical Database in Japan. J Hepatobiliary Pancreat Sci. 2021;28(4):305–16.
14. Ruys AT, van Beem BE, Engelbrecht MR, Bipat S, Stoker J, Van Gulik TM. Radiological staging in patients with hilar cholangiocarcinoma: a systematic review and meta-analysis. Br J Radiol. 2012;85(1017):1255–62.
15. Chung MJ, Lee KJ, Bang S, Park SW, Kim KS, Lee WJ, et al. Preoperative serum CA 19-9 level as a predictive factor for recurrence after curative resection in biliary tract cancer. Ann Surg Oncol. 2011;18(6):1651–6.

16. Kondo N, Murakami Y, Uemura K, Sudo T, Hashimoto Y, Sasaki H, et al. Elevated perioperative serum CA 19-9 levels are independent predictors of poor survival in patients with resectable cholangiocarcinoma. J Surg Oncol. 2014;110(4):422–9.
17. Bolm L, Petrova E, Weitz J, Rückert F, Wittel UA, Makowiec F, et al. Prognostic relevance of preoperative bilirubin-adjusted serum carbohydrate antigen 19–9 in a multicenter subset analysis of 179 patients with distal cholangiocarcinoma. HPB. 2019;21(11):1513–9.
18. Wang J-K, Hu H-J, Shrestha A, Ma W-J, Yang Q, Liu F, et al. Can preoperative and postoperative CA19-9 levels predict survival and early recurrence in patients with resectable hilar cholangiocarcinoma? Oncotarget. 2017;8(28):45335–44.
19. Yamashita S, Passot G, Aloia TA, Chun YS, Javle M, Lee JE, et al. Prognostic value of carbohydrate antigen 19–9 in patients undergoing resection of biliary tract cancer. Br J Surg. 2017;104(3):267–77.
20. Kim BH, Kim E, Kim K, Jang J-Y, Kim SW, Oh D-Y, et al. The impact of perioperative CA19-9 change on the survival and recurrence patterns after adjuvant chemoradiotherapy in resectable extrahepatic cholangiocarcinoma. J Surg Oncol. 2018;117(3):380–8.
21. Lee JW, Lee JH, Park Y, Kwon J, Lee W, Song KB, et al. Prognostic impact of perioperative CA19-9 levels in patients with resected perihilar cholangiocarcinoma. J Clin Med. 2021;10(7):1345.
22. Tempero MA, Uchida E, Takasaki H, Burnett DA, Steplewski Z, Pour PM. Relationship of carbohydrate antigen 19–9 and Lewis antigens in pancreatic cancer. Cancer Res. 1987;47(20):5501–3.
23. Yamamoto R, Sugiura T, Okamura Y, Ito T, Yamamoto Y, Ashida R, et al. Utility of remnant liver volume for predicting posthepatectomy liver failure after hepatectomy with extrahepatic bile duct resection. BJS Open. 2021;5(1):zraa049. https://doi.org/10.1093/bjsopen/zraa049
24. Ebata T, Hirano S, Konishi M, Uesaka K, Tsuchiya Y, Ohtsuka M, et al. Randomized clinical trial of adjuvant gemcitabine chemotherapy versus observation in resected bile duct cancer. Br J Surg. 2018;105(3):192–202.
25. Nakachi K, Konishi M, Ikeda M, Mizusawa J, Eba J, Okusaka T, et al. A randomized Phase III trial of adjuvant S-1 therapy vs observation alone in resected biliary tract cancer: Japan Clinical Oncology Group Study (JCOG1202, ASCOT). Jpn J Clin Oncol. 2018;48(4):392–5.
26. Sugiura T, Uesaka K, Okamura Y, Ito T, Yamamoto Y, Ashida R, et al. Adjuvant chemoradiotherapy for positive hepatic ductal margin on cholangiocarcinoma. Ann Gastroenterol Surg. 2020;4(4):455–63.
27. Del Villano BC, Brennan S, Brock P, Bucher C, Liu V, McClure M, et al. Radioimmunometric assay for a monoclonal antibody-defined tumor marker, CA 19–9. Clin Chem. 1983;29(3):549–52.
28. Lin Y. Robust inference for responder analysis: Innovative clinical trial design using a minimum p-value approach. Contemp Clin Trials Commun. 2016;3:65–9.
29. Sugiura T, Okamura Y, Ito T, Yamamoto Y, Ashida R, Ohgi K, et al. Left Hepatectomy with combined resection and reconstruction of right hepatic artery for bismuth type I and II perihilar cholangiocarcinoma. World J Surg. 2019;43(3):894–901.
30. Dindo D, Demartines N, Clavien PA. Classification of surgical complications: a new proposal with evaluation in a cohort of 6336 patients and results of a survey. Ann Surg. 2004;240(2):205–13.
31. Sobin LH, Gospodarowicz MK, Wittekind C. International union against cancer (UICC) TNM classification of malignant tumours. 7th ed. New York: Wiley-Liss; 2010.
32. Yoshimasu T, Maebeya S, Suzuma T, Bessho T, Tanino H, Arimoto J, et al. Disappearance curves for tumor markers after resection of intrathoracic malignancies. Int J Biol Markers. 1999;14(2):99–105.

16

Update on perioperative management of patients undergoing surgery for liver cancer

Masaki Kaibori[1] | Kosuke Matsui[1] | Mitsuo Shimada[2] | Shoji Kubo[3] | Kiyoshi Hasegawa[4]

[1]Department of Surgery, Kansai Medical University, Osaka, Japan

[2]Department of Surgery, Tokushima University, Tokushima, Japan

[3]Department of Hepato-Biliary-Pancreatic Surgery, Osaka City University Graduate School of Medicine, Osaka, Japan

[4]Hepato-Biliary-Pancreatic Surgery Division, Department of Surgery, Graduate School of Medicine, The University of Tokyo, Tokyo, Japan

Correspondence
Masaki Kaibori, Department of Surgery, Kansai Medical University, 2-5-1 Shinmachi, Hirakata, Osaka 573-1191, Japan.
Email: kaibori@hirakata.kmu.ac.jp

Abstract

Hepatocellular carcinoma is often accompanied by chronic hepatitis or cirrhosis. Preoperative evaluation of liver function and postoperative nutritional management are critical in patients with hepatocellular carcinoma who undergo liver surgery. Although the incidence of postoperative complications and death has declined in Japan over the last 10 years, postoperative complications have not been fully overcome. Therefore, surgical procedures and perioperative management must be improved. Accurate preoperative evaluations of liver function, nutrition, inflammation, and body skeletal muscle are required. Determination of the optimal surgical procedure should consider not only tumor characteristics but also the physical reserve of the patient. Nutritional management of chronic liver disorders, especially maintaining protein synthesis for postoperative protein/energy, is important. Prophylactic antibiotics are recommended for short-term use within 24 hours after surgery. Abdominal drainage is recommended for patients with cirrhosis who may develop large amounts of ascites, who are at risk of postoperative bleeding, or who may have bile leakage due to a large resection area. Postoperative exercise therapy may improve insulin resistance in patients with chronic liver damage. Implementation of an early/enhanced recovery after surgery program is recommended to reduce biological invasive responses and achieve early independence of physical activity and nutrition intake. We review the latest information on the perioperative management of patients undergoing liver resection for hepatocellular carcinoma.

KEYWORDS
liver cancer, perioperative management, review, surgery

1 | INTRODUCTION

Hepatocellular carcinoma (HCC) is the fifth most common cancer worldwide.[1] Although most affected patients are in Asia and Africa, HCC incidence and mortality rates are increasing in North America and Europe.[2,3] In Japan, most HCCs occur in patients with chronic hepatitis and liver cirrhosis induced by hepatitis B or C virus infection. Because of advances in perioperative management, anesthesia, and operative techniques, hepatectomy for HCC has become more common.[4] However, the postoperative mortality rate remains higher than in patients with cirrhosis or chronic hepatitis undergoing other types of surgery. The morbidity rate of patients with cirrhosis undergoing liver resection has been reported to range from 20% to 70%, with mortality rates of 5%-21%.[5-10] Mortality rates at high-volume centers in Japan are usually much lower, <2%,[11-13] although morbidity rates remain relatively high. The postoperative course of these patients does not always proceed as expected, owing to various types of intraoperative stress, including blood loss and ischemia. These findings emphasize the importance of improving both surgical techniques and perioperative care in reducing the mortality and morbidity of patients with HCC undergoing liver resection. In this review, we outline the current status of and topics regarding the perioperative management of patients undergoing surgery for liver cancer based on recent evidence.

2 | ALGORITHM FOR THE TREATMENT OF HCC AND APPROPRIATE EVALUATION OF LIVER FUNCTION BEFORE HEPATECTOMY

With regard to the therapeutic strategy for HCC, the Barcelona Clinic Liver Cancer (BCLC) staging system recommended by the American Association for the Study of Liver Diseases and the European Association for the Study of the Liver is used worldwide.[14] In Japan, the "treatment algorithm" described in the Clinical Guidelines for HCC is widely used to select the optimum treatment based on liver function and tumor status (Figure 1).[15] The Japanese treatment algorithm differs markedly from the BCLC system with regard to HCC with concomitant portal hypertension.[16] In the BCLC system, liver resection is not indicated if portal hypertension is present, and liver transplantation and radiofrequency ablation (RFA) are recommended. In contrast, liver resection is recommended based on the indocyanine green (ICG) retention rate at the 15-min (ICGR15) level in the Japanese treatment algorithm, and favorable outcomes have been reported.[17] Liver resection for HCC is chosen based on the balance between tumor status and liver function. Resection exceeding the hepatic functional reserve with the goal of cancer cure may lead to liver failure, whereas insufficient resection due to excessive safety concerns may have a high risk of early recurrence. Therefore, it is important to select the optimum surgical procedure based on the extent of the tumor and the acceptable liver resection range. As the liver reserve classification for preoperative liver function evaluation, the Child classification and its modified Child-Pugh classification have been widely used worldwide. In particular, the presence or absence of ascites is used as an index of the degree of portal hypertension, and poor control of ascites is not indicated for surgery. In Europe and the United States, it has been common that B and C cases of the Child-Pugh classification are not indicated for surgery, and even in cases of Child-Pugh classification A, if portal hypertension coexists, hepatectomy is not indicated. This standard is adopted in the liver cancer treatment guidelines in Europe and the United States.[14] In contrast, reports from Europe and the United States have stated that portal hypertension is not a contraindication for hepatectomy with more than two sections.[18] It has been reported in Japan that reduced hepatectomy with portal hypertension is not contraindicated, because no increase in postoperative complications was observed.[17] The ICG loading test and technetium-99m-garactosyl human serum albumin (^{99m}Tc-GSA) liver scintigraphy are the main quantitative preoperative evaluations of liver function for hepatectomy. Many studies of ICG load have found that it is a useful predictor of postoperative mortality.[5,19] The ICG retention rate at 15 minutes (ICGR15) has been adopted as a factor in the evaluation of liver damage by the Japan Liver Cancer Study Group[20] and has become a standard evaluation of preoperative liver function. Yamanaka et al reported that the prediction score for the occurrence of postoperative liver failure as a surgical indication criterion, which consists of the ICGR15, amount of resection, and age, could accurately predict postoperative mortality.[21,22] Takasaki et al proposed a standard that set a different permissible amount of hepatectomy for each value of the ICG loading test.[23] Postoperative liver failure and death within the permissible hepatectomy criteria were 2% and 0%, respectively, whereas for non-permissible hepatectomy, they were 23% and 1%, respectively.[24] The Makuuchi standard,[25] which is widely used in Japan, clearly indicates whether hepatectomy is indicated and the allowable range of resection based on ascites, total serum bilirubin level, and ICGR15 (Figure 2). It has been reported that 0% of surgical deaths occurred in 1056 patients who underwent hepatectomy in compliance with this standard.[26] Kokudo et al reported that the Albumin-Indocyanine Green Evaluation (ALICE) grade using the serum albumin level and ICGR15 is useful for predicting the occurrence of postoperative liver failure and survival.[27] The ALICE grade is superior to the Child-Pugh classification in predicting outcomes after hepatectomy and may be a more useful liver function evaluation classification when combined with the presence or absence of portal hypertension.[28,29] It has been reported that ^{99m}Tc-GSA liver scintigraphy was superior to the ICGR15 in the histologic evaluation of liver damage.[30] Evaluation of functional residual liver volume calculated from ^{99m}Tc-GSA liver scintigraphy was more informative than residual liver volume evaluation from computed tomography (CT) for predicting postoperative complications and death in patients with HCC and liver damage.[31] However, ^{99m}Tc-GSA liver scintigraphy has facility restrictions due to the use of nuclides. In the evaluation of preoperative liver function to decide the surgical indication, in addition to information such as the Child-Pugh classification obtained in daily clinical practice, including blood tests, many reports recommend the ICG load test as a quantitative test.[15] For hepatectomy, it is considered appropriate to determine the indication based on the balance between the degree of liver damage estimated from the ICGR15 and the range of hepatectomy (the amount of resection required).

3 | NUTRITIONAL STATUS OF PATIENTS WITH LIVER CANCER

3.1 | Evaluation by biochemical and physical factors

Recent studies have proposed markers based on several nutritional or inflammation-based prognostic indicators of HCC. Nutritional- or inflammation-based markers include the prognostic nutritional

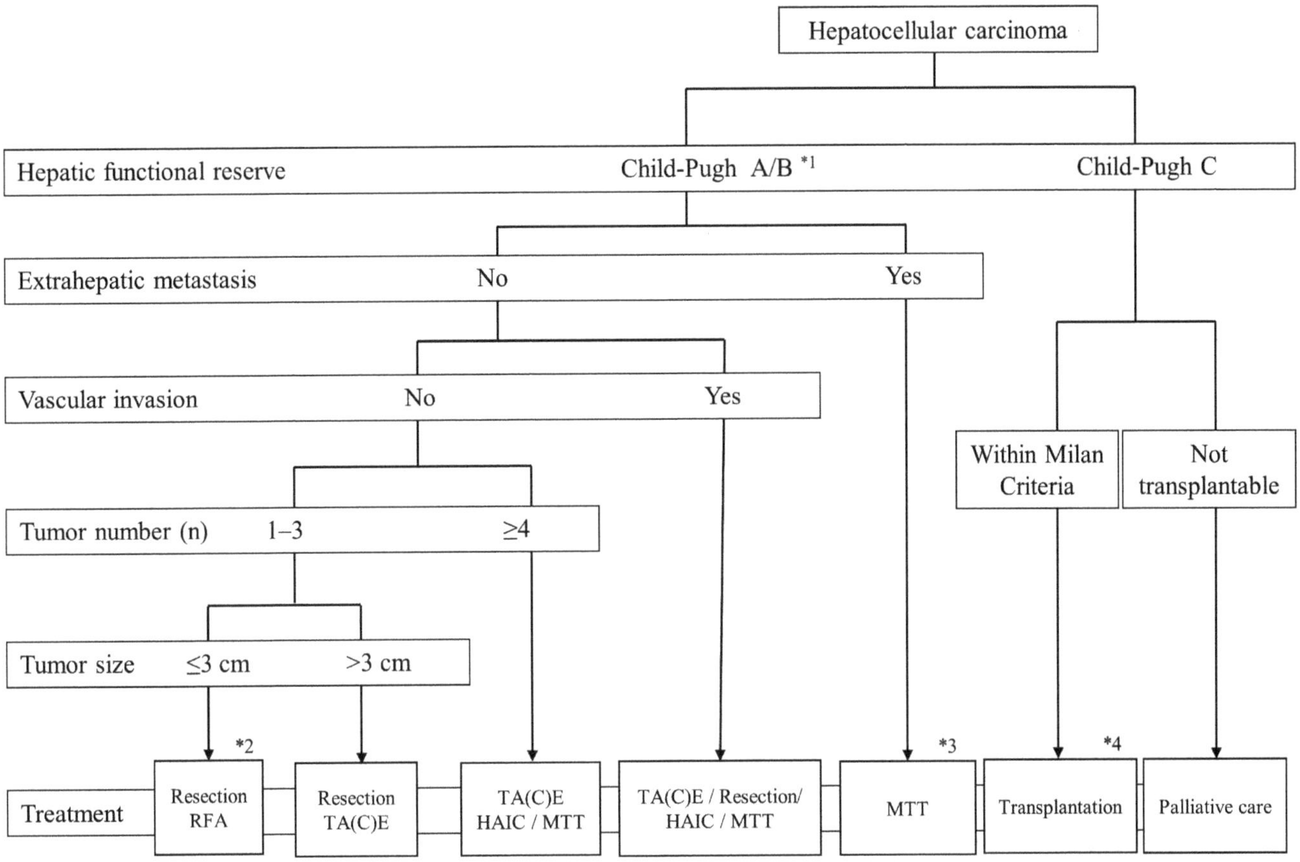

FIGURE 1 Algorithm for treatment in Japanese guidelines for hepatocellular carcinoma.[15] This algorithm is simple and easy to memorize, consisting of five factors: (a) hepatic functional reserve; (b) extrahepatic metastasis; (c) vascular invasion, (d) tumor number; and (e) tumor size. *1: Assessment based on liver damage is recommended in the case of hepatectomy. *2: For a solitary hepatocellular carcinoma, resection is recommended as first-line therapy, and ablation as second-line therapy. *3: Patients with Child-Pugh A only. *4: Patients aged ≤65 y. HAIC, hepatic arterial infusion chemotherapy; MTT, molecular-targeted therapy; RFA, radiofrequency ablation; TA(C)E, transcatheter arterial (chemo) embolization

index,[32-34] controlling nutritional status (CONUT) score,[35-37] Glasgow prognostic score,[38] C-reactive protein (CRP)-to-albumin ratio (CAR),[39] neutrophil-to-lymphocyte ratio (NLR),[40] platelet-to-lymphocyte ratio (PLR),[41,42] lymphocyte-to-monocyte ratio (LMR),[43,44] and CRP-albumin-lymphocyte index.[45] Table 1 shows combined indices that can reportedly be used to estimate the nutritional or inflammatory status relevant to short- and long-term outcomes after hepatectomy for HCC. While some of the algorithms are complicated, CRP and serum albumin measurements are used more often as components of combined indices.[39]

The use of sarcopenia to predict outcomes in patients with cancer has attracted more attention, including those with HCC[46-48] or colorectal liver metastases (CRLM)[49,50] undergoing hepatic resection. Previous studies also demonstrated that sarcopenia increased the risk of postoperative morbidity and longer hospital stay, as well as readmission rates, after partial liver resection for CRLM.[51,52] Those studies focused only on skeletal muscle mass, as assessed by CT of skeletal muscle area. In contrast, a few reports have described the deterioration of muscle quality associated with muscle fat deposition. The usefulness of intramuscular adipose tissue content in hepatectomy for HCC[53,54] and CRLM[55] has been reported. Preoperative sarcopenia and/or intramuscular adipose tissue content might be considered a new selection criterion for hepatectomy in patients with liver cancer.

3.2 | Nutrition therapy

Because many cases of hepatectomy for HCC coexist with chronic hepatitis and cirrhosis, these patients often have energy/substrate metabolic disorders. Specifically, it has been reported that nutritional disorders occur frequently in patients with liver cirrhosis; 84% and 95% of patients with Child-Pugh classifications B and C, respectively, are undernourished, and 45% of patients with Child-Pugh classification A are also undernourished.[56] The main characteristic of nutritional disorders in patients with liver cirrhosis is malnutrition of protein and energy, and a decrease in the burning ratio of glucose as an energy-burning source and an increase in the burning ratio of fat are observed.[57] These nutritional disorders in patients with cirrhosis are closely related to the incidence of complications after hepatectomy, and the importance of perioperative nutrition therapy has been noted.[58] In principle, oral and enteral nutrition should be

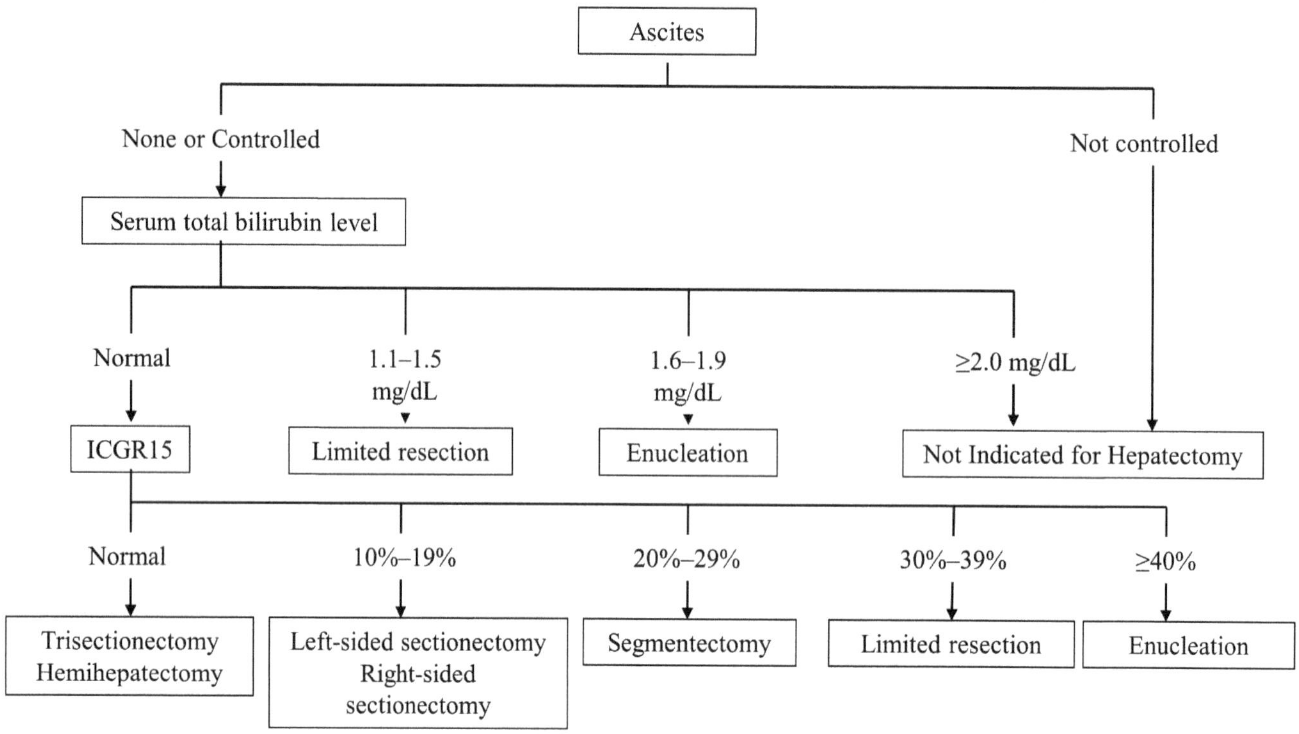

FIGURE 2 "Makuuchi's criteria" as a surgical decision tree for liver resection. Makuuchi's criteria include three factors: ascites, total serum bilirubin, and the ICGR15 (indocyanine green 15-min retention rate). This algorithm shows the maximal area for which an operation can be performed safely (modified ref. 25)

prioritized in nutrition therapy to maintain intestinal function. The European Society for Clinical Nutrition and Metabolism (ESPEN) guidelines also recommend early oral nutrition for surgical patients to restore intestinal function, and early postoperative nutrition therapy for patients with liver cirrhosis to prevent postoperative complications.[59] The results of some studies on branched-chain amino acid (BCAA) administration and immunonutrition therapy (immunonutrition) in liver surgery complicated with liver cirrhosis are described as follows. Fan et al[58] reported a randomized controlled trial (RCT) of 124 patients who underwent hepatectomy for HCC who were divided into a perioperative nutrition therapy group that received an infusion of an emulsion of dextrose, BCAA, and medium-chain triglycerides and a non-nutrition therapy group. The frequency of postoperative complications was significantly reduced in the nutrition therapy group, and the incidence of infectious complications was 17% and 37% ($P = .02$) in the nutrition therapy and non-nutrition therapy groups, respectively. Furthermore, the effect of these nutrition therapies on postoperative complications was remarkable in patients with cirrhosis who underwent major hepatectomy. Shirabe et al reported an RCT of 26 patients who underwent hepatectomy in which nutritional components containing BCAAs were administered by intravenous or enteral routes. The incidence of infectious complications was 31% in the intravenous route group and 8% in the enteral route group, demonstrating the superiority of the enteral route as a nutritional route after hepatectomy.[60] Enteral nutrition may induce retention of the intestinal mucosa, activation of the immune system in the mesenteric lymph nodes, and increased IgA production in patients with liver cirrhosis at high risk of bacterial translocation; therefore, the authors recommended enteral nutrition early after surgery. Recently, preoperative administration of BCAA in patients undergoing hepatic resection was shown to be effective for preventing ascites, plural effusion, or both, as well as for improving albumin metabolism and reducing the risk of complications and duration of hospital stay.[61,62] Previous reports have addressed the effects of BCAA on HCC recurrence after surgery[63,64]; however, no definitive conclusions have been reached. Hachiya et al reported the long-term prognosis of BCAA administration for patients with HCC who underwent hepatectomy.[65] They demonstrated that oral BCAA supplementation could not reduce the risk of recurrence after hepatic resection in HCC; however, the results suggested that BCAA supplementation may be beneficial for selected patients who were younger and had mildly impaired glucose tolerance.

Four studies on the efficacy of probiotics and prebiotics for patients who undergo hepatic resection have been published.[66-69] A meta-analysis including these studies showed that administration of probiotics and/or prebiotics prior to the day of surgery decreases the infection rate post-liver resection and could shorten the duration of hospitalization and antibiotic use.[70] However, as the quality of the evidence was low, further research is required. There were three reports of perioperative immunonutrition therapy with omega-3 fatty acids.[71-73] Two RCTs showed that intravenous administration of omega-3 lipids for 5 days after hepatectomy improved postoperative liver function and suppressed the occurrence of complications.[72] However, one RCT did not show these effects.[73]

TABLE 1 Combined indices estimating nutritional or inflammatory status for liver cancer surgery

Index	Components (serum levels)	Results
PNI	Albumin, lymphocyte	PNI <44 was associated with higher transfusion rates and surgical outcomes,[32] PNI <45 was the most powerful predictor of complications after hepatic resection.[33] Patients with PNI <37 were at high risk for early recurrence and poor survival.[34]
CONUT	Albumin, lymphocyte, total cholesterol	Early postoperative CONUT score >8 was identified as a risk factor for postoperative complication III-V.[35] Preoperative CONUT scores >4 was predictive of worse OS and RFS.[36] High CONUT score was an independent predictor of in-hospital mortality after hepatectomy[37]
GPS	Albumin, C-reactive protein	An elevated GPS was an independent prognostic indicator for OS after hepatectomy[38]
CRP/ALB ratio (CAR)	Albumin, C-reactive protein	High CAR (>0.027) was correlated with both poor OS and DFS[39]
NLR	Neutrophil, lymphocyte	Preoperative plus postoperative ratio was a prognostic factor for OS[40]
PLR	Platelet, lymphocyte	High PLR level (≥150) is a good indicator to predict recurrence beyond the Milan criteria.[41] High PLR indicates a higher rate of extrahepatic metastasis of HCC.[42]
LMR	Lymphocyte, monocyte	Both LMR and NLR might be preferable independent prognostic factors for DFS.[43] Elevated preoperative LMR (≥4.01) was independently associated with poor OS and DFS[44]
CRP-albumin-lymphocyte index	C-reactive protein, albumin, lymphocyte	OS and RFS were worse with an index of 5 or higher[45]

Abbreviations: CAR, C-reactive protein (CRP) to albumin ratio; CONUT, controlling nutritional status; DFS, disease-free survival; GPS, Glasgow prognostic score; LMR, lymphocyte to monocyte ratio; OS, overall survival; PFS, progression-free survival; PLR, platelet to lymphocyte ratio; PNI, prognostic nutritional index.

4 | PROPHYLACTIC ANTIBIOTICS

Hirokawa et al[74] reported the results of an RCT of the administration of prophylactic antibiotics to patients scheduled to undergo liver resection. The non-postoperative antibiotic group (n = 95) received 1.0 g of flomoxef sodium (FMOX) 30 minutes before surgery but was not given FMOX after surgery. The antibiotic group (n = 95) was given intravenous FMOX 1.0 g every 12 hours for 3 days after surgery. The groups did not differ significantly for signs of infection (21.3% vs 25.5%, $P = .61$), incidence of systemic inflammatory response syndrome (11.7% vs 17.0%, $P = .41$), infectious complications (7.5% vs 17.0%, $P = .07$), surgical site infection (SSI; 10.6% vs 13.8%, $P = .66$), and remote site infection (2.1% vs 8.5%, $P = .10$). Takayama et al[75] reported that the incidence of SSI was 9.5% and 9.8%, respectively, in a non-inferiority study comparing 232 patients who received 1 g of FMOX up to 6 hours after surgery (1-day group) and 235 patients who received it for up to 2 days (3-day group; $P = .001$ for non-inferiority). In a retrospective study, after propensity score matching, there was no difference in the incidence of SSI and distant site infections when comparing administration of FMOX up to 24 hours after surgery and administration for 3 days after surgery in patients undergoing open and laparoscopic hepatic resection.[76] Based on these results, it is recommended that prophylactic antibiotics be administered within 24 hours after hepatectomy.

5 | PROPHYLACTIC ABDOMINAL DRAINAGE

Routine prophylactic abdominal drainage was unnecessary or contraindicated for patients who underwent elective hepatectomy in RCTs, because drain placement increased the frequency of drain-related complications, wound complications, sepsis and infectious fluid retention, and significantly increased the length of hospital stay.[77-80] On the other hand, in patients with liver cirrhosis accompanied by portal hypertension, one report recommended drain placement, because abdominal drainage reduced complications related to postoperative ascites and shortened the length of hospital stay.[81] It was also reported that abdominal drainage should not be placed in patients unless they were at high risk of bleeding and bile leakage.[82] Late-onset bile leakage, which could lead to serious complications, such as sepsis, occurred in patients without abdominal drainage.[83] Intra-abdominal infection should also be treated as soon as possible, because it may induce refractory bile leakage with serious complications. Some reports recommended drain placement in cases of therapeutic usefulness for bile leakage and intraperitoneal fluid retention due to drainage,[84,85] for the possibility of predicting bile leakage by monitoring the bilirubin concentration in drainage,[85,86] for patients at high risk of bile leakage, such as those with biliary tract reconstruction, exposure of major Glisson's capsule, and with bile leakage observed during surgery.[87] It was also reported that prophylactic abdominal drainage was not essential for living-donor liver transplant donor hepatectomy.[88] Unlike other abdominal organ resections, hepatectomy is often associated with chronic liver damage, and it is necessary to pay attention to bleeding, bile leakage, and intractable ascites. Regarding the pros and cons of drain placement during elective hepatectomy, RCTs have been performed since the 1990s, but they had some limitations, such as a small number of patients and the methods used for evaluation. Therefore, it was necessary to consider the degree of coexisting liver damage and the surgical procedure. More careful consideration is required for abdominal drainage in living-donor liver transplant donor surgery performed on healthy people, and it is also necessary to consider the pros and cons of drain placement in laparoscopic hepatectomy, which has been increasing in recent years. It is currently considered that the presence or absence of abdominal drainage in elective hepatectomy should be determined in consideration of the risk of bleeding and bile leakage. The Centers for Disease Control and Prevention (CDC) guidelines for prevention of SSI recommend "if a drain is needed, use a closed drain and remove it as soon as possible."[89] Some reports demonstrated that it is desirable to remove the drain within 2-3 days after surgery if there is no problem with the drainage properties.[85,90,91]

6 | EXERCISE THERAPY

Dynamic assessment of preoperative exercise capacity may be a useful predictor of short- and long-term postoperative prognosis. Cardiopulmonary exercise (CPX) testing measures oxygen uptake at increasing levels of work and predicts cardiopulmonary performance under stress, such as after surgery. Among older patients undergoing major abdominal surgical procedures, most deaths from cardiopulmonary complications occur in those with an anaerobic threshold (AT) <11 mL/min/kg.[92,93] The AT is defined as the point during exercise at which oxygen demand outstrips oxygen delivery, and metabolism starts to become anaerobic. The AT is a measure of the ability of the cardiopulmonary system to deliver adequate oxygen to tissues, and it has the advantage of being independent of patient motivation. To date, few studies have examined the usefulness of pre- and postoperative CPX testing in patients undergoing hepatectomy.[94,95] Recently, Kaibori et al reported that in patients with HCC and hepatic impairment undergoing liver resection, exercise significantly decreased body mass and fat mass, as well as insulin resistance, 6 months postoperatively.[96] Maintenance of postoperative physical strength and earlier resumption of daily activities could be possible by intensifying perioperative and postoperative exercise. An exercise program was tailored for each patient. Exercise was started as soon as possible after diagnosis, up to 1 month preoperatively, and was resumed from 1 week postoperatively and continued for 6 months. The program consisted of three 60-minute exercise sessions per week. Each session included 5 minutes of stretching exercises, 30 minutes of walking at an intensity based on the AT of each patient, 20 minutes of targeted stretching exercises, and 5 minutes of cooling down with stretching. Patients with HCC (N = 51) were randomized to receive diet therapy alone (n = 25) or exercise in addition to diet therapy (n = 26). Whole body mass and fat mass in the exercise group compared with the diet group were significantly decreased at 6 months postoperatively. Fasting serum insulin and the homeostasis model assessment score were also significantly decreased (Figure 3). At 6 months, the AT and peak oxygen consumption were significantly increased, while serum insulin and insulin resistance significantly improved in a high frequency exercise subgroup compared with a low frequency group (Figure 2).

7 | ENHANCED RECOVERY AFTER SURGERY

Fast-track or enhanced recovery after surgery (ERAS) programs following surgical interventions are now within the standard of care for patients with several surgical indications.[97-101] These programs use a multimodal approach to maximize effectiveness and minimize cost, thus optimizing perioperative care pathways.[102] ERAS programs have been associated with reductions in complications, duration of hospital stay, and hospital costs in colorectal surgery.[97] Recently, ERAS programs have also been introduced in liver surgery. Wang et al demonstrated in a meta-analysis that the implementation of ERAS programs in liver surgery appears to be feasible and efficient and could significantly reduce overall morbidity, hospital stay and costs, intraoperative blood loss, and time to bowel function recovery without increasing rates of mortality, readmission, or transfusion.[103] They also found that ERAS programs reduced morbidity in open and laparoscopic surgery equally, whereas hospital stays were reduced more obviously in laparoscopic surgery. However, it is unclear why the implementation of ERAS programs resulted in the reduction of intraoperative blood loss, which is largely dependent on the surgical technique.

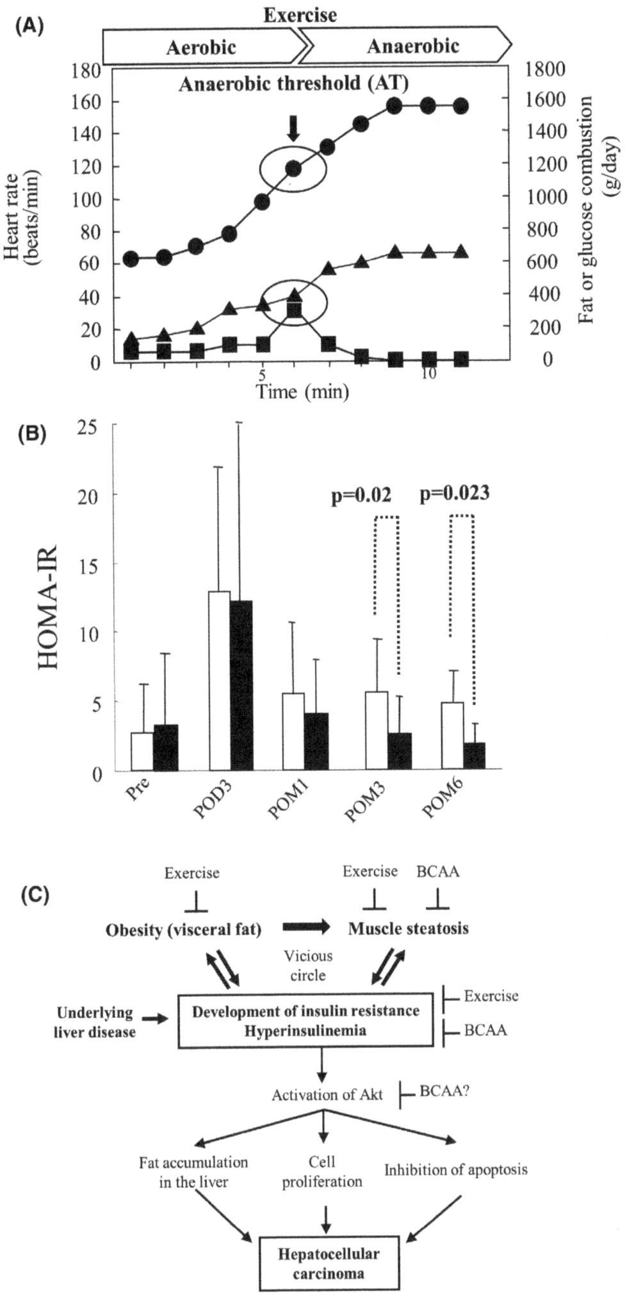

FIGURE 3 Exercise therapy. (A) Cardiopulmonary exercise test. The anaerobic threshold (AT) was set at the break point between carbon dioxide production and Vo_2, or the point at which the ventilatory equivalent for oxygen and end-tidal oxygen partial pressure curves reached their respective nadirs before beginning to increase again. Thus, the AT was set at a maximum point of fat combustion. ● heart rate; ▲ glucose combustion; ■ fat combustion. (B) Effect of exercise on insulin resistance in patients with HCC with hepatic impairment. HOMA-IR in the diet group (□) and the exercise group (■). HOMA-IR, homeostasis model for assessment of insulin resistance; POD, postoperative day; POM, postoperative month. (C) Estimating the mechanism of hepatocellular carcinoma development due to exacerbation of insulin resistance. There is a vicious cycle among obesity, muscle steatosis, and the development of insulin resistance in patients with liver diseases. Exercise and/or BCAA therapy is considered to suppress the deterioration of the condition. Akt; protein kinase B; BCAA; branched-chain amino acid

We consider that laparoscopic surgery, unlike open surgery, is effective for reduction in surgical bleeding because it requires minimal peeling due to the magnifying effect and reduces damage to tissues around the liver. The results of RCT and meta-analysis have shown that the introduction of ERAS programs reduced the frequency of complications as well as improved early postoperative recovery.[103-107] Among programs, pain management is an important factor, and Hausken et al reported that intravenous patient-controlled analgesia (IV-PCA) was non-inferior to epidural anesthesia.[106] Most of the patients in these studies underwent hepatectomy for colorectal liver metastases. Few studies have analyzed the effect of ERAS programs on patients with diseased livers who underwent hepatectomy for HCC. Kaibori et al[105] compared clinicopathologic factors, surgical factors, and outcomes of patients who underwent extended hepatectomy (defined as resection of more than two sections) for HCC coexistent with chronic hepatitis and cirrhosis, before and after the introduction of an ERAS program. Operating time and postoperative hospital stay were significantly shorter, and total volume infused during surgery was significantly lower for the ERAS group than for the control group. Although the percentage of patients with retention of abdominal drainage was significantly smaller in the ERAS group, the frequency of abdominal paracentesis in patients without intraoperative abdominal drainage was higher. Oral dietary intake and ability to walk stably occurred significantly earlier in the ERAS group. Postoperative serum concentrations of albumin and cholinesterase were significantly higher in the ERAS group than in the control group. We concluded that a multimodal ERAS program was feasible and effective for patients with chronic liver diseases undergoing extended liver resection for HCC.

We speculate that the spread of ERAS programs in hepatectomy in Japan will be as follows. There are 15 ERAS items essential for liver surgery: "Pre-admission counseling," "No bowel preparation," "Fluid and CHO-loading/no fasting," "No pre-anesthetic medication," "No routine nasogastric tubes postoperatively," "Epidural analgesia," "Short-acting anesthetic agent," "Avoidance of sodium/fluid overload," "Short incision," "Warm air body heating in theatre," "Early mobilization (routine mobilization care pathway)," "Non-opiate oral analgesics/NSAIDs," "Early feeding (stimulation of gut motility and perioperative oral nutrition)," and "Early removal of catheters." However, "No surgical drains," "Prevention of nausea and vomiting," and "Audit of compliance/outcome" are not yet widespread components of ERAS programs in Japan (Figure 4).

8 | CONCLUSIONS

This review summarizes a series of unique approaches to the perioperative management of patients with HCC undergoing liver resection based on the available evidence, with the goal of achieving "no

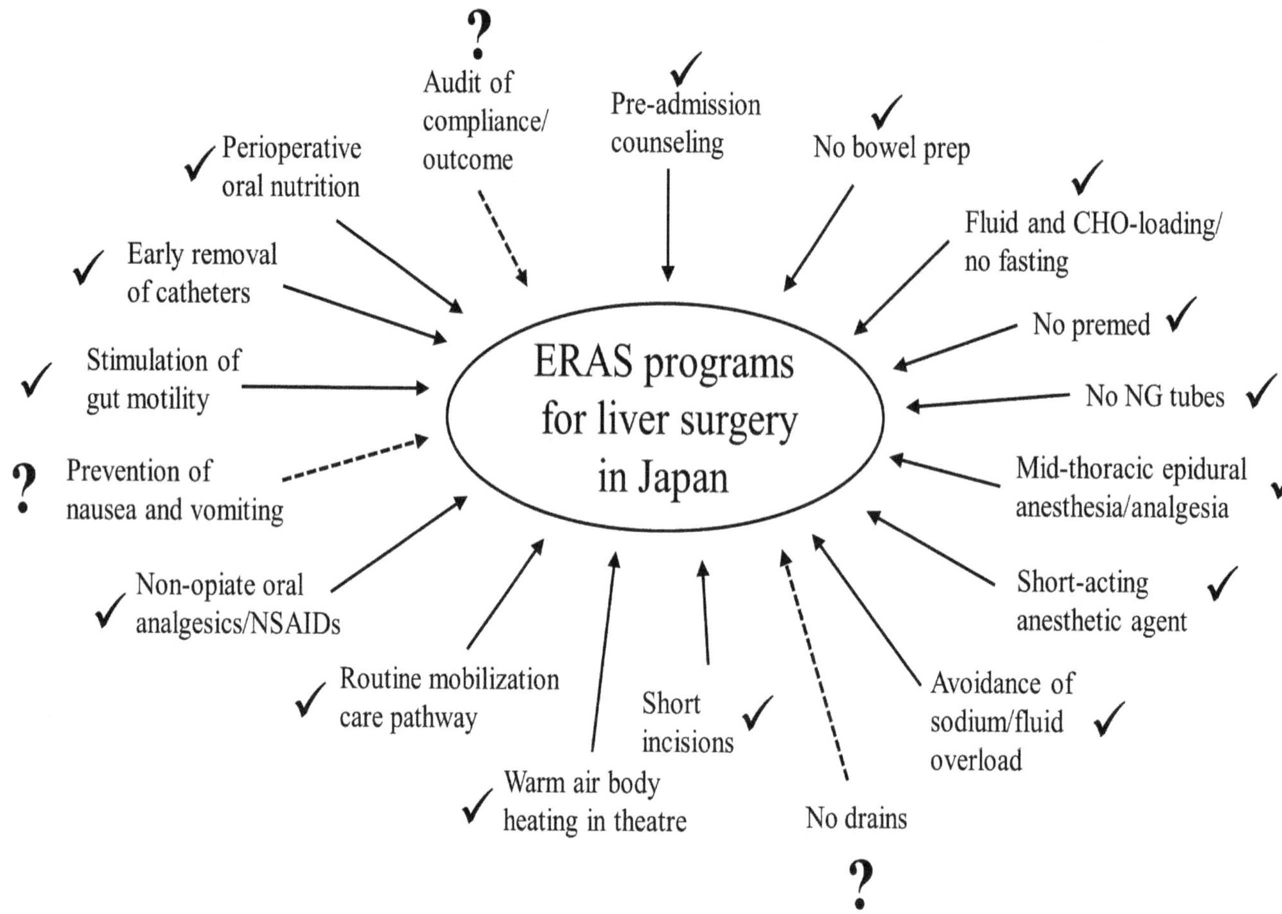

FIGURE 4 Enhanced recovery after surgery (ERAS) program items performed in patients undergoing hepatectomy in Japan. ERAS program items that have already been implemented at many facilities in Japan are marked with a check mark, and items that have not yet been implemented sufficiently are marked as question marks

mortality" and "minimal postoperative complications." We believe that general perioperative management of patients undergoing surgery for liver cancer is basically the same, even when there is a wide variety of patient and surgical factors. Whether the associated liver disease is normal vs severe cirrhosis, and whether the surgery is laparoscopic vs open hepatectomy, we perform the perioperative management described above in the same way. New methods for the improvement of preoperative liver function and perioperative management are likely to facilitate expansion of the indication for liver resection.

ACKNOWLEDGEMENTS

We are indebted to the following surgeons for their excellent collection and management of the manuscripts: Satoru Imura (Department of Surgery, Tokushima University) and Shogo Tanaka (Department of Hepato-Biliary-Pancreatic Surgery, Osaka City University Graduate School of Medicine).

DISCLOSURE

Author Contribution: MK drafted and wrote the manuscript. KM, MS, SK, and KH participated in the study design and helped draft the manuscript. All authors contributed to the interpretation of the findings, read, and approved the final manuscript.

REFERENCES

1. Bosch X, Ribes J, Borras J. Epidemiology of primary liver cancer. Semin Liver Dis. 1999;19:271–85.
2. Taylor-Robinson SD, Foster GR, Arora S, Hargreaves S, Thomas HC. Increase in primary liver cancer in the UK 1979–94. Lancet. 1997;350:1142–3.
3. El-Serag HB, Mason AC. Rising incidence of hepatocellular carcinoma in the United States. N Engl J Med. 1999;340:745–50.
4. Nanashima A, Nagayasu T. Development and clinical usefulness of the liver hanging maneuver in various anatomical hepatectomy procedures. Surg Today. 2016;46:398–404.
5. Fan ST, Lai EC, Lo CM, Ng IO, Wong J. Hospital mortality of major hepatectomy for hepatocellular carcinoma associated with cirrhosis. Arch Surg. 1995;130:198–203.
6. Tung-Ping Poon R, Fan ST, Wong J. Risk factors, prevention, and management of postoperative recurrence after resection of hepatocellular carcinoma. Ann Surg. 2000;232:10–24.

7. Yeh CN, Chen MF, Lee WC, Jeng LB. Prognostic factors of hepatic resection for hepatocellular carcinoma with cirrhosis: univariate and multivariate analysis. J Surg Oncol. 2002;81:195–202.
8. Benzoni E, Cojutti A, Lorenzin D, Adani GL, Baccarani U, Favero A, et al. Liver resective surgery: a multivariate analysis of postoperative outcome and complication. Langenbecks Arch Surg. 2007;392:45–54.
9. Chiappa A, Zbar AP, Audisio RA, Leone BE, Biella F, Staudacher C. Factors affecting survival and long-term outcome in the cirrhotic patient undergoing hepatic resection for hepatocellular carcinoma. Eur J Surg Oncol. 2000;26:387–92.
10. Farges O, Malassagne B, Flejou JF, Balzan S, Sauvanet A, Belghiti J. Risk of major liver resection in patients with underlying chronic liver disease: a reappraisal. Ann Surg. 1999;229:210–5.
11. Mizuguchi T, Kawamoto M, Meguro M, Okita K, Ota S, Ishii M, et al. Impact of aging on morbidity and mortality after liver resection: a systematic review and meta-analysis. Surg Today. 2015;45:259–70.
12. Makuuchi M. Remodeling the surgical approach to hepatocellular carcinoma. Hepatogastroenterology. 2002;49:36–40.
13. Taketomi A, Kitagawa D, Itoh S, Harimoto N, Yamashita Y, Gion T, et al. Trends in morbidity and mortality after hepatic resection for hepatocellular carcinoma: an institute's experience with 625 patients. J Am Coll Surg. 2007;204:580–7.
14. Bruix J, Sherman M. American Association for the Study of Liver Diseases. Management of hepatocellular carcinoma: an update. Hepatology. 2011;53:1020–2.
15. Kokudo N, Takemura N, Hasegawa K, Takayama T, Kubo S, Shimada M, et al. Clinical practice guidelines for hepatocellular carcinoma: the Japan Society of Hepatology 2017 (4th JSH-HCC guidelines) 2019 update. Hepatol Res. 2019;49:1109–13.
16. Nakayama H, Takayama H. Role of surgical resection for hepatocellular carcinoma based on Japanese clinical guidelines for hepatocellular carcinoma. World J Hepatol. 2015;7:261–9.
17. Ishizawa T, Hasegawa K, Aoki T, Takahashi M, Inoue Y, Sano K, et al. Neither multiple tumors nor portal hypertension are surgical contraindications for hepatocellular carcinoma. Gastroenterology. 2008;134:1908–16.
18. Cucchetti A, Ercolani G, Vivarelli M, Cescon M, Ravaioli M, Ramacciato G, et al. Is portal hypertension a contraindication to hepatic resection? Ann Surg. 2009;250:922–8.
19. Lau H, Man K, Fan ST, Yu WC, Lo CM, Wong J. Evaluation of preoperative hepatic function in patients with hepatocellular carcinoma undergoing hepatectomy. Br J Surg. 1997;84:1255–9.
20. Liver Cancer Study Group of Japan. The general rules for the clinical and pathological study of primary liver cancer (4th, Japanese ed.). Kanehara-Shuppan; 2000.
21. Yamanaka N, Okamoto E, Kuwata K, Tanaka N. A multiple regression equation for prediction of posthepatectomy liver failure. Ann Surg. 1984;200:658–63.
22. Yamanaka N, Okamoto E, Oriyama T, Fujimoto J, Furukawa K, Kawamura E, et al. A prediction scoring system to select the surgical treatment of liver cancer. Further refinement based on 10 years of use. Ann Surg. 1994;219:342–6.
23. Takasaki K, Kobayashi S, Suzuki S, Muto H, Marada M, Yamana Y, et al. Predeterming postoperative hepatic function for hepatectomies. Int Surg. 1980;65:309–13.
24. Ariizumi S, Yamamoto M, Takasaki K. Right hepatectomy for hepatocellular carcinoma in patients with an indocyanine green retention rate at 15 minutes of 10% or higher. Dig Surg. 2009;26:135–42.
25. Makuuchi M, Kosuge T, Takayama T, Yamazaki S, Kakazu T, Miyagawa S, et al. Surgery for small liver cancers. Semin Surg Oncol. 1993;9:298–304.
26. Imamura H, Seyama Y, Kokudo N, Maema A, Sugawara Y, Sano K, et al. One thousand fifty-six hepatectomies without mortality in 8 years. Arch Surg. 2003;138:1198–206.
27. Kokudo T, Hasegawa K, Amikura K, Uldry E, Shirata C, Yamaguchi T, et al. Assessment of preoperative liver function in patients with hepatocellular carcinoma - The Albumin-Indocyanine Green Evaluation (ALICE) Grade. PLoS One. 2016;11:e0159530.
28. Russolillo N, Forchino F, Conci S, Mele C, Langella S, Ruzzenente A, et al. Validation of the albumin-indocyanine green evaluation model in patients with resected hepatocellular carcinoma and comparison with the albumin-bilirubin score. J Hepatobiliary Pancreat Sci. 2019;26:51–7.
29. Shirata C, Kokudo T, Arita J, Akamatsu N, Kaneko J, Sakamoto Y, et al. Albumin-Indocyanine Green Evaluation (ALICE) grade combined with portal hypertension to predict post-hepatectomy liver failure. Hepatol Res. 2019;49:942–9.
30. Kwon AH, Ha-Kawa SK, Uetsuji S, Inoue T, Matsui Y, Kamiyama Y. Preoperative determination of the surgical procedure for hepatectomy using technetium-99m-galactosyl human serum albumin (^{99m}Tc-GSA) liver scintigraphy. Hepatology. 1997;25:426–9.
31. Hayashi H, Beppu T, Okabe H, Kuroki H, Nakagawa S, Imai K, et al. Functional assessment versus conventional volumetric assessment in the prediction of operative outcomes after major hepatectomy. Surgery. 2015;157:20–6.
32. Sim JH, Kim SH, Jun IG, Kang SJ, Kim B, Kim S, et al. The association between prognostic nutritional index (PNI) and intraoperative transfusion in patients undergoing hepatectomy for hepatocellular carcinoma: a retrospective cohort study. Cancers (Basel). 2021;13:2508.
33. Nagata S, Maeda S, Nagamatsu S, Kai S, Fukuyama Y, Korematsu S, et al. Prognostic nutritional index considering resection range is useful for predicting postoperative morbidity of hepatectomy. J Gastrointest Surg. 2021;25:2788–2795.
34. Tanemura A, Mizuno S, Hayasaki A, Gyoten K, Fujii T, Iizawa Y, et al. Onodera's prognostic nutritional index is a strong prognostic indicator for patients with hepatocellular carcinoma after initial hepatectomy, especially patients with preserved liver function. BMC Surg. 2020;20:261. doi:10.1186/s12893-020-00917-2
35. Li L, Liu C, Yang J, Wu H, Wen T, Wang W, et al. Early postoperative controlling nutritional status (CONUT) score is associated with complication III-V after hepatectomy in hepatocellular carcinoma: A retrospective cohort study of 1,334 patients. Sci Rep. 2018;8:13406. doi:10.1038/s41598-018-31714-w
36. Harimoto N, Yoshizumi T, Inokuchi S, Itoh S, Adachi E, Ikeda Y, et al. Prognostic significance of preoperative controlling nutritional status (CONUT) score in patients undergoing hepatic resection for hepatocellular carcinoma: a multi-institutional study. Ann Surg Oncol. 2018;25:3316–23.
37. Takagi K, Umeda Y, Yoshida R, Nobuoka D, Kuise T, Fushimi T, et al. Preoperative controlling nutritional status score predicts mortality after hepatectomy for hepatocellular carcinoma. Dig Surg. 2019;36:226–32.
38. Abe T, Tashiro H, Kobayashi T, Hattori M, Kuroda S, Ohdan H. Glasgow prognostic score and prognosis after hepatectomy for hepatocellular carcinoma. World J Surg. 2017;41:1860–70.
39. Yamamoto M, Kobayashi T, Kuroda S, Hamaoka M, Okimoto S, Honmyo N, et al. Verification of inflammation-based prognostic marker as a prognostic indicator in hepatocellular carcinoma. Ann Gastroenterol Surg. 2019;3:667–75.
40. Wu M, Yang S, Feng X, Yu F, Liu X, Dong J. Oncol Lett. 2020;20:375. doi:10.3892/ol.2020.12238
41. Kaida T, Nitta H, Kitano Y, Yamamura K, Arima K, Higashi T, et al. Preoperative platelet-to-lymphocyte ratio can predict recurrence beyond the Milan criteria after hepatectomy for patients with hepatocellular carcinoma. Hepatol Res. 2017;47:991–9.
42. Chen Y, Zeng J, Guo P, Zeng J, Liu J. Prognostic significance of platelet-to-lymphocyte ratio (PLR) in extrahepatic metastasis of hepatocellular carcinoma after curative resection. Cancer Manag Res. 2021;13:1395–405.

43. Yang T, Zhu J, Zhao L, Mai K, Ye J, Huang S, et al. Lymphocyte to monocyte ratio and neutrophil to lymphocyte ratio are superior inflammation-based predictors of recurrence in patients with hepatocellular carcinoma after hepatic resection. J Surg Oncol. 2017;115:718–28.
44. Yang YT, Jiang JH, Yang HJ, Wu ZJ, Xiao ZM, Xiang BD. The lymphocyte-to-monocyte ratio is a superior predictor of overall survival compared to established biomarkers in HCC patients undergoing liver resection. Sci Rep. 2018;8:2535. doi:10.1038/s41598-018-20199-2
45. Iida H, Tani M, Komeda K, Nomi T, Matsushima H, Tanaka S, et al. Superiority of CRP-albumin-lymphocyte index (CALLY index) as a non-invasive prognostic biomarker after hepatectomy for hepatocellular carcinoma. HPB (Oxford). 2021. doi:10.1016/j.hpb.2021.06.414.. Online ahead of print.
46. Berardi G, Antonelli G, Colasanti M, Meniconi R, Guglielmo N, Laurenzi A, et al. Association of sarcopenia and body composition with short-term outcomes after liver resection for malignant tumors. JAMA Surg. 2020;155:e203336. doi:10.1001/jamasurg.2020.3336
47. Kobayashi A, Kaido T, Hamaguchi Y, Okumura S, Shirai H, Yao S, et al. Impact of sarcopenic obesity on outcomes in patients undergoing hepatectomy for hepatocellular carcinoma. Ann Surg. 2019;269:924–31.
48. Xu L, Jing Y, Zhao C, Zhang Q, Zhao X, Yang J, et al. Preoperative computed tomography-assessed skeletal muscle index is a novel prognostic factor in patients with hepatocellular carcinoma following hepatectomy: a meta-analysis. J Gastrointest Oncol. 2020;11:1040–53.
49. Runkel M, Diallo TD, Lang SA, Bamberg F, Benndorf M, Fichtner-Feigl S. The role of visceral obesity, sarcopenia and sarcopenic obesity on surgical outcomes after liver resections for colorectal metastases. World J Surg. 2021;45:2218–26.
50. Liu YW, Lu CC, Chang CD, Lee KC, Chen HH, Yeh WS, et al. Prognostic value of sarcopenia in patients with colorectal liver metastases undergoing hepatic resection. Sci Rep. 2020;10:6459. doi:10.1038/s41598-020-63644-x
51. Peng PD, van Vledder MG, Tsai S, de Jong MC, Makary M, Ng J, et al. Sarcopenia negatively impacts short-term outcomes in patients undergoing hepatic resection for colorectal liver metastasis. HPB (Oxford). 2011;13:439–46.
52. Lodewick TM, van Nijnatten TJ, van Dam RM, van Mierlo K, Dello SA, Neumann UP, et al. Are sarcopenia, obesity and sarcopenic obesity predictive of outcome in patients with colorectal liver metastases? HPB (Oxford). 2015;17:438–46.
53. Hamaguchi Y, Kaido T, Okumura S, Ito T, Fujimoto Y, Ogawa K, et al. Preoperative intramuscular adipose tissue content is a novel prognostic predictor after hepatectomy for hepatocellular carcinoma. J Hepatobiliary Pancreat Sci. 2015;22:475–85.
54. Kaibori M, Ishizaki M, Iida H, Matsui K, Sakaguchi T, Inoue K, et al. Effect of intramuscular adipose tissue content on prognosis in patients undergoing hepatocellular carcinoma resection. J Gastrointest Surg. 2015;19:1315–23.
55. Horii N, Sawda Y, Kumamoto T, Tsuchiya N, Murakami T, Yabushita Y, et al. Impact of intramuscular adipose tissue content on short- and long-term outcomes of hepatectomy for colorectal liver metastasis: a retrospective analysis. World J Surg Oncol. 2020;18:68. doi:10.1186/s12957-020-01836-5
56. Cheung K, Lee SS, Raman M. Prevalence and mechanisms of malnutrition in patients with advanced liver disease, and nutrition management strategies. Clin Gastroenterol Hepatol. 2012;10:117–25.
57. Dudrick SJ, Kavic SM. Hepatobiliary nutrition: history and future. J Hepatobiliary Pancreat Surg. 2002;9:459–68.
58. Fan ST, Lo CM, Lai EC, Chu KM, Liu CL, Wong J, et al. Perioperative nutritional support in patients undergoing hepatectomy for hepatocellular carcinoma. N Engl J Med. 1994;331:1547–52.
59. Plauth M, Cabré E, Riggio O, Assis-Camilo M, Pirlich M, Kondrup J, et al. ESPEN Guidelines on Enteral Nutrition: Liver disease. Clin Nutr. 2006;25:285–94.
60. Shirabe K, Matsumata T, Shimada M, Takenaka K, Kawahara N, Yamamoto K, et al. A comparison of parenteral hyperalimentation and early enteral feeding regarding systemic immunity after major hepatic resection–the results of a randomized prospective study. Hepatogastroenterology. 1997;44:205–9.
61. Mizuguchi T, Kawamoto M, Meguro M, Nakamura Y, Harada K, Kukita K, et al. Prognostic impact of preoperative the branched-chain amino acid to the tyrosine ratio in hepatocellular carcinoma patients after initial hepatectomy. J Gastrointest Surg. 2011;15:1433–9.
62. Kikuchi Y, Hiroshima Y, Matsuo K, Kawaguchi D, Murakami T, Yabushita Y, et al. A randomized clinical trial of preoperative administration of branched-chain amino acids to prevent postoperative ascites in patients with liver resection for hepatocellular carcinoma. Ann Surg Oncol. 2016;23:3727–35.
63. Togo S, Tanaka K, Morioka D, Sugita M, Ueda M, Miura Y, et al. Usefulness of granular BCAA after hepatectomy for liver cancer complicated with liver cirrhosis. Nutrition. 2005;21:480–6.
64. Ichikawa K, Okabayashi T, Maeda H, Namikawa T, Iiyama T, Sugimoto T, et al. Oral supplementation of branched-chain amino acids reduces early recurrence after hepatic resection in patients with hepatocellular carcinoma: a prospective study. Surg Today. 2013;43:720–6.
65. Hachiya H, Aoki T, Iso Y, Shimizu T, Tago K, Park KH, et al. Effects of branched-chain amino acids on postoperative tumor recurrence in patients undergoing curative resection for hepatocellular carcinoma: A randomized clinical trial. J Hepatobiliary Pancreat Sci. 2020;27:819–29.
66. Sugawara G, Nagino M, Nishio H, Ebata T, Takagi K, Asahara T, et al. Perioperative synbiotic treatment to prevent postoperative infectious complications in biliary cancer surgery: a randomized controlled trial. Ann Surg. 2006;244:706–14.
67. Kanazawa H, Nagino M, Kamiya S, Komatsu S, Mayumi T, Takagi K, et al. Synbiotics reduce postoperative infectious complications: a randomized controlled trial in biliary cancer patients undergoing hepatectomy. Langenbecks Arch Surg. 2005;390:104–13.
68. Usami M, Miyoshi M, Kanbara Y, Aoyama M, Sakaki H, Shuno K, et al. Effects of perioperative synbiotic treatment on infectious complications, intestinal integrity, and fecal flora and organic acids in hepatic surgery with or without cirrhosis. JPEN J Parenter Enteral Nutr. 2011;35:317–28.
69. Rayes N, Pilarski T, Stockmann M, Bengmark S, Neuhaus P, Seehofer D. Effect of pre- and probiotics on liver regeneration after resection: a randomised, double-blind pilot study. Benef Microbes. 2012;3:237–44.
70. Gan Y, Su S, Li B, Fang C. Efficacy of probiotics and prebiotics in prevention of infectious complications following hepatic resections: systematic review and meta-analysis. J Gastrointestin Liver Dis. 2019;28:205–11.
71. Wu Z, Qin J, Pu L. Omega-3 fatty acid improves the clinical outcome of hepatectomized patients with hepatitis B virus (HBV)-associated hepatocellular carcinoma. J Biomed Res. 2012;26:395–9.
72. Gong Y, Liu Z, Liao Y, Mai C, Chen T, Tang H, et al. Effectiveness of ω-3 polyunsaturated fatty acids based lipid emulsions for treatment of patients after hepatectomy: a prospective clinical trial. Nutrients. 2016;8:357. doi:10.3390/nu8060357
73. Seguin P, Locher C, Boudjema K, Hamon C, Mouchel C, Malledant Y, et al. Effect of a perioperative nutritional supplementation with oral impact in patients undergoing hepatic surgery for liver cancer: A prospective, placebo-controlled, randomized, double-blind study. Nutr Cancer. 2016;68:464–72.
74. Hirokawa F, Hayashi M, Miyamoto Y, Asakuma M, Shimizu T, Komeda K, et al. Evaluation of postoperative antibiotic prophylaxis

after liver resection: a randomized controlled trial. Am J Surg. 2013;206:8–15.

75. Takayama T, Aramaki O, Shibata T, Oka M, Itamoto T, Shimada M, et al. Antimicrobial prophylaxis for 1 day versus 3 days in liver cancer surgery: a randomized controlled non-inferiority trial. Surg Today. 2019;49:859–69.
76. Shinkawa H, Tanaka S, Takemura S, Amano R, Kimura K, Nishioka T, et al. Giving short-term prophylactic antibiotics in patients undergoing open and laparoscopic hepatic resection. Ann Gastroenterol Surg. 2019;3:506–14.
77. Belghiti J, Kabbej M, Sauvanet A, Vilgrain V, Panis Y, Fekete F. Drainage after elective hepatic resection. A randomized trial. Ann Surg. 1993;218:748–53.
78. Liu CL, Fan ST, Lo CM, Wong Y, Ng IO-L, Lam C-M, et al. Abdominal drainage after hepatic resection is contraindicated in patients with chronic liver diseases. Ann Surg. 2004;239:194–201.
79. Sun HC, Qin LX, Lu L, Wang L, Ye QH, Ren N, et al. Randomized clinical trial of the effects of abdominal drainage after elective hepatectomy using the crushing clamp method. Br J Surg. 2006;93:422–6.
80. Kim YI, Fujita S, Hwang VJ, Nagase Y. Comparison of abdominal drainage and no—drainage after elective hepatectomy: a randomized study. Hepatogastroenterology. 2014;61:707–11.
81. Fuster J, Llovet JM, Garcia-Valdecasas JC, Grande L, Fondevila C, Vilana R, et al. Abdominal drainage after liver resection for hepatocellular carcinoma in cirrhotic patients: a randomized controlled study. Hepatogastroenterology. 2004;51:536–40.
82. Arita J, Sakamaki K, Saiura A, Konishi M, Sakamoto Y, Hashimoto M, et al. Drain placement after uncomplicated hepatic resection increases severe postoperative complication rate: A Japanese multi-institutional randomized controlled trial (ND-trial). Ann Surg. 2021;273:224–31.
83. Kaibori M, Shimizu J, Hayashi M, Nakai T, Ishizaki M, Matsui K, et al. Late-onset bile leakage after hepatic resection. Surgery. 2015;157:37–44.
84. Kyoden Y, Imamura H, Sano K, Beck Y, Sugawara Y, Kokudo N, et al. Value of prophylactic abdominal drainage in 1269 consecutive cases of elective liver resection. J Hepatobiliary Pancreat Sci. 2010;17:186–92.
85. Tanaka K, Kumamoto T, Nojiri K, Takeda K, Endo I. The effectiveness and appropriate managemnet of abdominal drains in patients undergoing elective liver resection: a retrospective analysis and prospective case series. Surg Today. 2013;43:372–80.
86. Torzilli G, Olivari N, Del Fabbro D, Gambetti A, Leoni P, Gendarini A, et al. Bilirubin level fluctuation in drain discharge after hepatectomies justifies long-term drain maintenance. Hepatogastroenterology. 2005;52:1206–10.
87. Hirokawa F, Hayashi M, Miyamoto Y, Asakuma M, Shimizu T, Komeda K, et al. Re-valuation of the necessity of prophylactic drainage after liver resection. Am Surg. 2011;77:539–44.
88. Liu CL, Fan ST, Lo CM, Chan SC, Yong BH, Wong J. Safety of donor right hepatectomy without abdominal drainage: a prospective evaluation in 100 consecutive liver donors. Liver Transpl. 2005;11:314–9.
89. Mangram AJ, Horan TC, Pearson ML, Silver LC, Jarvis WR. Guideline for prevention of surgical site infection. Hospital infection control practices advisory committee. Infect Control Hosp Epidemiol. 1999;1999(20):250–78.
90. Mitsuka Y, Yamazaki S, Yoshida N, Masamichi M, Higaki T, Takayama T. Prospective validation of optimal drain management "the 3×3 rule" after liver resection. World J Surg. 2016;40:2213–20.
91. Hokuto D, Nomi T, Yasuda S, Kawaguchi C, Yoshikawa T, Ishioka K, et al. The safety of the early removal of prophylactic drainage after liver resection based solely on predetermined criteria: a propensity score analysis. HPB (Oxford). 2017;19:359–64.
92. Older P, Hall A, Hader R. Cardiopulmonary exercise testing as a screening test for perioperative management of major surgery in the elderly. Chest. 1999;116:355–62.
93. Older P, Smith R, Courtney P, Hone R. Preoperative evaluation of cardiac failure and ischemia in elderly patients by cardiopulmonary exercise testing. Chest. 1993;104:701–4.
94. Dunne DF, Jack S, Jones RP, Jones L, Lythgoe DT, Malik HZ, et al. Randomized clinical trial of prehabilitation before planned liver resection. Br J Surg. 2016;103:504–12.
95. Kasivisvanathan R, Abbassi-Ghadi N, McLeod AD, Oliver A, Rao Baikady R, Jhanji S, et al. Cardiopulmonary exercise testing for predicting postoperative morbidity in patients undergoing hepatic resection surgery. HPB (Oxford). 2015;17:637–43.
96. Kaibori M, Ishizaki M, Matsui K, Nakatake R, Yoshiuchi S, Kimura Y, et al. Perioperative exercise for chronic liver injury patients with hepatocellular carcinoma undergoing hepatectomy. Am J Surg. 2013;206:202–9.
97. Adamina M, Kehlet H, Tomlinson GA, Senagore AJ, Delaney CP. Enhanced recovery pathways optimize health outcomes and resource utilization: A meta-analysis of randomized controlled trials in colorectal surgery. Surgery. 2011;149:830–40.
98. Lassen K, Soop M, Nygren J, Cox PB, Hendry PO, Spies C, et al. Consensus review of optimal perioperative care in colorectal surgery: Enhanced Recovery After Surgery (ERAS) Group recommendations. Arch Surg. 2009;144:961–9.
99. Leibman BD, Dillioglugil O, Abbas F, Tanli S, Kattan MW, Scardino PT. Impact of a clinical pathway for radical retropublic prostatectomy. Urology. 1998;52:94–9.
100. Niino T, Hata M, Sezai A, Yoshitake I, Unosawa S, Shimura K, et al. Optimal clinical pathway for the patient with type B acute aortic dissection. Circ J. 2009;73:264–8.
101. Spanjersberg WR, Reurings J, Keus F, van Laarhoven CJ. Fast track surgery versus conventional recovery strategies for colorectal surgery. Cochrane Database Syst Rev. 2011;(2):CD007635. doi:10.1002/14651858
102. Hall TC, Dennison AR, Biku DK, Metcalfe MS, Garcea G. Enhanced recovery programmes in hepatobiliary and pancreatic surgery: A systematic review. Ann R Coll Surg Engl. 2012;94:318–26.
103. Wang C, Zheng G, Zhang W, Zhang F, Lv S, Wang A, et al. Enhanced recovery after surgery programs for liver resection: a meta-analysis. J Gastrointest Surg. 2017;21:472–86.
104. Noba L, Rodgers S, Chandler C, Balfour A, Hariharan D, Yip VS. Enhanced recovery after surgery (ERAS) reduces hospital costs and improve clinical outcomes in liver surgery: a systematic review and meta-Analysis. J Gastrointest Surg. 2020;24:918–32.
105. Kaibori M, Matsui K, Ishizaki M, Iida H, Yoshii K, Asano H, et al. Effects of implementing an "enhanced recovery after surgery" program on patients undergoing resection of hepatocellular carcinoma. Surg Today. 2017;47:42–51.
106. Hausken J, Fretland ÅA, Edwin B, Andersen MH, Dagenborg VJ, Bjørnelv GMW, et al. Intravenous patient-controlled analgesia versus thoracic epidural analgesia after open liver surgery: a prospective, randomized, controlled, noninferiority trial. Ann Surg. 2019;270:193–9.
107. Melloul E, Hübner M, Scott M, Snowden C, Prentis J, Dejong CH, et al. Guidelines for Perioperative Care for Liver Surgery: Enhanced Recovery After Surgery (ERAS) Society Recommendations. World J Surg. 2016;40:2425–40.

17

Significance of the Glasgow prognostic score for short-term surgical outcomes: A nationwide survey using the Japanese National Clinical Database

Yoshihiro Hiramatsu[1,2,3] | Hiraku Kumamaru[4] | Hirotoshi Kikuchi[1,2] | Shiyori Usune[4] | Kinji Kamiya[1,2] | Hiroaki Miyata[4] | Hiroyuki Konno[1,5] | Yoshihiro Kakeji[6] | Yuko Kitagawa[1] | Hiroya Takeuchi[1,2]

[1]The Japanese Society of Gastroenterological Surgery, Minato-ku, Japan

[2]Department of Surgery, Hamamatsu University School of Medicine, Hamamatsu, Japan

[3]Department of Perioperative Functioning Care and Support, Hamamatsu University School of Medicine, Hamamatsu, Japan

[4]Department of Healthcare Quality Assessment, Graduate School of Medicine, University of Tokyo, Bunkyo-ku, Japan

[5]Hamamatsu University School of Medicine, Hamamatsu, Japan

[6]Database Committee, The Japanese Society of Gastroenterological Surgery, Minato-ku, Japan

Correspondence
Hiroya Takeuchi, Department of Surgery, Hamamatsu University School of Medicine, 1-20-1 Handayama, Higashi-ku, Hamamatsu-shi, Shizuoka, 431-3192, Japan.
Email: takeuchi@hama-med.ac.jp

Abstract

Aim: Preoperative inflammation-based Glasgow prognostic score (GPS) is a useful tool for predicting long-term prognosis in cancer patients. However, its association with postoperative short-term outcomes remains unknown. The aim of this study is to investigate the association between GPS and postoperative morbidity and mortality among patients undergoing surgery for various gastrointestinal malignancies.

Methods: Using the Japanese National Clinical Database, we analyzed the records of 312 357 patients with gastrointestinal malignancy who underwent six typical elective surgeries, including esophagectomy, distal gastrectomy, total gastrectomy, right hemicolectomy, low anterior resection, and pancreaticoduodenectomy, between January 2015 and December 2018. We assigned GPS of 0, 1, or 2 to patients with no, one, or both decreased albumin and elevated C-reactive protein levels, respectively. We investigated the relationship of GPS with operative morbidity and mortality for each procedure with adjustments for patients' demographics, preoperative status, comorbidities, and cancer stages.

Results: Crude operative morbidity was significantly higher for GPS 1 and 2 than GPS 0 patients in all procedures except pancreaticoduodenectomy. The postoperative length of hospital stay was significantly longer for GPS 1 and 2 patients in all procedures ($P < .001$). Operative mortality was also higher for GPS 1 and 2 patients in all procedures. The associations remained significant after adjustments for potential confounders of age, sex, physical status, tumor classification, use of preoperative therapy, and comorbidities.

Conclusion: This nationwide study provides solid evidence on the strong association between GPS and postoperative outcomes.

KEYWORDS

gastrointestinal malignancies, gastrointestinal neoplasms, Japanese National Clinical Database, prognostic factors, surgical outcomes

1 | INTRODUCTION

The systemic inflammatory response has been associated with poor clinical outcomes in many cancer types.[1-3] Elevated C-reactive protein (CRP) concentration is the most common measure of the systemic inflammatory response in cancer patients due to its sensitivity, specificity, and reproducibility in hospital laboratories. Furthermore, the magnitude of the increase in CRP concentrations has been shown to be associated with poorer survival in cancer patients, independent of performance status, weight loss, tumor stage, and other high-risk pathological features.[4-6] A correlation between hypoalbuminemia and poor prognosis in patients with malignancies is also well-recognized.[7,8] In cancer patients, malnutrition is often associated with anorexia-cachexia syndrome, characterized by decreased food intake, hypoalbuminemia, weight loss, and muscle tissue wasting.[9] Nutrition becomes the foremost concern as preoperative malnutrition is also an important risk factor for postoperative morbidity and mortality.[10]

Forrest et al developed the inflammation-based Glasgow prognostic score (GPS) consisting of two simple components: serum levels of CRP and albumin.[11] The GPS is one of the most useful indexes for predicting long-term prognosis in various cancers.[12-17] However, the relationship between GPS and postoperative short-term outcomes remains controversial.[18-22] Preoperative serum levels of CRP and albumin have been reported as the risk factors for postoperative complications and mortality.[23-32] Despite advances in surgical techniques and devices, some patients who undergo the procedure experience clinically relevant postoperative complications, resulting in a protracted recovery period, delayed administration of adjuvant chemotherapy, and impaired quality of life.[33-39] Therefore, risk management using a prediction tool based on preoperatively determining factors is important to obtain appropriate informed consent and perioperative management, as well as to minimize the medical cost burden.[40]

Several other predictive tools for cancer surgery prognosis have been developed, for example the prognostic nutritional index (PNI), the controlling nutritional status (CONUT) score, the CRP/Albumin ratio, and others.[20-21] These tools use a variety of factors that can be measured through standard clinical laboratory tests. However, since the Japanese National Clinical Database (NCD), from which data for this study were obtained, does not store data for factors such as total cholesterol, neutrophil count, and lymphocyte count, we excluded a number of these tools for use in this study. Furthermore, exact values for serum albumin and CRP levels were not available in the database for patients whose serum levels of these two markers fell within normal range. The modified GPS (mGPS), developed and used in various studies, does not show a clear superiority over the GPS for surgical outcome,[18,20,41] and would have greatly reduced the number of score 1s in this study. We therefore elected to use the original GPS as the predictive tool to analyze in this study.

Based on previous reports,[18-32] we hypothesized that the preoperative GPS could predict the postoperative short-term outcomes as well as long-term prognosis in various cancers. The present study aimed to investigate the significance of preoperative GPS in predicting postoperative morbidity and mortality in patients with gastrointestinal carcinoma. To our knowledge, this is the first study to demonstrate the impact of GPS on postoperative morbidity and mortality using extensive data from a nationwide database.

2 | METHODS

2.1 | The nationwide database system

The Japanese NCD, which started its data registration in 2011, has grown into a large nationwide database covering more than 95% of the surgeries performed by general surgeons in Japan.[39] As of the end of December 2019, 5276 facilities have enrolled in the NCD, and about 1 500 000 cases are registered every year.[39] The NCD is a nationwide project linked to the board certification system for surgery in Japan. The submission of cases to the NCD is a prerequisite for all member institutions of both the Japan Surgical Society and the Japanese Society of Gastrointestinal Surgery, and only registered cases can be used for board certification reviews. The data are evaluated annually using a web-based data management system to ensure data traceability. The data are also validated against medical charts via audits to randomly selected institutions.[42] The most recent laboratory data for each patient, obtained 90 days or less prior to surgery, are registered in the NCD.

The data from the NCD were provided to analysis teams after anonymization. Patients were provided with the opportunities to opt-out from their clinical information being used for research. The approval by the Ethics Committee of Hamamatsu University School of Medicine was obtained before starting data analysis, and this study was registered at the UMIN Clinical Trials Registry as UMIN 000036761.

2.2 | Patients

We analyzed data from a total of 312 357 patients who underwent six typical procedures of gastroenterological surgery (esophagectomy [Eso], distal gastrectomy [DG], total gastrectomy [TG], right hemicolectomy [RHC], low anterior resection [LAR], and pancreaticoduodenectomy [PD]) between 1 January 2015 and 31 December 2018. We only included patients who underwent surgical procedures for malignancy (Eso for esophageal cancer; TG and DG for gastric cancer; RHC for colon cancer; LAR for rectal cancer; PD for pancreatic cancer). The exclusion criteria were as follows: (a) cases with distant metastasis or disseminated cancer; (b) emergent surgery cases; (c) cases with concomitant major surgery; (d) cases in which artificial respiration management was performed before surgery; (e) cases with coexisting preoperative sepsis, pneumonia, or open wounds; (f) patients who regularly used steroids before surgery; and (g) missing values for preoperative serum CRP and albumin (Table S1).

2.3 | Assessment of GPS

We assessed patients' GPS as follows: patients with both elevated CRP (>10 mg/L) and hypoalbuminemia (<35 g/L) levels were allocated a score of 2; patients with only one of the biochemical abnormalities were allocated a score of 1; patients with neither of these abnormalities were allocated a score of 0.[11]

2.4 | Study outcomes

We assessed the occurrence of postoperative complications categorized as grade III or above based on the Clavien-Dindo (CD) classification,[43] operative mortality, and the length of hospital stay after surgery. Postoperative complications included surgical site infection, wound dehiscence, anastomotic leakage, pancreatic fistula, bile leakage, pneumonia, unplanned intubation, pulmonary embolism, ventilator-assisted respiration longer than 48 hours, progressive renal insufficiency, acute renal failure, urinary tract infection, cerebrovascular accident with neurological deficit, coma longer than 24 hours, peripheral nerve injury, cardiac arrest requiring cardiopulmonary resuscitation, myocardial infarction, bleeding complications defined by transfusions over one unit of blood, deep venous thrombosis, and sepsis. Detailed descriptions of the postoperative complications associated with individual cancers have been provided previously.[27-39] Operative mortality was defined as death during the index hospitalization, regardless of the length of hospital stay, as well as death after hospital discharge in ≤30 days from the surgery date.

2.5 | Statistical analysis

We tabulated the characteristics of the patients by GPS separately for each type of surgical procedure. We assessed the incidences of postoperative complications and operative mortality by GPS score for each procedure type and estimated the median and 10th-90th percentiles for the length of postoperative hospital stay. We compared the postoperative length of stay across the three GPS groups using the Kruskal-Wallis test. For each procedure type, relative odds for postoperative morbidity and mortality were estimated for GPS 1 and 2 groups as compared to GPS 0 group using multivariable logistic regression models, adjusting for patients' age; sex; American Society of Anesthesiologists-Physical Status (ASA-PS); T classification; N classification; use of preoperative chemo-, radiation-, or other therapy; and comorbidities including diabetes mellitus, hypertension, chronic obstructive pulmonary disease, cardiac disease, cerebrovascular disease, and kidney dysfunction. Tests were all two-sided and *P*-values <.05 were considered statistically significant. All statistical analyses were conducted using SAS 9.4 (SAS Institute).

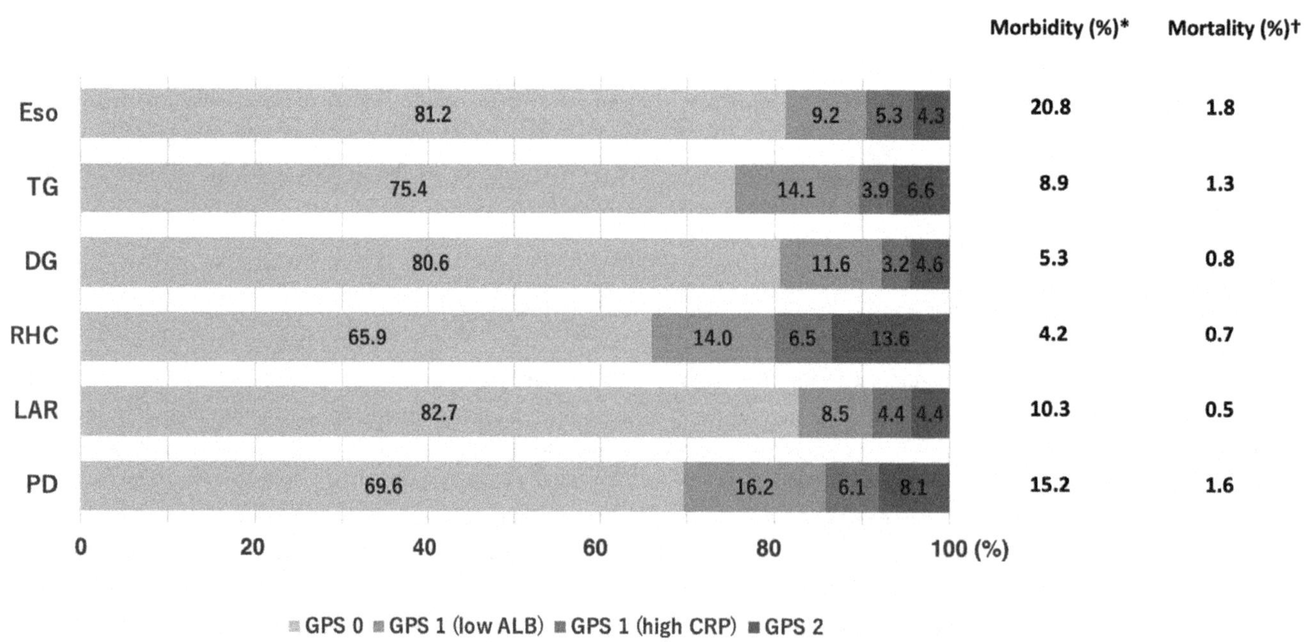

FIGURE 1 Glasgow Prognostic Score (GPS) distribution in the surgical procedures (%). *Operative morbidity included complications of grade 3 and greater according to Clavien-Dindo classification. †Operative mortality included all deaths occurring within the index hospitalization period, regardless of the length of hospital stay, or after hospital discharge (within 30 d after surgery). Eso, esophagectomy; TG, total gastrectomy; DG, distal gastrectomy; RHC, right hemicolectomy; LAR, low anterior resection; PD, pancreaticoduodenectomy; ALB, albumin; CRP, C-reactive protein

3 | RESULTS

The study population selection process for each procedure is summarized in Table S1. After subject selection, there were 20 541 Eso patients, 41 435 TG patients, 109 244 DG patients, 58 476 RHC patients, 62 693 LAR patients, and 19 968 PD patients.

3.1 | GPS distribution

Figure 1 shows the GPS distribution of all patients whose data were analyzed, together with the overall incidence of postoperative mortality and morbidity (CD-3 and above). Overall, 65.9%-82.7% of the procedures were performed on patients with GPS 0. GPS distribution varied by the procedure type, but the proportion of patients with GPS 2 did not exceed 10% in any procedure except RHC, in which the proportion of patients with GPS 2 was 13.6%. The proportion of patients with GPS 2 was the smallest in Eso (4.3%), which had the highest operative morbidity rate among the six procedures examined. Despite high invasiveness and morbidity in PD, the proportion of patients with GPS 1 or 2 was over 30% and higher than other procedures similar to RHC, which is generally considered less invasive. We saw no clear association between the GPS distribution and procedure's overall incidence of operative morbidity and mortality. In the GPS 1 group, patients with lower albumin levels were predominant for all procedures.

Table 1 summarizes the demographic and comorbidity parameters of patients who underwent each procedure. The mean age of patients in all procedures was approximately 70 years (67.3-73.7 years). Gender was disease-specific and varied widely depending on each surgical procedure. Age, ASA-PS, and clinical stage (cT, tumor invasion depth; and cN, lymph node metastasis) increased with an

TABLE 1 Clinical characteristics of study patients

	GPS	Number of patients	Age (y) (mean ± SD)	Sex (%) (Male ratio)	ASA-PS (%)[a]	cT (%)[b]	cN (%)[c]
Eso		20 541	67.3 ± 8.9	82.0	8.4	59.5	52.7
	0	16 672	66.8 ± 8.9	81.6	7.3	55.4	50.7
	1	2988	68.7 ± 8.4	83.3	11.8	75.6	59.9
	2	881	70.5 ± 8.2	85.0	18.8	84.0	64.5
TG		41 435	70.5 ± 10.4	74.2	11.8	70.8	50.7
	0	31 252	69.2 ± 10.4	73.6	8.9	65.9	46.0
	1	7466	73.9 ± 9.3	74.8	19.6	84.1	63.5
	2	2717	75.4 ± 8.5	79.6	24.4	89.9	69.0
DG		109 244	70.6 ± 11.2	66.6	11.8	45.4	32.4
	0	88 071	69.2 ± 11.1	66.5	8.9	39.1	27.4
	1	16 204	75.8 ± 9.5	66.7	22.8	69.5	51.7
	2	4969	77.5 ± 8.8	67.8	28.8	79.4	57.4
RHC		58 476	73.7 ± 10.7	49.5	15.1	85.2	39.5
	0	38 538	72.2 ± 10.5	50.5	10.6	79.9	35.9
	1	12 010	76.3 ± 10.5	48.8	21.8	94.4	45.7
	2	7928	77.1 ± 10.5	45.5	26.5	97.2	47.8
LAR		62 693	67.3 ± 11.3	65.3	9.8	80.6	37.7
	0	51 831	66.4 ± 11.2	65.2	7.8	78.4	36.3
	1	8088	71.4 ± 10.7	65.9	18.4	89.9	44.2
	2	2774	72.3 ± 10.4	66.5	21.4	93.9	43.5
PD		19 968	69.5 ± 9.7	56.2	13.0	82.1	47.0
	0	13 901	68.7 ± 10.0	55.4	11.2	78.3	43.4
	1	4450	71.1 ± 8.7	58.2	16.4	90.2	54.3
	2	1617	72.3 ± 8.3	56.9	19.7	92.7	58.5

Abbreviations: ASA-PS, American Society of Anesthesiologists-Physical Status; cN, preoperative diagnosis of lymph node metastasis; cT, preoperative diagnosis of tumor invasion depth; DG, distal gastrectomy; Eso, esophagectomy; GPS, Glasgow Prognostic Score; LAR, low anterior resection; PD, pancreaticoduodenectomy; RHC, right hemicolectomy; SD, standard deviation; TG, total gastrectomy.

[a]Represents proportion of patients with ASA-PS class 3 and above.

[b]Represents proportion of patients with stage T2 and above.

[c]Represents proportion of patients with stage N1 and above.

increase in GPS. Full tabulation of patients' characteristics, preoperative treatment, and comorbidities are presented in the supporting information material (Tables S2-S7). In summary, patients with high GPS had higher frequencies of receiving preoperative treatment and had more preoperative comorbidities. Table S8 shows the breakdown of preoperative treatments administered to patients for the different procedure types.

3.2 | Influence of GPS on operative morbidity and postoperative hospital stay

Table 2 shows the incidences of operative morbidity as well as the relative odds for operative morbidity from the logistic regression models for all procedures. The incidences of operative morbidity were higher for patients in higher GPS groups. The operative morbidity for patients with GPS 1 or GPS 2 was significantly higher than that for patients with GPS 0, for all procedures except PD. A remarkable difference was observed especially in the patients with GPS 2 in all procedures (odds ratio, 1.31-1.68; $P < .0001$), except in PD (odds ratio, 1.15; $P = .0577$) from the multivariable logistic regression models. As shown in Tables S9-S14, the confidence intervals of odds ratios for GPS 1 and 2 patients had little or no overlap between these two groups in the operative morbidity for all procedures except in PD, suggesting significant difference. The odds ratios were higher for surgical procedures with relatively lower overall complication rates, such as DG, RHC, and LAR. On the contrary, the odds ratios were lower in those surgical procedures that had a higher incidence of postoperative morbidities, such as Eso and PD, and no significant difference was observed in PD. The full list of estimates from the multivariable regression analyses is presented in Tables S9-S14. Together with GPS, poor physical health, advanced cancer stages as well as comorbidities such as past cerebrovascular or cardiovascular diseases, kidney dysfunction, and COPD were identified as strong risk predictors of complications after surgeries. The length of hospital stay after surgery also significantly increased with an increase in GPS in all procedures, including PD ($P < .0001$; Table 3). Table S15 shows the five most frequent postoperative complications in each surgical procedure.

3.3 | Influence of GPS on operative mortality

The crude operative mortality by GPS groups as well as the relative odds for postoperative death for GPS 1 and 2 vs 0 are shown in Table 4. There was almost no overlap in confidence intervals for odds ratios of operative mortality between GPS 1 and 2, and the higher GPS score was associated with higher operative mortality for

TABLE 2 Operative morbidity for different elective procedures

	GPS	Number of patients	Operative morbidity[a] n	%	OR[b]	95% CI	*P*-value[b]
Eso	0	16 672	3312	19.9			
	1	2988	701	23.5	1.15	(1.04-1.26)	.0049
	2	881	253	28.7	1.42	(1.22-1.66)	<.0001
TG	0	31 252	2565	8.2			
	1	7466	779	10.4	1.11	(1.02-1.22)	.0158
	2	2717	350	12.9	1.31	(1.16-1.48)	<.0001
DG	0	88 071	4105	4.7			
	1	16 204	1233	7.6	1.26	(1.17-1.35)	<.0001
	2	4969	468	9.4	1.43	(1.29-1.60)	<.0001
RHC	0	38 538	1324	3.4			
	1	12 010	596	5.0	1.27	(1.15-1.41)	<.0001
	2	7928	529	6.7	1.68	(1.50-1.88)	<.0001
LAR	0	51 831	4968	9.6			
	1	8088	1057	13.1	1.32	(1.22-1.42)	<.0001
	2	2774	433	15.6	1.58	(1.42-1.77)	<.0001
PD	0	13 901	2063	14.8			
	1	4450	697	15.7	1.06	(0.96-1.16)	.2624
	2	1617	275	17.0	1.15	(0.99-1.32)	.0577

Abbreviations: CI, confidence interval; DG, distal gastrectomy; Eso, esophagectomy; GPS, Glasgow Prognostic Score; LAR, low anterior resection; OR, odds ratio; PD, pancreaticoduodenectomy; RHC, right hemicolectomy; TG, total gastrectomy.

[a]Including grade 3 and grater according to Clavien-Dindo classification.

[b]Compared to GPS 0.

all procedures (Table 4 and S9-S14). The association between GPS and the incidence of operative mortality was more pronounced than that between GPS and the incidence of operative morbidity, and it was more noticeable for patients with GPS 2 (Eso, 2.62; TG, 3.07; DG, 3.83; RHC, 5.63; LAR, 5.59; PD, 2.06; $P < .0001$). Similar to the analysis of operative morbidity, the odds ratio for mortality was higher in the high GPS groups among patients undergoing procedures that had low mortality such as TG, DG, RHC, and LAR. In these four procedure types, with crude mortality of ≤0.7% for patients with GPS 0, the mortality of GPS 2 patients was more than three times higher. Associations between factors such as age, advanced cancer stage, and comorbidities with mortality after surgeries were stronger compared with those with incidences of post-surgical complications (Tables S9-S14).

4 | DISCUSSION

We conducted a large-scale study on the association between GPS and short-term operative outcomes in gastroenterological surgery, using data accumulated in the NCD in Japan. This nationwide survey confirmed that GPS is a strong risk predictor of operative morbidity and mortality and has a similar impact across different procedures in the field of gastrointestinal surgery.

Several previous studies have investigated the causal relationship between GPS and short-term surgical outcomes, such as morbidity and mortality after surgery in various fields, including gastroenterology.[18-22,25] However, according to the literature, the effects of GPS on postoperative morbidity and mortality vary among operative procedures and even for the same procedure, so the influence of GPS on operative short-term outcomes was controversial. In addition, while the sample size in the previous reports had been limited to approximately 1000 patients, the number of patients in this study was much greater than the previous studies, allowing us to separately evaluate data from different gastroenterological procedures at once.

Operative morbidity was significantly higher in patients with higher GPS for all procedures except PD. Interestingly, the procedures associated with the highest increase in operative morbidity were DG and RHC, which are generally considered to be less invasive and twice as safe as other procedures. On the contrary, Eso and PD, which had high morbidity in patients with GPS 0, had a smaller impact on the association of GPS with morbidity, and no significant difference was observed in PD. In a highly invasive surgery with high operative morbidity, it may be considered that patients with poor preoperative conditions were not indicated and appropriate alternative treatment was selected. It is also possible that PD has variables related to its morbidity that are more significant than GPS. Thus, as a risk factor for postoperative complications in PD, not only the preoperative condition of the patient, but also the surgical procedure itself may have a large impact. However, it was shown that the postoperative hospital stay was prolonged as the GPS increased in all surgical procedures including PD. In this study, we defined operative morbidity as grade III or higher complications of CD classification; however, GPS might have an effect on the incidence of postoperative complications less than grade III. The results of the previous studies were conflicting about the effect of GPS on operative morbidity, but those of the present study allowed us to conclude that high morbidity is predicted for patients with high GPS for almost all the procedures evaluated.

TABLE 3 Postoperative length of hospital stay

	GPS	Postoperative hospital stay (d) median (10th-90th percentiles)	P-value
Eso	0	14 (23-62)	<.0001
	1	15 (26-79)	
	2	15 (28-90)	
TG	0	15 (9-36)	<.0001
	1	17 (10-49)	
	2	20 (11-57)	
DG	0	12 (8-27)	<.0001
	1	15 (9-42)	
	2	18 (10-56)	
RHC	0	11 (7-22)	<.0001
	1	14 (8-33)	
	2	15 (8-43)	
LAR	0	14 (8-35)	<.0001
	1	17 (9-48)	
	2	20 (10-55)	
PD	0	24 (14-51)	<.0001
	1	26 (14-56)	
	2	26 (14-59)	

Abbreviations: DG, distal gastrectomy; Eso, esophagectomy; GPS, Glasgow Prognostic Score; LAR, low anterior resection; PD, pancreaticoduodenectomy; RHC, right hemicolectomy; TG, total gastrectomy.

Operative mortality was also significantly increased in patients with higher GPS for all procedures. The highest increase in operative mortality, i.e. by 5.63 of the odds ratio, was observed for RHC, while that for PD increased by 2.06 of the odds ratio. The impact of GPS on mortality was greater than the impact on morbidity in all surgical procedures evaluated, even in patients with GPS 1. Interestingly, the influence of GPS on operative mortality was also greater in procedures which are generally considered to be less invasive and relatively safe, such as DG, RHC, and LAR, than the influence in the procedures which had high morbidity for patients with GPS 0, such as Eso and PD. Therefore, it is suggested that an appropriate preoperative risk assessment is important even for less invasive procedures, and in some cases modified surgery, multistep surgery, or alternative therapy needs to be considered. Previous studies that have evaluated the influence of GPS on short-term postoperative outcomes have a small sample size,[18-22,25] and few have investigated the relationship between GPS and operative mortality.[19,22] The

TABLE 4 Operative mortality for different elective procedures

	GPS	Number of patients	Operative mortality[a] n	%	OR[b]	95% CI	P-value[b]
Eso	0	16 672	226	1.4			
	1	2988	87	2.9	1.57	(1.20-2.04)	.0010
	2	881	52	5.9	2.62	(1.88-3.65)	<.0001
TG	0	31 252	232	0.7			
	1	7466	185	2.5	2.11	(1.71-2.59)	<.0001
	2	2717	115	4.2	3.07	(2.40-3.92)	<.0001
DG	0	88 071	359	0.4			
	1	16 204	292	1.8	2.21	(1.87-2.62)	<.0001
	2	4969	188	3.8	3.83	(3.14-4.67)	<.0001
RHC	0	38 538	95	0.2			
	1	12 010	117	1.0	2.59	(1.94-3.44)	<.0001
	2	7928	187	2.4	5.63	(4.28-7.42)	<.0001
LAR	0	51 831	150	0.3			
	1	8088	80	1.0	2.11	(1.58-2.80)	<.0001
	2	2774	77	2.8	5.59	(4.15-7.54)	<.0001
PD	0	13 901	166	1.2			
	1	4450	108	2.4	1.68	(1.30-2.16)	<.0001
	2	1617	53	3.3	2.06	(1.49-2.85)	<.0001

Abbreviations: CI, confidence interval; DG, distal gastrectomy; Eso, esophagectomy; GPS, Glasgow Prognostic Score; LAR, low anterior resection; OR, odds ratio; PD, pancreaticoduodenectomy; RHC, right hemicolectomy; TG, total gastrectomy.

[a]Including all deaths occurring within the index hospitalization period, regardless of the length of hospital stay, or after hospital discharge (within 30 d after surgery).

[b]Compared to GPS 0.

results of this study indicate that the GPS can predict the risk of short-term postoperative mortality.

McMillan et al developed the mGPS and demonstrated that it was significantly associated with overall and cancer-specific survival for patients with colorectal cancer.[41] However, some studies showed that the GPS reflected the prognosis of patients with curable gastric cancer more accurately than the mGPS.[18,20] In these studies, the number of patients with hypoalbuminemia in the absence of an elevated CRP concentration who changed from GPS 1 to mGPS 0 was different, with the former being 16/109 (14.7%) and the latter being 52/92 (56.5%). Compared to other preoperative evaluation indicators such as PNI and CONUT, GPS tends to increase the number of patients in the normal group (GPS 0). Using mGPS, the number of patients with a 0 score is even higher than the number of patients using the GPS. In this study, the number of patients with lower albumin levels was predominant in the GPS 1 group, so the percentage of the normal group in the mGPS analysis was even greater.

While GPS is recognized as one of the most useful indicators for predicting long-term prognosis in various cancers,[12-17] its usefulness as a predictor in the short-term outcomes of patients undergoing surgery remains unclear.[18-22,25] Our multivariable analysis revealed that while the common risk factors of perioperative morbidity or mortality, including age, gender, ASA-PS, tumor depth, lymph node metastasis, and preoperative comorbidity, were consistently valuable predicting factors, the GPS was also an independent risk predictor of operative morbidity and mortality in patients who underwent surgical treatment for gastroenterological malignancies. Since the GPS has the advantage of being easy to obtain prior to surgical intervention, it may be a useful tool for routine evaluation during gastrointestinal cancer treatment planning. The GPS provides a preoperative means to predict short-term postoperative outcomes. Postoperative complications have been reported to worsen long-term prognosis after surgery,[44] and their incidence has been reportedly reduced by the intervention of the multidisciplinary perioperative management team.[45] Thus, it is important to pay attention to perioperative care for patients with an elevated GPS for the reduction of postoperative complications and improvement of long-term prognosis. Some research has reported that exercise and/or nutrition prehabilitation is associated with positive effects for weight maintenance and surgical complications.[46-47] However, a recent systematic review demonstrated the lack of strong evidence to determine the most optimal methods of preoperative support for patients undergoing gastrointestinal cancer resection.[46-47] There is also no evidence that an improvement of GPS prior to surgery will result in better short-term outcomes in gastroenterological surgeries. It would be important and interesting for a future investigation to assess the optimal protocol for preoperative intervention and clarify whether a preoperative improvement of GPS correlates with an improved surgical outcome.

This study has the advantage of involving a large number of patients nationwide. However, there are limitations due to its observational design. While we adjusted for various risk factors for postoperative complications and mortality, there may be residual confounding from factors not included in the model. Certain details such as tumor location, surgery time, intraoperative bleeding, and the extent of lymphadenectomy were not assessed. In addition, the outcomes obtained in this study were influenced by various factors including hospital volume, training status and compliance, surgical specialization, resource utilization, and procedure-specific variables, which may influence the clinical outcomes of the surgical procedures. However, our study highlights the correlation between the GPS and operative morbidity and mortality, and the GPS is expected to be a useful tool to preoperatively predict the short-term outcomes of various gastroenterological surgeries.

In conclusion, we investigated the relationship of GPS with clinical outcomes of several gastroenterological surgical procedures based on data from 312 357 patients obtained from a Japanese nationwide database. This study demonstrated the significant and strong association between GPS and operative morbidity, as well as operative mortality for all surgical procedures investigated. This Japanese nationwide study provides novel evidence that the GPS is a significant risk predictor for short-term outcomes after gastrointestinal surgery.

ACKNOWLEDGEMENTS

The authors thank all the data managers and hospitals for participating in the NCD project and for their great efforts in entering data. They also thank the working members of the Japanese Society of Gastroenterological Surgery data committee (Drs. H Ueno, S Eguchi, T Goi, A Saiura, A Sasaki, S Takiguchi, T Tanaka, M Hashimoto, N Hiki, A Horiguchi, S Marubashi, and H Yamamoto).

DISCLOSURE

Author Contributions: All listed authors have contributed significantly to, and are in agreement with, the content of the manuscript. Each author's contribution is as follows. Study conception and design: Yoshihiro Hiramatsu, Hiroyuki Konno, and Hiroya Takeuchi. Acquisition of data: Yoshihiro Kakeji and Yuko Kitagawa. Analysis and interpretation of data: Yoshihiro Hiramatsu, Hiraku Kumamaru, Hirotoshi Kikuchi, Shiyori Usune, Kinji Kamiya, Hiroaki Miyata and Hiroya Takeuchi. Participation in drafting the article or revising it critically for important intellectual content: All authors. Final approval of the version to be published: All authors.

REFERENCES

1. Scott HR, McMillan DC, Forrest LM, Brown DJF, McArdle CS, Milroy R. The systemic inflammatory response, weight loss, performance status and survival in patients with inoperable non-small cell lung cancer. Br J Cancer. 2002;87(3):264–7.
2. Hilmy M, Bartlett JM, Underwood MA, McNicol A-M, Underwood MA, McMillan DC. The relationship between the systemic inflammatory response and survival in patients with transitional cell carcinoma of the urinary bladder. Br J Cancer. 2005;92(9):625–7.
3. Fearon KC, Voss AC, Hustead DS. Definition of cancer cachexia: effect of weight loss, reduced food intake, and systemic inflammation on functional status and prognosis. Am J Clin Nutr. 2006;83(6):1345–50.
4. O'Gorman P, McMillan DC, McArdle CS. Prognostic factors in advanced gastrointestinal cancer patients with weight loss. Nutr Cancer. 2000;37(1):36–40.
5. McMillan DC, Elahi MM, Sattar N, Angerson WJ, Johnstone J, McArdle CS. Measurement of the systemic inflammatory response predicts cancer-specific and non-cancer survival in patients with cancer. Nutr Cancer. 2001;41(1–2):64–9.
6. Maltoni M, Caraceni A, Brunelli C, Broeckaert B, Christakis N, Eychmueller S, et al. Prognosis factors in advanced cancer patients: evidence-based clinical recommendations – a study by the Steering Committee of the European Association for Palliative Care. J Clin Oncol. 2005;23(25):6240–8.
7. McMillan DC, Watson WS, O'Gorman P, Preston T, Scott HR, McArdle CS. Albumin concentrations are primarily determined by the body cell mass and the systemic inflammatory response in cancer patients with weight loss. Nutr Cancer. 2001;39(2):210–3.
8. Oñate-Ocaña LF, Aeillo-Crocifoglio V, Gallardo-Rincón D, Herrera-Goepfert R, Brom-Valladares R, Carrillo JF, et al. Serum albumin as a significant prognostic factor for patients with gastric carcinoma. Ann Surg Oncol. 2007;14(2):381–9.
9. Muliawati Y, Haroen H, Rotty LW. Cancer anorexia – cachexia syndrome. Acta Med Indones. 2012;44(2):154–62.
10. Cerantola Y, Grass F, Cristaudi A, Demartines N, Schäfer M, Hübner M. Perioperative nutrition in abdominal surgery: recommendations and reality. Gastroenterol Res Pract. 2011;2011:1–8.
11. Forrest LM, McMillan DC, McArdle CS, Angerson WJ, Dunlop DJ. Evaluation of cumulative prognosis scores based on the systemic inflammatory response in patients with inoperative non-small-cell lung cancer. Br J Cancer. 2003;89(6):1028–30.
12. Ishizuka M, Nagata H, Takagi H, Horie T, Kubota K. Inflammation-based prognostic score is a novel predictor of postoperative outcome in patients with colorectal cancer. Ann Surg. 2007;246(6):1047–51.
13. Crumley AB, McMillan DC, McKernan M, McDonald AC, Stuart RC. Evaluation of an inflammation-based prognostic score in patients with inoperable gastro-oesophageal cancer. Br J Cancer. 2006;94(5):637–41.
14. Ramsey S, Lamb GW, Aitchison M, Graham J, McMillan DC. Evaluation of an inflammation-based prognostic score in patients with metastatic renal cancer. Cancer. 2007;109(2):205–12.
15. Murri AMAI, Bartlett JMS, Canney PA, Doughty JC, Wilson C, McMillan DC. Evaluation of an inflammation-based prognostic score (GPS) in patients with metastatic breast cancer. Br J Cancer. 2006;94(2):227–30.
16. Glen P, Jamieson NB, McMillan DC, Carter R, Imrie CW, McKay CJ. Evaluation of an inflammation-based prognostic score in patients with inoperable pancreatic cancer. Pancreatology. 2006;6(5):450–3.
17. Brown DJ, Milroy R, Preston T, McMillan DC. The relationship between an inflammation-based prognostic score (Glasgow Prognostic Score) and changes in serum biochemical variables in patients with advanced lung and gastrointestinal cancer. J Clin Pathol. 2007;60(6):705–8.

18. Kubota T, Hiki N, Nunobe S, Kumagai K, Aikou S, Watanabe R, et al. Significance of the inflammation-based Glasgow Prognostic Score for short- and long-term outcomes after curative resection of gastric cancer. J Gastrointest Surg. 2012;16(11):2037–44.
19. Melling N, Grüning A, Tachezy M, Nentwich M, Reeh M, Uzunoglu FG, et al. Glasgow prognostic score may be a prognostic index for overall and perioperative survival in gastric cancer without perioperative treatment. Surgery. 2016;159(6):1548–56.
20. Inaoka K, Kanda M, Uda H, Tanaka Y, Tanaka C, Kobayashi D, et al. Clinical utility of the platelet-lymphocyte ratio as a predictor of postoperative complications after radical gastrectomy for clinical T2–4 gastric cancer. World J Gastroenterol. 2017;23(14):2519–26.
21. Man W, Lin H, Liu Z, Jin L, Wang J, Zhang J, et al. Usefulness of inflammation-based prognostic score for predicting the risk of complications after radical resection of colorectal carcinoma. Cancer Manag Res. 2020;12:1029–38.
22. Hsueh SW, Liu KH, Hung CY, et al. Significance of the Glasgow Prognostic Score in predicting the postoperative outcome of patients with stage III gastric cancer. J Clin Med. 2019;8(9):1448.
23. Deans DAC, Tan BH, Wigmore SJ, Kuo YC, Tsai CY, Hsu JT, et al. The influence of systemic inflammation, dietary intake and stage of disease of rate of weight loss in patients with gastro-oesophageal cancer. Br J Cancer. 2009;100(1):63–9.
24. Gokel I, Dirksen K, Messow CM, Junginger T. Significance of preoperative C-reactive protein as a parameter of the perioperative course and long-term prognosis in squamous cell carcinoma and adenocarcinoma of the oeshophagus. World J Gastroenterol. 2006;12(23):3746–50.
25. Moyes LH, Leitch EF, McKee RF, Anderson JH, Horgan PG, McMillan DC. Preoperative systemic inflammation predicts postoperative infectious complications in patients undergoing curative resection of colorectal cancer. Br J Cancer. 2009;100(8):1236–9.
26. Winter JM, Cameron JL, Yeo CJ, Alao B, Lillemoe KD, Campbell KA, et al. Biochemical markers predict morbidity and mortality after pancreaticoduodenectomy. J Am Coll Surg. 2007;204(5):1029–36.
27. Kunisaki C, Miyata H, Konno H, Saze Z, Hirahara N, Kikuchi H, et al. Modeling preoperative risk factors for potentially lethal morbidities using a nationwide Japanese web-based database of patients undergoing distal gastrectomy for gastric cancer. Gastric Cancer. 2017;20(3):496–507.
28. Kikuchi H, Miyata H, Konno H, Kamiya K, Tomotaki A, Gotoh M, et al. Development and external validation of preoperative risk models for operative morbidities after total gastrectomy using a Japanese web-based nationwide registry. Gastric Cancer. 2017;20(6):987–97.
29. Aoki S, Miyata H, Konno H, Gotoh M, Motoi F, Kumamaru H, et al. Risk factors of serious postoperative complications after pancreaticoduodenectomy and risk calculators for predicting postoperative complications: a nationwide study of 17,564 patients in Japan. J Hepatobiliary Pancreat Sci. 2017;24(5):243–51.
30. Yoshida T, Miyata H, Konno H, Kumamary H, Tangoku A, Furukita Y, et al. Risk assessment of morbidities after hemicolectomy based on the National Clinical Database in Japan. Ann Gastroenterol Surg. 2018;2(3):220–30.
31. Watanabe T, Miyata H, Konno H, Kawai K, Ishihara S, Sunami E, et al. Prediction model for complications after low anterior resection based on data from 33,411 Japanese patients included in the National Clinical Database. Surgery. 2017;161(6):1597–608.
32. Ohkura Y, Miyata H, Konno H, Udagawa H, Ueno M, Shindoh J, et al. Development of a model predicting the risk of eight major postoperative complications after esophagectomy based on 10 826 cases in the Japan National Clinical Database. J Surg Oncol. 2020;121(2):313–21.
33. Kurita N, Miyata H, Dotoh M, Shimada M, Imura S, Kimura W, et al. Risk model for distal gastrectomy when treating gastric cancer on the basis of data from 33,917 Japanese patients collected using a nationwide web-based data entry system. Ann Surg. 2015;262(2):295–303.
34. Watanabe M, Miyata H, Gotoh M, Baba H, Kimura W, Tomita N, et al. Total gastrectomy risk model: data from 20,011 Japanese patients in a nationwide internet-based database. Ann Surg. 2014;260(6):1034–9.
35. Takeuchi H, Miyata H, Gotoh M, Kitagawa Y, Baba H, Kimura W, et al. A risk model for esophagectomy using data of 5354 patients included in a Japanese nationwide web-based database. Ann Surg. 2014;260(2):259–66.
36. Kimura W, Miyata H, Gotoh M, Hirai I, Kenjo A, Kitagawa Y, et al. A pancreaticoduodenectomy risk model derived from 8575 cases from a nationwide singe-race population (Japanese) using a web-based data entry system: The 30-day and in-hospital mortality rates for pancreaticoduodenectomy. Ann Surg. 2014;259(4):773–80.
37. Matsubara N, Miyata H, Gotoh M, Tomita N, Baba H, Kimura W, et al. Mortality after common rectal surgery in Japan: a study on low anterior resection from a newly established nationwide large-scale clinical database. Dis Colon Rectum. 2014;57(9):1075–81.
38. Kobayashi H, Miyata H, Gotoh M, Baba H, Kimura W, Kitagawa Y, et al. Risk model for right hemicolectomy based on 19,070 Japanese patients in the nationwide clinical database. J Gastroenterol. 2014;49(6):1047–55.
39. Kakeji Y, Takahashi A, Hasegawa H, Ueno H, Eguchi S, Endo I, et al. Surgical outcomes in gastroenterological surgery in Japan: report of the National Clinical Database 2011–2018. Ann Gastroenterol Surg. 2020;4(3):250–74.
40. Meguid RA, Bronsert MR, Juarez-Colunga E, Hammermeister KE, Henderson WG. Surgical risk preoperative assessment system (SURPAS): III. Accurate preoperative prediction of 8 advanced outcomes using 8 predictor variables. Ann Surg. 2016;264(1):23–31.
41. McMillan DC, Crozier JE, Canna K, Angerson WJ, McArdle CS. Evaluation of an inflammation-based prognostic score (GPS) in patients undergoing resection for colon and rectal cancer. Int J Colorectal Dis. 2007;22(8):881–6.
42. Kanaji S, Takahashi A, Miyata H, Marubashi S, Kakeji Y, Konno H, et al. Initial verification of data from a clinical database of gastroenterological surgery in Japan. Surg Today. 2019;49(4):328–33.
43. Dindo D, Demartines N, Clavien PA. Classification of surgical complications: a new proposal with evaluation in a cohort 6336 patients and results of a survey. Ann Surg. 2004;240(2):205–13.
44. Kataoka K, Takeuchi H, Mizusawa ME, Igaki H, Ozawa S, Abe T, et al. Prognostic impact of postoperative morbidity after esophagectomy for esophageal cancer: exploratory analysis of JCOG9907. Ann Surg. 2017;265(6):1152–7.
45. Kawata S, Hiramatsu Y, Takeuchi H, Watanabe K, Nagafusa T, Matsumoto T, et al. Multidisciplinary team management for prevention of pneumonia and long-term weight loss after esophagectomy: a single-center retrospective study. Esophagus. 2020;17(3):270–8.
46. Minnella EM, Awasthi R, Loiselle SE, Agnihotram RV, Ferri LE, Carli F. Effect of exercise and nutrition prehabilitation on functional capacity in esophagogastric cancer surgery: a randomized clinical trial. JAMA Surg. 2018;153(12):1081–9.
47. Deftereos I, Kiss N, Isenring E, Carter VM, Yeung JMC. A systematic review of the effect of preoperative nutrition support on nutritional status and treatment outcomes in upper gastrointestinal cancer resection. Eur J Surg Oncol. 2020;46(8):1423–34.

18

Alteration of prognostic efficacy of albumin-bilirubin grade and Child-Pugh score according to liver fibrosis in hepatocellular carcinoma patients with Child-Pugh A following hepatectomy

Tatsunori Miyata[1] | Yo-ichi Yamashita[1] | Kota Arima[1] | Takaaki Higashi[1] | Hiromitsu Hayashi[1] | Katsunori Imai[1] | Hidetoshi Nitta[2] | Akira Chikamoto[1] | Toru Beppu[1,3] | Hideo Baba[1]

[1]Department of Gastroenterological Surgery, Graduate School of Life Sciences, Kumamoto University, Kumamoto, Japan

[2]Department of Surgery, Saiseikai Kumamoto Hospital, Kumamoto, Japan

[3]Department of Surgery, Yamaga City Medical Center, Kumamoto, Japan

Correspondence
Hideo Baba, Department of Gastroenterological Surgery, Graduate School of Life Sciences, Kumamoto University, 1-1-1 Honjo, Chuo-ku, Kumamoto 860-0811, Kumamoto, Japan.
Email: hdobaba@kumamoto-u.ac.jp

Abstract

Background: The albumin-bilirubin (ALBI) grade was developed to predict the prognosis of patients with hepatocellular carcinoma (HCC), which can stratify the prognosis even in HCC patients with Child-Pugh A. We evaluated the prognostic efficacy of the ALBI grade and Child-Pugh classification in HCC patients with Child-Pugh A stratified by the presence or absence of advanced fibrosis or a preoperative biomarker for advanced fibrosis.

Methods: We retrospectively analyzed 490 consecutive HCC patients with Child-Pugh A who underwent initial hepatectomies. The accuracy of prognostic prediction using both models was compared by the presence or absence of advanced fibrosis (F3-4) and its predictor, the preoperative platelet count (PLT).

Results: The prognostic accuracy of the ALBI grade was better in patients without advanced fibrosis (F3-4; likelihood ratio: 4.39, corrected Akaike information criterion [AICc]: 453.0, $P = .074$), but Child-Pugh score was better in the advanced fibrosis group (likelihood ratio: 10.67, AICc: 915.2, $P = .0014$). In the high PLT group ($\geq 140 \times 10^3/\mu L$), the prognostic accuracy using the ALBI grade was better in overall survival (OS) and relapse-free survival (RFS), but in the low PLT group, the Child-Pugh score was the more accurate model in OS and RFS.

Conclusions: Depending on the degree of fibrosis or preoperative PLT, the ALBI grade and Child-Pugh score may provide more accurate prognoses after initial hepatectomy in HCC patients with Child-Pugh A.

KEYWORDS
advanced fibrosis, Child-Pugh score, HCC, prognosis, The ALBI grade

1 | INTRODUCTION

Hepatocellular carcinoma (HCC), which comprises approximately 90% of liver cancers, is the fourth-leading deadly cancer worldwide.[1] Hepatectomy is obviously the most effective treatment to achieve a cure in selected HCC cases; however, 70% of cases have recurrence within 5 years after hepatectomy.[2,3] Many studies have demonstrated that repeat hepatectomy for recurrent HCC is a promising therapeutic strategy to improve a patient's prognosis.[4] For initial and repeat hepatectomy, preoperative liver function is an essential factor to determine an indication of hepatectomy or resectable liver volume for HCC, to allow safe hepatectomy without postoperative complications, including death.[2,5]

The Child-Pugh classification is one of the most common assessment models for liver function in decision-making processes for the treatment of HCC worldwide. It was originally developed to evaluate prognoses in patients with portal hypertension and cirrhosis following treatment for variceal bleeding.[6,7] Because of this background, most patients who were considered for hepatectomy were categorized by Child-Pugh A; however, it includes a wide range of liver function so that the Child-Pugh classification does not always correctly reflect the prognosis after hepatectomy.[8-10] Because of these issues, the albumin-bilirubin (ALBI) grade was developed in 2015, and its prognostic value was validated using several large international cohorts with HCC.[8,11-13] Even in HCC patients with Child-Pugh A following hepatectomy, the ALBI grade stratified patient prognoses.[8,13,14] Therefore, the ALBI grade might be a better assessment model for predicting a prognosis than the Child-Pugh classification.[12]

However, given the history of the development of the Child-Pugh classification,[6,7] it might be appropriate for assessing cirrhosis or advanced fibrosis, but not for assessing the prognosis after hepatectomy in HCC patients with relatively mild fibrosis.

We hypothesized that the prognostic accuracy of the ALBI grade and Child-Pugh score would be different in patients with or without advanced fibrosis. In addition, we thought that it would be useful in clinical practice to use both models to predict prognosis according to the biomarkers of fibrosis before hepatectomy. The aim of this study was to investigate the prognostic accuracy of the ALBI grade and Child-Pugh score depending on the presence or absence of advanced fibrosis, or its biomarker in HCC patients with Child-Pugh A following hepatectomy.

2 | PATIENTS AND METHODS

2.1 | Patients

Between January 2000 and December 2015, 531 consecutive patients underwent initial and curative hepatectomy for HCC at the Department of Gastroenterological Surgery, Kumamoto University, Kumamoto, Japan. Of these patients, we excluded patients with Child-Pugh B ($n = 18$) and those with unavailable pathological fibrosis data ($n = 23$). Finally, 490 patients were enrolled in this study. The pathologists histologically confirmed all tumors as HCC. Written informed consent was obtained from all patients before treatment. This study was approved by the Human Ethics Review Committee of the Graduate School of Medicine, Kumamoto University, Kumamoto, Japan.

2.2 | Surgical indications and procedures

Each hepatectomy was performed based on the tumor location, extent of the tumor invasion, parenchymal liver function, and the patient's general condition, as described previously.[15] Before hepatectomy, patients underwent liver function tests, including bilirubin, albumin, prothrombin time, and indocyanine green retention rate at 15 minutes. Major hepatectomy was defined as resection of three or more liver segments.

2.3 | Data collection and patient follow-up

Preoperative data were collected within 1 month before each hepatectomy. The ALBI grade formula is as follows: ALBI grade = 0.669 $\log_{10}$ (total bilirubin [μmol/L]) − 0.085 (albumin [g/L]). The ALBI grade is stratified as grade 1 (−2.60 or less), grade 2 (−2.59 to −1.39), and grade 3 (greater than −1.39).[8] Tumor stage was assessed according to the 8th edition of the AJCC staging system.[16] All patients were followed up with a physical examination, determination of α-fetoprotein (AFP) and des-γ-carboxyprothrombin (DCP) levels, and an imaging examination every 3 months for 2 years after hepatectomies, and every half a year thereafter. Recurrence was defined as the appearance of a lesion with radiological features typical of HCC. If recurrence was detected, the patient underwent additional treatments with hepatectomy, local ablation therapy, or transarterial chemoembolization according to recurrence patterns, their general condition, and remnant liver functions. Overall survival (OS) was defined from hepatectomy to death or last follow-up. Relapse-free survival (RFS) was defined from hepatectomy to recurrence, death, or last follow-up. The patients were followed until death or December 31, 2019. Postoperative complications were classified by the Clavien-Dindo Classification (CD)[17]; we defined CD IIIa or more as a postoperative complication.

2.4 | Histological assessments

We utilized the New Inuyama Classification[18] to evaluate histological liver fibrosis. The fibrosis severity (F score) was classified into five subgroups: F0 (no fibrosis); F1 (mild fibrosis), fibrous portal expansion; F2 (moderate fibrosis), bridging fibrosis; F3 (severe fibrosis), bridging fibrosis with distorted acinar architecture; and F4, cirrhosis. All resected specimens were evaluated by pathologists who were blinded to the outcome of patients with HCC. We defined F3 and F4 as advanced fibrosis. If each case was diagnosed as intermediate between each category, it was classified as a severe category (e.g. F4 for F3-4).

2.5 | Statistical analysis

Continuous variables were presented as medians (interquartile ranges [IQRs]). Survival outcome was estimated using the Kaplan-Meier method and compared using the generalized Wilcoxon test. To assess interactions among the preoperative factors, the ALBI grade and Child-Pugh score were cross-correlated with another variable of interest via an univariable Cox proportional hazard model, and the interaction was evaluated using the Wald test. We compared the prognostic accuracy of the ALBI grade and Child-Pugh score by assessing their homogeneity (likelihood ratio chi square values, related to the generalized Wilcoxon test) and discriminatory ability (corrected Akaike information criterion [AICc], related to univariate Cox analyses). More accurate models showed higher likelihood ratio chi square values and lower AICc values. The platelet count threshold was calculated using a receiver operating characteristic (ROC) curve for advanced fibrosis (F3-4). All results with two-tailed values of $P < .05$ were considered statistically significant. All statistical analyses were performed using JMP software (Version 12; SAS Institute).

3 | RESULTS

3.1 | Patient characteristics

Among 490 HCC patients with Child-Pugh A, the median age was 67 years, and 382 were men (77.8%). Eighty-two patients had Child-Pugh scores of 6 (16.7%), and 195 patients were ALBI grade 2 (39.9%). There were no patients with ALBI grade 3 in this cohort. The numbers of patients classified by the ALBI grade and Child-Pugh score are shown in Table S1. Histological assessment showed 277 patients (56.5%) had advanced fibrosis (F3-4). The other perioperative factors and tumor-related factors are shown in Table 1. In particular, in the association between tumor-related factors, which have been reported to be associated with prognosis, and the ALBI grade and Child-Pugh score, AFP was higher in patients with ALBI grade 2 than those with grade 1 ($P = .0029$). On the other hand, there was no significant difference in Child-Pugh score (Table S2). The median observation period in this cohort was 8.8 years. During the follow-up of 490 patients, there were 269 recurrences (54.9%) and 144 deaths (29.4%), and the 5-year OS rate was 73.5%.

TABLE 1 The characteristics of this cohort

Variables	All (n = 490)
Clinical factors	
Age (years)	67 (61-74)
Male	382 (77.8%)
HBs-Ag positive	128 (26.1%)
HCV-Ab positive	236 (48.2%)
Total bilirubin (mg/dL)	0.8 (0.6-1.0)
Albumin (g/dL)	4.0 (3.7-4.3)
Prothrombin time (%)	95 (86-104)
Platelet count ($\times 10^3/\mu L$)[a]	146 (112-190)
Child-Pugh score 6	82 (16.7%)
ALBI grade 2	195 (39.9%)
ICG R15 (%)	11.7 (7.8-16.8)
AFP (ng/mL)	12.8 (4.8-149)
DCP (mU/mL)	86 (24-785)
Perioperative factors	
Major hepatectomy	135 (27.6%)
Anatomical resection	351 (71.6%)
Blood loss (ml)	395 (180-726)
Blood transfusion	64 (13.1%)
Operating time (min)	396 (324-476)
Postoperative complication (CD ≥ III)	90 (18.4%)
Tumor-related factors	
Tumor size > 5 (34)	127 (25.9%)
Multiple tumors	139 (28.4%)
Microvascular invasion	181 (36.9%)
Poorly differentiation[b]	100 (20.7%)
Advanced fibrosis (F3-4)	277 (56.5%)
AJCC Stage I/II/III	239/194/57

Abbreviations: AFP, alpha-fetoprotein; ALBI, albumin-bilirubin; CD, Clavian-Dindo classification; DCP, des-gamma-carboxy prothrombin; HBs-Ag, hepatitis B surface antigen; HCV-Ab, hepatitis C virus antibody; ICG R15, indocyanine green retention rate at 15 min.
[a]Five patients' data were unavailable. [b]Seven patients' data were unavailable.

3.2 | The prognosis according to the ALBI grade and Child-Pugh score

As many studies have already demonstrated,[8] in this study, the ALBI grade stratified the prognosis in HCC patients with Child-Pugh A in OS ($P = .0003$; Figure S1A). The Child-Pugh score (5 or 6) also stratified the prognosis in OS ($P < .0001$; Figure S1B). In addition, the subgroup analysis showed that the ALBI grade and Child-Pugh score were significant prognostic factors in OS, but each preoperative factor did not modify the risk in OS in both models (Figure S2). For RFS, as well as OS, the ALBI grade ($P = .0018$) and the Child-Pugh score ($P = .0039$) also stratified the prognosis in HCC patients with Child-Pugh A (Figure S1C,D).

3.3 | The ALBI grade in patients with Child-Pugh score 5

Next, we examined whether the ALBI grade could stratify patients with the most favorable liver function, classified as Child-Pugh score 5 (n = 408). Patient characteristics related to liver function (total bilirubin, albumin, prothrombin) were significantly worse in the ALBI grade 2 group (n = 122) than in the ALBI grade 1 group (n = 286). In addition, in the ALBI grade 2 group, the platelet count was lower ($135 \times 10^3/\mu L$ vs $157 \times 10^3/\mu L$, $P = .021$), the AFP level was higher (17.2 ng/mL vs 10.2 ng/mL, $P = .018$), the rates of anatomical resection were lower (64.8% vs 76.6%, $P = .018$), and advanced fibrosis was higher (63.1% vs 49.0%, $P = .018$) than those in the ALBI grade 1 group (Table 2). However, there was no significant difference in OS ($P = .074$) and RFS ($P = .076$) between the two groups (Figure S3A,B). Median survival time in the grade 1 and grade 2 groups was 11.0 and 8.4 years in OS, 3.6 and 1.9 years in RFS, respectively.

3.4 | Preoperative prognostic efficacy of the ALBI grade and Child-Pugh score according to the presence or absence of advanced fibrosis

Next, to evaluate our hypotheses that the ALBI grade was a more suitable model to predict prognosis in patients with a moderate or low degree of fibrosis (F0-2), we compared the prognostic accuracy of both models according to the presence or absence of advanced fibrosis (F3-4).

In the F0-2 group (n = 213), the numbers of patients classified into worsened categories by the ALBI grade and Child-Pugh score were 64 (30.0%) and 22 (10.3%), respectively. The homogeneity

TABLE 2 The clinicopathological characteristics, tumor-related factors, and perioperative factors of patients with Child-Pugh score 5 (n = 408) according to the ALBI grade

	ALBI		
Variables	**Grade 1 (n = 286)**	**Grade 2 (n = 122)**	***P***
Clinical factors			
Age (y)	7.5 (61-74)	67.0 (59-74)	.52
Male	228 (79.7%)	88 (72.1%)	.12
HBs-Ag positive	74 (25.9%)	35 (28.7%)	.63
HCV-Ab positive	125 (43.7%)	61 (50.0%)	.28
Total bilirubin (mg/dL)	0.7 (0.6-0.9)	0.9 (0.7-1.1)	<.0001
Albumin (g/dL)	4.3 (4.1-4.5)	3.7 (3.7-3.9)	<.0001
Prothrombin time (%)	99 (91-106)	83 (91-98)	<.0001
Platelet count ($\times 10^3/\mu L$)[a]	157 (123-193)	135 (107-179)	**.021**
ICG R15 (%)	10.3 (6.8-13.7)	14.7 (9.2-21.0)	<.0001
AFP (ng/mL)	10.2 (4.0-144)	17.2 (7.0-149)	**.018**
DCP (mU/mL)	75 (23-584)	109 (24-1169)	.52
Perioperative factors			
Major hepatectomy	83 (29.0%)	35 (28.7%)	1.0
Anatomical resection	219 (76.6%)	79 (64.8%)	**.015**
Blood loss (mL)	380 (173-736)	381 (180-674)	.79
Blood transfusion	26 (9.1%)	16 (13.1%)	.29
Operating time (min)	399 (327-467)	397 (311-466)	.61
Postoperative complication (CD ≥ III)	51 (17.8%)	18 (14.8%)	.48
Tumor-related factors			
Tumor size > 5 (cm)	78 (27.3%)	27 (22.1%)	.32
Multiple tumors	79 (27.6%)	37 (30.3%)	.63
Microvascular invasion	115 (40.2%)	38 (31.2%)	.094
Poorly differentiation[b]	60 (21.1%)	21 (17.4%)	.42
Advanced fibrosis (F3-4)	140 (49.0%)	77 (63.1%)	**.0094**
AJCC Stage I/II/III	136/114/36	63/47/12	.64

Abbreviations: AFP, alpha-fetoprotein; ALBI, albumin-bilirubin; DCP, des-gamma-carboxy prothrombin; HBs-Ag, hepatitis B surface antigen; HCV-Ab, hepatitis C virus antibody; ICG R15, indocyanine green retention rate at 15 min.

[a]Five patients' data were unavailable. [b]Three patients' data were unavailable.

(likelihood ratio) and discriminatory ability (AICc) of the ALBI grade were better than those of the Child-Pugh score (likelihood ratio: 4.39 [P = .036] vs 4.19 [P = .041], AICc: 453.0 [P = .074] vs 453.8 [P = .13], ALBI vs Child-Pugh score; Figure 1A,B).

Next, in the F3-4 group (n = 277), the numbers of patients classified into worsened categories by each biomarker were 131 (47.3%) by the ALBI grade and 60 (21.7%) by Child-Pugh score. Contrary to the F0-2 group, the likelihood ratio and AICc of Child-Pugh score were better than those of the ALBI grade (likelihood ratio: 5.91 [P = .015] vs 10.67 [P = .0005], AICc: 918.4 [P = .0083] vs 915.2 [P = .0014], ALBI vs Child-Pugh score; Figure 1C,D). Thus, the prognostic accuracy between the ALBI grade and Child-Pugh score may depend on the presence of advanced fibrosis.

3.5 | The platelet count level was associated with fibrosis

Next, we evaluated how to apply the characteristics of these two models in clinical practice because they are important to evaluate liver function and prognosis in decision-making processes for treatment strategies. Accumulating evidence has demonstrated that liver fibrosis is associated with the platelet count.[19,20] Therefore, we decided to use the preoperative platelet count (PLT) as a biomarker for advanced fibrosis. In the context of the threshold, ROC curve analysis showed 140 × $10^3/\mu L$ was the best to predict advanced fibrosis (AUC: 0.744, P < .0001, sensitivity: 65.6%, specificity: 88.3%; Figure S4). Using this threshold, patients were categorized into two groups: those with high PLT (n = 263, 54.2%) or low PLT (n = 222, 45.8%).

3.6 | Preoperative prognostic efficacy of the ALBI grade and Child-Pugh classification according to the preoperative platelet count level

For the OS, in the high PLT group (PLT ≥ 140 × $10^3/\mu L$), the numbers of patients classified into worsened categories by the ALBI grade and Child-Pugh score were 83 (31.6%) and 31 (11.8%), respectively. The likelihood ratio and AICc of the ALBI grade were better than those of the Child-Pugh score (likelihood ratio: 4.53 [P = .033] vs 2.36 [P = .12], AICc: 585.3 [P = .041] vs 588.2 [P = .26], ALBI vs Child-Pugh score; Figure 2A,B). In the low PLT group (PLT < 140 × $10^3/\mu L$), the numbers of patients classified into worsened categories by the ALBI grade and Child-Pugh score were 109 (49.1%) and 51 (23.0%), respectively. The likelihood ratio and AICc of the Child-Pugh score were better than those of the ALBI grade (likelihood ratio: 4.99 [P = .026] vs 13.15 [P = .0003], AICc: 747.8 [P = .067] vs 738.0 [P = .0003], ALBI vs Child-Pugh score; Figure 2C,D).

For RFS, as with the OS, the likelihood ratio for the ALBI grade and AICc were better than those for Child-Pugh score in the high PLT group (likelihood ratio: 10.3 [P = .013] vs 5.05 [P = .025]; AICc: 1386.0 [P = .0003] vs 1395.5 [P = .065], ALBI versus Child-Pugh score; Figure S5A,B). In the low PLT group, the likelihood ratio and AICc of the Child-Pugh score were better than those of the ALBI grade, although not significantly different in each model (likelihood ratio: 0.45 [P = .50] vs 1.96 [P = .16]; AICc: 1331.8 [P = .55] vs 1329.4 [P = .093], ALBI vs Child-Pugh score; Figure S5C,D). Thus, the ALBI grade and Child-Pugh score may have different prognostic accuracy depending on the preoperative PLT.

4 | DISCUSSION

To the best of our knowledge, this is the first study to assess the prognostic accuracy of the ALBI grade and Child-Pugh score in HCC patients with Child-Pugh A following hepatectomy depending on the presence of advanced fibrosis. Our data suggested that the preoperative prognostic efficacy of the ALBI grade and Child-Pugh score varied depending on the presence of advanced fibrosis (F3-4). In addition, considering the clinical application of the results of this analysis, we also demonstrated that it might be important to use the models differently depending on the preoperative PLT. Taken together, our results suggested the prognostic value of both models might be affected depending on the status of liver fibrosis.

In this study, we found that the ALBI grade had better prognostic efficacy than the Child-Pugh score in HCC patients without advanced fibrosis (F0-2) or with a PLT ≥ 140 × $10^3/\mu L$ (Figures 2 and 3). This indicated that for patients with preserved liver function, the Child-Pugh score was not able to determine a liver injury, whereas the ALBI grade may be able to identify such liver dysfunction. This may be due to the wide range of changes in each parameter that affects the Child-Pugh score. In addition, Child-Pugh includes subjective evaluations. In this study, both OS and RFS could not be stratified by the ALBI grade in patients with Child-Pugh score 5 (Figure S3); however, in view of the survival curve, it seems necessary to increase the number of patients to verify the results. The ALBI grade might detect patients with relatively low liver function and even those with a Child-Pugh score of 5 (Table 2), suggesting it may be able to predict patients' prognoses.

Of note, the ALBI grade was not always better than the Child-Pugh score. In patients with advanced fibrosis or a PLT < 140 × $10^3/\mu L$, Child-Pugh score had a better prognostic efficacy after hepatectomy than the ALBI grade. Interestingly, the differences in homogeneity and discriminatory ability between the ALBI grade and Child-Pugh score in patients with advanced fibrosis or a PLT < 140 × $10^3/\mu L$ were more obvious than in patients without advance fibrosis (F0-2) or with a PLT ≥ 140 × $10^3/\mu L$. This suggested that the Child-Pugh score more accurately sorted patients with a poor prognosis than the ALBI grade in patients with advanced fibrosis. This may be due to the large value range of each parameter leading to an altered Child-Pugh score, which may increase the sensitivity of the Child-Pugh score as well as the specificity as fibrosis progresses. Taken together, the ALBI grade may identify prognostic hepatic dysfunction earlier, but as fibrosis progresses, Child-Pugh

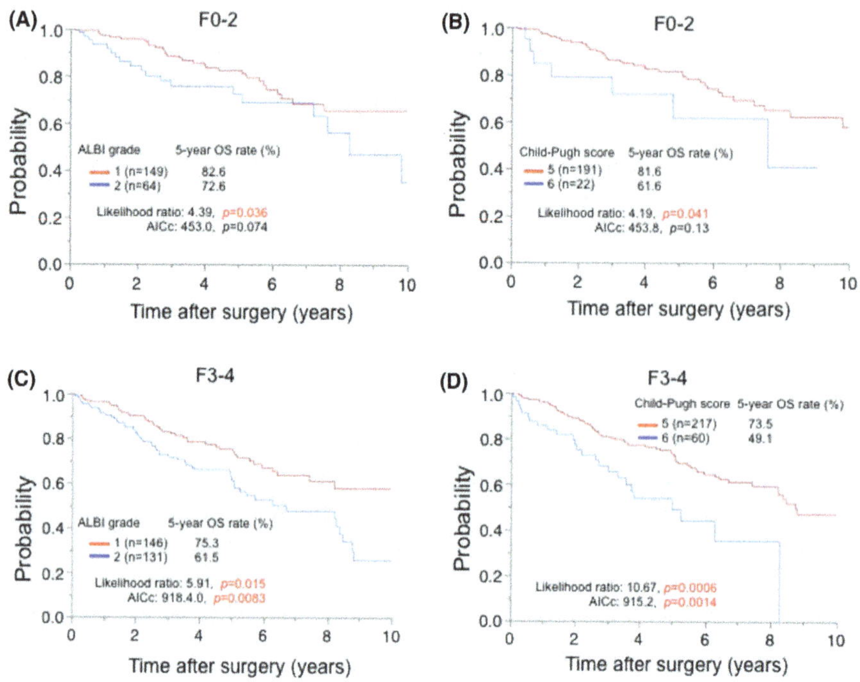

FIGURE 1 The ALBI grade and the Child-Pugh score stratified overall survival both in HCC patients with F0-2 and F3-4. The prognostic efficacy of the ALBI grade was better in patients with F0-2 (n = 213) (A, B), whereas that of the Child-Pugh score was more accurate in those with F3-4 (n = 277) (C, D). ALBI, albumin-bilirubin; AICc, Corrected Akaike information criterion; OS, overall survival

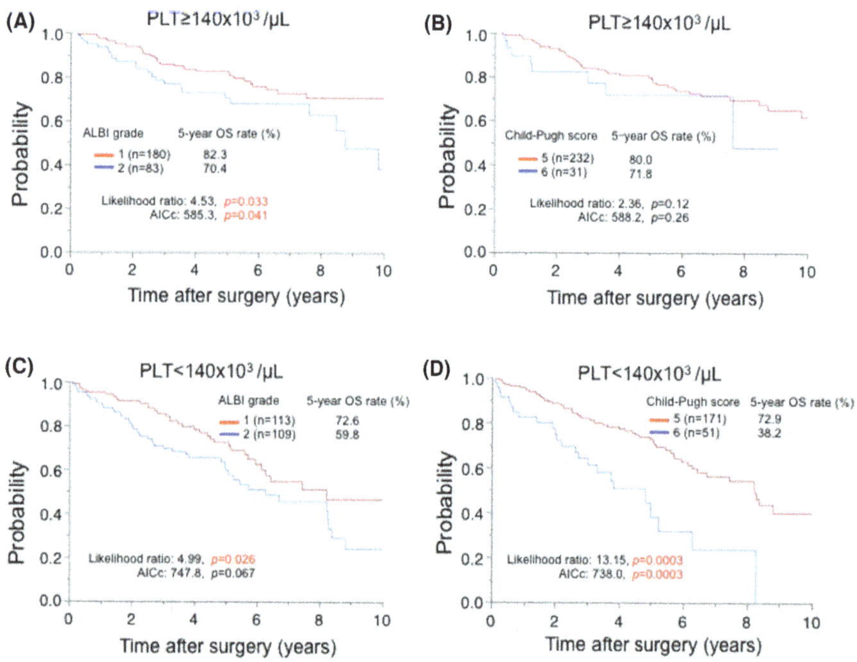

FIGURE 2 The different prognostic efficacy of the ALBI grade and the Child-Pugh score was shown according to the platelet count (PLT). The prognostic efficacy of the ALBI grade was better in patients with PLT ≥ 140 x 10^3/μL (n = 263) (A, B), whereas that of the Child-Pugh score was better in those with PLT < 140 x 10^3/μL (n = 222) (C, D). Five patients' data were unavailable. ALBI, albumin-bilirubin; AICc, Corrected Akaike information criterion; OS, overall survival

score may identify more prognostic hepatic dysfunction in patients with Child-Pugh A (Figure 3).

Our results also demonstrated that the ALBI grade identified patients with liver disorders that were not detected by the Child-Pugh score (Table 2). Indeed, only six patients (11.0%) were ALBI grade 1 in patients with a Child-Pugh score of 6. However, of patients with a Child-Pugh score of 5, 70.1% were classified as ALBI grade 1 (Table S1), suggesting a Child-Pugh score of 5 and 6 indicated a different category of liver function when compared with the ALBI grade even though they are in the same category in Child-Pugh classification. In addition, the ALBI grade could stratify HCC patients with a Child-Pugh score of 5 in the assessment of liver function and fibrosis (Table 2). Thus, HCC patients with Child-Pugh A themselves were a heterogeneous group that included a variety of liver functions.

This study also showed that the patients with the ALBI grade 2 displayed higher levels of AFP than those with ALBI grade 1, but this difference was not seen in the Child-Pugh score (Table S2). Meanwhile, contrary to our result, the two previous studies demonstrated that AFP was not significantly different according to the ALBI grade in patients with Child-Pugh A.[21,22] Thus, most tumor-related factors may be independent of the ALBI grade and Child-Pugh score; however, to conclude, the association between the ALBI grade and

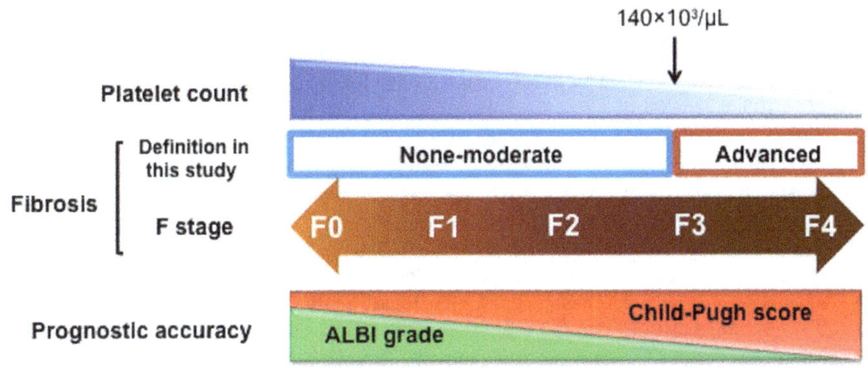

FIGURE 3 The platelet count, a biomarker of fibrosis, may make a difference in the prognostic accuracy of the ALBI grade and the Child-Pugh classification. ALBI, albumin-bilirubin

AFP seems to be difficult now because the number of patients was not enough.

Liver biopsy is the gold standard for diagnosing fibrosis, but it is not performed routinely to evaluate fibrosis because of its notable risks.[23] In this study, we applied PLT as a non-invasive biomarker to identify advanced fibrosis.[20,24] Udell et al[20] demonstrated a PLT of $160 \times 10^3/\mu L$ was the most accurate threshold to distinguish cirrhosis with a sensitivity of 0.74 and a specificity of 0.88. Bashour et al[24] also demonstrated that patients with cirrhosis or advanced fibrosis had a mean platelet level of $144.6 \times 10^3/\mu L$. Compared with previous studies, our cohort included more patients with hepatitis B or C virus (n = 364, 72.3%), which might have had an impact on the lower PLT.[25] Therefore, our threshold of PLT $140 \times 10^3/\mu L$ for advanced fibrosis might be reasonable. Recently, useful serum biomarkers for fibrosis have been identified including the fibrosis-4 (FIB-4) index, the aspartate transaminase to platelet ratio index (APRI), and the Mac-2 binding protein glycosylation isomer.[23,26,27] Imaging tests can also predict fibrosis.[28] We were unable to examine patients using these interesting serum or imaging biomarkers; however, the application of them may better reflect our proposed concept of using different biomarkers to assess key liver functions depending on the degree of fibrosis.

This study had several limitations. First, this study was retrospective in design. Second, we did not have enough data on preoperative blood test data such as AST and ALT, preoperative diagnostic imaging for liver fibrosis, the therapies used to treat hepatitis or recurrent HCC, and causes of death. Third, we applied the New Inuyama Classification for the histological evaluation of fibrosis, which was not a common tool worldwide. However, this study was performed in a single institution without bias of surgical procedure with 490 patients with HCC. Therefore, our results might have an important impact on clinical practice.

In conclusion, the ALBI grade and Child-Pugh score were useful prognosis prediction biomarkers for HCC patients following curative hepatectomy. It may be necessary to use each assessment model while taking into account the level of PLT or degree of fibrosis. Further studies using large-scale cohorts are needed to validate our findings.

ACKNOWLEDGEMENTS

We thank the Wordvice for editing a draft this manuscript.

DISCLOSURE

Ethical Statement: Written informed consent was obtained from all patients before treatment. This study was approved by the Human Ethics Review Committee of the Graduate School of Medicine, Kumamoto University, Kumamoto, Japan.

REFERENCES

1. Bray F, Ferlay J, Soerjomataram I, Siegel RL, Torre LA, Jemal A. Global cancer statistics 2018: GLOBOCAN estimates of incidence and mortality worldwide for 36 cancers in 185 countries. CA Cancer J Clin. 2018;68(6):394–424.
2. El-Serag HB. Hepatocellular carcinoma. N Engl J Med. 2011;365(12):1118–27.
3. Hasegawa K, Kokudo N, Makuuchi M, Izumi N, Ichida T, Kudo M, et al. Comparison of resection and ablation for hepatocellular carcinoma: a cohort study based on a Japanese nationwide survey. J Hepatol. 2013;58(4):724–9.
4. Roayaie S, Bassi D, Tarchi P, Labow D, Schwartz M. Second hepatic resection for recurrent hepatocellular cancer: a Western experience. J Hepatol. 2011;55(2):346–50.
5. EORTC. EASL Clinical Practice Guidelines: management of hepatocellular carcinoma. J Hepatol. 2012;56(4):908–43.
6. Pugh RN, Murray-Lyon IM, Dawson JL, Pietroni MC, Williams R. Transection of the oesophagus for bleeding oesophageal varices. Br J Surg. 1973;60(8):646–9.
7. Kok B, Abraldes JG. Child-pugh classification: time to abandon? Semin Liver Dis. 2019;39(1):96–103.
8. Johnson PJ, Berhane S, Kagebayashi C, Satomura S, Teng M, Reeves HL, et al. Assessment of liver function in patients with hepatocellular carcinoma: a new evidence-based approach-the ALBI grade. J Clin Oncol. 2015;33(6):550–8.
9. The Cancer of the Liver Italian Program (Clip) Investigators. A new prognostic system for hepatocellular carcinoma: a retrospective study of 435 patients: the Cancer of the Liver Italian Program (CLIP) investigators. Hepatology. 1998;28(3):751–5.
10. Kokudo N, Hasegawa K, Akahane M, Igaki H, Izumi N, Ichida T, et al. Evidence-based Clinical Practice Guidelines for Hepatocellular Carcinoma: The Japan Society of Hepatology 2013 update (3rd JSH-HCC Guidelines). Hepatology Research. 2015;45(2).
11. Hiraoka A, Kumada T, Kudo M, Hirooka M, Tsuji K, Itobayashi E, et al. Albumin-Bilirubin (ALBI) Grade as Part of the Evidence-Based Clinical Practice Guideline for HCC of the Japan Society of Hepatology: a comparison with the liver damage and Child-Pugh classifications. Liver Cancer. 2017;6(3):204–15.
12. Peng Y, Wei Q, He Y, Xie Q, Liang Y, Zhang L, et al. ALBI versus child-pugh in predicting outcome of patients with HCC: A systematic review. Expert Rev Gastroenterol Hepatol. 2020;14(5):383–400.

13. Wang YY, Zhong JH, Su ZY, Huang JF, Lu SD, Xiang BD, et al. Albumin-bilirubin versus Child-Pugh score as a predictor of outcome after liver resection for hepatocellular carcinoma. Br J Surg. 2016;103(6):725–34.
14. Zhao S, Wang M, Yang Z, Tan K, Zheng D, Du X, et al. Comparison between Child-Pugh score and Albumin-Bilirubin grade in the prognosis of patients with HCC after liver resection using time-dependent ROC. Ann Transl Med. 2020;8(8):539.
15. Beppu T, Ishiko T, Chikamoto A, Komori H, Masuda T, Hayashi H, et al. Liver hanging maneuver decreases blood loss and operative time in a right-side hepatectomy. Hepatogastroenterology. 2012;59(114):542–5.
16. Amin MB, Greene FL, Edge SB, Compton CC, Gershenwald JE, Brookland RK, et al. The Eighth Edition AJCC Cancer Staging Manual: Continuing to build a bridge from a population-based to a more "personalized" approach to cancer staging. CA Cancer J Clin. 2017;67(2):93–9.
17. Dindo D, Demartines N, Clavien PA. Classification of surgical complications: a new proposal with evaluation in a cohort of 6336 patients and results of a survey. Ann Surg. 2004;240(2):205–13.
18. Ichida F, Tsuji T, Omata M, Ichida T, Inoue K, Kamimura T, et al. New Inuyama classification; new criteria for histological assessment of chronic hepatitis. Int Hepatol Commun. 1996;6(2):112–9.
19. Afdhal N, McHutchison J, Brown R, Jacobson I, Manns M, Poordad F, et al. Thrombocytopenia associated with chronic liver disease. J Hepatol. 2008;48(6):1000–7.
20. Udell JA, Wang CS, Tinmouth J, FitzGerald JM, Ayas NT, Simel DL, et al. Does this patient with liver disease have cirrhosis? JAMA. 2012;307(8):832–42.
21. Amisaki M, Uchinaka E, Morimoto M, Tokuyasu N, Sakamoto T, Honjo S, et al. Post-operative albumin-bilirubin grade predicts long-term outcomes among Child-Pugh grade A patients with hepatocellular carcinoma after curative resection. Hepatobiliary Pancreat Dis Int. 2018;17(6):502–9.
22. Sonohara F, Yamada S, Tanaka N, Suenaga M, Takami H, Hayashi M, et al. Perioperative and prognostic implication of albumin-bilirubin-TNM score in Child-Pugh class A hepatocellular carcinoma. Ann Gastroenterol Surg. 2019;3(1):65–74.
23. Agbim U, Asrani SK. Non-invasive assessment of liver fibrosis and prognosis: an update on serum and elastography markers. Expert Rev Gastroenterol Hepatol. 2019;13(4):361–74.
24. Bashour FN, Teran JC, Mullen KD. Prevalence of peripheral blood cytopenias (hypersplenism) in patients with nonalcoholic chronic liver disease. Am J Gastroenterol. 2000;95(10):2936–9.
25. Tejima K, Masuzaki R, Ikeda H, Yoshida H, Tateishi R, Sugioka Y, et al. Thrombocytopenia is more severe in patients with advanced chronic hepatitis C than B with the same grade of liver stiffness and splenomegaly. J Gastroenterol. 2010;45(8):876–84.
26. Nishikawa H, Enomoto H, Yoh K, Iwata Y, Sakai Y, Kishino K, et al. Combined albumin-bilirubin grade and Mac-2 binding protein glycosylation isomer as a useful predictor in compensated liver cirrhosis. Medicine. 2019;98(50):e18366.
27. Toshima T, Shirabe K, Ikegami T, Yoshizumi T, Kuno A, Togayachi A, et al. A novel serum marker, glycosylated Wisteria floribunda agglutinin-positive Mac-2 binding protein (WFA(+)-M2BP), for assessing liver fibrosis. J Gastroenterol. 2015;50(1):76–84.
28. Xiao G, Zhu S, Xiao X, Yan L, Yang J, Wu G. Comparison of laboratory tests, ultrasound, or magnetic resonance elastography to detect fibrosis in patients with nonalcoholic fatty liver disease: a meta-analysis. Hepatology. 2017;66(5):1486–501.

19

The influence and countermeasure of obesity in laparoscopic colorectal resection

Hideya Kashihara | Mitsuo Shimada | Kozo Yoshikawa | Jun Higashijima | Takuya Tokunaga | Masaki Nishi | Chie Takasu | Toshiaki Yoshimoto

Department of Surgery, Tokushima University, Tokushima, Japan

Correspondence
Hideya Kashihara, Department of Surgery, Tokushima University, 3-18-15 Kuramoto-cho, Tokushima 770-8503, Japan.
Email: kashihara.hideya@tokushima-u.ac.jp

Abstract

Background: The aim of this study was to investigate the influence of obesity and the usefulness of a preoperative weight loss program (PWLP) for obese patients undergoing laparoscopic colorectal resection (LCR).

Methods: Study 1: 392 patients who underwent LCR for colorectal cancer were divided into two groups: those with a body mass index (BMI) ≥25 kg/m^2 (n = 113) and those with a BMI <25 kg/m^2 (n = 279). The influence of BMI on LCR was investigated. Study 2: Patients with a BMI ≥28 kg/m^2 who were scheduled to undergo LCR (n = 7, mean body weight 87.0 kg, mean BMI 33.9 kg/m^2) undertook a PWLP including caloric restriction and exercise for 29.6 (15–70) days. The effects of this program were evaluated.

Results: Study 1: The BMI ≥25 kg/m^2 group had a prolongation of operation time and hospital stay than the BMI <25 kg/m^2 group. Study 2: The patients achieved a mean weight loss of 6.9% (−6.0 kg). The mean visceral fat area was significantly decreased by 18.0%, whereas the skeletal muscle mass was unaffected. The PWLP group had a significantly lower prevalence of postoperative complications compared with the BMI ≥25 kg/m^2 group.

Conclusion: Obesity affected the surgical outcomes in LCR. A PWLP may be useful for obese patients undergoing LCR.

KEYWORDS

colorectal cancer, laparoscopic colorectal resection, obesity, preoperative weight loss program

1 | INTRODUCTION

The prevalence of obesity is currently very high in Western countries, and has also increased in Asian countries, including Japan.[1] In laparoscopic surgery, obesity may reduce technical feasibility, prolong operative time, and increase operative blood loss. Therefore, obesity is a major risk factor for complications in laparoscopic surgery.[2–4]

Some authors have reported that laparoscopic colectomy can be safely performed in overweight and obese patients.[5] However, others have reported that obese patients have a greater conversion rate to laparotomy, greater anastomotic leakage rate, and greater rate of complications compared with nonobese patients.[2,6] Furthermore, studies have reported that laparoscopic surgery for colorectal cancer is technically more difficult in obese patients than in nonobese patients.[2,7,8]

Previous studies have reported that obesity is a risk factor for complications after rectal surgery. Heus et al[9] evaluated the influence of visceral obesity and muscle mass on postoperative complications in rectal surgery, and found that visceral obesity is correlated with a worse outcome after surgery for rectal cancer than body mass index (BMI), subcutaneous fat, and skeletal muscle area. Yamamoto et al[10] reported that an increased BMI might be a potential risk factor for anastomotic leakage after laparoscopic surgery for rectal cancer using a stapling technique. Anastomotic leakage is reportedly associated with poor oncologic outcomes, especially regarding disease-free survival.[11]

Therefore, obesity is an important risk factor of the severe complications and poor oncological outcomes after laparoscopic colorectal surgery. Thus, there is a need for preoperative intervention for obese patients with colorectal cancer.

Regarding preoperative weight loss before cancer surgery, Inoue et al[12] reported that the preoperative 20-day very low-calorie diet weight loss program showed weight loss, reduction of visceral fat mass, and severe postoperative morbidity before laparoscopic gastrectomy for gastric cancer. In bariatric surgery, preoperative weight loss reduced the risk of postoperative complications and contributed to postoperative weight loss [13]. However, there were only a few reports about preoperative weight loss in colorectal surgery. The effect of preoperative weight loss remains unclear, especially in cancer surgery.

To minimize these issues in obese patients undergoing laparoscopic colorectal resection (LCR), a preoperative weight loss program (PWLP) was started in our department. The aim of the present study was to investigate the influence of obesity on complications in LCR, and to investigate the usefulness of a PWLP for obese patients undergoing LCR.

2 | METHODS

2.1 | Study 1: The influence of BMI in laparoscopic anterior resection

From January 2007 to December 2015, 630 patients (open; n = 176, laparoscopy; n = 454) were referred to Tokushima University Hospital for the treatment of colorectal cancer. At first, 176 laparotomy cases were excluded. In 454 laparoscopy cases, the patients who underwent laparoscopic abdominoperineal resection (n = 38), Hartmann's operation (n = 4), total colectomy (n = 1), or temporary diverting stoma (n = 19) were excluded in this series. In total, 392 patients who underwent LCR with D2 or D3 lymph node dissection for colorectal cancer were enrolled in this study. All cancers were staged based on the Japanese Classification of Colorectal, Appendiceal, and Anal Carcinoma.[14]

The patients were divided into two groups: those with a BMI of ≥25 kg/m^2 (BMI ≥25 kg/m^2 group; n = 113) and those with a BMI of <25 kg/m^2 (BMI < 25 kg/m^2 group; n = 279). The patient background data are shown in Table 1.

2.2 | Study 2: Evaluation of a PWLP for laparoscopic colorectal resection

To improve the operative outcomes in obese patients, a PWLP was started in the Department of Surgery, Tokushima University, with the approval of a suitably constituted Ethics Committee of Tokushima University Hospital (Figure 1).

The indications for a PWLP at Tokushima University Hospital were a BMI ≥28 kg/m^2, early colorectal cancer (tumor depth ≤muscularis propria), and a planned LCR. Written informed consent was provided by each patient before surgery. The exclusion criteria were conditions associated with poor compliance (e.g., psychiatric illness). There were no dropped out patients in this study.

The PWLP comprised caloric restriction (total 1200 kcal per day) and exercise (matched age and activities of daily living) for 29.6 (15–70) days. The exercise in the PWLP comprised standing exercises, leg presses, calf raises, ergometer cycling, and self-training in the Department of Rehabilitation.

The primary endpoint was the minimization or exclusion of postoperative complications. The secondary endpoints were: weight loss, visceral fat area (VFA), body fat mass, skeletal muscle mass, obesity-related nutritional parameters, operative time, intraoperative blood loss, and length of hospital stay. The data regarding VFA, body fat mass, and skeletal muscle mass were obtained by the InBody 770 (Cerritos, CA).

Table 2 shows the characteristics of the patients in the PWLP. The PWLP participants were patients with a BMI of ≥28 kg/m^2 who were scheduled to undergo LCR (n = 7, mean body weight 87.0 kg, mean BMI 33.9 kg/m^2). These PWLP participants were enrolled from 2016 to 2019. To confirm the tumor progression in PWLP, we checked tumor marker, computed tomography, and colonoscopy in pre- and post-PWLP. There was no tumor progression in all patients who underwent PWLP.

General clinical and clinicopathological data from each eligible patient were retrieved from the medical reports. All data were reviewed retrospectively, and the Clavien-Dindo classification was used to evaluate the short-term complication rate during hospitalization.

2.3 | Statistical analysis

The unpaired/paired Student's *t*-test or the Mann-Whitney *U*-test was used for the statistical analysis of the continuous variables, while the chi-square test was used for the categorical variables. In all three statistical tests, $P < .05$ was considered to represent a significant difference. The values for each of the continuous variables are expressed as the mean ± standard deviation.

To test the independence of risk factor for postoperative complication and anastomotic leakage, all factors in univariate analyses

TABLE 1 Patients' characteristics in BMI ≥25 and <25 groups in laparoscopic colorectal resection

Factors	BMI ≥ 25 (n = 113)	BMI < 25 (n = 279)	P value
Age (y.o.)	67.4 (37–85)	69.4 (34–92)	.10
Gender: Male/female	70/43	170/109	.85
BMI (kg/m^2)	26.6 (25.0–41.8)	21.6 (13.1–24.9)	<.01
Tumor location (C/A/T/D/S/R)	17/5/10/7/30/44	50/20/12/14/81/102	.44
Operation type (IC/Partial/RHC/LHC/S/HAR/LAR)	17/17/5/0/30/12/32	50/27/16/3/81/19/83	.21
fStage: 0/I/II/III/IV/Others	5/34/32/32/6/4	11/83/73/74/22/16	.88

Note: The Mann-Whitney *U*-test was used for the statistical analysis of continuous variables, while the chi-square test was used for categorical variables. $P < .05$ was considered to indicate a significant difference. Continuous variables are expressed as the mean ± standard deviation.

Abbreviation: BMI, body mass index.

Preoperative Weight Loss Program (PWLP)

Indications;
- **BMI ≥28 kg/m^2**
- **Early colorectal cancer (tumor depth≤MP)**
- **Planned LCR**
- **Written informed consent**

Exclusion criteria
- **Poor compliance (e.g. psychiatric illness)**

Contents;
- **Caloric restriction (total 1,200 kcal / day)**
- **Exercise (standing exercises, leg presses, calf raises, ergometer cycling, and self-training)**

Primary endpoint;
- **Minimization or exclusion of postoperative complications**

Secondary endpoints
weight loss, VFA, body fat mass, skeletal muscle mass, obesity-related nutritional parameters, operative time, intraoperative blood loss, and length of hospital stay

FIGURE 1 Preoperative weight loss program (PWLP)

were included in a final model of logistic regression. All statistical analyses were performed using JMP software (SAS Institute, Cary, NC).

3 | RESULTS

3.1 | Study 1: The influence of BMI in laparoscopic anterior resection

Table 3 shows the operation times and intraoperative blood loss in the BMI ≥25 kg/m^2 and BMI <25 kg/m^2 groups. The operation time of the BMI ≥25 kg/m^2 group was significantly longer than that of the BMI <25 kg/m^2 group. Postoperative complications of Clavien-Dindo grade II and anastomotic leakage did not significantly differ between the two groups. The duration of postoperative hospitalization of the BMI ≥25 kg/m^2 group was significantly longer than that of the BMI <25 kg/m^2 group.

TABLE 2 Patient characteristics in the PWLP group

Factors	n = 7
Age (y.o.)	65.7 (53–80)
Gender: Male/female	3/4
BMI (kg/m^2)	33.9 (30.7–43.7)
Body weight (kg)	87.0 (73.9–109)
Comorbidity (+/−)	4/3
Duration of PWLP (days)	29.6 (15–70)
Tumor location (A/T/D/S/R)	1/1/1/3/1
Operation type (IC/partial resection/HAR)	1/4/2
fStage (I/II)	6/1

Note: Continuous variables are expressed as the mean ± standard deviation.

Abbreviation: PWLP, preoperative weight loss program.

TABLE 3 Operative outcomes in BMI ≥25 and <25 groups in laparoscopic colorectal resection

Factors	BMI ≥ 25 (n = 113)	BMI < 25 (n = 279)	P value
Operation time (min)	231.0 (102–510)	207 (50–551)	<.05
Blood loss (mL)	20.0 (0–650)	20 (0–2260)	.84
Postoperative complications (CD ≥ grade 2)	14.2%	12.9%	.74
	Ileus (n = 4, 3.5%)	Ileus (n = 8, 2.9%) Ascites (n = 4, 1.4%)	.26
Anastomotic leakage	8.0%	5.0%	.26
Hospital stay (days)	23.6 (6–382)	17.6 (6–85)	<.05

Note: The Mann-Whitney *U*-test was used for the statistical analysis of continuous variables. $P < .05$ was considered to indicate a significant difference. Continuous variables are expressed as the mean ± standard deviation.

Abbreviation: BMI, body mass index.

TABLE 4 Comparison of with and without postoperative complication and anastomotic leakage in laparoscopic colorectal resection

Factors	Complications (n = 52)	No complications (n = 340)	P value	Anastomotic leakage (n = 23)	No anastomotic leakage (n = 369)	P value
Age (y.o.): <70/70≤	27/25	183/157	.80	16/7	194/175	.11
Gender: Male/female	37/15	203/137	.11	18/5	222/147	.08
BMI (kg/m^2): <25/25≤	36/16	243/97	.74	14/9	265/104	.26
Tumor location: Colon/rectum	24/28	222/118	<.01	6/17	240/129	<.01
Operation time (min): <300/300≤	38/14	301/39	<.01	15/8	323/46	<.01
Blood loss (mL): <100/100≤	39/13	303/37	<.01	21/2	321/48	.59

Note: The chi-square test was used for categorical variables. $P < .05$ was considered to indicate a significant difference.
Abbreviation: BMI, body mass index.

TABLE 5 The independent risk factor of postoperative complications and anastomotic leakage

	Postoperative complications		Anastomotic leakage	
Factors	Hazard ratio	P value	Hazard ratio	P value
Age (y.o.): 70≤	0.41	.69	−1.29	.20
Gender: Male	1.17	.24	1.17	.24
BMI (kg/m^2): 25≤	0.46	.65	0.94	.35
Tumor location: Rectum	1.63	.11	2.32	<.05
Operation time (min): 300≤	1.70	.09	2.27	<.05
Blood loss (mL): 100≤	2.28	<.05	−0.99	.32

Note: To test the independence of risk factor for postoperative complication and anastomotic leakage; all factors in univariate analyses were included in a final model of logistic regression.
Abbreviation: BMI, body mass index.

TABLE 6 Obesity-related factors in pre- and post-PWLP

Factors	Pre-PWLP	Post-PWLP	P value
Body weight (kg)	87.0 (73.9–109)	81.0 (69.8–96.0)	<.05
BMI (kg/m^2)	33.9 (30.7–43.7)	31.6 (28.9–38.0)	<.05
Visceral fat area (m^2)	169.0 (114.5–217.0)	138.6 (91.5–212.0)	<.05
Body fat mass	40.7% (30.0–54.1)	36.9% (26.2–47.8)	<.05
Skeletal muscle	31.8% (21.9–48.7)	31.1 (21.8–44.6)	.26
AST (IU/L)	27.1 (14–45)	23.7 (13–39)	.53
ALT (IU/L)	24.9 (8–39)	18.4 (9–26)	.21
Total cholesterol (mg/dL)	214.9 (189–258)	167.8 (116–188)	<.05
Albumin (g/dL)	4.1 (3.6–4.4)	4.0 (3.6–4.3)	.39

Note: The Mann-Whitney *U*-test was used for the statistical analysis of continuous variables. $P < .05$ was considered to indicate a significant difference.
Abbreviation: PWLP, preoperative weight loss program.

Table 4 shows the comparison of with and without postoperative complication and anastomotic leakage in laparoscopic colorectal resection. In the complication group, there was a significantly higher prevalence of rectum, operation time ≥300 minutes, and blood loss ≥100 mL. In the anastomotic leakage group, there was a significantly higher prevalence of rectum and operation time ≥300 minutes were independent risk factors of anastomotic leakage. Regarding postoperative complication, blood loss ≥100 mL was an independent risk factor in multivariate analysis. Furthermore, rectum and operation time 300 ≥minutes were independent risk factors of anastomotic leakage (Table 5).

3.2 | Study 2: Evaluation of a PWLP for laparoscopic colorectal resection

The patients achieved a mean weight loss of 6.9% (−6.0 kg) after the PWLP. Compared with the pre-PWLP values, the mean post-PWLP VFA and body fat mass were significantly decreased (mean VFA decrease 18.0%; mean body fat mass decrease 9.3%), whereas the skeletal muscle mass was unchanged.

Regarding the obesity-related parameters, the mean total cholesterol was significantly decreased after the PWLP. However, the mean pre- and post-PWLP albumin values did not significantly differ (Table 6).

Table 7 shows the comparison of operative outcomes between the BMI ≥25 and PWLP group. In the BMI ≥25 group of Table 7, the cases of fStageIII, IV (n = 38) were excluded to match the tumor progression. The PWLP group showed a lower prevalence of postoperative complications (including anastomotic leakage) compared with the BMI ≥25 kg/m^2 group. There was no significant difference in operation time and postoperative hospital stay between the two groups (Table 7).

4 | DISCUSSION

The present study was designed to investigate the influence of obesity on LCR for colorectal cancer, and to evaluate the usefulness of

TABLE 7 Comparison of operative outcomes between the BMI >25 and PWLP group

Factors	BMI ≥25[a] (n = 75)	PWLP (n = 7)	P value
Operation time (min)	231.5 (102–510)	237.9 (159–305)	.92
Postoperative complication (CD > grade 2)	16.0%	0%	<.05
Anastomotic leakage	8.0%	0%	<.05
Hospital stay (days)	14.0 (6–382)	15.0 (9–28)	.56

Note: The Mann-Whitney *U*-test was used for the statistical analysis of continuous variables. $P < .05$ was considered to indicate a significant difference.

Abbreviations: BMI, body mass index; PWLP, preoperative weight loss program.

[a]Excluded the cases of fStage III, IV (n = 38).

a PWLP for obese patients undergoing LCR for colorectal cancer. The BMI ≥25 kg/m^2 group had a significantly longer operation time and postoperative hospital stay than the BMI <25 kg/m^2 group. The PWLP group achieved significant decreases in body weight and VFA. Furthermore, the PWLP group had a lower prevalence of postoperative complications compared with the BMI ≥25 kg/m^2 group.

For patients undergoing laparoscopic sleeve gastrectomy, a preoperative diet comprising immune-enhancing nutrition formulas reportedly achieves greater preoperative weight loss, lower postoperative pain, and lower levels of C-reactive protein and liver enzymes than high-protein formulas or a regular diet with similar caloric intakes.[15] However, one of the important problems with weight loss is the incidence of sarcopenia. A decrease in skeletal muscle, referred to as sarcopenia, is reportedly correlated with morbidity and mortality in patients undergoing digestive surgery. Thus, unintentional weight loss can be used to predict mortality and morbidity rates in colorectal surgery. In particular, preoperative weight loss is significantly associated with cardiopulmonary complications.[16] Kaido et al[17] reported that sarcopenia is closely related with postoperative mortality in patients undergoing living donor liver transplantation and that perioperative nutritional intervention is important for the survival of patients with sarcopenia. Sarcopenic obesity is defined using the criteria for sarcopenia and obesity by body fat mass (≥25% body fat for males, ≥35% body fat for females). In patients undergoing surgery for hepatocellular carcinoma, preoperative sarcopenic obesity is an independent risk factor for patient survival and postoperative recurrence.[18]

In preoperative weight loss, the prevention of sarcopenia is very important in decreasing perioperative complications. In the present study, the PWLP resulted in the maintenance of several nutritional parameters and did not cause a decrease in skeletal muscle mass. Yamamoto et al[19] reported that preoperative exercise and a nutritional support program for elderly sarcopenic patients with gastric cancer increased handgrip strength, gait speed, and skeletal muscle mass index. The intervention of nutrition and exercise was essential for the maintenance of skeletal muscle.

Patients with both visceral obesity and sarcopenia were reported to have a higher complication rate after colorectal cancer surgery.[20] In this report, age ≥65 years, visceral obesity, and sarcopenia were independent risk factors for total complications. Obesity with reduced muscle mass was related to higher 30-day morbidity and mortality rates.[21] In addition, postoperative complication, especially anastomotic leakage, was reported to be associated with poor oncologic outcomes.[11] Sarcopenia and fatty infiltration of the muscle (myosteatosis) were independent predictors of worse survival in Stage I to III colorectal cancer. And their joint effect was highly reduced oncologic survival.[22] Therefore, obesity and sarcopenia are associated with difficulty of surgical procedure, postoperative complication, and poor postoperative oncological outcomes. Thus, the preoperative intervention for obesity and sarcopenia is very important for improving short- and long-term surgical outcomes.

The progression of colorectal cancer during the PWLP may be a major problem. However, Brenkman et al[23] reported that a longer waiting time (even >8 weeks) before gastrectomy surgery for gastric cancer is not associated with a worse overall survival rate. In addition, Fujiya et al[24] also reported that a prolonged wait time (6 mo) for surgery was not related with survival of Stage I gastric cancer. Therefore, the duration of the PWLP may be reasonable for the purpose of decreasing postoperative complications.

The limitations of this study were that it was a retrospective study, single institution, and a small number of patients. In addition, the comparison between the PWLP group and the no-PWLP group in the same background was not done.

In conclusion, obesity affected the operative outcomes in LCR. A PWLP may be useful for obese patients undergoing LCR, and a PWLP may be useful in minimizing complications for obese patients undergoing LCR.

ACKNOWLEDGMENTS

The authors thank the staff at the Department of Surgery, Institute of Health Biosciences, Tokushima University, for their important contributions. We thank Kelly Zammit, BVSc, from the Edanz Group for editing a draft of this article.

REFERENCES

1. WHO, Expert Consultation. Appropriate bode-mass index for Asian populations and its implications for policy and intervention strategies. Lancet. 2004;363(9403):157–63.
2. Pikarsky AJ, Saida Y, Yamaguchi T, Martinez S, Chen W, Weiss EG, et al. Is obesity a high-risk factor for laparoscopic colorectal surgery? Surg Endosc. 2002;16(5):855–8.
3. Pandya S, Murray JJ, Coller JA, Rusin LC. Laparoscopic colectomy: Indications for conversion to laparotomy. Arch Surg. 1999;134(5):471–5.
4. Veldkamp R, Gholghesaei M, Bonjer HJ, Meijer DW, Buunen M, Jeekel J, et al. Laparoscopic resection of colon cancer: consensus of the European Association of Endoscopic Surgery (EAES). Surg Endosc. 2004;18(8):1163–85.
5. Tuech JJ, Regenet N, Hennekinne S, Pessaux P, Bergamaschi R, Arnaud JP. Laparoscopic colectomy for sigmoid diverticulitis in obese and nonobese patients. Surg Endosc. 2001;15(12):1427.
6. Senagore AJ, Delaney CP, Madboulay K, Brady KM, Fazio VW. Laparoscopic colectomy in obese and nonobese patients. J Gastrointest Surg. 2003;7(4):558–61.
7. Hazebroek EJ, Color Study G. COLOR: a randomized clinical trial comparing laparoscopic and open resection for colon cancer. Surg Endosc. 2002;16:949–53.
8. Marusch F, Gastinger I, Schneider C, Scheidbach H, Konradt J, Bruch HP, et al. Experience as a factor influencing the indications for laparoscopic colorectal surgery and the results. Surg Endosc. 2001;15(2):116–20.
9. Heus C, Bakker N, Verduin WM, Doodeman HJ, Houdijk AP. Impact of body composition on surgical outcome in rectal cancer patients, a retrospective cohort study. World J Surg. 2019;43(5):1370–6.
10. Yamamoto S, Fujita S, Akasu T, Inada R, Moriya Y. Risk factors for anastomotic leakage after laparoscopic surgery for rectal cancer using a stapling technique. Surg Laparosc Endosc Percutan Tech. 2012;22(3):239–43.
11. Noh GT, Ann YS, Cheong C, Han J, Cho MS, Hur H, et al. Impact of anastomotic leakage on long-term oncologic outcome and its related factors in rectal cancer. Medicine. 2016;95(30):e4367.
12. Inoue K, Yoshiuchi S, Yoshida M, Nakamura N, Nakajima S, Kitamura A, et al. Preoperative weight loss program involving a 20-day very low-calorie diet for obesity before laparoscopic gastrectomy for gastric cancer. Asian J Endosc Surg. 2019;12(1):43–50.
13. Anderin C, Gustafsson UO, Heijbel N, Thorell A. Weight loss before bariatric surgery and postoperative complications: data from the Scandinavian Obesity Registry (SOReg). Ann Surg. 2015;261(5):909–13.
14. Japanese Society for Cancer of the Colon and Rectum. Japanese classification of colorectal, appendiceal, and anal carcinoma: the 3rd English edition. J Anus Rectum Colon. 2019;3(4):175–95.
15. Ruiz-Tovar J, Zubiaga L, Diez M, Murcia A, Boix E, Muñoz JL, et al. Preoperative regular diet of 900 kcal/day vs balanced energy high-protein formula vs immunonutrition formula: effect on preoperative weight loss and postoperative pain, complications and analytical acute phase reactants after laparoscopic sleeve gastrectomy. Obes Surg. 2016;26(6):1221–7.
16. Moghadamyeghaneh Z, Hanna MH, Hwang G, Carmichael JC, Mills SD, Pigazzi A, et al. Outcome of preoperative weight loss in colorectal surgery. Am J Surg. 2015;210(2):291–7.
17. Kaido T, Ogawa K, Fujimoto Y, Ogura Y, Hata K, Ito T, et al. Impact of sarcopenia on survival in patients undergoing living donor liver transplantation. Am J Transplant. 2013;13(6):1549–56.
18. Kobayashi A, Kaido T, Hamaguchi Y, Okumura S, Shirai H, Yao S, et al. Impact of sarcopenic obesity on outcomes in patients undergoing hepatectomy for hepatocellular carcinoma. Ann Surg. 2019;269(5):924–31.
19. Yamamoto K, Nagatsuma Y, Fukuda Y, Hirao M, Nishikawa K, Miyamoto A, et al. Effectiveness of a preoperative exercise and nutritional support program for elderly sarcopenic patients with gastric cancer. Gastric Cancer. 2017;20(5):913–8.
20. Chen W-Z, Chen X-D, Ma L-L, Zhang F-M, Lin JI, Zhuang C-L, et al. Impact of visceral obesity and sarcopenia on short-term outcomes after colorectal cancer surgery. Dig Dis Sci. 2018;63(6):1620–30.
21. Malietzis G, Currie AC, Athanasiou T, Johns N, Anyamene N, Glynne-Jones R, et al. Influence of body composition profile on outcomes following colorectal cancer surgery. Br J Surg. 2016;103(5):572–80.
22. Hopkins JJ, Reif RL, Bigam DL, Baracos VE, Eurich DT, Sawyer MB. The impact of muscle and adipose tissue on long-term survival in patients with stage I to III colorectal cancer. Dis Colon Rectum. 2019;62(5):549–60.
23. Brenkman HJ, Visser E, van Rossum PS, Siesling S, van Hillegersberg R, Ruurda JP. Association between waiting time from diagnosis to treatment and survival in patients with curable gastric cancer: a population-based study in the Netherlands. Ann Surg Oncol. 2017;24(7):1761–9.
24. Fujiya K, Irino T, Furukawa K, Omori H, Makuuchi R, Tanizawa Y, et al. Safety of prolonged wait time for gastrectomy in clinical stage I gastric cancer. Eur J Surg Oncol. 2019;45(10):1964–8.

Which is the best predictor of clinically relevant pancreatic fistula after pancreatectomy: Drain fluid concentration or total amount of amylase?

Yasuyuki Fukami | Takuya Saito | Takaaki Osawa | Takaaki Hanazawa | Takehiro Kurahashi | Shintaro Kurahashi | Tatsuki Matsumura | Shunichiro Komatsu | Kenitiro Kaneko | Tsuyoshi Sano

Division of Gastroenterological Surgery, Department of Surgery, Aichi Medical University, Nagakute, Japan

Correspondence
Yasuyuki Fukami, Division of Gastroenterological Surgery, Department of Surgery, Aichi Medical University, 1-1 Yazakokarimata, Nagakute, Aichi 480-1195, Japan.
Email: yasuyuki490225@yahoo.co.jp

Abstract

Aim: Drain fluid amylase concentration (DFAC) has been reported as a predictor of clinically relevant postoperative pancreatic fistula (CR-POPF) after pancreatectomy. However, the clinical significance of measuring the total drain fluid amylase amount (DFAA) considering the daily drainage volume of CR-POPF remains unclear.

Methods: Data from 216 consecutive patients who underwent pancreaticoduodenectomy (PD) (n = 126) or distal pancreatectomy (DP) (n = 90) between August 2014 and November 2020 were reviewed. All drains were closed but not suctioned. DFAA was calculated by multiplying the DFAC and daily drainage fluid volume. DFAC and DFAA were recorded on d 1 and 3 after pancreatectomy. The cutoff value of CR-POPF was determined using the receiver operating characteristic curve.

Results: CR-POPF was found in 75 patients (35%) (PD: 30%, DP: 41%, $P = .111$); the mortality rate was zero. The cutoff value of DFAC-day 1 was 1757 U/L (sensitivity [SE]: 84%, specificity [SP]: 62%, and accuracy [AC]: 69%). The cutoff value of DFAA-day 1 was 139 U (SE: 71%, SP: 72%, and AC: 71%). The cutoff value of DFAC-day 3 was 1044 U/L (SE: 73%, SP: 79%, and AC: 78%). The cutoff value of DFAA-day 3 was 21 U (SE: 68%, SP: 72%, and AC: 70%). Multivariate analysis indicated that a nondilated pancreatic duct and high DFAC-day 3 were independently associated with CR-POPF after PD, indicating that a prolonged operative duration, massive blood loss, and high DFAC-day 3 are independently associated with CR-POPF after DP.

Conclusion: DFAC is more reliable than DFAA for predicting CR-POPF after both PD and DP.

KEYWORDS
distal pancreatectomy, drain amylase, pancreatectomy, pancreatic fistula, pancreaticoduodenectomy

1 | INTRODUCTION

Postoperative pancreatic fistula (POPF) remains one of the most common complications after pancreatic surgery, such as pancreaticoduodenectomy (PD) and distal pancreatectomy (DP). Despite modifications in surgical techniques and perioperative patient care to prevent POPF, the incidence of POPF has been reported to range from 3%–50%, even at high-volume centers.[1-4]

The International Study Group of Pancreatic Surgery (ISGPS) has developed and validated a universally applicable definition for POPF.[5,6] According to the classification, grade B or C POPF is regarded as clinically relevant POPF (CR-POPF) and requires major deviations in clinical management. CR-POPF can lead to more life-threatening complications, including intraabdominal abscess or intraabdominal bleeding and septicemia. As a result, CR-POPF is responsible for prolonged hospital stays and increased healthcare costs.

Many studies have demonstrated risk factors for CR-POPF, such as pancreatic texture, pancreatic duct size, body mass index (BMI), and massive intraoperative blood loss.[7,8] Recently, several studies have reported that the drain fluid amylase concentration (DFAC) on the 1st and 3rd d after pancreatectomy can be a reliable predictor of CR-POPF.[9-18] DFAC can reveal the optimal timing of drain removal after pancreatectomy by data-driven decisions. However, the value of the drain fluid amylase amount (DFAA) when considering the daily drainage volume has not been investigated, so it is unclear whether DFAC or DFAA is the more reliable predictor of CR-POPF after pancreatectomy. Therefore, this study aimed to investigate the practical significance of DFAA as a predictor of CR-POPF following pancreatectomy.

2 | PATIENTS AND METHODS

Between August 2014 and November 2020, 216 consecutive patients who underwent PD (n = 126) or DP (n = 90) at our institution were enrolled in the study. Patients undergoing hepatopancreaticoduodenectomy (n = 12), central pancreatectomy (n = 4), total pancreatectomy (n = 18), or partial pancreatectomy (n = 1) were excluded. The demographics, clinical characteristics, operative details, and postoperative outcomes of patients with and without CR-POPF were retrospectively analyzed. All patients provided written informed consent before undergoing therapy. This study was approved by the Institutional Review Board of our institution (No. 2020-119) and was performed in accordance with the 1964 Declaration of Helsinki and its later amendments or comparable ethical standards.

2.1 | Surgical procedure

After review by a multidisciplinary board, all pancreatic disease cases were assessed by pancreatic surgeons to determine resectability and the most appropriate surgical procedure. The subtotal stomach-preserving method was the standard procedure for PD. In patients with malignant disease, lymph nodes are dissected at the hepatoduodenal ligament, around the common hepatic artery, around the superior mesenteric artery (SMA), and around the pancreatic head. Transection of the pancreatic parenchyma was performed with an electric scalpel. A modified Child method, with duct-to-mucosa pancreatojejunostomy, was chosen for organ reconstruction in all cases. The modified Blumgart mattress suture was the procedure of choice for pancreatic remnant reconstruction when feasible.[19,20] In all cases, a 4-Fr polyethylene tube was placed through the pancreatojejunal anastomotic site as an external stent. Three silastic flexible drains were routinely placed adjacent to the anastomosis and at both the cranial and caudal sites of the pancreatojejunostomy and choledochojejunostomy.

In the case of DP, transection of the pancreatic parenchyma was performed with a stapler from 2017 on. A silastic flexible drain was placed at the pancreatic stump. However, in the case of radical antegrade modular pancreatosplenectomy (RAMPS) for pancreatic ductal adenocarcinoma (PDAC), an additional drain was placed at the left subphrenic space.

Energy devices, such as LigaSure (TM) (Covidien, Japan) was used only during laparoscopic surgery. All drains were closed but not suctioned. Prophylactic octreotide to prevent POPF was not administered in either PD or DP.

2.2 | Definition of DFAC and DFAA

Amylase levels in the drainage fluid were routinely measured on postoperative d (PODs) 1 and 3 (ie, DFAC-day 1 and DFAC-day 3). If there were multiple drains, the highest DFAC-day 1 value was defined as analysis drain. DFAA-day 1 was calculated by multiplying DFAC-day 1 and the 24-h drainage volume from the morning of POD 1. In the same way, DFAA-day 3 was calculated by multiplying DFAC-day 3 and the 24-h drainage volume from the morning of POD 3.

The drain was removed on POD 4 or 5 if the drainage fluid was clear and pancreatic fistula and bacterial contamination were absent. In the case that bacterial contamination was detected based on a bacterial culture test of drain fluid, or suspected by nonserous (turbid) fluid of the drain, drains were replaced on POD 7.

2.3 | Postoperative complications

Any complications that developed within 90 d after the operation were included. No patients were lost to follow-up. CR-POPF included grade B or C POPF based on the definition of ISGPS.[6] Bile leakage was defined according to International Study Group of Liver Surgery (ISGLS) criteria.[21] Intraabdominal bleeding and delayed gastric emptying (DGE) were also defined by ISGPS criteria.[22,23] Surgical mortality was defined as perioperative death within the first 90 d following surgery.

2.4 | Statistical analysis

The continuous data are expressed as the medians (ranges). The statistical analyses were performed using chi square tests, Mann–Whitney *U*-tests, or Fisher's exact probability tests, as appropriate. The predictive ability of DFAC and DFAA for the occurrence of CR-POPF was assessed by calculating the area under the receiver operating characteristic (ROC) curve. The variables identified as potentially significant by univariate analysis were selected for multivariate analysis with a logistic regression model to identify the independent predictors of CR-POPF. All *P* values were 2-sided, and $P < .05$ was considered to indicate a statistically significant difference. All statistical calculations were performed using the IBM SPSS Statistics 27 software package (IBM Japan).

3 | RESULTS

3.1 | Patient characteristics and surgical outcomes

The patient demographics and clinical characteristics are shown in Table 1. CR-POPF was found in 75 patients (35%). Among the CR-POPF patients, grade C POPF occurred in only two patients (3%) who underwent PD, and the remaining 73 patients (97%) had grade B POPF. The CR-POPF group had a significantly higher BMI than the no CR-POPF group ($P < .001$). The CR-POPF group had a significantly lower incidence of PDAC than the no CR-POPF group ($P < .001$). The median age, sex, preoperative albumin concentration, and incidence of comorbidities did not differ between the two groups.

The laparoscopic approach was performed in 24 cases during DP. Among the 126 cases of PD, the incidence of patients who underwent the modified Blumgart method was 79% (100 cases). Table 2 shows the surgical outcomes after pancreatectomy. The type of pancreatectomy, operative duration, and total blood loss volume did not differ between the two groups. There were significant differences between the two groups in terms of the pancreatic duct size <3 mm (53% in the no CR-POPF group vs 85% in the CR-POPF group) and soft pancreatic texture rate (62% in the no CR-POPF group vs 80% in the CR-POPF group). The median DFAC-day 1, DFAA-day 1, DFAC-day 3, and DFAA-day 3 were significantly higher in the CR-POPF group than in the no CR-POPF group. On the other hand, the median drainage volumes on POD 1 and POD 3 were significantly lower in the CR-POPF group than in the no CR-POPF group (Figure S1). There were significant differences between the two groups in terms of intraabdominal bleeding (0% in the no CR-POPF group vs 5% in the CR-POPF group) and median postoperative hospital stays (12 d

TABLE 1 Patient characteristics

	CR-POPF		
	No (n = 141)	Yes (n = 75)	*P*
Age (y)	70 (28–89)	69 (24–88)	.147
Sex (male/female)	62/79	40/35	.201
BMI (kg/m^2)	20.8 (13.3–35.0)	22.8 (14.6–32.0)	<.001
Albumin (g/dL)	3.6 (2.4–4.8)	3.8 (1.7–4.8)	.103
ASA status (I/II/III)	83/57/1	56/17/2	.021
Comorbidity			
Cardiovascular disease	17 (12%)	7 (9%)	.652
Cerebrovascular disease	8 (6%)	1 (1%)	.167
Pulmonary disease	10 (7%)	6 (8%)	.791
Chronic kidney disease	7 (5%)	3 (4%)	1.000
Diabetes mellitus	36 (26%)	11 (15%)	.083
Previous intraabdominal operation	23 (16%)	8 (11%)	.312
Disease			
PDAC	81 (57%)	22 (29%)	<.001
Cancer excepting PDAC[a]	15 (11%)	17 (23%)	
IPMN	15 (11%)	6 (8%)	
NET	6 (4%)	10 (13%)	
Others	24 (17%)	20 (27%)	

Note: Expressed as N (%) or median (range).

Abbreviations: ASA, American Society of Anesthesiologists; BMI, body mass index; CR-POPF, clinically relevant postoperative pancreatic fistula; IPMN, intraductal papillary mucinous neoplasm; NET, neuroendocrine tumor, PDAC, pancreatic ductal adenocarcinoma.

[a]Includes duodenal, ampullary of the pancreas, and bile duct cancer.

TABLE 2 Surgical outcome

	CR-POPF		
	No (n = 141)	Yes (n = 75)	*P*
Type of pancreatectomy			
Pancreaticoduodenectomy	88 (70%)	38 (30%)	.111
Distal pancreatectomy	53 (59%)	37 (41%)	
Operative duration (min)	334 (124-660)	362 (109-598)	.944
Total blood loss (mL)	320 (3-4514)	458 (3-4250)	.324
Pancreatic duct size (<3 mm)	75 (53%)	64 (85%)	<.001
Pancreatic texture			
Soft	87 (62%)	60 (80%)	.006
Hard	54 (38%)	15 (20%)	
Postoperative day 1 drain status			
DFAC (U/L)	981 (11-32 048)	5559 (90-30 017)	<.001
Drainage volume (mL)	54 (3-658)	39 (3-740)	.018
DFAA (U)	50 (1-2832)	180 (8-2014)	<.001
Postoperative day 3 drain status			
DFAC (U/L)	268 (8-14 500)	3271 (31-142 458)	<.001
Drainage volume (mL)	42 (1-633)	15 (1-352)	<.001
DFAA (U)	11 (1-499)	36 (3-712)	<.001
Morbidity other than CR-POPF			
Bile leakage	3 (2%)	1 (1%)	1.000
Intraabdominal abscess	14 (10%)	3 (4%)	.184
Intraabdominal bleeding	0	5 (7%)	.005
Delayed gastric emptying	8 (6%)	2 (3%)	.724
Septicemia	1 (1%)	3 (4%)	.122
Mortality	0	0	–
Postoperative hospital stays (d)	12 (6-138)	30 (13-90)	<.001

Note: Expressed as N (%) or median (range).

Abbreviations: CR-POPF, clinically relevant postoperative pancreatic fistula; DFAA, drain fluid amylase amount; DFAC, drain fluid amylase concentration.

in the no CR-POPF group vs 30 d in the CR-POPF group). The in-hospital and 90-d postoperative mortality rates were zero in both groups.

3.2 | Cutoff values of DFAC/DFAA-day 1 and day 3 for predicting CR-POPF

The ROC curves for generating cutoff values of DFAC/DEAA-day 1 and day 3 for rates of CR-POPF for all patient groups are shown in Figure 1 and Table 3. The cutoff value of DFAC-day 1 was 1757 U/L, with a sensitivity of 84%, specificity of 62%, and accuracy of 69%. The cutoff value of DFAA-day 1 was 139 U, with a sensitivity of 71%, specificity of 72%, and accuracy of 71%. The cutoff value of DFAC-day 3 was 1044 U/L, with a sensitivity of 73%, specificity of 79%, and accuracy of 78%. The cutoff value of DFAA-day 3 was 21 U, with a sensitivity of 68%, specificity of 72%, and accuracy of 70%. Altogether, the results indicated that the most reliable predictor of CR-POPF after pancreatectomy was DFAC-day 3, which had the highest area under the ROC curve (AUC) value (0.843; optimal cutoff value 1044 U/L).

3.3 | Subgroup analysis of DFAC/DFAA according to the type of pancreatectomy and predictors of CR-POPF

Subgroup analysis of CR-POPF according to the type of pancreatectomy was performed. The median operative duration was 424 min, and total blood loss was 495 mL following PD. The median operative duration was 245 min, and total blood loss was 178 mL following DP. CR-POPF was found in 38 patients (30%) after PD and 37 patients (41%) after DP (*P* = .111). The ROC curves for generating cutoff values of DFAC/DEAA-day 1 and day 3 for rates of CR-POPF after PD are shown in Figure S2 and Table 4. The most reliable predictors of CR-POPF after PD were DFAC-day 1 (AUC = 0.855; optimal cutoff value 1773 U/L) and DFAC-day 3 (AUC = 0.855; optimal cutoff value 713 U/L). The multivariate

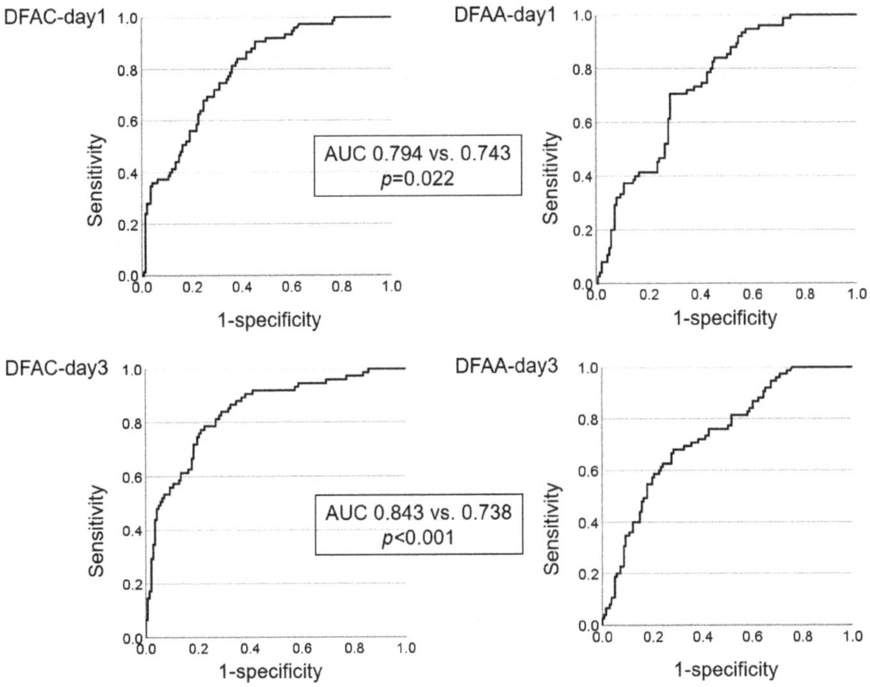

FIGURE 1 ROC curve of DFAC/DEAA-day 1 and day 3 for rates of CR-POPF for all patient groups

TABLE 3 Accuracy of DFAC/DFAA-day 1 and day 3 to predict CR-POPF

Variable	Cutoff value	AUC	Sensitivity	Specificity	PPV	NPV	Accuracy
DFAC-day 1	1757 (U/L)	0.794	84%	62%	54%	88%	69%
DFAA-day 1	139 (U)	0.743	71%	72%	57%	82%	71%
DFAC-day 3	1044 (U/L)	0.843	73%	79%	66%	87%	78%
DFAA-day 3	21 (U)	0.738	68%	72%	56%	81%	70%

Abbreviations: AUC, area under the ROC curve; CR-POPF, clinically relevant postoperative pancreatic fistula; DFAA, drain fluid amylase amount; DFAC, drain fluid amylase concentration; NPV, negative predictive value; PPV, positive predictive value.

TABLE 4 Accuracy of DFAC/DFAA-day 1 and day 3 to predict CR-POPF after PD

Variable	Cutoff value	AUC	Sensitivity	Specificity	PPV	NPV	Accuracy
DFAC-day 1	1773 (U/L)	0.855	84%	80%	64%	92%	81%
DFAA-day 1	67 (U)	0.793	79%	71%	54%	89%	73%
DFAC-day 3	713 (U/L)	0.855	84%	80%	64%	92%	81%
DFAA-day 3	13 (U)	0.754	74%	69%	51%	86%	71%

Abbreviations: AUC, area under the ROC curve; CR-POPF, clinically relevant postoperative pancreatic fistula; DFAA, drain fluid amylase amount; DFAC, drain fluid amylase concentration; NPV, negative predictive value; PD, pancreaticoduodenectomy; PPV, positive predictive value.

analysis results indicated that pancreatic duct size <3 mm (odds ratio [OR]: 4.20, 95% confidence interval [CI]: 1.47–11.94, $P = .007$) and DFAC-day 3 value >713 U/L (OR: 15.66, 95% CI: 5.38–45.60, $P < .001$) were independently associated with CR-POPF after PD (Table 5).

The ROC curves for generating cutoff values of DFAC/DEAA-day 1 and day 3 for rates of CR-POPF after DP are shown in Figure S3 and Table 6. The most reliable predictor of CR-POPF after DP was DFAC-day 3 (AUC = 0.819; optimal cutoff value 3506 U/L). The multivariate analysis results indicated that an operative duration >300 min (OR: 3.79, 95% CI: 1.04–13.86, $P = .044$), total blood loss >400 mL (OR: 3.63, 95% CI: 1.03–12.72, $P = .044$), and DFAC-day 3 value ≥3506 U/L (OR: 40.57, 95% CI: 9.80–167.92, $P < .001$) were independently associated with CR-POPF after DP (Table 7).

4 | DISCUSSION

Pancreatic surgery has become safer, especially in high-volume centers, due to advances in technology and perioperative management. Nevertheless, CR-POPF is the most common complication and subsequently triggers other infectious complications, which is concerning for both patients and surgeons. Many studies have reported risk factors for CR-POPF, including not only pancreas-related factors (eg,

TABLE 5 Uni- and multivariate predictors of CR-POPF after PD

Variable	Univariate OR	Univariate 95% CI	Univariate P	Multivariate OR	Multivariate 95% CI	Multivariate P
Age (y)						
>70 (n = 73)	1.66	0.56-4.90	.357			
<70 (n = 53)	1					
Sex						
Female (n = 70)	1.21	0.40-3.63	.740			
Male (n = 56)	1					
BMI (kg/m^2)						
>24 (n = 36)	2.38	0.76-7.45	.138			
<24 (n = 90)	1					
Operative duration (min)						
>480 (n = 35)	1.89	0.46-7.74	.378			
<480 (n = 91)	1					
Total blood loss (mL)						
>1000 (n = 24)	1.97	0.38-10.28	.422			
<1000 (n = 102)	1					
Pancreatic duct size (mm)						
<3 (n = 58)	3.74	1.07-13.12	.039	4.20	1.47-11.94	.007
>3 (n = 68)	1			1		
Pancreatic texture						
Soft (n = 73)	1.49	0.39-5.67	.557			
Hard (n = 53)	1					
DFAA-day 3 (U)						
>13 (n = 54)	0.734	0.21-2.57	.628			
<13 (n = 72)	1					
DFAC-day 3 (U/L)						
>713 (n = 50)	27.36	6.00-124.74	<.001	15.66	5.38-45.60	<.001
<713 (n = 76)	1			1		

Abbreviations: BMI, body mass index; CR-POPF, clinically relevant postoperative pancreatic fistula; DFAA, drain fluid amylase amount; DFAC, drain fluid amylase concentration; PD, pancreaticoduodenectomy.

TABLE 6 Accuracy of DFAC/DFAA-day 1 and day 3 to predict CR-POPF after DP

Variable	Cutoff value	AUC	Sensitivity	Specificity	PPV	NPV	Accuracy
DFAC-day 1	9401 (U/L)	0.715	51%	94%	86%	74%	77%
DFAA-day 1	139 (U)	0.674	78%	55%	55%	78%	64%
DFAC-day 3	3506 (U/L)	0.819	62%	93%	85%	78%	80%
DFAA-day 3	21 (U)	0.711	76%	66%	61%	80%	70%

Abbreviations: AUC, area under the ROC curve; CR-POPF, clinically relevant postoperative pancreatic fistula; DFAA, drain fluid amylase amount; DFAC, drain fluid amylase concentration; DP, distal pancreatectomy; NPV, negative predictive value; PPV, positive predictive value.

pancreatic texture and pancreatic duct size) but also perioperative factors (eg, massive intraoperative blood loss and DFAC).[7-18]

DFAC can help to determine the optimal timing of drain removal after pancreatectomy with data-driven decisions. However, various DFAC cutoff values have been proposed in the literature. Molinari et al[15] demonstrated that a DFAC-day 1 value ≥5000 U/L was a significant predictive factor of POPF after PD and DP. Ansorge et al[17] reported that a DFAC-day 1 value ≥1322 U/L was a significant predictive factor of CR-POPF after PD. Maggino et al[10] reported that a DFAC-day 1 value ≥2000 U/L was a significant predictive factor of

TABLE 7 Uni- and multivariate predictors of CR-POPF after DP

	Univariate			Multivariate		
Variable	OR	95% CI	P	OR	95% CI	P
Age (y)						
>70 (n = 39)	0.67	0.19–2.38	.553			
<70 (n = 51)	1					
Sex						
Female (n = 44)	0.82	0.18–3.74	.799			
Male (n = 46)	1					
BMI (kg/m^2)						
>24 (n = 19)	0.85	0.20–3.67	.827			
<24 (n = 71)	1					
Stump closure method						
Stapler (n = 49)	0.43	0.11–1.64	.217			
Handsewn (n = 41)	1					
Operative duration (min)						
>300 (n = 20)	3.90	0.95–15.97	.059	3.79	1.04–13.86	.044
<300 (n = 70)	1			1		
Total blood loss (mL)						
>400 (n = 25)	2.33	0.49–11.09	.290	3.63	1.03–12.72	.044
<400 (n = 65)	1			1		
Pancreatic duct size (mm)						
<3 (n = 9)	1.67	0.20–13.72	.634			
>3 (n = 81)	1					
Pancreatic texture						
Soft (n = 74)	0.63	0.14–2.73	.533			
Hard (n = 16)	1					
DFAA-day 3 (U)						
>21 (n = 46)	2.12	0.51–8.72	.299			
<21 (n = 44)	1					
DFAC-day 3 (U/L)						
>3506 (n = 27)	23.31	4.61–117.85	<.001	40.57	9.80–167.92	<.001
<3506 (n = 63)	1			1		

Abbreviations: BMI, body mass index; CR-POPF, clinically relevant postoperative pancreatic fistula; DFAA, drain fluid amylase amount; DFAC, drain fluid amylase concentration; DP, distal pancreatectomy.

CR-POPF after DP. According to the systematic review and meta-analysis by Yang et al,[18] a DFAC-day 1 value ≥1300 U/L was a risk factor for POPF after pancreatectomy. Few studies have reported DFAC-day 3 data in predicting CR-POPF[12,13]. Noji et al[12] showed that a DFAC-day 3 value ≥3000 U/L was the best cutoff value of CR-POPF after pancreaticoenteral anastomosis, and DFAC-day 3 was more useful than DFAC-day 1. In our study, the most reliable predictor of CR-POPF after pancreatectomy was DFAC-day 3, which had the highest area under the ROC curve (AUC) value (0.843; optimal cutoff value 1044 U/L). Thus, the best cutoff value of the DFAC remains unclear, but once identified, it can provide a reference for institution-specific early drain removal strategies.

Even with the same surgery, postoperative drainage output varies from case to case. If the drainage volume is large, including serous ascites, DFAC will be diluted and therefore lowered. Prior to this study, we considered DFAC to be of limited utility because the drainage quantity was not being considered. However, the results of this study revealed DFAC to be more reliable than DFAA as a predictor of CR-POPF after pancreatectomy. One of the reasons for this result was the difference in the drainage volume between the CR-POPF group and the no CR-POPF group. The median drainage volumes on POD 1 and POD 3 were significantly lower in the CR-POPF group than in the no CR-POPF group. The exact reason for this is unclear, but the CR-POPF group was more turbid, and the drainage efficiency by nonsuctioned (gravity) drains may have been low. Leakage of the pancreatic juice potentially elicits local inflammatory changes around the pancreatic stump or pancreatojejunostomy, which is related to the dense adhesion of the surrounding tissue. This may be the cause of the difference in fluid volume between the cases with and those without CR-POPF. On the other hand, Molinari et al[15] reported that there was no significant difference in drainage volume between the POPF group and the no POPF group following pancreatectomy. Further investigation into the drainage volume after pancreatectomy based on the type and method of drainage is needed.

In this study, subgroup analysis of CR-POPF according to the type of pancreatectomy was performed. The cutoff value of DFAC-day 3 after PD was 713 U/L, while the cutoff value of DFAC-day 3 after DP was 3506 U/L. Previous reports have also tended to report higher cutoff values for DP than for PD.[10,12,15,17] Since DP does not include pancreaticoenteral anastomosis, CR-POPF may not develop, even if a biochemical leak occurs. Therefore, the drain removal strategy should be adjusted according to the surgical procedure. The patients with normal DFAC-day1 level after DP may be able to remove the drain within POD 1, because of DP is less likely to have more serious complications than PD.

Although early drain removal following pancreatectomy resulted in a reduction in CR-POPF, most surgeons continued to remove drains late, even when DFAC was low, which was associated with inferior outcomes. Seykora et al[24] reported that the early drain removal (on or before POD 3) rate after DP was only 15.2% in a retrospective cohort study of the American College of Surgeons' National Surgical Quality Improvement Program (ACS-NSQIP) registry. Additionally, DFAC was not assessed in most cases by surgeons who removed drains late. Some surgeons believe they will control POPF and intraabdominal abscess via drain placement following pancreatic resection. However, prolonged drains interfere with adjacent structures and introduce bacteria into sterile pancreatic fluid collection, increasing the incidence of CR-POPF and intraabdominal abscesses. Although both pancreas-related risk factors and perioperative risk factors, including DFAC, should be considered, serous (nonturbid) fluid visible to the naked eye indicates that the drain should be removed as soon as possible. On the other hand, Ohgi et al[25] reported that latent pancreatic fistula (LPF) with initially normal DFAC occurred 10%, and LPF was significantly associated with severe complication and worse outcome after PD.

This study has some limitations that should be mentioned. First, this was a single-center retrospective study, and a propensity score matching analysis was not possible because the number of patients with CR-POPF was too small. However, the strength of this study is that surgical techniques and postoperative management were unified. Second, the cutoff values of DFAC and DFAA were derived from nonsuctioned drains. There were no data on the type of drain suction used after pancreatectomy in our institution. However, Kone et al[26] recently analyzed closed suction vs closed gravity drainage after pancreatectomy in a large sample. They showed that the type of drain is not associated with increased CR-POPF or other postoperative outcomes. In the future, large-series multicenter studies evaluating the clinical impact of DFAC will help to compensate for the limitations of this study.

In conclusion, the results of our study indicate that DFAC is more reliable than DFAA as a predictor of CR-POPF after pancreatectomy. Routine postoperative assessment of DFAC could provide more meticulous follow-up after pancreatectomy. DFAC can indicate the optimal timing of drain removal after pancreatectomy. However, the cutoff value of DFAC may vary slightly between institutions. Therefore, we propose an early drain removal strategy based on institution-specific DFAC values, along with consideration of other risk factors for CR-POPF.

DISCLOSURE

Author Contributions: Fukami designed the study and wrote the initial draft of the article. Sano contributed to interpretation of the data and the critical revision of the article for important intellectual content. All the other authors (TS, TO, TH, TK, SK, TM, SK, and KK) contributed to the data collection and interpretation and critically reviewed the article. All the authors have read and approved the final version of the article and have agreed to be accountable for all aspects of the study, ensuring that any questions related to the accuracy or integrity of any part of the work are resolved.

REFERENCES

1. Andrianello S, Marchegiani G, Malleo G, Masini G, Balduzzi A, Paiella S, et al. Pancreaticojejunostomy with externalized stent vs pancreaticogastrostomy with externalized stent for patients with high-risk pancreatic anastomosis: a single-center, phase 3, randomized clinical trial. JAMA Surg. 2020;155:313–21.
2. Zhang H, Zhu F, Shen M, Tian R, Shi CJ, Wang X, et al. Systematic review and meta-analysis comparing three techniques for pancreatic remnant closure following distal pancreatectomy. Br J Surg. 2015;102:4–15.
3. Kawai M, Tani M, Terasawa H, Ina S, Hirono S, Nishioka R, et al. Early removal of prophylactic drains reduces the risk of intra-abdominal infections in patients with pancreatic head resection: prospective study for 104 consecutive patients. Ann Surg. 2006;244:1–7.
4. Xiong JJ, Tan CL, Szatmary P, Huang W, Ke NW, Hu WM, et al. Meta-analysis of pancreaticogastrostomy versus pancreaticojejunostomy after pancreaticoduodenectomy. Br J Surg. 2014;101:1196–208.
5. Bassi C, Dervenis C, Butturini G, Fingerhut A, Yeo C, Izbicki J, et al. Postoperative pancreatic fistula: an international study group (ISGPF) definition. Surgery. 2005;138:8–13.
6. Bassi C, Marchegiani G, Dervenis C, Sarr M, Abu Hilal M, Adham M, et al. The 2016 update of the International Study Group (ISGPS) definition and grading of postoperative pancreatic fistula: 11 years after. Surgery. 2017;161:584–91.
7. Gaujoux S, Cortes A, Couvelard A, Noullet S, Clavel L, Rebours V, et al. Fatty pancreas and increased body mass index are risk factors of pancreatic fistula after pancreaticoduodenectomy. Surgery. 2010;148:15–23.
8. Mathur A, Pitt HA, Marine M, Saxena R, Schmidt CM, Howard TJ, et al. Fatty pancreas: a factor in postoperative pancreatic fistula. Ann Surg. 2007;246:1058–64.

9. Newhook TE, Vega EA, Vreeland TJ, Prakash L, Dewhurst WL, Bruno ML, et al. Early postoperative drain fluid amylase in risk-stratified patients promotes tailored post-pancreatectomy drain management and potential for accelerated discharge. Surgery. 2020;167:442–7.
10. Maggino L, Malleo G, Bassi C, Allegrini V, Beane JD, Beckman RM, et al. Identification of an optimal cut-off for drain fluid amylase on postoperative day 1 for predicting clinically relevant fistula after distal pancreatectomy: a multi-institutional analysis and external validation. Ann Surg. 2019;269:337–43.
11. Giglio MC, Spalding DR, Giakoustidis A, Zarzavadjian Le Bian A, Jiao LR, Habib NA, et al. Meta-analysis of drain amylase content on postoperative day 1 as a predictor of pancreatic fistula following pancreatic resection. Br J Surg. 2016;103:328–36.
12. Noji T, Nakamura T, Ambo Y, Suzuki O, Nakamura F, Kishida A, et al. Clinically relevant pancreas-related infectious complication after pancreaticoenteral anastomosis could be predicted by the parameters obtained on postoperative day 3. Pancreas. 2012;41:916–21.
13. Kanda M, Fujii T, Takami H, Suenaga M, Inokawa Y, Yamada S, et al. Novel diagnostics for aggravating pancreatic fistulas at the acute phase after pancreatectomy. World J Gastroenterol. 2014;20:8535–44.
14. Mintziras I, Maurer E, Kanngiesser V, Bartsch DK. C-reactive protein and drain amylase accurately predict clinically relevant pancreatic fistula after partial pancreaticoduodenectomy. Int J Surg. 2020;76:53–8.
15. Molinari E, Bassi C, Salvia R, Butturini G, Crippa S, Talamini G, et al. Amylase value in drains after pancreatic resection as predictive factor of postoperative pancreatic fistula: results of a prospective study in 137 patients. Ann Surg. 2007;246:281–7.
16. Shinchi H, Wada K, Traverso LW. The usefulness of drain data to identify a clinically relevant pancreatic anastomotic leak after pancreaticoduodenectomy? J Gastrointest Surg. 2006;10:490–8.
17. Ansorge C, Nordin JZ, Lundell L, Strömmer L, Rangelova E, Blomberg J, et al. Diagnostic value of abdominal drainage in individual risk assessment of pancreatic fistula following pancreaticoduodenectomy. Br J Surg. 2014;101:100–8.
18. Yang J, Huang Q, Wang C. Postoperative drain amylase predicts pancreatic fistula in pancreatic surgery: a systematic review and meta-analysis. Int J Surg. 2015;22:38–45.
19. Grobmyer SR, Kooby D, Blumgart LH, Hochwald SN. Novel pancreaticojejunostomy with a low rate of anastomotic failure-related complications. J Am Coll Surg. 2010;210:54–9.
20. Fujii T, Sugimoto H, Yamada S, Kanda M, Suenaga M, Takami H, et al. Modified Blumgart anastomosis for pancreaticojejunostomy: technical improvement in matched historical control study. J Gastrointest Surg. 2014;18:1108–15.
21. Koch M, Garden OJ, Padbury R, Rahbari NN, Adam R, Capussotti L, et al. Bile leakage after hepatobiliary and pancreatic surgery: a definition and grading of severity by the International Study Group of Liver Surgery. Surgery. 2011;149:680–8.
22. Wente MN, Veit JA, Bassi C, Dervenis C, Fingerhut A, Gouma DJ, et al. Postpancreatectomy hemorrhage (PPH): an International Study Group of Pancreatic Surgery (ISGPS) definition. Surgery. 2007;142:20–5.
23. Wente MN, Bassi C, Dervenis C, Fingerhut A, Gouma DJ, Izbicki JR, et al. Delayed gastric emptying (DGE) after pancreatic surgery: a suggested definition by the International Study Group of Pancreatic Surgery (ISGPS). Surgery. 2007;142:761–8.
24. Seykora TF, Liu JB, Maggino L, Pitt HA, Vollmer CM Jr. Drain management following distal pancreatectomy: characterization of contemporary practice and impact of early removal. Ann Surg. 2020;272:1110–7.
25. Ohgi K, Yamamoto Y, Sugiura T, Okamura Y, Ito T, Ashida R, et al. The clinical impact and risk factors of latent pancreatic fistula after pancreatoduodenectomy. J Hepatobiliary Pancreat Sci. 2020;27:1002–10.
26. Kone LB, Maker VK, Banulescu M, Maker AV. Should drains suck? A propensity score analysis of closed-suction versus closed-gravity drainage after pancreatectomy. J Gastrointest Surg. 2020. https://doi.org/10.1007/s11605-020-04613-7. Online ahead of print. PMID: 32394123

21

Overall survival after recurrence in stage I–III colorectal cancer patients in accordance with the recurrence organ site and pattern

Hiroshi Sawayama[1] | Yuji Miyamoto[1] | Yukiharu Hiyoshi[2] | Katsuhiro Ogawa[1] | Rikako Kato[1] | Takahiko Akiyama[1] | Yuki Kiyozumi[2] | Naoya Yoshida[1] | Hideo Baba[1]

[1]Department of Gastroenterological Surgery, Graduate School of Medical Sciences, Kumamoto University, Kumamoto, Japan

[2]Department of Gastroenterological Surgery, Cancer Institute Hospital of Japanese Foundation for Cancer Research, Tokyo, Japan

Correspondence
Hideo Baba, Department of Gastroenterological Surgery, Graduate School of Medical Sciences, Kumamoto University, 1-1-1, Honjo, Chuo-ku, Kumamoto 860-8556, Japan.
Email: hdobaba@kumamoto-u.ac.jp

Abstract

Aim: This study aimed to investigate the prognosis after recurrence in patients with stage I–III colon cancer (CC) and rectal cancer (RC).

Methods: Cancer recurred in 116 (15.2%) out of 763 patients with stage I–III colorectal cancer. The overall survival (OS) after recurrence was evaluated based on the recurrence organs and patterns.

Results: The first recurrence occurred in the lungs, livers, lymph nodes, and other sites in 32, 22, 12, and 2 patients, respectively. It was localized, disseminated, and involved two or more organs in 14, 9, and 25 patients, respectively. Patients with CC had a shorter OS after recurrence as compared to those with RC ($P = .0103$). Compared to other organ metastasis, liver metastasis was associated with an earlier recurrence ($P = .0026$) and shorter OS after recurrence (hazard ratio [HR]: 2.216; 95% confidence interval [CI]: 1.052–4.459; $P = .0370$). Lung metastasis was associated with a more favorable prognosis as compared to other organ recurrences (HR: 0.338; 95% CI: 0.135–0.741; $P = .0057$). One-organ recurrence and oligometastasis were observed in 78.4% and 49.1% of the patients, respectively. The 5-y OS rates of patients with one-organ recurrence and oligometastasis were 47.5% and 71.7%, respectively. Invasive treatment was associated with a favorable prognosis ($P < .0001$).

Conclusions: Liver metastasis and dissemination were associated with a shorter OS after recurrence. Approximately 50% of the patients experienced oligometastasis, which was associated with a favorable prognosis. Hence, to improve patient prognosis it is better to perform invasive treatments when possible.

KEYWORDS
colorectal cancer, oligometastasis, prognosis, recurrence organ, recurrence pattern

1 | INTRODUCTION

Colorectal cancer (CRC) is the second and third most commonly diagnosed malignancy in women and men worldwide, respectively.[1] Recurrence has been observed in 18.7% of the patients with stage I–III CRC; the recurrence organ was reportedly associated with the primary lesion in accordance with the Japanese Society for Cancer of the Colon and Rectum guidelines. Patients with colon cancer (CC) reportedly experienced peritoneal metastasis more frequently as compared to those with rectal cancer (RC). Conversely, patients with RC reportedly experienced lung metastasis and local recurrence more frequently as compared to those with CC. Patients with stage II–III CRC experienced an earlier recurrence as compared to those with stage I CRC. The cumulative incidence of recurrence, accordance to the recurrence site, was demonstrated in a previous study[2]; however, there was no evidence of an association between the recurrence organ site and pattern and the overall survival (OS) after recurrence.[3]

In a previous study, the OS of patients with stage IV CRC was difficult to estimate based on the metastatic lesions, because the degree of progression of CRC differed in each patient. Various triggers were diagnosed as CRC with distant metastasis, such as stenosis of the primary lesion, bleeding, and detection of fecal occult blood. The metastatic organ sites and number of metastases are known to vary, and the treatment strategy for metastatic lesions differs according to the status of distant metastasis. In our study, patients with stage I–III CRC who underwent surgery were followed up in accordance with the treatment guidelines.[2] Recurrence was diagnosed during the early phase of widespread metastasis. The metastatic organ site and the number of metastases can be estimated with precision using diagnostic imaging.

The concept of oligometastasis was reported by Hellman and Weichselbaum.[4] Sentinel lymph nodes (LN) may be the first site of recurrence from the primary lesion. Metastatic lesions are initially detected in a limited area of a distant organ; they then metastasize to involve multiple organs. Oligometastasis is an intermediate state between localized disease and widespread metastases. There have been a few reports on oligometastasis in CRC.[5] The aim of this retrospective study was to investigate the prognosis of CRC patients with recurrence, in terms of the recurrence organs, recurrence patterns, number of recurrence organs, and treatment for the recurrence sites.

2 | MATERIALS AND METHODS

2.1 | Patients

In this study we included 763 patients with stage I–III CRC who underwent primary resection at the Kumamoto University Hospital between April 2005 and March 2019. These patients were analyzed for the recurrence organ, recurrence pattern, and number of recurrences. The clinical and pathological characteristics of the patients were retrieved from the medical record database to analyze the association between the prognosis and recurrence organs and patterns. Recurrence occurred in 116 of the 763 patients. Hence, 116 patients were available for the analysis of first organ recurrence and survival after recurrence. In this study surgical resection (n = 44), radiofrequency ablation (n = 2), and radiation therapy (n = 5) were considered invasive treatments, while palliative surgery and palliative radiation therapy (n = 6) were not. Therefore, 51 patients underwent invasive treatments. Of the remaining 65 patients, 29 underwent chemotherapy after recurrence in our hospital, 11 underwent neither chemotherapy nor invasive treatment, and 25 were not followed up for chemotherapy in detail. Further, we defined both one-organ recurrence and the presence of fewer than five lesions in the organ as oligometastasis, in accordance with previous studies.[6] Data on the number of lesions in a recurrent organ and on invasive treatment were unavailable for 10 patients with one-organ recurrence and 8 patients, respectively. Hence, these patients were excluded from the analysis of oligometastasis and invasive treatment. Written informed consent was obtained from all patients.

2.2 | Clinicopathological characteristics of the patients

We observed that right-sided CC was proximal to the splenic flexure and left-sided CC was distal to the splenic flexure, without the involvement of the rectum; this was in accordance with recent reports.[7] Tumor location was classified in accordance with the Japanese classification of colorectal, appendiceal, and anal carcinoma.[8] Therefore, the rectal sigmoid (defined as the segment from the height of the sacral promontory to the inferior border of the second sacral vertebra) was considered the rectum. Clinical data, including age, sex, body mass index, TNM stage, preoperative carcinoembryonic antigen titer, and preoperative carbohydrate antigen 19-9 titer, were retrospectively available for 116 patients. The cutoff value for each was based on the recommendations of the measuring kits adopted by our institute.

2.3 | Treatment strategy and follow-up evaluation

The treatment strategy and follow-up evaluation were in accordance with the Japanese colorectal cancer guidelines. Primary resection with LN dissection was recommended for Stage I–III CRC. Of the 116 patients, 3 (2.6%), 17 (14.6%), and 96 (82.8%) patients underwent D1, D2, and D3 LN dissection, respectively. After the surgery, the patients were followed up at 3-mo intervals. Recurrence was confirmed by clinical examinations including computed tomography (CT). Tumor marker levels were measured every 3 mo, and CT scanning studies from the neck to the pelvis were performed at least twice a year for 5 y after the surgery.

2.4 | Adjuvant chemotherapy

For adjuvant chemotherapy, stage III and high-risk stage II patients received monotherapy (UFT/UZEL, Capecitabine or S-1) or doublet therapy (CAPOX or SOX regimen) for 3–6 mo. None of the 10 stage I patients received adjuvant chemotherapy. Of the 40 stage II patients, four (10%) and one (2.5%) patients received monotherapy and doublet therapy, respectively. Furthermore, of the 66 stage III patients, 20 (30.3%) and 19 (28.8%) patients received monotherapy and doublet therapy, respectively. In the case of eight patients, it was unclear whether they received adjuvant chemotherapy or not.

2.5 | Statistical analyses

The relationship between primary lesions and the clinicopathological characteristics of the patients was determined using the chi-squared test. Mortality was estimated using the recurrence rate and the OS after recurrence. The Wilcoxon signed-rank test was used to evaluate early recurrence. The log-rank test and univariate Cox proportional hazard regression analysis were used to analyze the OS, and the Kaplan–Meier estimator was used to assess the distribution of survival time. All *P* values were two-sided, and statistical significance was set at $P < .05$. The results are presented as hazard ratios (HRs) and 95% confidence intervals (CIs). All data were processed and analyzed using the JMP 11 software (SAS Institute, Cary, NC).

3 | RESULTS

3.1 | Incidence of recurrence and overall survival

A total of 763 patients underwent surgery for stage I–III CRC. Over a median follow-up of 36.4 mo, 116 (15.2%) cases experienced recurrence. The incidence of recurrence varied according to the site of the primary lesion. Recurrence was detected in 11.0% (26/236), 13.3% (33/248), and 20.4% (57/279) of the patients with right-sided primary lesions, left-sided primary lesions, and primary lesions in the rectum, respectively. The recurrence rates in stage I, stage II, and stage III patients were 3.7% (10/267), 14.9% (40/268), and 28.9% (66/228), respectively. The 5-y OS rate in all 763 patients was 81.9%.

3.2 | Association between tumor location and prognosis

A total of 488 patients (64.0%) had CC (right-sided: 247 [32.4%], left-sided: 241 [31.6%]), while 275 patients (36.0%) had RC. Univariate analysis revealed that RC was significantly associated with a younger age ($P < .0001$), advanced tumor stage ($P = .0031$), and the presence of LN metastasis ($P = .0007$) (Table S1). The 5-y recurrence rate was higher in patients with RC (23.3%) than in patients with CC (14.1%) ($P = .0018$; Figure S1A and Table S2). However, the 5-y OS tended to be longer in patients with RC (84.3%) than in those with CC (80.6%) ($P = .0652$; Figure S1B and Table S3). Multivariate analysis also revealed that the recurrence rate was higher in patients with RC than in those with CC (Table S2); however, no significant differences in the OS rate were noted between patients with RC and CC (Table S3).

3.3 | Recurrence organs and survival according to the primary tumor location

The 116 patients with recurrence were evaluated on the basis of the primary tumor location and recurrence organ sites. Patients with recurrent RC were significantly younger than those with recurrent right- or left-sided CC ($P = .0245$). Other clinicopathological characteristics were not associated with the primary lesion location (Table 1). Patients with right- or left-sided CC had an earlier recurrence (Wilcoxon test, $P = .0489$) and a shorter OS after recurrence ($P = .0103$) as compared to those with RC (Figure 1). The first recurrence occurred at one site in 91 cases (78.4%), two sites in 20 cases (17.2%), three sites in three cases (2.6%), and four sites in two cases (1.7%) (Table 2). The recurrence organ site was more frequently localized in RC ($P = .0408$) as compared to in right- or left-sided CC, and tended to accompany lung recurrence when the patients had two or more organ recurrences ($P = .0618$). The liver was the more frequent recurrence organ site in right- or left-sided CC ($P = .0313$) as compared to in RC, and was accompanied by dissemination when the patients had two or more organ recurrences ($P = .0073$; Table 3 and Table S4).

3.4 | Evaluation of the association between recurrence organ site and survival

Liver, as the first recurrence site, was associated with an earlier recurrence after surgery as compared to other organ recurrences ($P = .0026$); local recurrence was detected later than other organ recurrences ($P = .0536$; Figure 2). Compared to the absence of liver metastasis, the presence of liver metastasis as the first recurrence was associated with a shorter OS after recurrence (HR: 2.216; 95% CI: 1.052–4.459; $P = .0370$). Compared to the absence of lung metastasis, the presence of lung metastasis as the first recurrence was associated with a longer OS after recurrence (HR: 0.338; 95% CI: 0.135–0.741; $P = .0057$; Figure 3). Of the 17 disseminations noted, eight (47.1%) were accompanied by other organ recurrences, and recurrences with accompanying dissemination were associated with a shorter OS after recurrence as compared to those without dissemination (HR: 2.962; 95% CI: 1.381–5.805; $P = .0069$; Figure S2).

3.5 | Prognosis according to the recurrence patterns, invasive treatments, and adjuvant chemotherapy after primary resection

The difference in the number of recurrence organ sites between right- or left-sided CC and RC was not determined ($P = .5853$), but

TABLE 1 Association between the primary lesion and clinicopathological factors

Factors	Total N	Colon N = 59	[R/L]		Rectum N = 57		P-value
Age							
≤70	61	25	[13/12]	(42.4%)	36	(63.2%)	.0245[a]
>70	55	34	[22/12]	(57.6%)	21	(36.8%)	
Gender							
Male	56	27	[13/14]	(45.8%)	29	(50.9%)	.5815
Female	60	32	[22/10]	(54.2%)	28	(49.1%)	
Body mass index							
<18.5	18	11	[8/3]	(18.6%)	7	(12.3%)	.6326
18.5-25	74	36	[19/17]	(61.0%)	38	(66.7%)	
>25	24	12	[8/4]	(20.3%)	12	(21.1%)	
CEA							
≤3.4	47	21	[13/8]	(35.6%)	26	(45.6%)	.2714
>3.4	69	38	[22/16]	(64.4%)	31	(54.4%)	
CA19-9							
≤37	92	44	[24/20]	(74.6%)	48	(84.2%)	.1982
>37	24	15	[11/4]	(25.4%)	9	(15.8%)	
Stage							
I	10	6	[3/3]	(10.2%)	4	(7.0%)	.5055
II	40	18	[5/13]	(30.5%)	22	(38.6%)	
III	66	35	[25/10]	(59.3%)	31	(54.4%)	
ASA performance status							
1-2	86	42	[23/19]	(71.2%)	44	(77.2%)	.5107
3-	19	11	[8/3]	(18.6%)	8	(14.0%)	
Unknown	11	6	[2/4]	(59.3%)	5	(8.8%)	
Adjuvant chemotherapy							
None	64	34	[16/18]	(57.6%)	30	(52.6%)	.5899
Monotherapy	24	12	[8/4]	(20.3%)	12	(21.1%)	
Doublet therapy	20	8	[6/2]	(13.6%)	12	(21.1%)	
Unknown	8	5	[3/2]	(8.5%)	3	(5.3%)	
Palliative chemotherapy							
None	32	19	[9/10]	(32.2%)	13	(22.8%)	0.2076
Done	53	21	[13/8]	(35.6%)	32	(56.1%)	
Unknown	31	19	[11/8]	(32.2%)	12	(21.1%)	

Abbreviations: ASA, American Society of Anesthetists; CA19-9, carbohydrate antigen 19-9; CEA, carcinoembryonic antigen; L, left-sided colon; R, right-sided colon.
[a]Significant difference.

oligometastasis was observed more frequently in cases of RC than in those of right-or left-sided CC ($P = .0513$; Figure 4A,B). Patients with recurrence in multiple-organ sites were associated with a shorter OS after recurrence as compared to those with recurrence in one-organ sites (HR: 3.084; 95% CI: 1.597–5.707; $P = .0012$). Further, compared to those with oligometastasis, patients with multiple-organ site metastasis were also associated with a shorter OS after recurrence (HR: 7.373; 95% CI: 3.608–16.360; $P < .0001$). The 5-y OS rates of the patients with one recurrent organ site and oligometastasis were 47.5% and 71.7%, respectively (Figure 5A,B).

Invasive treatments tended to be performed more frequently for metastatic lesions in RC than for those in right-or left-sided CC ($P = .0658$), (Figure 4C). Patients who underwent invasive treatment for metastatic lesions had a longer OS after recurrence as compared to those who did not (HR: 0.184; 95% CI: 0.090–0.353; $P < .0001$; Figure 5C). A significant relationship between surgical procedures and prognosis was shown ($P <.0001$; Figure 5D).

The 5-y OS after recurrence in patients who underwent invasive treatment was 71.9%. The median survival time in patients who

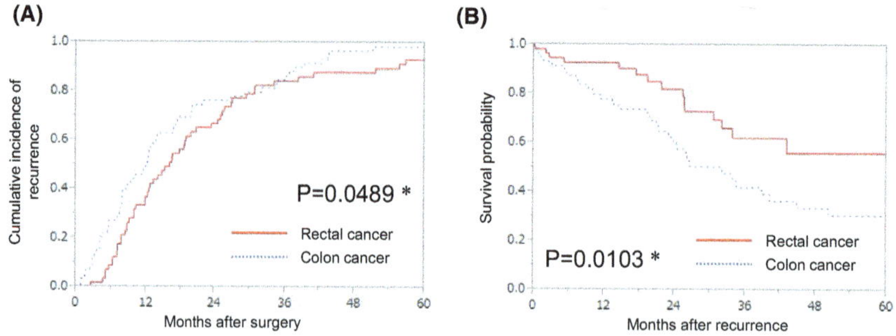

FIGURE 1 Recurrence rate and survival after recurrence according to the primary lesion. Kaplan–Meier survival curve for the recurrence rate (*P* value was estimated using the Wilcoxon signed-rank test) (A). Kaplan–Meier curve for the overall survival after recurrence (*P* value was estimated using the log-rank test) (B). *Statistically significant

TABLE 2 Number of recurrence organ sites in accordance with primary lesion

Number of recurrence organ sites	Total N = 116		Colon N = 59	[R/L]		Rectum N = 57		*P*-value
One	91	(78.4%)	44	[24/20]	(74.6%)	47	(82.5%)	
Two	20	(17.2%)	12	[8/4]	(20.3%)	8	(14.0%)	.5401
Three or more	5	(4.3%)	3	[3/0]	(5.1%)	2	(3.5%)	

Abbreviations: L, left-sided colon; R, right-sided colon.

TABLE 3 Association between primary lesion and recurrence organ site

Recurrence organ	Total N = 91	Colon N = 44	[R/L]		Rectum N = 47		*P*-value
Lung							
Present	32	13	[7/6]	(29.5%)	19	(40.4%)	.2763
Absent	59	31	[17/14]	(70.5%)	28	(59.6%)	
Liver							
Present	22	15	[8/7]	(34.1%)	7	(14.9%)	.0313[a]
Absent	69	29	[16/13]	(65.9%)	40	(85.1%)	
Local recurrence							
Present	14	3	[0/3]	(6.8%)	11	(23.4%)	.0408[a,b]
Absent	77	41	[24/17]	(93.2%)	36	(76.6%)	
Lymph node							
Present	12	6	[4/2]	(13.6%)	6	(12.8%)	.9024
Absent	79	38	[20/18]	(86.4%)	41	(87.2%)	
Dissemination							
Present	9	7	[5/2]	(15.9%)	2	(4.3%)	.0838[b]
Absent	82	37	[19/18]	(84.1%)	45	(95.7%)	
Other organ							
Present	2	0	[0/0]	(0.0%)	2	(4.3%)	.4950[b]
Absent	89	44	[24/20]	(100.0%)	45	(95.7%)	

Abbreviations: L, left-sided colon; R, right-sided colon.

[a]Statistically significant.

[b]Fisher's exact test.

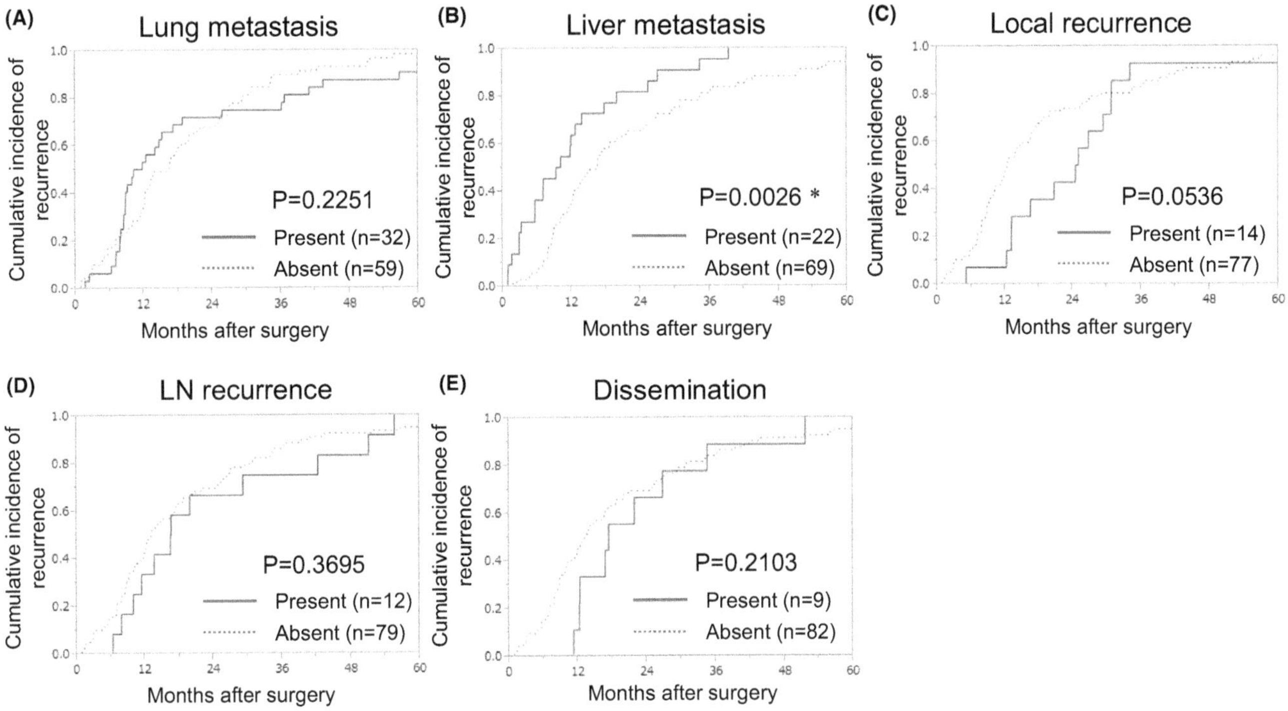

FIGURE 2 Recurrence rate according to the first recurrence organ (*P* value was estimated using the Wilcoxon signed-rank test). Lung metastasis (A), liver metastasis (B), local recurrence (C), LN recurrence (D), and dissemination (E). LN, lymph node. *Statistically significant

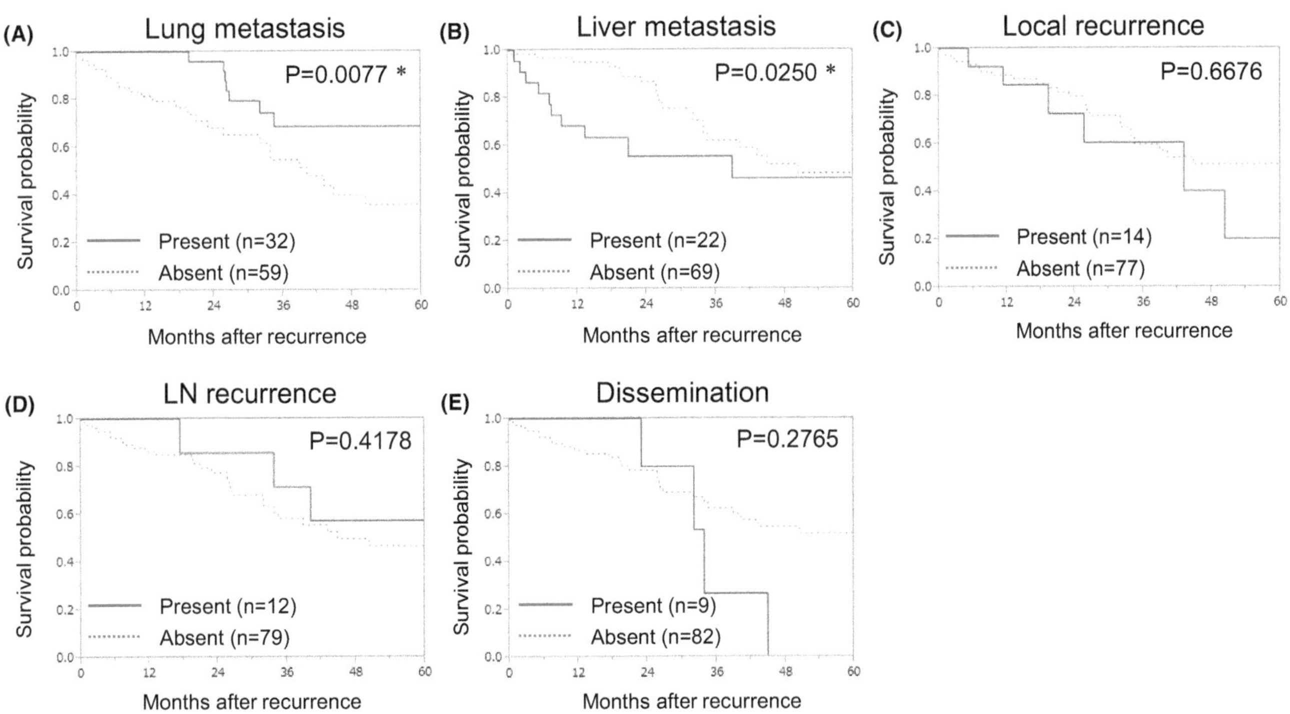

FIGURE 3 Overall survival after recurrence according to the first recurrence organ (*P* value was estimated using the log-rank test). Lung metastasis (A), liver metastasis (B), local recurrence (C), LN recurrence (D), and dissemination (E). LN, lymph node. *Statistically significant

underwent chemotherapy without invasive treatment was 24.3 mo and in patients who underwent neither invasive treatment nor chemotherapy was 8.6 mo (Figure S3).

The relationship between survival after recurrence and adjuvant chemotherapy after primary lesion resection was analyzed. Stage III patients who received adjuvant chemotherapy had a longer OS

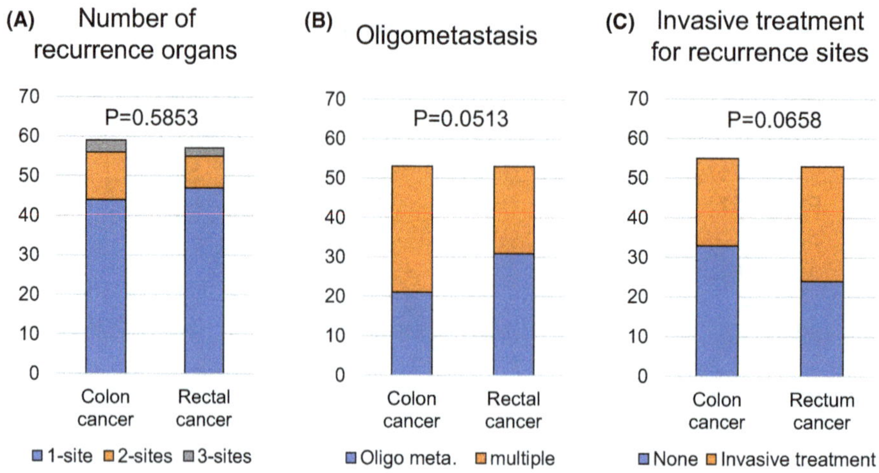

FIGURE 4 The number of patients according to the primary lesion. The number of recurrence organs (n = 116) (A), oligometastasis (n = 106; data on the number of lesions in a recurrent organ were unavailable for 10 patients with one-organ recurrence) (B), and invasive treatment for recurrence sites (n = 108; data on invasive treatment were unavailable for eight patients) (C). Meta., metastasis

FIGURE 5 Kaplan–Meier survival curve according to the number of recurrence organs (n = 116) (A), oligometastasis (n = 106; data on the number of lesions in a recurrent organ were unavailable for 10 patients with one-organ recurrence) (B), invasive treatment for recurrence sites (n = 108; data on invasive treatment were unavailable for eight patients) (C), and treatment procedures (n = 108) (D). *Statistically significant

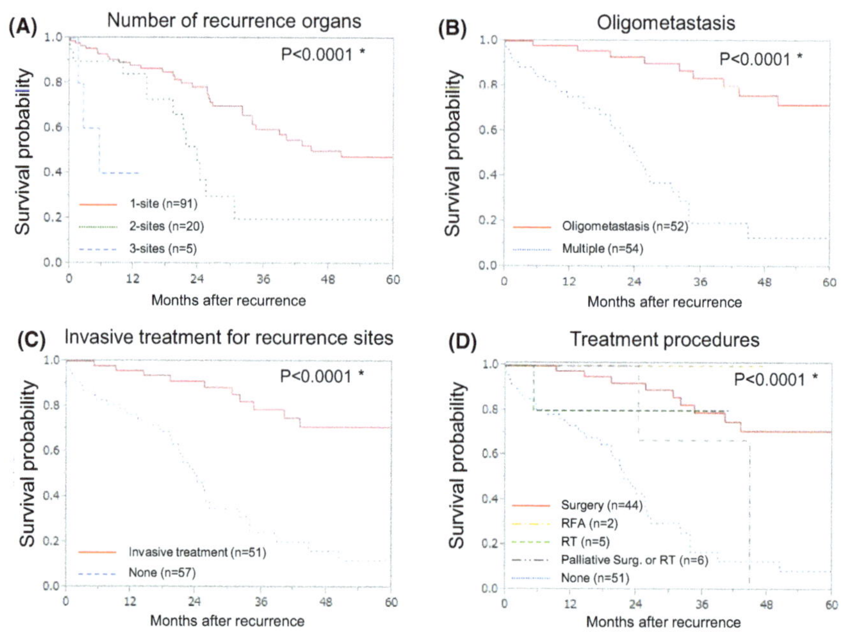

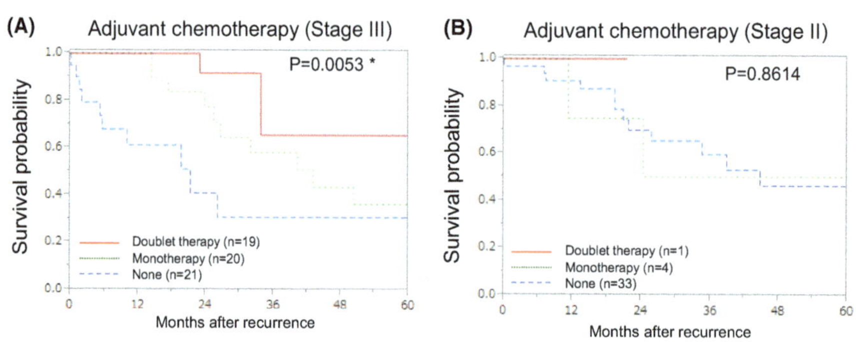

FIGURE 6 Kaplan–Meier survival curve according to adjuvant chemotherapy. Adjuvant chemotherapy for stage III patients (n = 60; data on adjuvant chemotherapy were unavailable for six patients) (A), adjuvant chemotherapy for Stage II patients (B) (n = 38; data on adjuvant chemotherapy were unavailable for two patients). *Statistically significant

TABLE 4 Invasive treatment for recurrence in accordance with recurrence organ site

	Total	Initial treatment	Secondary treatment							Third treatment						
Rec. Organ	N	N	N	Liver	Lung	Local	LN	Diss.	Other	N	Liver	Lung	Local	LN	Diss.	Other
Lung	32	20 (62.5%)	10 (31.3%)	0	9	1	0	0	0	2 (6.3%)	0	1	1	0	0	0
Liver	22	11 (50.0%)	5 (22.7%)	3	2	0	0	0	0	1 (4.5%)	0	0	1	0	0	0
Local	14	9 (64.3%)	1 (7.1%)	0	1	0	0	0	0	1 (7.1%)	0	0	1	0	0	0
LN	12	5 (41.7%)	2 (16.7%)	1	0	0	1	0	0	0 (0.0%)	0	0	0	0	0	0
Diss.	9	1 (11.1%)	1 (11.1%)	0	1	0	0	0	0	0 (0.0%)	0	0	0	0	0	0
Site ≥ 2	25	3 (12.0%)	0 (0.0%)	0	0	0	0	0	0	0 (0.0%)	0	0	0	0	0	0

Note: Two patients were other site recurrence.

Abbreviations: diss., dissemination; LN, lymph node.

after recurrence as compared to stage III patients who did not receive adjuvant chemotherapy (P = .0053; Figure 6A). Survival after recurrence in Stage II patients did not differ with respect to adjuvant chemotherapy administration (Figure 6B).

3.6 | Invasive treatments according to the recurrence organ

Invasive treatments for recurrence sites and the recurrence patterns after invasive treatment were evaluated according to the recurrence organ. Of the 14 patients with local recurrence, nine (64.3%) underwent an initial invasive treatment; one of these underwent a secondary invasive treatment for the lungs. Of the 32 patients with lung recurrence, 20 (62.5%) underwent invasive treatment and 10 (31.3%) underwent secondary treatment for re-recurrence. Of these 10 patients, nine were treated for lung metastasis. Lung recurrence can be managed using several invasive treatments (Table 4), but recurrence accompanied by dissemination is difficult to treat, and only one patient underwent invasive treatment for this in our study (Table S5).

4 | DISCUSSION

In this study the OS after recurrence in stage I–III CRC was evaluated with respect to the recurrence sites and patterns. Patients with recurrent RC had a longer OS after recurrence as compared to those with recurrent CC. The first recurrence of CC was more frequent in the liver as compared to that of RC and was accompanied by dissemination. However, liver metastasis and dissemination were associated with a poor prognosis after recurrence, and hence, treatment for recurrent lesions may focus on controlling tumor progression in the organs. On appropriate follow-up, 50% of the recurrences were found to be oligometastases, which had favorable prognoses. Hence, for patients with oligometastasis, it is better to perform an aggressive treatment when possible.

The prognosis after recurrence of CRC was reported with respect to the primary lesions, stage at the primary surgery, and organ recurrence. O'Connell et al[9] reported that the OS after recurrence was shorter in stage III CRC than in stage II CRC and that early recurrence was associated with a more unfavorable prognosis as compared to late recurrence. With respect to the primary lesion, the interval until recurrence was longer in cases of RC (26.0 ± 24.2 mo) as compared to in cases of CC (17.1 ± 11.0 mo; P = .03).[10] Pugh et al[3] also reported the prognosis after recurrence with respect to the stage of primary lesion, site of primary lesion, and site of recurrence; they found that an initial stage (P = .005) and the site of primary lesion influenced post-recurrence survival. The results of our study were similar to those of previous studies with respect to the prognosis after recurrence and the primary location; however, the association between OS after recurrence and the first recurrence organ observed in our study offers a new insight. Local recurrence and lung metastasis are usually associated with RC. These recurrence patterns are likely due to the invasive and secondary treatments administered for re-recurrence. Invasive treatments for local recurrence and lung metastasis may lead to a favorable prognosis for recurrent RC.

The prognosis after treatment of a recurrent organ, with respect to a metastatic lesion, has been reported previously. In previous meta-analyses, the 5-y OS rate following liver resection was approximately 38% (median survival: 3.6 y)[11]; it was 27%–68% after complete resection of lung metastasis[12] and 36.4% after R0 resection for metachronous peritoneal metastasis.[13] The risk factors associated with organ recurrence were also reported in these articles; however, the prognosis in relation to the first recurrence organ was not clear. We demonstrated that the OS after recurrence differed with the first organ recurrence. The prognosis of lung metastasis recurrence was favorable, and that of liver metastasis recurrence and accompanying dissemination was unfavorable. These data indicate that liver metastasis and dissemination may require the development of a more effective novel treatment strategy. Twelve patients experienced distant LN recurrence, 10 and 8 of which underwent D3 LN dissection and adjuvant chemotherapy, respectively. Biomarkers for predicting distant LN recurrence and a novel treatment strategy may be required for reducing LN recurrence. In a previous study, out of 119 recurrences, 93 (78%) involved a single organ and 26 (22%) involved multiple organs.[14] These data were also similar to the data in our study with respect to the number of first recurrence organs. The interval from surgery to recurrence may be associated with first organ recurrence. In our study, liver metastasis occurred at an earlier stage as compared to other metastases. Roth et al[15] reported that none of the patients had bone metastasis as the first metastatic lesion. Metastasis of CRC may occur in a limited area of an organ and then progress to various other organs.

We also evaluated the number of recurrences and the status of oligometastasis. Oligometastasis was a state of limited metastatic lesions. Treatment for all known metastatic lesions may lead to a cure, and further distant progression could be avoided.[16] The impact of invasive treatment for oligometastasis was reported in several randomized controlled trails (RCTs). In one RCT, compared to conventional treatment, stereotactic ablative radiotherapy (SABR) improved the prognosis for solid tumors (median OS [control group vs. SABR group]: 28 mo [95% CI: 19–33 mo] vs. 41 mo [95% CI: 26–not reached]; hazard ratio: 0.57, 95% CI: 0.30–1.10; $P = .090$).[17] The inclusion criteria in this RCT were the presence of controlled primary tumors and up to five metastases. In our study, the primary lesion was resected and we defined both one-organ recurrence and the presence of fewer than five lesions in the organ as oligometastasis. It has been reported that metastasis-directed therapy also improves prognosis of oligometastasis in prostate cancer.[18] In that study, the number of patients with one recurrence organ site and oligometastasis was 91/116 (78.4%) and 52/106 (49.1%), respectively. Half of the patients who experienced recurrence were diagnosed with oligometastasis based on the follow-up guidelines in the study. Furthermore, the 5-y OS rates of the patients with one recurrence organ site and oligometastasis were 47.5% and 71.7%, respectively. The survival curve of patients with oligometastasis was closer to the survival curve of patients with stage III CRC than to the curve of those with stage IV CRC. These data support the use of aggressive treatments in patients with oligometastasis when possible.

This study has some limitations. First, it was a retrospective study, and the treatment strategy employed for the recurrence site was at the personal discretion of our medical team. Second, although we noted treatments performed in accordance with the treatment guidelines, the treatment outcomes differed between the institutions.

In conclusion, we found that with respect to the first recurrence site, liver metastasis was associated with an earlier recurrence in patients with stage I–III CRC. Patients with recurrence in the liver and accompanying dissemination had a shorter OS after recurrence as compared to those with other organ recurrences. Patients with recurrences in the lung had a more favorable prognosis as compared to those with other organ recurrences. The number of metastatic organs and invasive treatments were associated with patient prognosis. Future investigation into treatment strategies with respect to the number and organ of first recurrence may be useful in improving the prognosis of CRC patients after recurrence.

ACKNOWLEDGMENTS

The authors thank Dr. Kenichi Iyama and Yoshiki Mikami for their pathological diagnoses.

REFERENCES

1. Torre LA, Bray F, Siegel RL, Ferlay J, Lortet-Tieulent J, Jemal A. Global cancer statistics, 2012. CA Cancer J Clin. 2015;65(2):87–108.
2. Hashiguchi Y, Muro K, Saito Y, Ito Y, Ajioka Y, Hamaguchi T, et al. Japanese Society for Cancer of the Colon and Rectum (JSCCR) guidelines 2019 for the treatment of colorectal cancer. Int J Clin Oncol. 2020;25(1):1–42.
3. Pugh SA, Shinkins B, Fuller A, Mellor J, Mant D, Primrose JN. Site and stage of colorectal cancer influence the likelihood and distribution of disease recurrence and postrecurrence survival: data from the FACS randomized controlled trial. Ann Surg. 2016;263(6):1143–7.
4. Hellman S, Weichselbaum RR. Oligometastases. J Clin Oncol. 1995;13(1):8–10.
5. Poon I, Erler D, Dagan R, Redmond KJ, Foote M, Badellino S, et al. Evaluation of definitive stereotactic body radiotherapy and outcomes in adults with extracranial oligometastasis. JAMA Netw Open. 2020;3(11):e2026312.
6. Takeda A, Sanuki N, Kunieda E. Role of stereotactic body radiotherapy for oligometastasis from colorectal cancer. World J Gastroenterol. 2014;20(15):4220–9.
7. Holch JW, Ricard I, Stintzing S, Modest DP, Heinemann V. The relevance of primary tumour location in patients with metastatic colorectal cancer: a meta-analysis of first-line clinical trials. Eur J Cancer. 2017;70:87–98.
8. Japanese classification of colorectal, appendiceal, and anal carcinoma: the 3d English Edition [Secondary Publication]. J Anus Rectum Colon. 2019;3(4):175–95.
9. O'Connell MJ, Campbell ME, Goldberg RM, Grothey A, Seitz JF, Benedetti JK, et al. Survival following recurrence in stage II and III colon cancer: findings from the ACCENT data set. J Clin Oncol. 2008;26(14):2336–41.
10. Sadahiro S, Suzuki T, Ishikawa K, Nakamura T, Tanaka Y, Masuda T, et al. Recurrence patterns after curative resection

of colorectal cancer in patients followed for a minimum of ten y. Hepatogastroenterology. 2003;50(53):1362–6.
11. Kanas GP, Taylor A, Primrose JN, Langeberg WJ, Kelsh MA, Mowat FS, et al. Survival after liver resection in metastatic colorectal cancer: review and meta-analysis of prognostic factors. Clin Epidemiol. 2012;4:283–301.
12. Gonzalez M, Poncet A, Combescure C, Robert J, Ris HB, Gervaz P. Risk factors for survival after lung metastasectomy in colorectal cancer patients: a systematic review and meta-analysis. Ann Surg Oncol. 2013;20(2):572–9.
13. Sato H, Maeda K, Kotake K, Sugihara K, Takahashi H. Factors affecting recurrence and prognosis after R0 resection for colorectal cancer with peritoneal metastasis. J Gastroenterol. 2016;51(5): 465–72.
14. Ding P, Liska D, Tang P, Shia J, Saltz L, Goodman K, et al. Pulmonary recurrence predominates after combined modality therapy for rectal cancer: an original retrospective study. Ann Surg. 2012;256(1):111–6.
15. Roth ES, Fetzer DT, Barron BJ, Joseph UA, Gayed IW, Wan DQ. Does colon cancer ever metastasize to bone first? a temporal analysis of colorectal cancer progression. BMC Cancer. 2009;9:274.
16. Palma DA, Louie AV, Rodrigues GB. New strategies in stereotactic radiotherapy for oligometastases. Clin Cancer Res. 2015;21(23):5198–204.
17. Palma DA, Olson R, Harrow S, Gaede S, Louie AV, Haasbeek C, et al. Stereotactic ablative radiotherapy versus standard of care palliative treatment in patients with oligometastatic cancers (SABR-COMET): a randomised, phase 2, open-label trial. Lancet. 2019;393(10185):2051–8.
18. Phillips R, Shi WY, Deek M, Radwan N, Lim SJ, Antonarakis ES, et al. Outcomes of observation vs. stereotactic ablative radiation for oligometastatic prostate cancer: the ORIOLE phase 2 randomized clinical trial. JAMA Oncol. 2020;6(5):650–9.

22

Superiority of laparoscopic liver resection to open liver resection in obese individuals with hepatocellular carcinoma

Atsushi Ishihara[1] | Shogo Tanaka[1] | Hiroji Shinkawa[1] | Hisako Yoshida[2] | Shigekazu Takemura[1] | Ryosuke Amano[1] | Kenjiro Kimura[1] | Go Ohira[1] | Kohei Nishio[1] | Shoji Kubo[1]

[1]Department of Hepato-Biliary-Pancreatic Surgery, Osaka City University Graduate School of Medicine, Osaka, Japan

[2]Department of Medical Statistics, Osaka City University Graduate School of Medicine, Osaka, Japan

Correspondence
Shogo Tanaka, Department of Hepato-Biliary-Pancreatic Surgery, Osaka City University Graduate School of Medicine, 1-4-3 Asahimachi, Abeno-ku, Osaka 545-8585, Japan.
Email: m8827074@msic.med.osaka-cu.ac.jp

Abstract

Aim: This study aimed to elucidate the effects of laparoscopic liver resection (LLR) vs open liver resection (OLR) for major complications (Clavien-Dindo classification grade ≥ IIIa) in obese individuals with hepatocellular carcinoma (HCC).

Methods: The clinical records of 339 and 733 patients who underwent LLR and OLR, respectively, for HCC between 2000 and 2019 were retrospectively reviewed. Body mass index (BMI) groups were classified according to the definitions of the World Health Organization: underweight group, BMI ≤ 18.4 kg/m^2 (LLR vs OLR: 27 vs 47); normal weight, BMI 18.5-24.9 kg/m^2 (211 vs 483); overweight, BMI 25.0-29.9 kg/m^2 (85 vs 181); and obese, BMI ≥ 30.0 kg/m^2 (16 vs 22). The effects of obesity on major complications after LLR and OLR were investigated.

Results: In total, 18 (5.3%) and 127 (17.3%) patients presented with major complications after LLR and OLR, respectively. There was no significant difference in the incidence of major complications after OLR in the four BMI groups. However, a stepwise decrease in the incidence of major complications after LLR was observed from the underweight to the obese group. In addition, a multivariate analysis revealed that increased BMI was an independent preventive factor for major complications after LLR (P = .026, odds ratio: 0.84). The estimated adjusted risk of major postoperative complications decreased with increased BMI in the LLR group, while the risk did not decrease in the OLR group (P for interaction = .048).

Conclusion: Laparoscopic liver resection is beneficial for obese patients and is superior to OLR.

KEYWORDS

body mass index, hepatectomy, laparoscopic liver resection, obesity, postoperative complication

1 | INTRODUCTION

The prevalence of obesity and its associated diseases is still increasing worldwide. The prevalence of obesity (body mass index [BMI] of ≥30 kg/m^2) is 40% in the United States[1] and approximately 20% in Europe.[2] In Japan, obesity is defined by a BMI of ≥25 kg/m^2.[3] As of 2018, 32.2% of men and 21.9% of women of ≥20 years of age were classified as obese.[4] Obesity is correlated with comorbidities and technical difficulties in surgery and is considered a risk factor for postoperative complications in several surgical fields.[5,6] Furthermore, several reports have shown that obese patients are at high risk of developing hepatocellular carcinoma (HCC).[7,8] Thus, a higher prevalence of obesity and expansion of the indications for liver resection could increase the number of liver resection procedures among obese patients with HCC in the future. Obesity is associated with an increased risk of postoperative morbidity in individuals undergoing open liver resection (OLR).[9,10] Recently, laparoscopic liver resection (LLR) has been widely performed and is correlated with low morbidity and mortality.[11,12] However, the superiority of LLR to OLR was not evaluated according to BMI. Thus, previous reports cannot support the efficacy and safety of LLR for obese individuals.[13,14]

The current study investigated the effects of obesity on major complications (≥grade IIIa based on the Clavien-Dindo classification system[15]) after LLR and OLR for HCC based on BMI (from underweight to obese). Moreover, the superiority of LLR to OLR in terms of major postoperative complications based on BMI was evaluated.

2 | MATERIALS AND METHODS

2.1 | Study design and participants

In total, 1072 consecutive patients with HCC who underwent liver resection in our department between January 2000 and December 2019 were included in this study. Patient's height and weight were assessed preoperatively, and BMI was calculated as weight in kilograms (kg) divided by height in meters squared (m^2). The patients were allocated to one of four groups based on BMI, as defined by the World Health Organization[16]: underweight group, BMI of ≤18.4 kg/m^2; normal weight group, 18.5 ≤ BMI ≤ 24.9 kg/m^2; overweight group, 25.0 ≤ BMI ≤ 29.9 kg/m^2; and obesity group, BMI of ≥30.0 kg/m^2. The local institutional review board of our institution approved this study (registration no. 1646).

2.2 | Surgical procedure

In total, 923 and 149 patients who underwent their first and second hepatic procedure, respectively, were included in the analysis. LLR was performed on 339 patients (LLR group) and OLR on 733 patients (OLR group). As described in our previous study on OLR,[17] in most patients who underwent segmentectomy or more, after Glissonean sheath transection or clamping, an ultrasonic surgical aspirator was used for hepatic dissection during total or unilateral clamping of the hepatic vascular inflow. In the majority of patients who underwent partial hepatic resection, as resection of less than a segmentectomy, an ultrasonic surgical aspirator and bipolar or monopolar forceps was utilized for hepatic dissection with the Pringle maneuver. The major branches of the Glissonean sheath and the hepatic vein were sutured using non-absorbent sutures. Patients who underwent LLR were placed in supine or left-lateral decubitus position and on an average five trocars according to tumor location were used. Hepatic transection was performed using a laparoscopic ultrasonic surgical aspirator and a vessel sealing system with soft coagulation.[18] In general, the Pringle maneuver was applied. Hand-assisted laparoscopy, or the so-called hybrid procedure or laparoscopy-assisted resection, was performed on patients with tumors that are challenging to evaluate via pure laparoscopy due to limited visualization and heavy bleeding. In this study, LLR was defined as all laparoscopic surgeries. Further, the surgical procedures were classified into partial resection, segmentectomy, sectionectomy, and resection of two or more sections according to the Brisbane 2000 Terminology of Liver Anatomy and Resections.[19]

2.3 | Indication for laparoscopic liver resection

We performed LLR for ≤5-cm solitary lesions located in the peripheral liver segments 2-6 according to the Louisville consensus.[20] Thereafter, we extended the indication for more difficult procedures including major hepatectomy. However, LLR was selected according to tumor location, types of operative procedures, tumor size, proximity to major vessels, and liver function.

2.4 | Clinicopathological characteristics and surgical outcomes

The clinical data of all patients were collected prospectively, as shown in Table 1. The date of follow-up was on March 31, 2020.

2.5 | Definitions

Patients were diagnosed with diabetes mellitus (DM), hypertension, and dyslipidemia according to the guidelines of the Japan Diabetes Society,[21] Japanese Society of Hypertension,[22] and Japan Atherosclerosis Society,[23] respectively. DM was defined as a fasting plasma glucose level of ≥126 mg/dL, hemoglobin A1c level of ≥6.5%, or need for hypoglycemic drugs or insulin. Hypertension was defined as a systolic blood pressure of ≥140 mmHg, diastolic blood pressure of ≥90 mmHg, or need for antihypertensive drugs. Dyslipidemia was defined as a serum low-density lipoprotein cholesterol level of ≥140 mg/dL, high-density lipoprotein cholesterol level of <40 mg/dL, and/or triglyceride level of ≥150 mg/dL or a need for

TABLE 1 Clinicopathological characteristics and surgical outcomes of laparoscopic and open liver resection in patients with hepatocellular carcinoma (n = 1072)

Variables	Study cohort (n = 1072)	Laparoscopic liver resection group (n = 339)	Open liver resection group (n = 733)	P value
BMI, kg/m^2; median (range)	23.2 (12.4-40.2)	23.6 (12.4-40.2)	23.0 (15.0-38.2)	.080
BMI groups, underweight/normal/ overweight/obesity, n	74/694/266/38	27/211/85/16	47/483/181/22	.357
Age, years; median (range)	69 (19-87)	70 (21-87)	69 (19-87)	.288
Sex, male/female, n	832/240	242/97	590/143	.001
Comorbidities and/or previous medical history, n (%)				
Diabetes mellitus	351 (32.7)	121 (35.7)	230 (31.4)	.162
Hypertension	525 (49.9)	183 (54.0)	342 (46.7)	.026
Dyslipidemia	196 (18.3)	79 (23.3)	117 (16.0)	.004
Ischemic heart diseases	51 (4.8)	15 (4.4)	36 (4.9)	.728
Alcohol abuse (≥60 g/d), n (%)	317 (29.6)	109 (32.2)	317 (43.2)	.208
Underlying hepatic disease, n (%)				
HBV	177 (16.5)	66 (19.5)	111 (15.1)	.248
HCV	572 (53.4)	180 (53.1)	392 (53.5)	
HBV + HCV	11 (1.0)	4 (1.2)	7 (0.9)	
Non-B, non-C	310 (28.9)	89 (26.3)	223 (30.4)	
Pathologically confirmed cirrhosis	324 (30.2)	91 (26.8)	233 (31.8)	.101
Laboratory tests				
Total bilirubin level, mg/dL; median (range)	0.7 (0.7-2.7)	0.6 (0.2-2.3)	0.7 (0.1-2.7)	<.001
Albumin level, g/dL; median (range)	4.0 (2.3-5.3)	4.1 (2.3-5.3)	3.9 (2.6-5.0)	<.001
Prothrombin time, %; median (range)	93 (13-147)	93 (57-144)	94 (13-147)	.816
Child-Pugh score, A/B, n	1035/37	710/23	325/14	.408
Platelet count, ×10^4/μL; median (range)	14.8 (1.3-46.2)	14.0 (4.0-35.5)	15.1 (1.3-46.2)	<.001
AST level, IU/L; median (range)	37 (11-201)	32 (11-201)	39 (12-187)	<.001
ALT level, IU/L; median (range)	31 (5-270)	26 (6-166)	34 (5-270)	<.001
Surgery-related factors, n (%)				
Recurrence	277 (25.8)	95 (28.0)	182 (24.8)	.267
Repeat liver resection	149 (13.9)	43 (12.7)	106 (14.5)	.434
Types of liver resection				
Partial resection	669 (62.4)	278 (82.0)	391 (53.3)	<.001
Segmentectomy	98 (9.1)	14 (4.1)	84 (11.5)	
Sectionectomy	170 (15.9)	34 (10.0)	136 (18.6)	
Resection of two or more sections	135 (12.6)	13 (3.8)	122 (16.6)	
Conversion, n (%)	5 (0.5)	5 (1.5)		-
Operative time, min; median (range)	276 (75-915)	259 (75-750)	276 (75-915)	<.001
Volume of blood loss, mL; median (range)	340 (0-7460)	100 (0-3025)	500 (0-7460)	<.001
Non-curative surgery	25 (2.3)	2 (0.6)	23 (3.1)	.008
Tumor-related factors				
AFP level, ≥ 20 ng/mL; n (%)	412 (38.4)	114 (33.6)	298 (40.7)	.028
Tumor size, cm; median (range)	2.7 (0.4-21.0)	2.2 (0.4-9.5)	3.1 (0.5-21.0)	
Number, solitary/multiple; n (%)	798/274	286/53	512/221	<.001
Macrovascular invasion, n (%)	118 (11.0)	17 (5.0)	101 (13.8)	<.001

(Continues)

TABLE 1 (Continued)

Variables	Study cohort (n = 1072)	Laparoscopic liver resection group (n = 339)	Open liver resection group (n = 733)	P value
UICC stage, n (%)				
Ia	274 (25.6)	130 (38.3)	144 (19.6)	<.001
Ib	461 (43.0)	146 (43.1)	315 (43.0)	
II	246 (22.9)	60 (17.7)	186 (25.4)	
IIIa	44 (4.1)	1 (0.3)	43 (5.9)	
IIIb	42 (3.9)	2 (0.6)	40 (5.5)	
IVa	1 (0.1)	0	1 (0.1)	
IVb	4 (0.4)	0	4 (0.5)	
Pathology				
Poor HCC, n (%)	267 (24.9)	53 (15.6)	214 (29.1)	<.001
Number, solitary/multiple; n (%)	765/307	274/65	491/242	<.001
Microvascular invasion, n (%)	337 (31.4)	76 (22.4)	261 (35.6)	<.001
Postoperative complications, n (%)				
Overall	329 (30.7)	59 (17.4)	270 (36.8)	<.001
Major†	145 (13.5)	18 (5.3)	127 (17.3)	<.001
In-hospital death	4 (0.4)	0	4 (0.5)	.173
Hospital stay, days; median (range)	13 (4-212)	9 (4-88)	15 (5-212)	<.001

Abbreviations: AFP, alpha fetoprotein; ALT, alanine aminotransferase; AST, aspartate aminotransferase; BMI, body mass index; COPD, chronic obstructive pulmonary disease; HBV, hepatitis B virus; HCC, hepatocellular carcinoma; HCV, hepatitis C virus; UICC, Union for International Cancer Control.

†≥Grade IIIa based on the Clavien-Dindo classification system.

lipid-lowering drugs. Regarding postoperative complications, wound infection was defined as the presence of bacteria in the wound exudate. Bile leakage was defined as a bilirubin concentration of at least three times the serum bilirubin concentration in the drainage fluid on or after postoperative day (POD) 3 or a need for radiological or surgical intervention for biliary collection or bile peritonitis.[24] Intractable ascites was defined as drainage of 1 L/day for more than 2 days or ascites in the whole abdomen. Intractable pleural effusion was diagnosed when thoracentesis was performed.[25] Pneumonia and atelectasis were considered respiratory complications.[26] Liver failure was defined as the presence of prolonged hyperbilirubinemia (total serum bilirubin concentration of ≤3.0 mg/dL) on or after POD 5 and a need for fresh frozen plasma to decrease prothrombin time (≤50%) based on the modified definitions proposed by the International Study Group of Liver Surgery[27] and Balzan et al.[28] The severity of postoperative complications was graded according to the Clavien-Dindo classification system.[15] In this study, major complication was defined as ≥grade IIIa based on the Clavien-Dindo classification system.

2.6 | Outcomes

The primary outcome was the effect of BMI on major complications after LLR and OLR. Patients who underwent LLR and OLR initially presented with risk factors for major complications. Finally, to evaluate the superiority of LLR to OLR in patients with increased BMI, the difference in major complications between patients who underwent LLR and OLR was analyzed via a multivariate analysis.

2.7 | Statistical analyses

Categorical variables were presented as numbers and percentages and were compared between groups using the Fisher's exact test or the χ^2 test, as appropriate. Continuous variables were expressed as median (range) and were compared using the Kruskal-Wallis test. The Holm's method[29] was used to adjust *P* values for multiple comparisons of demographic variables among the different groups. We performed the Cochran-Armitage trend test[30] to assess the categorical variables and the Jonckheere-Terpstra trend test[31] to assess the continuous variables. Univariate and multivariate logistic regression analyses were performed to evaluate the relative risk for major postoperative complications. A nonlinear restricted cubic spline was contained to consider the nonlinear effect of BMI on the risk for major postoperative complications. All statistical inferences were assessed using a two-sided significance level of 5%, except for the interaction (cross-product term) analysis. Variables with a *P* value of <.05 in the univariate analysis (Cox's proportional hazard model) were included in the multivariate analysis. A *P* value <.05

TABLE 2 Clinicopathological characteristics of patients with hepatocellular carcinoma (n = 1072) after laparoscopic or open liver resection according to body mass index

	Laparoscopic liver resection group						Open liver resection group					
	Underweight group	Normal weight group	Overweight group	Obese group			Underweight group	Normal weight group	Overweight group	Obese group		
Variables	(n = 27)	(n = 211)	(n = 85)	(n = 16)	*P* value	*P* value for trend	(n = 47)	(n = 483)	(n = 181)	(n = 22)	*P* value	*P* value for trend
BMI, kg/m^2; median (range)	17.4 (12.4-18.4)	22.6 (18.5-24.9)	26.9 (25.0-29.7)	33.0 (30.1-40.2)	<.001	<.001	17.4 (15.0-18.4)	22.1 (18.5-24.9)	26.5 (25.0-29.9)	31.2 (30.0-38.1)	<.001	<.001
Age, years; median (range)	70 (46-83)	71 (21-85)	71 (47-87)	65 (44-73)	.093		72 (19-82)	69 (20-87)	69 (37-85)	70 (44-78)	0.299	
Sex, male/female, n	14/13	153/58	63/22	12/4	.133		34/13	398/85	144/37	14/8	0.066	
Comorbidities and/or previous history, n (%)												
Diabetes mellitus	7 (25.9)	72 (34.1)	31 (36.5)	11 (68.8)	.029	.019	9 (19.1)	138 (28.6)	69 (38.1)	14 (63.6)	<.001	<.001
Hypertension	11 (40.7)	111 (52.6)	53 (62.4)	8 (50.0)	.206		11 (23.4)	213 (44.1)	102 (56.4)	16 (72.7)	<.001	<.001
Dyslipidemia	4 (14.8)	46 (21.8)	24 (28.2)	5 (31.3)	.380		2 (4.3)	65 (13.5)	45 (24.9)	5 (22.7)	<.001	<.001
Ischemic heart disease	0	11 (5.2)	4 (4.7)	0	.509		1 (2.1)	25 (5.2)	10 (5.5)	0	0.545	
Alcohol abuse (≥ 60 g/d), n (%)	7 (25.9)	70 (33.2)	25 (29.4)	7 (43.8)	.602		10 (21.3)	135 (28.0)	56 (30.9)	7 (31.8)	0.589	
Underlying hepatic diseases, n (%)												
HBV	6 (22.2)	39 (18.5)	17 (20.0)	4 (25.0)	.412		8 (17.0)	72 (14.9)	28 (15.5)	3 (13.6)	<.001	<.001
HCV	15 (55.6)	116 (55.0)	45 (52.9)	4 (25.0)			31 (66.0)	278 (57.6)	80 (44.2)	3 (13.6)		
HBV + HCV	0	4 (1.9)	0	0			1 (2.1)	4 (0.8)	2 (1.1)	0		
Non-B, non-C	6 (22.2)	52 (24.6)	23 (27.1)	6 (37.5)			7 (14.9)	129 (26.7)	71 (39.2)	16 (72.7)		
Pathologically confirmed cirrhosis	7 (25.9)	48 (22.7)	31 (36.5)	5 (31.3)	.112		15 (31.9)	143 (29.6)	64 (35.4)	11 (50.0)	.139	
Laboratory tests												
Total bilirubin level, mg/dL; median (range)	0.6 (0.3-1.5)	0.6 (0.2-2.2)	0.6 (0.2-2.3)	0.8 (0.3-2.3)	.124		0.6 (0.2-1.4)	0.7 (0.1-2.7)	0.7 (0.1-2.2)	0.6 (0.2-2.0)	.4	.041
Albumin level, g/dL; median (range)	4.1 (3.4-5.3)	4.1 (2.3-5.1)	4.2 (3.1-4.8)	4.0 (3.6-4.5)	.940		3.9 (3.2-4.6)	3.9 (2.6-5.0)	4.0 (2.1-5.0)	3.7 (2.9-4.3)	<.001	
Prothrombin time, %; median (range)	100 (71-122)	93 (62-144)	93 (57-138)	89 (69-114)	.083		91 (67-123)	93 (13-141)	94 (40-130)	95 (71-147)	.856	
Child-Pugh score, A/B; n (%)	27/0	202/9	82/3	14/2	.253		46/1	464/19	179/2	21/1	.288	

(Continues)

TABLE 2 (Continued)

	Laparoscopic liver resection group						Open liver resection group					
	Underweight group	Normal weight group	Overweight group	Obese group			Underweight group	Normal weight group	Overweight group	Obese group		
Variables	(n = 27)	(n = 211)	(n = 85)	(n = 16)	*P* value	*P* value for trend	(n = 47)	(n = 483)	(n = 181)	(n = 22)	*P* value	*P* value for trend
Platelet count, $\times 10^4/\mu L$; median (range)	13.6 (6.0-25.2)	13.6 (4.0-35.5)	14.9 (4.1-32.1)	15.3 (5.7-29.7)	.488		16.0 (7.9-34.0)	14.9 (2.2-42.8)	15.3 (1.3-46.2)	16.4 (1.7-31.8)	.854	
AST level, IU/L; median (range)	34 (23-201)	32 (11-159)	32 (15-163)	39 (11-98)	.107		45 (14-123)	40 (12-187)	35 (13-105)	38 (14-110)	.005	<.001
ALT level, IU/L; median (range)	24 (13-96)	26 (6-166)	28 (8-162)	34 (13-91)	.478		32 (6-113)	37 (8-270)	31 (5-172)	28 (11-104)	.037	.022
Surgery-related factors, n (%)												
Recurrence	8 (29.6)	60 (28.4)	22 (25.9)	5 (31.3)	.955		12 (25.5)	115 (23.8)	53 (29.3)	2 (9.1)	.163	
Repeat liver resection	3 (11.1)	30 (14.2)	10 (11.8)	0	.408		7 (14.9)	65 (13.5)	32 (17.7)	2 (9.1)	.488	
Types of liver resection												
Partial resection	21 (77.8)	166 (78.7)	77 (90.6)	14 (87.5)	.279		27 (57.4)	249 (51.6)	103 (56.9)	12 (54.5)	.548	
Segmentectomy	2 (7.4)	11 (5.2)	0 (0.0)	1 (6.3)			5 (10.6)	63 (13.0)	15 (8.3)	1 (4.5)		
Sectionectomy	4 (14.8)	24 (11.4)	5 (5.9)	1 (6.3)			8 (17.0)	84 (17.4)	39 (21.5)	5 (22.7)		
Resection of two or more sections	0	10 (4.7)	3 (3.5)	0			7 (14.9)	87 (18.0)	24 (13.3)	4 (18.2)		
Conversion, n (%)	2 (7.4)	1 (0.5)	1 (1.2)	1 (6.3)	.014	.826						
Operative time, min; median (range)	284 (135-605)	253 (75-750)	262 (87-704)	270 (90-593)	.614		271 (93-610)	276 (75-915)	276 (84-662)	345 (105-640)	.028	.062
Volume of blood loss, mL; median (range)	70 (0-1850)	90 (0-1625)	100 (5-3025)	130 (10-1540)	.247	.147	330 (10-5100)	490 (0-7460)	550 (0-5050)	1230 (90-6265)	.001	.002
Non-curative surgery	0	2 (0.9)	0	0	.748		1 (2.1)	16 (3.3)	4 (2.2)	2 (9.1)	.35	

(Continues)

TABLE 2 (Continued)

	Laparoscopic liver resection group						Open liver resection group					
	Underweight group	Normal weight group	Overweight group	Obese group			Underweight group	Normal weight group	Overweight group	Obese group		
Variables	(n = 27)	(n = 211)	(n = 85)	(n = 16)	*P* value	*P* value for trend	(n = 47)	(n = 483)	(n = 181)	(n = 22)	*P* value	*P* value for trend
Tumor-related factors												
AFP level, ≥ 20 ng/mL, n (%)	10 (37.0)	75 (35.5)	25 (29.4)	4 (25.0)	.637		21 (44.7)	197 (40.8)	69 (38.1)	11 (50.0)	.66	
Tumor size, cm; median (range)	2.0 (0.7-7.8)	2.1 (0.4-7.0)	2.5 (0.7-9.0)	2.6 (1.7-9.5)	.075		2.7 (0.6-15.0)	3.0 (0.7-20.0)	3.1 (0.5-21.0)	5.1 (2.2-12.0)	.004	.104
Number, solitary/multiple; n (%)	24/3	174/37	72/13	16/0	.265		35/12	337/146	124/57	16/6	.869	
Macrovascular invasion, n (%)	1 (3.7)	13 (6.2)	3 (3.5)	0	.590		6 (12.8)	67 (13.9)	22 (12.2)	6 (27.3)	.282	
UICC stage, n (%)												
Ia	14 (51.9)	86 (40.8)	27 (27.8)	3 (18.8)	.135		11 (23.4)	100 (20.7)	33 (18.2)	0	.245	
Ib	10 (37.0)	81 (38.4)	42 (42.4)	13 (81.3)			21 (44.7)	201 (41.6)	80 (44.2)	13 (59.1)		
II	3 (11.1)	41 (19.4)	16 (16.8)	0			9 (19.1)	124 (25.7)	49 (27.1)	4 (18.2)		
IIIa	0	1 (0.5)	0	0			3 (6.4)	26 (5.4)	12 (6.6)	2 (9.1)		
IIIb	0	2 (0.9)	0	0			3 (6.4)	30 (6.2)	5 (2.8)	2 (9.1)		
IVa	0	0	0	0			0	1 (0.2)	0 (0.0)	0		
IVb	0	0	0	0			0	1 (0.2) (0.0)	2 (1.1)	1 (4.5)		
Pathology												
Poor HCC, n (%)	4 (14.8)	33 (15.6)	13 (13.3)	3 (18.8)	.987		16 (34.0)	137 (28.4)	52 (28.7)	9 (40.9)	.537	
Number, solitary/multiple; n (%)	24/3	164/47	70/15	16/0	.095		33/14	325/158	117/64	16/6	.797	
Microvascular invasion, n (%)	4 (14.8)	54 (25.6)	16 (18.8)	2 (12.5)	.301		17 (36.2)	178 (36.9)	58 (32.0)	8 (36.4)	.719	

Abbreviations: AFP, alpha fetoprotein; AST, aspartate aminotransferase; ALT, alanine aminotransferase; BMI, body mass index; COPD, chronic obstructive pulmonary disease; HBV, hepatitis B virus; HCC, hepatocellular carcinoma; HCV, hepatitis C virus; UICC, Union for International Cancer Control.

was considered statistically significant. All statistical analyses were performed using the Statistical Package for the Social Sciences® software version 26.0 (IBM Corp.) and EZR (Saitama Medical Center, Jichi Medical University, Saitama, Japan), which is a graphic user interface for the R software version 3.5.1 (The R Foundation for Statistical Computing).[32]

3 | RESULTS

3.1 | Characteristics of patients who underwent laparoscopic liver resection and open liver resection

There was no significant difference in terms of median BMI among patients who underwent LLR and OLR (Table 1). Among the patients who underwent LLR/OLR, 27/47, 211/483, 85/181, and 16/22 patients were classified into the underweight, normal weight, overweight, and obese groups, respectively. In the LLR group, the proportion of female patients, patients with HT, and patients with DL was higher when compared with the OLR group. The preoperative serum concentrations of total bilirubin, albumin, aspartate aminotransferase (AST), and alanine aminotransferase (ALT) were better in the LLR group than in the OLR group. However, the distribution of the Child-Pugh scores among the two groups did not significantly differ. The proportion of patients who underwent partial liver resection was higher in the LLR group than in the OLR group, who had a shorter operative time and lower volume of blood loss. Based on tumor-related factors or pathology, the OLR group had a more advanced HCC than the LLR group. The rate of incidence of overall and major postoperative complications was lower in the LLR group than in the OLR group, who had a shorter hospital stay.

3.2 | Clinical characteristics of patients who underwent LLR and OLR according to BMI status

The clinicopathological characteristics of patients (n = 1072) after LLR or OLR according to BMI are shown in Table 2. In the LLR group, the proportion of patients with DM had a stepwise increase from the underweight to obese group. However, there was no significant difference in terms of other background characteristics, liver function test results, and tumor-related factors among the four BMI groups. Moreover, type of liver resection, operative time, and volume of blood loss did not differ among the four groups. However, the conversion rate from laparoscopic to open surgery was high in the underweight group ($P = .014$). That is, the procedure was converted to open surgery in two (7.4%) patients in the underweight group because bleeding could not be controlled due to a narrow working space and in two patients in the normal weight and overweight groups because of injury in the major hepatic vein. Moreover, in one (6.3%) patient in the obesity group, the surgery was converted because of cancer invasion to the diaphragm (n = 1). By contrast, in the OLR group, the proportion of patients with DM, hypertension,

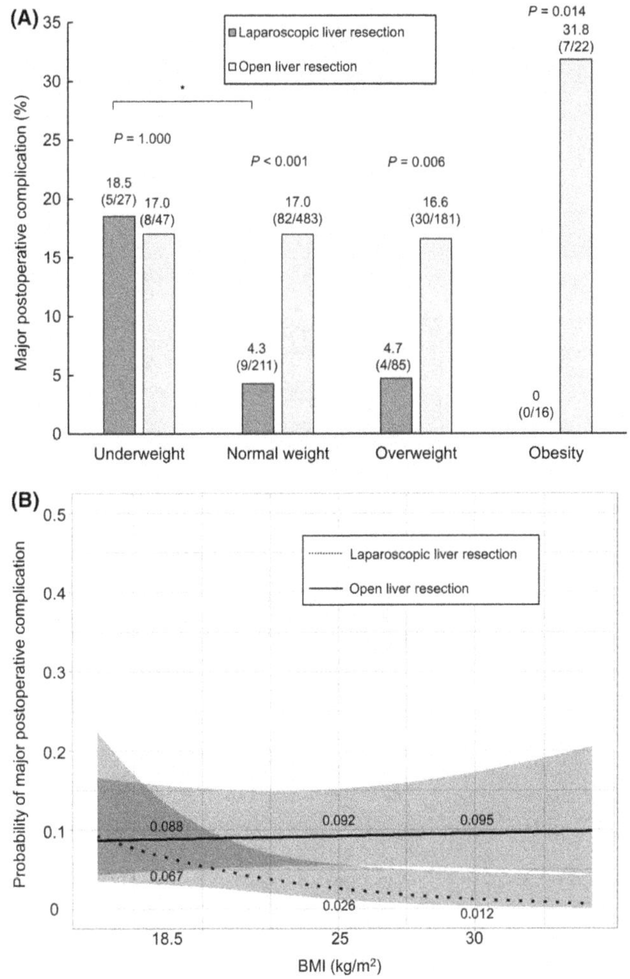

FIGURE 1 (A) Incidence of major postoperative complications according to BMI in patients who underwent LLR and OLR. The incidence of major postoperative complications had a stepwise decrease from underweight to obese patients in the LLR group ($P = .013$, Cochran-Armitage trend test, $P = .037$), but not in the OLR group ($P = .342$). Underweight, BMI of ≤18.4 kg/m^2; normal weight, 18.5 kg/m^2 ≤ BMI ≤ 24.9 kg/m^2; overweight, 25.0 kg/m^2 ≤ BMI ≤ 29.9 kg/m^2; and obesity, 30.0 kg/m^2 ≤ BMI. BMI, body mass index; LLR, laparoscopic liver resection; OLR, open liver resection. *$P < .01$ using the Holm's method. (B) Risk of major postoperative complications after LLR and OLR according to BMI after adjusting for confounding variables via a multivariate analysis. A linear line with area represents the risk (mean with 95% confidence intervals). There was no difference in terms of the risk of major postoperative complications in patients with a BMI of 18.5 kg/m^2. However, among patients with a BMI of 25.0 and 30.0 kg/m^2, the risk was lower in the LLR group than in the OLR group. In addition, there was significant effect of interaction between patients who underwent LLR and those who underwent OLR according to increase in BMI value (P for interaction = .048). BMI, body mass index; LLR, laparoscopic liver resection; OLR, open liver resection. Major complication, ≥grade IIIa based on the Clavien-Dindo classification system

dyslipidemia, and non-B non-C hepatitis indicated a stepwise increase from the underweight to obesity groups. There was a significant difference in the serum concentrations of albumin, AST, and

TABLE 3 Postoperative course in patients with hepatocellular carcinoma (n = 1072) after laparoscopic or open liver resection according to body mass index

	Laparoscopic liver resection group					Open liver resection group				
	Underweight group	Normal weight group	Overweight group	Obese group		Underweight group	Normal weight group	Overweight group	Obese group	
Variables	(n = 27)	(n = 211)	(n = 85)	(n = 16)	*P* value	(n = 47)	(n = 483)	(n = 181)	(n = 22)	*P* value
Postoperative complications										
Overall	7 (25.9)	35 (16.6)	16 (18.8)	1 (6.3)	.397	17 (36.2)	179 (37.1)	64 (35.4)	10 (45.5)	.828
Wound infection	0	1 (0.5)	0	0	.894	2 (4.3)	22 (4.6)	8 (4.4)	1 (4.5)	1.000
Intra-abdominal infection†	2 (7.4)	2 (0.9)	1 (1.2)	0	.065	4 (8.5)	38 (7.9)	12 (6.6)	1 (4.5)	.888
Bile leakage†	2 (7.4)	3 (1.4)	3 (3.5)	0	.197	3 (6.4)	30 (6.2)	8 (4.4)	4 (18.2)	.091
Ascites†	0	1 (0.5)	0	0	.894	0	21 (4.3)	3 (1.7)	1 (4.5)	.193
Pleural effusion†	1 (3.7)	1 (0.5)	2 (2.4)	0	.312	2 (4.3)	27 (5.6)	8 (4.4)	2 (9.1)	.780
Bleeding†	1 (3.7)	1 (0.5)	0	0	.164	1 (2.1)	2 (0.4)	0	0	.237
Gastrointestinal bleeding†	0	2 (0.9)	0	0	.748	0	2 (0.4)	1 (0.6)	1 (4.5)	.075
Respiratory complications†	0	2 (0.9)	0	0	.748	2 (4.3)	8 (1.7)	0	0	.110
Liver failure‡	0	1 (0.5)	0	0	.894	1 (2.1)	9 (1.9)	1 (0.6)	0	.574
Grade (A/B/C)	0/0/0	0/1/0	0/0/0	0/0/0		0/0/1	1/3/5	0/0/1	0/0/0	
Ileus†	0	0	1 (1.2)	0	.392	0	1 (0.2)	0	0	.915
Others†	1 (3.7)	1 (0.5)	0	0	.164	1 (2.1)	5 (1.0)	1 (0.6)	0	.744
In-hospital death	0	0 0	0	-		1 (2.1)	3 (0.6)	0	0	.343
Hospital stay, days; median (range)	10 (6-88)	9 (4-79)	9 (5-86)	8 (6-17)	.366	16 (6-67)	15 (6-212)	15 (5-102)	14 (6-134)	.901

†≥ Grade IIIa based on the Clavien-Dindo classification. ‡International Study Group of Liver Surgery definition.

TABLE 4 Univariate and multivariate analyses of risk factors associated with major complications after laparoscopic and open liver resection

	Laparoscopic liver resection group				Open liver resection group			
	Univariate analysis		Multivariate analysis		Univariate analysis		Multivariate analysis	
Variables	*P* value	Odds ratio (95% CI)	*P* value	Odds ratio (95% CI)	*P* value	Odds ratio (95% CI)	*P* value	Odds ratio (95% CI)
BMI, per 1 kg/m^2 increase	.044	0.87 (0.75-0.996)	.026	0.84 (0.73-0.98)	.670	1.01 (0.96-1.07)	.845	1.01 (0.95-1.07)
Age, per 1 year increase	.220	1.04 (0.98-1.09)	.258	1.04 (0.73-1.53)	.342	1.01 (0.99-1.03)	.072	1.02 (0.998-1.05)
Sex, male/female	.259	2.07 (0.59-7.32)	.519	1.59 (0.39-6.48)	.097	1.57 (0.92-2.69)	.207	1.45 (0.82-2.58)
Comorbidities and/or previous history								
Diabetes mellitus	.474	0.68 (0.24-1.96)			.055	1.48 (0.99-2.20)		
Hypertension	.728	0.85 (0.33-2.18)			.464	1.15 (0.79-1.69)		
Dyslipidemia	.645	1.28 (0.44-3.72)			.384	0.78 (0.45-1.36)		
Ischemic heart diseases	.275	0.32 (0.04-2.49)			.036	2.20 (1.06-4.60)	.149	1.81 (0.81-4.06)
Alcohol abuse	.359	0.59 (0.19-1.83)			.283	1.25 (0.83-1.89)		
Viral hepatitis	.880	0.92 (0.32-2.66)			.178	0.76 (0.51-1.13)		
Pathologically confirmed cirrhosis	.324	0.53 (0.15-1.87)			.111	1.38 (0.93-2.06)		
Laboratory tests								
Total bilirubin per 1 g/dL increase	.437	0.55 (0.12-2.51)			.638	0.88 (0.51-1.52)		
Albumin per 1 g/dL increase	.269	0.56 (0.20-1.56)			.021	0.60 (0.38-0.92)	.151	0.68 (0.40-1.15)
Prothrombin activity per 1% increase	.188	1.02 (0.99-1.05)			.039	0.99 (0.97-0.99)	.267	0.99 (0.98-1.01)
Child-Pugh score, B to A	.999	-			.030	2.65 (1.10-6.39)	.467	1.51 (0.50-4.61)
		-						
Platelet count per 1 × 10^4/mL increase	.931	0.996 (0.92-1.08)			.054	1.03 (1.00-1.06)		
AST per 1 IU/L increase	.156	1.01 (0.996-1.03)			.588	1.002 (0.995-1.01)		
ALT per 1 IU/L increase	.933	1.001 (0.98-1.02)			.888	1.00 (0.99-1.01)		
Surgery-related factors								
Recurrence	.607	1.30 (0.48-3.58)			.578	1.13 (0.73-1.75)		
Repeat liver resection	.837	0.85 (0.19-3.85)			.705	0.90 (0.51-1.57)		
Sectionectomy or more	.003	4.47 (1.64-12.20)	0.707	1.31 (0.32-5.46)	<.001	2.16 (1.46-3.18)	0.549	1.17 (0.70-1.95)
Operative time per 1 h increase	<.001	1.70 (1.37-2.12)	0.011	1.47 (1.09-1.99)	<.001	1.34 (1.23-1.46)	<.001	1.27 (1.11-1.46)
Bleeding per 1 mL increase	<.001	4.21 (2.05-8.63)	0.125	2.22 (0.80-6.12)	<.001	1.59 (1.36-1.86)	.071	1.23 (0.98-1.53)
Non-curative surgery	.999	-	-		.583	0.71 (0.21-2.42)		

(Continues)

TABLE 4 (Continued)

Variables	Laparoscopic liver resection group				Open liver resection group			
	Univariate analysis		Multivariate analysis		Univariate analysis		Multivariate analysis	
	P value	Odds ratio (95% CI)	P value	Odds ratio (95% CI)	P value	Odds ratio (95% CI)	P value	Odds ratio (95% CI)
Tumor-related factors								
AFP level (≥ 20 ng/mL)	.978	0.986 (0.36-2.70)			0.638	1.10 (0.75-1.62)		
Tumor size per 1 cm increase	.003	1.47 (1.14-1.89)	.753	1.06 (0.73-1.53)	.016	1.07 (1.01-1.14)	.091	0.93 (0.86-1.01)
Number, multiple to solitary	.590	0.66 (0.15-2.97)			.716	1.08 (0.71-1.63)		
Macrovascular invasion	.999	-			.017	1.82 (1.11-2.99)	.749	1.12 (0.57-2.20)
UICC stage per 1 stage increase	.179	1.48 (0.84-2.62)			.011	1.24 (1.05-1.46)	.834	0.98 (0.77-1.32)
Pathology								
Poor HCC	.901	1.08 (0.30-3.88)			.656	0.91 (0.59-1.39)		
Number, multiple to solitary	.380	0.51 (0.12-2.28)			.988	1.003 (0.67-1.51)		
Microvascular invasion	.093	2.32 (0.87-6.22)			.571	1.12 (0.76-1.67)		

Abbreviations: AFP, alpha fetoprotein; AST, aspartate aminotransferase; ALT, alanine aminotransferase; BMI, body mass index; CI, confidence interval; COPD, chronic obstructive pulmonary disease; HBV, hepatitis B virus; HCC, hepatocellular carcinoma; HCV, hepatitis C virus; UICC, Union for International Cancer Control.

ALT. However, the distribution of Child-Pugh scores did not remarkably differ among the four groups. Although there was no difference in the type of liver resection among the four BMI groups, the proportion of patients who experienced bleeding indicated a stepwise increase from the underweight to obesity groups. In each BMI group, the proportion of patients who had intraoperative bleeding was higher in the OLR group than in the LLR group ($P = .011$ in the underweight group and $P < .001$ in the normal weight, overweight, and obesity groups).

3.3 | Major complications after LLR and OLR according to BMI status

The incidence of major complications after LLR indicated a stepwise decrease from the underweight to obese groups (Cochran-Armitage trend test, $P = .037$, Figure 1A). A multiple analysis using Holm's test indicated that the incidence in the underweight group was higher than that in the normal weight group; however, there were no significant differences among the normal weight, overweight, and obese groups. The incidence of wound infection and intra-abdominal infection did not differ among the four groups, and none of the patients presented with complex venous thromboembolism (Table 3). There was no significant difference in the incidence of each complication among the four BMI groups with zero in-hospital death. In patients who underwent OLR, there was no difference in the incidence of overall or major complications among the four groups (Figure 1A). The incidence of wound infection and abdominal infection did not differ among the four groups, and only one (0.6%) patient in the overweight group had complex venous thromboembolism. One patient in the underweight group and three in the normal weight group died of liver failure. In the normal weight, overweight, and obesity groups, the incidence of major complications was higher in patients who underwent OLR than in those who underwent LLR (underweight group, $P = .871$; normal weight group, $P < .001$; overweight group, $P = .006$; and obesity group, $P < .001$).

3.4 | Risk factors for major complications after LLR and OLR

In all the cohorts including the LLR and the OLR groups, univariate and multivariate logistic regression analyses showed that age, operative time, volume of blood loss, serum albumin concentration, and LLR were independent predictive factors for major postoperative complications (Table S1). Meanwhile, BMI was not associated with major postoperative complications in all the cohorts including the LLR and OLR groups. However, in the LLR group, an increased BMI was considered an independent favorable factor and long operative time was a risk factor for postoperative complications (Table 4). On the contrary, among patients who underwent OLR, BMI was not a risk for postoperative major complication; however, long operative time was a risk factor.

After adjusting for age, sex, liver function test, and surgery- and tumor-related factors between the LLR and OLR groups, the risk of major postoperative complications in the LLR group decreased with increased BMI, while that in the OLR group increased with greater BMI (Figure 1B). In patients with a BMI of 25 and 30, but not 18.5, kg/m^2, the risk was lower in the LLR group than in the OLR group. In addition, there was significant effect of interaction between patients who underwent LLR and those who underwent OLR according to increase in BMI value (*P* for interaction = .048, Figure 1B).

4 | DISCUSSION

Countermeasures for the depth of surgical field and large volume of intraperitoneal fat are important in abdominal surgery, including liver resection, in overweight and obese patients.[33,34] In this study, a high BMI was associated with operative time and volume of blood loss in the OLR group, but not in the LLR group. Despite a large skin incision and compression of the gastrointestinal tract and greater omentum in OLR, liver parenchyma dissection and treatment of hepatic hilum are sometimes challenging, and this can be associated with long operative time and large volume of blood loss. This finding was in accordance with that of other reports.[9,35-38] In contrast, in LLR, pneumoperitoneum, head up position, and high magnification—even at deep portions in the caudal view—can provide sufficient free space to control the forceps, even in overweight and obese patients.[39,40] These conditions cannot affect operative time or volume of blood loss in overweight and obese patients. Even after adjusting for confounding variables, the risk of major postoperative complications was higher in overweight and obese patients (BMI of 25 and 30 kg/m^2, respectively) in the OLR group than in the LLR group. Based on these data, the physical characteristics of overweight and obese patients can be risk factors for major complications after OLR compared with LLR. We showed a stepwise decrease in the incidence of major postoperative complications according to increasing BMI. Hence, LLR should be recommended for eligible overweight and obese patients to prevent major postoperative complications. Obesity is a high-risk factor for several complications such as infections, venous thromboembolism, and respiratory complications after OLR.[10,41,42] In this study, there was no significant difference in terms of complications associated with OLR among the four BMI groups despite a greater proportion of comorbidities, including DM. This phenomenon can be attributed to controlling comorbidities before surgery and preventing surgical site infection.[43,44]

Moreover, even after adjusting for confounding variables between the LLR and OLR groups, there was no difference in terms of the incidence of major complications among underweight patients in the LLR and OLR groups. Some studies have shown that the risk of postoperative complications after abdominal or non-abdominal surgery according to BMI has a reverse J-shape relationship, with underweight and morbidly obese individuals showing the highest rates and overweight and moderately obese individuals showing the lowest rates.[45-47] Yu et al[33] revealed that underweight patients who underwent LLR had a higher complication rate than normal body weight patients, which corresponded with our results. These phenomena are referred to as the obesity paradox, and its cause has not been fully elucidated. However, underweight-induced hypoalbuminemia, sarcopenia, frailty, malnutrition, and a poor immune function may be correlated with poor outcomes after surgery.[48-51] In this study, the albumin level was basically good because the liver function reserve (e.g. the Child-Pugh classification) was assessed before hepatectomy. In fact, there was no difference in albumin level among the BMI groups in patients who underwent LLR. In addition, we did not evaluate sarcopenia or frailty; thus, we could not elucidate the cause of the higher proportion of major complications in the underweight group after LLR in our own study. However, we could suggest that sufficient operative space could be obtained during LLR, even in overweight and obese patients, and that this was associated with surgical safety and a decreased incidence of major complications.

The current study had several limitations. That is, it has a retrospective design, and the number of patients was large. Moreover, the research was conducted at a single institution. A BMI of >40 kg/m^2 was considered a risk factor for in-hospital death.[52] However, none of the patients had a BMI of >40 kg/m^2. Further, LLR was safely performed on each eligible patient. LLR and OLR have different indications according to patient and tumor characteristics, both of which may act as independent risk factors for postoperative complications. Nevertheless, the results of this study should be validated by performing multicenter and international studies.

5 | CONCLUSION

Laparoscopic liver resection is superior to OLR in overweight and obese patients in regard to decrease in incidences of postoperative major complications.

ACKNOWLEDGEMENTS

This work was supported by JSPS KAKENHI (Grant Number 19K09152) and The Health, Labour and Welfare Policy Research Grants from the Ministry of Health, Labour, and Welfare of Japan (Policy Research for Hepatitis Measures [H30-Kansei-Shitei-003]).

DISCLOSURE

Author Contributions: Project development: A. Ishihara, S. Tanaka, H. Shinkawa, and S. Kubo; Acquisition of data: A. Ishihara, S. Tanaka, H. Shinkawa, H. Yoshida, S. Takemura, R. Amano, K. Kimura, G. Ohira, and K. Nishio. Analysis and interpretation of data: A. Ishihara, S. Tanaka, H. Shinkawa, H. Yoshida, S. Kubo. Drafting of the manuscript: A. Ishihara and S. Tanaka. Editing of the manuscript: All authors. All authors have approved the final manuscript and agree to be accountable for all aspects of the work.

REFERENCES

1. Hales CM, Fryar CD, Carroll MD, Freedman DS, Ogden CL. Trends in obesity and severe obesity prevalence in US youth and adults by sex and age, 2007–2008 to 2015–2016. JAMA. 2018;319(16):1723–5.
2. WHO Regional Office for Europe. Obesity - Data and statistics [Internet]. Copenhagen, Denmark. c2021 [cited July 12 2021]. Available from: https://www.euro.who.int/en/health-topics/noncommunicable-diseases/obesity/data-and-statistics
3. McCurry J. Japan battles with obesity. Lancet. 2007;369(9560):451–2.
4. Ministry of Health, Labour and Welfare of Japan. Report of national health and nutrition [Internet]. Tokyo, Japan; 2020 [cited 12 July 2021]. Available from: https://www.mhlw.go.jp/stf/seisakunitsuite/bunya/kenkou_iryou/kenkou/eiyou/h30-houkoku_00001.html
5. Dindo D, Muller MK, Weber M, Clavien P-A. Obesity in general elective surgery. Lancet. 2003;361(9374):2032–5.
6. Mullen JT, Davenport DL, Hutter MM, Hosokawa PW, Henderson WG, Khuri SF, et al. Impact of body mass index on perioperative outcomes in patients undergoing major intra-abdominal cancer surgery. Ann Surg Oncol. 2008;15(8):2164–72.
7. Larsson SC, Wolk A. Overweight, obesity and risk of liver cancer: a meta-analysis of cohort studies. Br J Cancer. 2007;97(7):1005–8.
8. Berentzen TL, Gamborg M, Holst C, Sørensen TIA, Baker JL. Body mass index in childhood and adult risk of primary liver cancer. J Hepatol. 2014;60(2):325–30.
9. Gedaly R, McHugh PP, Johnston TD, Jeon H, Ranjan D, Davenport DL. Obesity, diabetes, and smoking are important determinants of resource utilization in liver resection: a multicenter analysis of 1029 patients. Ann Surg. 2009;249(3):414–9.
10. Cucchetti A, Cescon M, Ercolani G, Di Gioia P, Peri E, Pinna AD. Safety of hepatic resection in overweight and obese patients with cirrhosis. Br J Surg. 2011;98(8):1147–54.
11. Tanaka S, Kawaguchi Y, Kubo S, Kanazawa A, Takeda Y, Hirokawa F, et al. Validation of index-based IWATE criteria as an improved difficulty scoring system for laparoscopic liver resection. Surgery. 2019;165(4):731–40.
12. Tanaka S, Kubo S, Kanazawa A, Takeda Y, Hirokawa F, Nitta H, et al. Validation of a difficulty scoring system for laparoscopic liver resection: a multicenter analysis by the endoscopic liver surgery study group in Japan. J Am Coll Surg. 2017;225(2):249–58.
13. Nomi T, Fuks D, Ferraz JM, Kawaguchi Y, Nakajima Y, Gayet B. Influence of body mass index on postoperative outcomes after laparoscopic liver resection. Surg Endosc. 2015;29(12):3647–54.
14. Toriguchi K, Hatano E, Sakurai T, Seo S, Taura K, Uemoto S. Laparoscopic liver resection in obese patients. World J Surg. 2015;39(5):1210–5.
15. Dindo D, Demartines N, Clavien PA. Classification of surgical complications: a new proposal with evaluation in a cohort of 6336 patients and results of a survey. Ann Surg. 2004;240(2):205–13.
16. World Health Organization. Obesity: preventing and managing the global epidemic: report of a WHO consultation. Geneva: World Health Organization; 2000.
17. Tanaka S, Hirohashi K, Tanaka H, Shuto T, Lee SH, Kubo S, et al. Incidence and management of bile leakage after hepatic resection for malignant hepatic tumors. J Am Coll Surg. 2002;195(4):484–9.
18. Tanaka S, Takemura S, Shinkawa H, Nishioka T, Hamano G, Kinoshita M, et al. Outcomes of pure laparoscopic versus open hepatic resection for hepatocellular carcinoma in cirrhotic patients: a case-control study with propensity score matching. Eur Surg Res. 2015;55(4):291–301.
19. Strasberg SM, Belghiti J, Clavien PA, Gadzijev E, Garden JO, Lau WY, et al. The Brisbane 2000 terminology of liver anatomy and resections. HPB (Oxford). 2000;2(3):333–9.
20. Buell JF, Cherqui D, Geller DA, O'Rourke N, Iannitti D, Dagher I, et al. The international position on laparoscopic liver surgery: the Louisville statement, 2008. Ann Surg. 2009;250(5):825–30.
21. Seino Y, Nanjo K, Tajima N, Kadowaki T, Kashiwagi A, Araki E, et al. Report of the committee on the classification and diagnostic criteria of diabetes mellitus: the committee of the Japan diabetes society on the diagnostic criteria of diabetes mellitus. J Diabetes Investig. 2010;1(5):212–28.
22. Umemura S, Arima H, Arima S, Asayama K, Dohi Y, Hirooka Y, et al. The Japanese society of hypertension guidelines for the management of hypertension (JSH 2019). Hypertens Res. 2019;42(9):1235–481.
23. Kinoshita M, Yokote K, Arai H, Iida M, Ishigaki Y, Ishibashi S, et al. Japan atherosclerosis society (JAS) guidelines for prevention of atherosclerotic cardiovascular diseases 2017. J Atheroscler Thromb. 2018;25(9):846–984.
24. Koch M, Garden OJ, Padbury R, Rahbari NN, Adam R, Capussotti L, et al. Bile leakage after hepatobiliary and pancreatic surgery: a definition and grading of severity by the international study group of liver surgery. Surgery. 2011;149(5):680–8.
25. Tanaka S, Kubo S, Tsukamoto T, Hirohashi K, Tanaka H, Shuto T, et al. Risk factors for intractable pleural effusion after liver resection. Osaka City Med J. 2004;50(1):9–18.
26. Tanaka S, Iida H, Ueno M, Hirokawa F, Nomi T, Nakai T, et al. Preoperative risk assessment for loss of independence following hepatic resection in elderly patients: a prospective multicenter study. Ann Surg. 2021;13(3):e253–61.
27. Rahbari NN, Garden OJ, Padbury R, Brooke-Smith M, Crawford M, Adam R, et al. Posthepatectomy liver failure: a definition and grading by the international study group of liver surgery (ISGLS). Surgery. 2011;149(5):713–24.
28. Balzan S, Belghiti J, Farges O, Ogata S, Sauvanet A, Delefosse D, et al. The "50-50 criteria" on postoperative day 5: an accurate predictor of liver failure and death after hepatectomy. Ann Surg. 2005;242(6):824–9.
29. Holm S. A simple sequentially rejective multiple test procedure. Scand J Stat. 1979;6(2):65–70.
30. Bansal S, Buring JE, Rifai N, Mora S, Sacks FM, Ridker PM. Fasting compared with nonfasting triglycerides and risk of cardiovascular events in women. JAMA. 2007;298(3):309–16.
31. Mikami S, Hamano T, Fujii N, Nagasawa Y, Isaka Y, Moriyama T, et al. Serum osteoprotegerin as a screening tool for coronary artery calcification score in diabetic pre-dialysis patients. Hypertens Res. 2008;31(6):1163–70.
32. Kanda Y. Investigation of the freely available easy-to-use software 'EZR' for medical statistics. Bone Marrow Transplant. 2013;48(3):452–8.
33. Yu X, Yu H, Fang X. The impact of body mass index on short-term surgical outcomes after laparoscopic hepatectomy, a retrospective study. BMC Anesthesiol. 2016;16(1):1–7.
34. WHO Expert Consultation. Appropriate body-mass index for Asian populations and its implications for policy and intervention strategies. Lancet. 2004;363(9403):157–63.
35. Tanaka S, Iimuro Y, Hirano T, Hai S, Suzumura K, Nakamura I, et al. Safety of hepatic resection for hepatocellular carcinoma in obese patients with cirrhosis. Surg Today. 2013;43(11):1290–7.
36. Langella S, Russolillo N, Forchino F, Lo Tesoriere R, D'Eletto M, Ferrero A. Impact of obesity on postoperative outcome of hepatic resection for colorectal metastases. Surgery. 2015;158(6):1521–9.
37. Balzan S, Nagarajan G, Farges O, Galleano CZ, Dokmak S, Paugam C, et al. Safety of liver resections in obese and overweight patients. World J Surg. 2010;34(12):2960–8.
38. Uchida H, Iwashita Y, Saga K, Takayama H, Watanabe K, Endo Y, et al. Benefit of laparoscopic liver resection in high body mass index patients. World J Gastroenterol. 2016;22(10):3015–22.
39. Soubrane O, Schwarz L, Cauchy F, Perotto LO, Brustia R, Bernard D, et al. A conceptual technique for laparoscopic right hepatectomy based on facts and oncologic principles: the caudal approach. Ann Surg. 2015;261(6):1226–31.
40. Tomishige H, Morise Z, Kawabe N, Nagata H, Ohshima H, Kawase J, et al. Caudal approach to pure laparoscopic posterior sectionec-

tomy under the laparoscopy-specific view. World J Gastrointest Surg. 2013;5(6):173–7.

41. Yang G, Staercke CD, Hooper WC. The effects of obesity on venous thromboembolism: a review. Open J Prev Med. 2012;02(04):499–509.
42. Yang T, Tu PA, Zhang H, Lu JH, Shen YN, Yuan SX, et al. Risk factors of surgical site infection after hepatic resection. Infect Control Hosp Epidemiol. 2014;35(3):317–20.
43. Vogt AP, Bally L. Perioperative glucose management: current status and future directions. Best Pract Res Clin Anaesthesiol. 2020;34(2):213–24.
44. Takayama T, Aramaki O, Shibata T, Oka M, Itamoto T, Shimada M, et al. Antimicrobial prophylaxis for 1 day versus 3 days in liver cancer surgery: a randomized controlled non-inferiority trial. Surg Today. 2019;49(10):859–69.
45. Mullen JT, Moorman DW, Davenport DL. The obesity paradox: body mass index and outcomes in patients undergoing nonbariatric general surgery. Ann Surg. 2009;250(1):166–72.
46. Tjeertes EK, Hoeks SE, Beks SB, Valentijn TM, Hoofwijk AG, Stolker RJ. Obesity–a risk factor for postoperative complications in general surgery? BMC Anesthesiol. 2015;15(1):112.
47. Benjamin ER, Dilektasli E, Haltmeier T, Beale E, Inaba K, Demetriades D. The effects of body mass index on complications and mortality after emergency abdominal operations: the obesity paradox. Am J Surg. 2017;214(5):899–903.
48. Wang H, Yang J, Zhang X, Yan L, Yang J. Liver resection in hepatitis B-related hepatocellular carcinoma: clinical outcomes and safety in overweight and obese patients. PLoS One. 2014;9(6):e99281.
49. Harimoto N, Shirabe K, Yamashita YI, Ikegami T, Yoshizumi T, Soejima Y, et al. Sarcopenia as a predictor of prognosis in patients following hepatectomy for hepatocellular carcinoma. Br J Surg. 2013;100(11):1523–30.
50. Ji F, Liang Y, Fu S, Chen D, Cai X, Li S, et al. Prognostic value of combined preoperative prognostic nutritional index and body mass index in HCC after hepatectomy. HPB (Oxford). 2017;19(8):695–705.
51. Tanaka S, Ueno M, Iida H, Kaibori M, Nomi T, Hirokawa F, et al. Preoperative assessment of frailty predicts age-related events after hepatic resection: a prospective multicenter study. J Hepatobiliary Pancreat Sci. 2018;25(8):377–87.
52. Saunders JK, Rosman AS, Neihaus D, Gouge TH, Melis M. Safety of hepatic resections in obese veterans. Arch Surg. 2012;147(4):331–7.

23

Long distance between the superior mesenteric artery root and bottom of the external anal sphincter is a risk factor for stoma outlet obstruction after total proctocolectomy and ileal-pouch anal anastomosis for ulcerative colitis

Ryota Mori[1] | Takayuki Ogino[1,2] | Yuki Sekido[1] | Tsuyoshi Hata[1] | Hidekazu Takahashi[1] | Norikatsu Miyoshi[1] | Mamoru Uemura[1] | Yuichiro Doki[1] | Hidetoshi Eguchi[1] | Tsunekazu Mizushima[1,2,3]

[1]Department of Gastroenterological Surgery, Graduate School of Medicine, Osaka University, Osaka, Japan

[2]Department of Therapeutics for Inflammatory Bowel Diseases, Graduate School of Medicine, Osaka University, Osaka, Japan

[3]Department of Surgery, Osaka Police Hospital, Osaka, Japan

Correspondence
Takayuki Ogino, Department of Gastroenterological Surgery, Graduate School of Medicine, Osaka University, Osaka, Japan.
Email: togino04@gesurg.med.osaka-u.ac.jp

Abstract

Background: Stoma outlet obstruction (SOO) is much more common after total proctocolectomy (TPC) and ileal-pouch anal anastomosis (IPAA) for ulcerative colitis (UC) compared to after rectal surgery for cancer. Few prior reports have evaluated anatomical risk factors for SOO. In this study we aimed to clarify the risk factors for SOO after IPAA, focusing on the anatomical perspective.

Methods: This study included 68 UC patients who underwent IPAA with diverting ileostomy. These cases were analyzed based on clinicopathological factors and computed tomography (CT)-based anatomical factors.

Results: SOO was identified in 18 patients (26.5%). We compared this SOO group with the non-SOO group. The two groups significantly differed in sex distribution, and patients in the SOO group tended to have a longer postoperative hospital stay. Regarding surgery-related factors, patients who underwent two-stage surgery and experienced high-output syndrome tended to develop SOO. Analysis of anatomical risk factors revealed that SOO was more common in patients with a longer distance between the root of their superior mesenteric artery and the bottom of the external anal sphincter (rSMA-bEAS). This tendency remained significant even with adjustment for patient height. In multivariate analyses, adjusted rSMA-bEAS (>191.0 mm/m) and male sex were independent risk factors associated with SOO.

Conclusion: A long rSMA-bEAS distance suggests that the mesentery is likely to be under tension. In such cases, surgeons should endeavor to avoid tension in the mesentery as much as possible.

KEYWORDS
ileal pouch-anal anastomosis, small bowel obstruction, stoma outlet obstruction, total proctocolectomy, ulcerative colitis

1 | INTRODUCTION

Ulcerative colitis (UC) is a chronic inflammatory disease of unknown cause, in which the large intestine repeatedly becomes inflamed, and which is affecting an increasing number of patients. The main treatments for UC are medications, such as amino salicylates, steroids, immunosuppressants, and antitumor necrosis factor (TNF)-α receptor antibody. However, a substantial number of patients require surgery due to toxic megacolon, failing to achieve remission, or tumor formation.[1]

Among patients with UC, the lifetime risk of operation is about 40%,[2] with the standard surgical procedures including total proctocolectomy (TPC) and ileal-pouch anal anastomosis (IPAA). Previous reports indicate that IPAA is associated with higher rates of postoperative complications than other types of abdominal surgery, particularly small bowel obstruction (SBO) related to diverting ileostomy.[3]

A diverting ileostomy is created to avoid the risk of anastomotic leakage; however, it sometimes leads to stoma-associated SBO, termed stoma outlet obstruction (SOO), due to angulations of the ileum near the stoma site. SOO occurs with incidence rates of 20%–40% after IPAA with diverting ileostomy, compared to less than 15% after low anterior resection for rectal cancer.[4] We reported that the high risk of SOO after IPAA with diverting ileostomy was associated with a short distance from the pouch to the diverting ileostomy, caused by excessive tension of the mesentery.[5]

Based on clinical experience and previous reports, we inferred that taut superior mesenteric vessels after IPAA with diverting ileostomy created a situation in which the ileum could be easily twisted and difficult to restore, due to excessive tension of the mesentery. To date, few studies have evaluated the anatomical risk factors for SOO. Thus, in the present study we aimed to clarify the risk factors for SOO after IPAA with diverting ileostomy, focusing on the anatomical perspective.

2 | METHODS

2.1 | Surgical procedure

TPC and hand-sewn IPAA were performed for UC with cancer or dysplasia, whereas TPC and stapled IPAA were performed for refractory or severe UC. Hand-sewn anastomosis with mucosectomy was performed in cases with severe inflammation around the anal canal. Some patients initially underwent subtotal colectomy (STC) as an emergency surgery for acute exacerbation, followed by residual rectum resection (RR) and IPAA as a secondary surgery. In accordance with Health and Labor Sciences Research Grants for research on intractable diseases from the Ministry of Health, Labor and Welfare of Japan, the operation could include up to three phases based on whether a diverting ileostomy was created and when closure was performed.

Most procedures involved the creation of a 15-cm-long ileal J-pouch, without dissection of the ileocecal artery (ICA), and a diverting ileostomy on the oral side 30–80 cm side from the IPAA. A diverting ileostomy was created at the umbilicus or right lower abdomen, at the surgeon's discretion. At the site of stoma, a lengthwise incision was made at the rectus muscle fascia, along with a fascial trephination large enough to allow passage of two fingers. Finally, a Turnbull loop ileostomy was fashioned without rotation, in a vertical orientation.

2.2 | Study population

This study included UC patients who underwent IPAA with a diverting ileostomy at Osaka University Hospital, Japan, between January 2010 and November 2020. Patients with insufficient imaging data were excluded. Informed consent was obtained from all patients

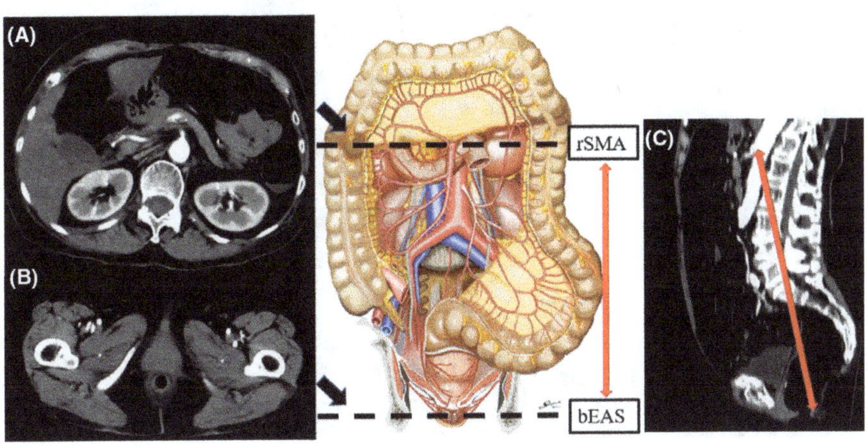

FIGURE 1 Methods of measuring the distance between the root of the superior mesenteric artery and the bottom of the external anal sphincter (rSMA-bEAS) on CT images. a: Axial image showing the location of the root of the superior mesenteric artery (rSMA). b: Axial image showing the location of the bottom of the external anal sphincter (bEAS). c: Sagittal image showing the fixed angle such that rSMA and bEAS are on the same slice

before the operation. The study protocol was approved by the Institutional Review Board of Osaka University Hospital (#15028).

2.3 | CT imaging and measurement of anatomical distances

Abdominal and pelvic computed tomography (CT) was performed using 64- or 320-detector row CT. Contrast-enhanced CT was performed during the portal venous phase (delay, 75 s), after injection of nonionic contrast material (dose, 100 mL of 300 mgI/mL). Axial 3- to 5-mm images were reconstructed and reviewed using a picture archiving and communication system monitor, by two board-certified gastroenterological surgeons. On the axial image, we identified the location of the root of the superior mesenteric artery (rSMA) and the bottom edge of the external anal sphincter (bEAS; Figure 1a,b). On the sagittal image, we fixed the angle for measurement (Figure 1c).

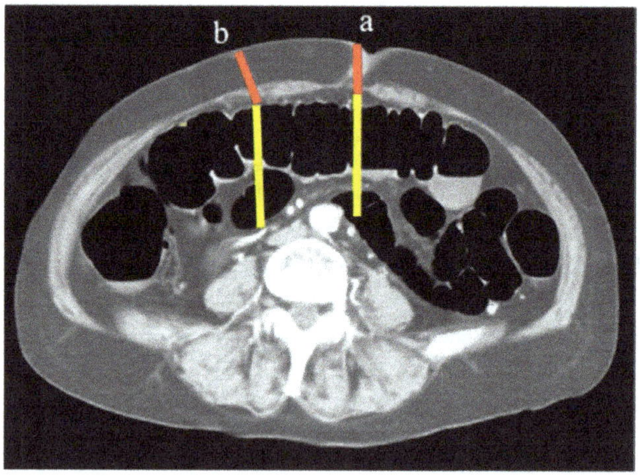

FIGURE 2 Methods of measuring the abdominal cavity depth and abdominal wall thickness at the site of stoma construction. a: In a case with a diverting ileostomy in the umbilicus. b: In a case with a diverting ileostomy in the lower abdomen

We then measured the distance between the root of their superior mesenteric artery and the bottom of the external anal sphincter (rSMA-bEAS). For this analysis, rSMA-bEAS was adjusted according to the patient's height (m) to exclude any influence of height. In the axial image, we also measured the depth of the abdominal cavity, and thickness of the abdominal wall at the stoma site (Figure 2).

2.4 | Definition of stoma outlet obstruction and high-output syndrome

Stoma outlet obstruction was defined as SBO that showed symptoms of intestinal obstruction, with caliber changes near the ileostomy detected by CT imaging, or recovered by insertion of a tube through the stoma (Figure 3a,b). High-output syndrome (HOS) was defined as stoma drainage of 2000 mL/d for more than 2 d, or 1500 mL/d for more than 3 d.

2.5 | Statistical analysis

All statistical analyses were performed using JMP pro 14.0.0 (SAS Institute, Cary, NC). Categorical variables were compared using the chi-squared test, and continuous variables using the Mann–Whitney *U*-test and Student's *t*-test. We assessed the univariate and multivariable associations between factors using binary logistic regression. The cutoff value was determined based on receiver operating characteristic (ROC) curve analysis. $P < .05$ was considered significant.

3 | RESULTS

3.1 | Patient characteristics

A total of 78 patients underwent IPAA for UC during the study period. We excluded seven patients without diverting ileostomy, and

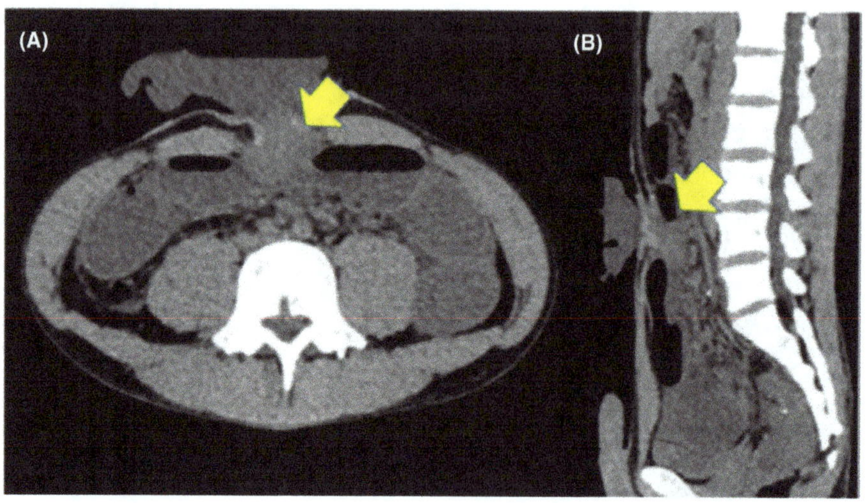

FIGURE 3 Representative CT images of stoma outlet obstruction (SOO). The arrow points to the area where the intestine was obstructed at the site of a diverting ileostomy. a: Axial image. b: Sagittal image

three patients with incomplete data, such that a total of 68 patients were analyzed in this study. Their clinical characteristics are shown in Table 1. The median age at surgery was 49 y, and mediate disease duration was 9.0 y. The extent of colitis was pancolitis in 57 patients (83.8%), and the main surgical indication was cancer/dysplasia in 27 patients (39.7%).

Among the 68 patients, SOO was identified in 18 (26.5%). SOO severity was assessed using the Clavien–Dindo classification.[6] Overall, 12 patients recovered by ileostomy tube drainage with intravenous feeding (Grade II), four patients needed ileus tube insertion (Grade IIIa), and two patients required early stoma closure to manage SOO (Grade IIIb).

We compared the patients in the SOO group (n = 18) with those in the non-SOO group (n = 50). In terms of patients' characteristics, sex distribution significantly differed between the two groups (*P* =.003; Table 2). We also assessed surgery-related and postoperative factors

TABLE 1 Clinical characteristics of participants

	n = 68
Sex	
Male	45 (66.2%)
Female	23 (33.8%)
Age at surgery, y	49.0 ± 16.5
Disease duration, y	9 ± 9.7
Body mass index, kg/m^2	20.8 ± 4.3
Height, m	165.1 ± 9.3
Body weight, kg	57.5 ± 14.2
Smoking	12 (17.6%)
Type 2 diabetes	5 (7.4%)
Extent of colitis	
Pancolitis	57 (83.8%)
Left-sided colitis	10 (14.7%)
Proctitis	0 (0.0%)
Others	1 (1.5%)
Surgical indication	
Cancer/Dysplasia	27 (39.7%)
Severe/Fulminant	19 (27.9%)
Refractory	22 (32.4%)
Nutritional status (Onodera PNI)	
>40	27 (39.7%)
≦40	41 (60.3%)
Preoperative CRP (mg/dL)	0.5 ± 3.5
Preoperative medication	
Amino salicylate	55 (80.9%)
Anti-TNFα antibody	26 (38.2%)
Steroid	46 (67.6%)
Immunosuppressant	33 (48.5%)

Note: Data are presented as n (%) or median ± SD.
Abbreviations: CRP, C-reactive protein; PNI, prognostic nutritional index; TNF, tumor necrosis factor.

TABLE 2 Comparison of clinical characteristics between SOO group and non-SOO group

	SOO group (n = 18)	Non-SOO group (n = 50)	P value
Sex			.003
Male	17 (94.4%)	28 (56.0%)	
Female	1 (5.6%)	22 (44.0%)	
Age at surgery, y	59.0 ± 21.4	48.5 ± 14.6	.4
Disease duration, y	5.5 ± 7.6	11.0 ± 14.6	.1
Body mass index, kg/m^2	20.8 ± 3.6	20.8 ± 4.6	.9
Height, cm	169.2 ± 7.2	162.0 ± 9.8	.09
Body weight, kg	60.1 ± 10.8	56.5 ± 15.3	.53
Smoking	3 (16.7%)	9 (18.0%)	.76
Type 2 diabetes	1 (5.6%)	4 (8.0%)	.65
Extent of colitis			.95
Pancolitis	15 (83.3%)	42 (84.0%)	
Left-sided colitis/ Others	3 (16.7%)	8 (16.0%)	
Surgical indication			.43
Cancer/Dysplasia	7 (38.9%)	20 (40.0%)	
Severe/Fulminant	3 (16.7%)	16 (32.0%)	
Refractory	8 (44.4%)	14 (28.0%)	
Nutritional status (Onodera PNI)			.93
>40	7 (38.9%)	20 (40.0%)	
≦40	11 (61.1%)	30 (60.0%)	
Preoperative CRP (mg/dL)	0.5 ± 3.3	0.5 ± 3.5	.91
Preoperative medication			
Amino salicylate	15 (83.3%)	40 (80.0%)	.76
Anti-TNFα antibody	10 (55.6%)	16 (32.0%)	.08
Steroid	11 (61.1%)	35 (70.0%)	.68
Immunosuppressant	12 (66.7%)	21 (42.0%)	.07

Note: Data are presented as n (%) or median ± SD.
Abbreviations: CRP, C-reactive protein; PNI, prognostic nutritional index; SOO, stoma outlet obstruction; TNF, tumor necrosis factor.

(Table 3). SOO development was significantly associated with undergoing two-stage surgery (*P* = .01) and experiencing HOS (*P* = .001). The two groups did not differ in terms of operative time (*P* = .23), blood loss (*P* = .86), location of the ileostomy (*P* = .23), or use of laparoscopy (*P* = .95). SOO incidence was not affected by the occurrence of intra-abdominal abscesses (*P* = .11).

In our analysis of anatomical risk factors, we found that patients with a longer rSMA-bEAS distance were more likely to develop SOO (*P* = .001; Table 4). This tendency remained significant even with adjustment for patient height (*P* = .002). SOO was not significantly correlated with abdominal wall thickness (*P* = .28) or abdominal cavity depth at the site of stoma (*P* = .73).

We performed univariate and multivariate analyses using four risk factors: sex, surgical strategy, HOS, and rSMA-bEAS (Table 5). The results showed that SOO was independently associated with

TABLE 3 Comparison of surgery-related and postoperative factors between SOO group and non-SOO group

	SOO group (n = 18)	Non-SOO group (n = 50)	P value
Surgery-related factors			
Operation time, min	385.5 ± 158.7	368.0 ± 179.4	.23
Blood loss (mL)	235.0 ± 979.7	179.4 ± 315.4	.86
Surgical approach			.95
Open	1 (5.6%)	3 (6.0%)	
Laparoscopy	17 (94.4%)	47 (94.0%)	
Anastomosis (IPAA)			.69
Hand-sewn	8 (44.4%)	25 (50.0%)	
Stapled	10 (55.6%)	25 (50.0%)	
Strategy			.01
2-stage surgery (TPC)	17 (94.4%)	32 (64.0%)	
3-stage surgery (STC + RR)	1 (5.6%)	18 (36.0%)	
Site of stoma construction			.23
Umbilicus	13 (72.2%)	28 (56.0%)	
Right lower abdomen	5 (27.8%)	22 (44.0%)	
Postoperative factors			
Intra-abdominal abscess	2 (11.1%)	1 (2.0%)	.11
High-output syndrome[a]	14 (77.8%)	17 (34.0%)	.002

Note: Data are presented as n (%) or median ± SD.

IPAA, ileal pouch-anal anastomosis; RR, residual rectal resection; SOO, stoma outlet obstruction; STC, subtotal proctocolectomy; TPC, total proctocolectomy.

[a]High-output syndrome: stoma drainage of 2000 mL/d for more than 2 d or 1500 mL/d for more than 3 d.

adjusted rSMA-bEAS (>191.0 mm/m; $P = .004$; odds ratio [OR]: 4.5; 95% confidence interval [CI]: 2.3–73.7) and male sex ($P = .01$; OR: 25.9; 95% CI: 2.1–318.5).

4 | DISCUSSION

UC is an inflammatory bowel disease that has shown a rising incidence and prevalence in industrialized countries over recent years.

The standard surgical procedure for UC is TPC. TPC procedures can be divided into three categories depending on the included stages. One-stage surgery is IPAA without ileostomy. Two-stage surgery includes TPC with ileostomy + stoma closure, or STC with ileostomy + RR without ileostomy. Three-stage surgery includes STC with ileostomy + RR with ileostomy + stoma closure. In a large-scale study, it was reported that about 75% of patients have a diverting ileostomy, and that one-stage surgery is not common.[5] In our hospital, about 90% of patients underwent creation of a diverting ileostomy. Overall, of the 68 patients in our study, 18 (26.5%) experienced SOO.

TABLE 4 Comparison of anatomical factors between SOO group and non-SOO group

	SOO group (n = 18)	Non-SOO group (n = 50)	P value
Thickness of abdominal wall (mm)	18.3 ± 11.7	23.4 ± 9.2	.28
Depth of the abdominal cavity (mm)	66.0 ± 17.8	62.2 ± 24.1	.73
rSMA-bEAS (mm)	322.2 ± 22.0	294.0 ± 22.1	.001
Height adjusted rSMA-bEAS (mm/m)	191.8 ± 9.0	180.5 ± 10.7	.002

Note: Data are presented as median ± SD.

Abbreviations: bEAS, bottom of the external anal sphincter; rSMA, the root of superior mesenteric artery; SOO, stoma outlet obstruction.

The most common reconstruction approach is IPAA using an ileal J-pouch.[7] IPAA can involve shortening of the intestinal tract, with correspondingly increased tension on the mesentery. The major difficulty in IPAA arises when the pouch does not quite reach the anal canal for anastomosis.[7] Some reports have demonstrated methods to resolve this situation, including sufficient mobilization of the small intestine, division of the serosa of the mesentery, and division of blood vessels to stretch the mesentery.[7,8] It has previously been reported that the distances from the rSMA to the terminal of the ICA (tICA), and from the tICA to the anal verge are associated with anastomosis difficulty.[7] These findings suggest that SMA could be an indicator of mesenteric length.

Previously reported risk factors for SBO (including SOO) after TPC have included laparoscopic surgery, loop ileostomy, low BMI, rectus abdominus wall thickness at the stoma-penetrating site, HOS, and the distance from the ileal pouch inlet to the loop-ileostomy (<30 cm).[4,5,9-11] The higher incidence of SBO after laparoscopic surgery for UC is in contrast with the lower incidence of SBO after laparoscopic surgery for colorectal cancer compared with open surgery.[12] This discrepancy is caused by the fact that the small intestine can more easily twist due to the increased movable space after TPC and decreased postoperative adhesions from laparoscopic surgery.[9,13] In our present study, very few patients underwent open surgery (5.9%), and thus there was no significant difference between the two groups.

Comparing clinical characteristics between the SOO group and the non-SOO group revealed that male sex, two-stage surgery, and experienced HOS were more common in the SOO group. Anatomical analysis showed that SOO development was more common in patients with a longer rSMA-bEAS distance. This tendency remained significant even with adjustment for patient height. Univariate and multivariable analysis revealed that SOO was independently

TABLE 5 Univariate and multivariate association with SOO

	SOO group (n = 18)	Non-SOO group (n = 50)	Univariate analysis		Multivariate analysis	
			P value	Odds ratio (95% CI)	*P* value	Odds ratio (95% CI)
Sex			0.003	13.4	0.01	25.9
Male	17 (94.4%)	28 (56.0%)		(1.6–108.3)		(2.1–318.5)
Female	1 (5.6%)	22 (44.0%)				
Strategy			0.01	9.6	0.09	9.1
2-stage procedure (TPC)	17 (94.4%)	32 (64.0%)		(1.2–77.9)		(0.7–114.8)
3-stage procedure (STC + RR)	1 (5.6%)	18 (36.0%)				
High-output syndrome			0.002	6.8	0.17	2.9
Yes	14 (77.8%)	17 (34.0%)		(1.9–23.9)		(0.6–13.5)
No	4 (22.2%)	33 (66.0%)				
Adjusted rSMA-bEAS, mm/m			0.001	6.3	0.004	13.1
>191.0	11 (61.1%)	10 (20.0%)		(1.9–20.3)		(2.3–73.7)
≤191.0	7 (38.9%)	40 (80.0%)				

Note: Data are presented as n (%).
bEAS, bottom of the external anal sphincter; RR, residual rectal resection; rSMA, root of superior mesenteric artery; SOO, stoma outlet obstruction; STC, subtotal proctocolectomy; TPC, total proctocolectomy.

associated with adjusted rSMA-bEAS (>191.0 mm/m) and male sex. Together with previous findings, our present results suggest that SMA is the defining factor of mesenteric length, and that mesenteric tension not only makes anastomosis more difficult but also increases the risk of developing SOO. After IPAA with diverting ileostomy, fixation of the mesentery with excessive tension and free movement of the small intestine will lead to a twisted ileum and make it difficult to restore the original position. The fact that women are less likely to suffer from postoperative SOO may be due to the fact that they are more prone to visceral ptosis.[14] This is the first study to identify a risk factor for SOO from the anatomical perspective.

Our study has several limitations. First, these results were based on a single-center retrospective study with a small sample size. Second, we estimated mesenteric tension based only on measurement of the rSMA-bEAS distance. Accurate estimation of the intestinal membrane tension would require measurement of the length of the blood vessels via 3D reconstruction. However, the aim of our present study was to predict the risk of SOO before surgery using simple imaging; therefore, we did not measure blood vessel lengths in this study.

In conclusion, in this study we demonstrated that male sex and longer rSMA-bEAS distance (indicating greater mesentery tension) were risk factors for SOO after IPAA with diverting ileostomy for UC. These findings suggest that surgeons should endeavor to reduce tension in the mesentery by using an applicable technique as much as possible.

ACKNOWLEDGMENTS

The authors thank San Francisco Edit for English language editing, and Shigeyuki Sakaguchi for providing anatomical drawings.

REFERENCES

1. Uchino M, Ikeuchi H, Hata K, Okada S, Ishihara S, Morimoto K, et al. Changes in the rate of and trends in colectomy for ulcerative colitis during the era of biologics and calcineurin inhibitors based on a Japanese nationwide cohort study. Surg Today. 2019;49(12):1066–73.
2. Yang Z, Wu Q, Wu K, Fan D. Meta-analysis: pre-operative infliximab treatment and short-term post-operative complications in patients with ulcerative colitis. Aliment Pharmacol Ther. 2010;31(4):486–92.
3. Truelove SC, Witts LJ. Cortisone in ulcerative colitis; final report on a therapeutic trial. Br Med J. 1955;2(4947):1041–8.
4. Okada S, Hata K, Emoto S, Murono K, Kaneko M, Sasaki K, et al. Elevated risk of stoma outlet obstruction following colorectal surgery in patients undergoing ileal pouch-anal anastomosis: a retrospective cohort study. Surg Today. 2018;48(12):1060–7.
5. Mizushima T, Kameyama H, Watanabe K, Kurachi K, Fukushima K, Nezu R, et al. Risk factors of small bowel obstruction following total proctocolectomy and ileal pouch anal anastomosis with diverting loop-ileostomy for ulcerative colitis. Ann Gastroenterol Surg. 2017;1(2):122–8.
6. Clavien PA, Sanabria JR, Strasberg SM. Proposed classification of complications of surgery with examples of utility in cholecystectomy. Surgery. 1992;111(5):518–26.
7. Ohira G, Miyauchi H, Narushima K, Kagaya A, Mutou Y, Saitou H, et al. Predicting difficulty in extending the ileal pouch to the anus in restorative proctocolectomy: investigation of a simple predictive method using computed tomography. Colorectal Dis. 2017;19(1):O34–8.
8. Uraiqat AA, Byrne CM, Phillips RK. Gaining length in ileal-anal pouch reconstruction: a review. Colorectal Dis. 2007;9(7):657–61.
9. Ohira G, Miyauchi H, Hayano K, Kagaya A, Imanishi S, Tochigi T, et al. Incidence and risk factor of outlet obstruction after construction of ileostomy. J Anus Rectum Colon. 2018;2(1):25–30.
10. Hara Y, Miura T, Sakamoto Y, Morohashi H, Nagase H, Hakamada K. Organ/space infection is a common cause of high output stoma and outlet obstruction in diverting ileostomy. BMC Surg. 2020;20(1):83.
11. Takeda M, Takahashi H, Haraguchi N, Miyoshi N, Hata T, Yamamoto H, et al. Factors predictive of high-output ileostomy: a retrospective single-center comparative study. Surg Today. 2019;49(6):482–7.

12. Matsuda T, Endo H, Inomata M, Hasegawa H, Kumamaru H, Miyata H, et al. Clinical outcome of laparoscopic vs open right hemicolectomy for colon cancer: a propensity score matching analysis of the Japanese National Clinical Database. Ann Gastroenterol Surg. 2020;4(6):693–700.
13. Dolejs S, Kennedy G, Heise CP. Small bowel obstruction following restorative proctocolectomy: affected by a laparoscopic approach? J Surg Res. 2011;170(2):202–8.
14. Hardisty RH. The management of visceroptosis. Can Med Assoc J. 1925;15(2):158–63.

Impact of reconstruction route on postoperative morbidity after esophagectomy: Analysis of esophagectomies in the Japanese National Clinical Database

Hirotoshi Kikuchi[1] | Hideki Endo[2] | Hiroyuki Yamamoto[2] | Soji Ozawa[3] | Hiroaki Miyata[2] | Yoshihiro Kakeji[4,5] | Hisahiro Matsubara[6,7] | Yuichiro Doki[7,8] | Yuko Kitagawa[9,10] | Hiroya Takeuchi[1]

[1]Department of Surgery, Hamamatsu University School of Medicine, Hamamatsu, Japan
[2]Department of Healthcare Quality Assessment, The University of Tokyo, Tokyo, Japan
[3]Department of Gastroenterological Surgery, Tokai University School of Medicine, Isehara, Japan
[4]Division of Gastrointestinal Surgery, Department of Surgery, Graduate School of Medicine, Kobe University, Kobe, Japan
[5]Database Committee, The Japanese Society of Gastroenterological Surgery, Tokyo, Japan
[6]Department of Frontier Surgery, Chiba University Graduate School of Medicine, Chiba, Japan
[7]The Japan Esophageal Society, Tokyo, Japan
[8]Department of Gastroenterological Surgery, Osaka University Graduate School of Medicine, Osaka, Japan
[9]Department of Surgery, Keio University School of Medicine, Tokyo, Japan
[10]The Japanese Society of Gastroenterological Surgery, Tokyo, Japan

Correspondence
Hiroya Takeuchi, MD, PhD, Department of Surgery, Hamamatsu University School of Medicine, 1-20-1 Handayama, Higashi-ku, Hamamatsu 431-3192, Japan.
Email: takeuchi@hama-med.ac.jp

Abstract

Background: Esophagectomy followed by gastric conduit reconstruction is a standard surgical procedure for esophageal cancer. However, there is no evidence of the superiority or inferiority of the posterior mediastinal (PM) versus the retrosternal (RS) reconstruction route with regard to short-term outcomes after esophagectomy. We aimed to elucidate whether the reconstruction route can affect the short-term outcomes after esophagectomy followed by gastric conduit reconstruction.

Methods: We reviewed the clinical data of patients who underwent esophagectomy between 2016 and 2018 from the Japanese National Clinical Database. This study included 9786 patients who underwent gastric conduit reconstruction through the PM or RS route with cervical anastomosis.

Results: Of the 9786 patients analyzed, 3478 and 6308 underwent gastric conduit reconstruction thorough the PM and RS routes, respectively. The incidence of anastomotic leak and surgical site infection (SSI) was significantly lower in the PM group than in the RS group (11.7% vs 13.8%, $P = .005$ and 8.4% vs 14.9%, $P < .001$, respectively), while the incidence of pneumonia was higher in the PM group (13.7% vs 12.2%, $P = .040$). Generalized estimating equation logistic regression analysis revealed a higher risk of anastomotic leak and SSI (odds ratio [OR], 1.32; 95% confidence interval [CI], 1.15–1.51; $P < .001$ and OR, 2.06; 95% CI, 1.78–2.38; $P < .001$, respectively) and a lower risk of pneumonia (OR, 0.86; 95% CI, 0.75–0.98; $P = .028$) in the RS group than in the PM group.

Conclusion: The findings of this study will help surgeons to design the reconstruction route following esophagectomy.

KEYWORDS

anastomotic leak, national clinical database, pneumonia, posterior mediastinal route, retrosternal route, surgical site infection

1 | INTRODUCTION

Esophageal cancer is one of the leading causes of cancer-related deaths worldwide.[1] Esophagectomy plays an important role in the multidisciplinary treatment strategies for esophageal cancer.[2-4] In the Asia-Pacific region, including Japan, the vast majority of esophageal cancers are squamous cell carcinomas (SCC) located at the upper to lower thoracic esophagus.[4-6] Surgical treatment of thoracic esophageal SCC generally consists of subtotal esophagectomy, two- or three-field lymphadenectomy, and reconstruction using organs such as the stomach.[6-8] Recent advances in surgical techniques and perioperative management have enabled us to safely perform one-stage esophagectomy with radical lymphadenectomy followed by reconstruction; however, esophagectomy remains a highly invasive procedure that can lead to severe morbidities such as anastomotic leak, respiratory complications, and cardiac events.[9-11]

The stomach is the most commonly used organ for reconstruction following esophagectomy.[3,6,8] Reconstruction using a gastric conduit can be performed via the posterior mediastinal (PM), retrosternal (RS), or subcutaneous (SC) route, among which PM and RS comprise the vast majority of reconstruction routes due to advantages over the SC route, such as shorter reconstruction route and fewer cosmetic changes after esophagectomy.[6,8] Esophagogastric anastomosis is generally made at the cervical incision in cases of RS reconstruction. Cervical or intrathoracic anastomosis can be used in cases of PM reconstruction, and cervical anastomosis is commonly performed in several Japanese institutes.[6] There are some controversies regarding the superiority or inferiority of PM reconstruction to RS reconstruction; however, there is no evidence on the impact of the reconstruction route on short-term outcomes after esophagectomy based on large-scale clinical data.

In this study we reviewed the clinical data of 17,478 patients who underwent esophagectomy followed by one-stage reconstruction using the National Clinical Database (NCD), a nationwide, web-based, data entry system in Japan.[10-14] We sought to elucidate whether the reconstruction route can affect the short-term outcomes after esophagectomy followed by gastric conduit reconstruction.

2 | MATERIALS AND METHODS

2.1 | NCD data registration

Details of the data registration system of the Japanese NCD are available elsewhere.[10-14] The NCD started data registration in January 2011, and ~1,500,000 cases are registered annually from over 5000 institutions, which corresponds to >95% of surgeries in Japan.[14] For the eight major gastroenterological surgery procedures, including esophagectomy, that were determined to represent the performance of surgery in each specialty, the input of detailed items, such as lab data and operative morbidities, are requested. Since January 2016, more detailed information, including the reconstruction organ, reconstruction route, and the location of anastomosis have been included in the requested items for esophagectomy cases. The Union for International Cancer Control TNM staging version 7 was adopted to classify the pretreatment tumor stages. All variables, definitions, and inclusion criteria for the NCD were accessible online by the participating institutions (http://www.ncd.or.jp/). The NCD supports an E-learning system that can be used by participants to enter consistent data. The patient variables in the NCD were almost identical to those used by the American College of Surgeons National Surgical Quality Improvement Program (ACS NSQIP).[15,16]

2.2 | Study design

This was a retrospective cohort study. We reviewed the clinical data of patients who underwent esophagectomy between 2016 and 2018 from the NCD Japan. According to the inclusion criteria, only thoracic esophageal cancer patients who underwent esophagectomy followed by gastric conduit reconstruction through the RS or PM route with cervical anastomosis were included in this study. Patients with metastatic or recurrent diseases, those with clinical T4, TX, NX, or M1 tumors, those who underwent emergency operation, those <18 y, and those with missing data were excluded from this study.

2.3 | Endpoints

The primary outcome measure was the incidence of major postoperative morbidities, including anastomotic leak; surgical site infection (SSI), including superficial incisional SSI, deep incisional SSI, and organ space SSI with or without leak; and pneumonia. The secondary endpoints included the 30-d and operative mortality rates, operation time, and bleeding. Operative mortality included all patients who died within the index hospitalization period, regardless of the length of hospital stay (up to 90 d), and any patient who died after hospital discharge (up to 30 d after surgery).

2.4 | Statistical analysis

For categorical variables, the proportion of patients experiencing the abovementioned outcomes was compared between the PM and RS groups using Pearson's chi-squared test, and continuous variables were compared using the Mann–Whitney *U*-test. Considering clustering of the patients at the hospital level, generalized estimating equation (GEE) logistic regression analysis was used for multivariable analysis of the impact of each clinical factor on short-term outcomes, including age at surgery (<59, 60–64, 65–69, 70–74, 75–79, and ≥80 y), sex (male vs female), body mass index (BMI; <25 vs ≥25 kg/m^2), weight loss (<10% vs ≥10%), smoking (yes vs no), habitual alcohol use (yes vs no), any respiratory distress (yes vs no), preoperative activities of daily living (ADL) with any assistance (yes vs no), American Society of Anesthesiologists physical status (ASA-PS; 1–2 vs ≥3), diabetes mellitus (DM) with insulin use (yes vs no), chronic obstructive pulmonary disease (COPD; yes vs no), hypertension (yes vs no), congestive heart failure (yes vs no), previous cardiovascular surgery (yes vs no), previous cerebrovascular disease (yes vs no), need for preoperative dialysis (yes vs no), chronic steroid use (yes vs no), serum albumin level (<2.5 vs ≥2.5 g/dL), creatinine level (<1.2 vs ≥1.2 mg/dL), clinical T stage (T0/Tis/T1a, T1b, T2, T3), clinical N stage (N0, N1, N2, N3), and histological type of cancer (SCC, adenocarcinoma, others). In addition, the use of thoracoscopy or mediastinoscopy for esophagectomy (minimally invasive esophagectomy: MIE), and the hospital esophagectomy case volume according to interquartile ranges (1–8, 9–18, 19–41, ≥42 cases/year) were included in the multivariable analysis based on our previous study.[17] All statistical tests were two-sided, and $P < .05$ was considered significant. All statistical analyses were performed using R v. 3.6.3 (2020; R Foundation for Statistical Computing, Vienna, Austria).

3 | RESULTS

3.1 | Study population

Between January 2016 and December 2018, the NCD registered 17,478 patients who underwent esophagectomy followed by one-stage reconstruction at Japanese institutes. According to the

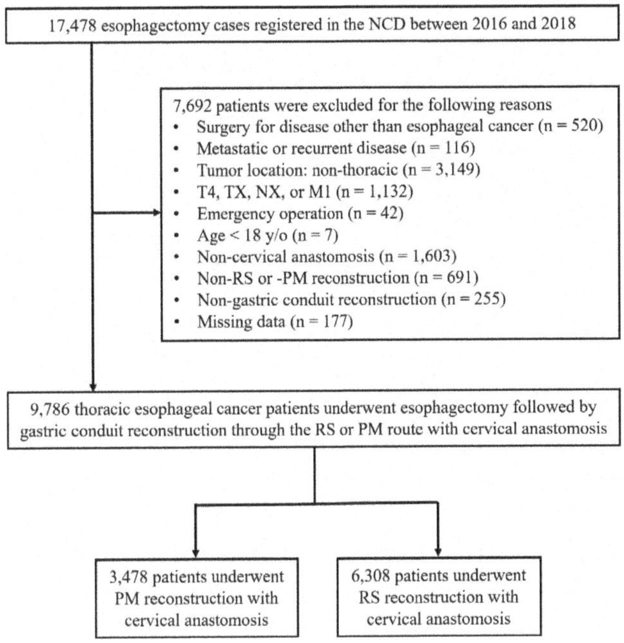

FIGURE 1 Selection process for the study population

inclusion and exclusion criteria, 9786 thoracic esophageal cancer patients who underwent esophagectomy followed by gastric conduit reconstruction through the RS or PM route with cervical anastomosis were included for analysis. Of the total analysis population, 3478 (35.5%) and 6308 (64.5%) patients underwent gastric conduit reconstruction thorough the PM route and RS route with cervical anastomosis, respectively (Figure 1).

3.2 | Risk profile

Of the 9786 thoracic esophageal cancer patients who underwent esophagectomy followed by gastric conduit reconstruction thorough either the PM or RS route with cervical anastomosis, 80.2% were male and 41.8% were elderly patients ≥70 y old. Among these patients, 36.6% had a smoking habit within 1 y, 0.9% needed assistance with ADL, 5.1% demonstrated weight loss of more than 10%, and 7.7% had an ASA-PS of grade ≥3. Preoperative comorbidities included DM with insulin use in 2.8% of patients, preoperative respiratory distress within 30 d in 0.8%, COPD in 7.6%, and history of cardiac surgery and cerebrovascular disease in 0.6% and 3.0%, respectively. Tumor histology was SCC in 95.1% and adenocarcinoma in 2.3%. Regarding the surgical procedure, MIE was performed in 78.4% of patients. A full demographic and risk profile of the study population is shown in Table 1.

3.3 | Background characteristics of the PM and RS groups

Most of the preoperative variables, such as age, BMI, ASA-PS, and previous cerebrovascular disease were equivalent between the PM and RS groups; however, the rates of DM with insulin use, congestive

TABLE 1 Comparison of preoperative variables between the PM and RS groups

	Total (n = 9786)		PM (n = 3478)		RS (n = 6308)		
Variables	n	%	n	%	n	%	*P*
Age							
<59 y	1675	17.1	546	15.7	1129	17.9	.053
60–64 y	1525	15.6	542	15.6	983	15.6	
65–69 y	2498	25.5	891	25.6	1607	25.5	
70–74 y	2175	22.2	783	22.5	1392	22.1	
75–79 y	1476	15.1	542	15.6	934	14.8	
≥80 y	437	4.5	174	5.0	263	4.2	
Male sex	7850	80.2	2791	80.2	5059	80.2	.976
BMI ≥25	8627	88.2	412	11.8	747	11.8	1
Weight loss, ≥10%	497	5.1	182	5.2	315	5.0	.64
Smoking	3586	36.6	1294	37.2	2292	36.3	.405
Habitual alcohol use	6759	69.1	2361	67.9	4398	69.7	.063
Respiratory distress	74	0.8	32	0.9	42	0.7	.205
ADL, any assistance	92	0.9	41	1.2	51	0.8	.088
ASA-PS grade ≥3	750	7.7	286	8.2	464	7.4	.133
DM with insulin use	275	2.8	122	3.5	153	2.4	.002
COPD	744	7.6	251	7.2	493	7.8	.303
Hypertension	3824	39.1	1386	39.9	2438	38.6	.253
Congestive heart failure	15	0.2	10	0.3	5	0.1	.024
Past cardiac surgery	55	0.6	42	1.2	13	0.2	<.001
Cerebrovascular disease	296	3.0	113	3.2	183	2.9	.368
Preoperative dialysis	14	0.1	6	0.2	8	0.1	.77
Chronic steroid use	87	0.9	30	0.9	57	0.9	.925
Serum albumin <2.5 g/dL	75	0.8	28	0.8	47	0.7	.838
Serum creatinine ≥1.2 mg/dL	622	6.4	259	7.4	363	5.8	.001
Clinical T stage							
T0, Tis, T1a	1218	12.4	468	13.5	750	11.9	.002
T1b	3242	33.1	1194	34.3	2048	32.5	
T2	1555	15.9	561	16.1	994	15.8	
T3	3771	38.5	1255	36.1	2516	39.9	
Clinical N stage							
N0	4840	49.5	1773	51.0	3067	48.6	.019
N1	2766	28.3	978	28.1	1788	8.3	
N2	1664	17.0	539	15.5	1125	17.8	
N3	516	5.3	188	5.4	328	5.2	
Histology type							
Squamous cell carcinoma	9306	95.1	3311	95.2	5995	95.0	.695
Adenocarcinoma	224	2.3	82	2.4	142	2.3	
Others	256	2.6	85	2.4	171	2.7	
Minimally invasive esophagectomy	7676	78.4	2986	85.9	4690	74.4	<.001
Hospital esophagectomy volume (per year)							
1–8 cases	2168	22.2	873	25.1	1295	20.5	<.001
9–18 cases	2489	25.4	1181	34.0	1308	20.7	
19–41 cases	2637	26.9	1067	30.7	1570	24.9	
≥42 cases	2492	25.5	357	10.3	2135	33.8	

Abbreviations: ADL, activities of daily living; ASA-PS, American Society of Anesthesiologists physical status; BMI, body mass index; COPD, chronic obstructive pulmonary disease; DM, diabetes mellitus; PM, posterior mediastinal route; RS, retrosternal route.

heart failure, and past cardiac surgery were significantly higher in the PM group than the RS group (3.5% vs 2.4%, $P = .002$; 0.3% vs 0.1%, $P = .024$; and 1.2% vs 0.2%, $P < .001$, respectively) (Table 1). Regarding preoperative lab data, the number of patients with serum creatinine ≥1.2 mg/dl was higher in the PM group than the RS group (7.4% vs 5.8%, $P = .001$) (Table 1). In contrast, clinical T stage and N stage were higher in the RS group than the PM group ($P = .002$ and .019, respectively) (Table 1). There was no significant difference in the histological type of esophageal cancer between the two groups ($P = .695$) (Table 1). MIE was performed more frequently in the PM group than the RS group ($P < .001$) (Table 1). The RS route was more commonly selected for reconstruction after esophagectomy in hospitals with a higher esophagectomy case volume per year ($P < .001$) (Table 1).

3.4 | Effect of reconstruction route on operation time and bleeding

The median operation time and bleeding in the 9786 patients who underwent esophagectomy followed by gastric conduit reconstruction with cervical anastomosis was 488 (427–549) min and 200 min (100–370) mL, respectively. The operation time was significantly longer in the PM group than in the RS group, although the median value was the same between the two groups (488 [427–610] min vs 488 [366–549] min, $P < .001$). The bleeding volume was lower in the PM group than in the RS group (166 [72–334] ml vs 220 [110–389] ml, $P < .001$) (Table 2).

3.5 | Effect of reconstruction route on postoperative morbidities

Major postoperative morbidities, including anastomotic leak, SSI, and pneumonia were observed in 13.0%, 12.6%, and 12.7%, respectively, of the 9786 patients who underwent esophagectomy followed by gastric conduit reconstruction with cervical anastomosis (Table 2). The rates of anastomotic leak and SSI were significantly lower in the PM group than the RS group (11.7% vs 13.8%, $P = .005$ and 8.4% vs 14.9%, $P < .001$, respectively). In contrast, the rate of pneumonia was higher in the PM group than the RS group (13.7% vs 12.2%, $P = .040$) (Table 2).

3.6 | Mortality

The mortality rates of esophagectomy followed by gastric conduit reconstruction are presented in Table 2. The 30-d mortality was 0.6%, and the overall operative mortality was 1.0%. There was no significant difference in either 30-d or operative mortality rates between the PM and RS groups (0.5% vs 0.7%, $P = .445$ and 0.9% vs 1.0%, $P = .835$, respectively).

3.7 | Risk comparison of postoperative morbidities between the PM and RS groups

As shown in Figure 2, GEE logistic regression analysis revealed that the risks of anastomotic leak and SSI were significantly greater in the RS group compared to the PM group (odds ratio [OR], 1.32; 95% confidence interval [CI], 1.15–1.51; $P < .001$, and OR, 2.06; 95% CI, 1.78–2.38; $P < .001$, respectively), whereas the risk of pneumonia was significantly lower in the RS group compared to the PM group (OR, 0.86; 95% CI, 0.75–0.98; $P = .028$).

4 | DISCUSSION

In this study we analyzed 9786 thoracic esophageal cancer patients in the NCD who underwent esophagectomy followed by gastric conduit reconstruction with cervical anastomosis. Our results demonstrated the RS route as a risk factor for anastomotic leak and SSI and the PM route as a risk factor for pneumonia. To the best of our knowledge, this is the first and largest comparison report based on a nationwide database, to elucidate the impact of reconstruction route on the short-term outcomes after esophagectomy.

In daily medical practice, the route used as the first choice for reconstruction after esophagectomy is dependent on the institutional policy or surgeons' preference. However, the final reconstruction route is generally decided based on the tumor stage and the patient's comorbidities, such as DM, which is a known risk factor for anastomotic leak and SSI,[11,18] and cardiac dysfunction, which may be affected by the stomach in the RS route.[19,20] The history of cardiac surgery can make it difficult to construct the RS route through

TABLE 2 Comparison of operative outcomes between the PM and RS groups

Variables	Total (n = 9786)	PM (n = 3478)	RS (n = 6308)	P
Operation time (median [IQR], min)	488 [427–549]	488 [427–610]	488 [366–549]	<.001
Bleeding (median [IQR], mL)	200 [100–370]	166 [72–334]	220 [110–389]	<.001
Anastomotic leak (%)	1276 (13.0)	408 (11.7)	868 (13.8)	.005
Surgical site infection (%)	1232 (12.6)	293 (8.4)	939 (14.9)	<.001
Pneumonia (%)	1244 (12.7)	475 (13.7)	769 (12.2)	.040
30-d mortality (%)	60 (0.6)	18 (0.5)	42 (0.7)	.445
Operative mortality (%)	97 (1.0)	33 (0.9)	64 (1.0)	.835

Abbreviations: IQR, interquartile range; PM, posterior mediastinal route; RS, retrosternal route.

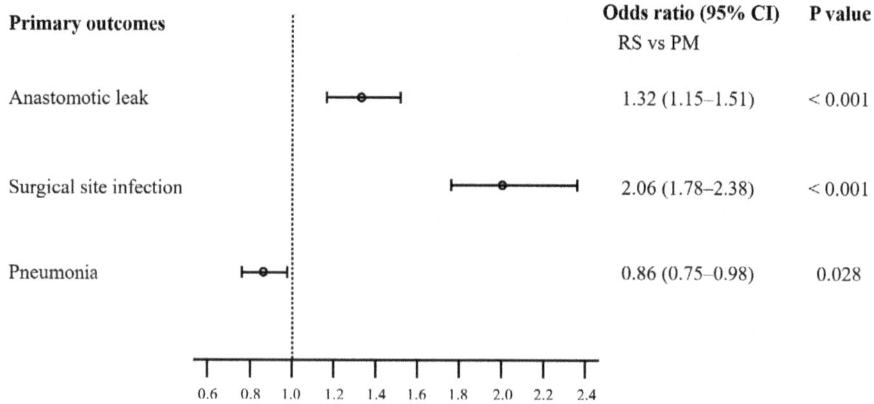

FIGURE 2 Risk comparison of postoperative morbidities between the posterior mediastinal (PM) and retrosternal (RS) groups. Circles represent the estimate of odds ratio and bars represent their 95% confidence interval (CI)

the front of the heart. In cases of local recurrence following PM reconstruction, tumors may invade the gastric conduit, leading to secondary complications, such as bleeding and stenosis, and difficulty in radiation therapy.[21] These general backgrounds in deciding the reconstruction route were reflected in the present study as the difference between the PM and RS groups is shown in Table 1.

In previous reports using NCD data, anastomotic leak and SSI were the most frequent surgical complications (approximately 13% and 14%, respectively), and pneumonia was the most frequent nonsurgical complication (approximately 15%) among major morbidities after esophagectomy.[10,11,22] In the present study, the rates and risks of anastomotic leak, SSI, and pneumonia were investigated as major morbidities after esophagectomy, as well as candidates of reconstruction route-related morbidities clinically.

Previous studies, including one randomized control trial (RCT) and five retrospective studies that enrolled a relatively small number of patients, have compared postoperative morbidities between the PM and RS routes in patients undergoing esophagectomy followed by gastric conduit reconstruction with cervical anastomosis.[21,23-27] Whereas two retrospective studies showed a higher incidence of anastomotic leak in the RS group,[24,25] the others showed no significant differences between the PM and RS routes,[21,23,26,27] and the impact of reconstruction route on anastomotic leak remained controversial. In the present study, anastomotic leak and SSI were more frequently observed in the RS group than the PM group, and multivariable analyses identified the RS route as an independent risk factor for anastomotic leak and SSI. The higher rate and risks of SSI appear to be affected by the higher incidence of anastomotic leak in the RS group. However, the mechanisms by which the RS route increased the risk of anastomotic leak are currently unclear. Although the length of reconstruction route may explain the risk of anastomotic leak, there are controversies surrounding the required conduit length between the PM and RS routes.[28-31] Furthermore, the size of the thoracic inlet (superior thoracic aperture) is reportedly associated with cervical anastomotic leak, both in the PM and RS reconstructions, suggesting that compression of the clavicular head and the sternoclavicular joint may impair blood flow of the gastric conduit.[32-34] However, it is unclear which route is more significantly affected by a narrow thoracic inlet, and whether this may lead to different risks of anastomotic leak between the two groups. The effect of the gastric conduit width (wide vs narrow) on anastomotic leak is another topic of clinical interest; however, there is currently no consensus on the superiority of either method.[35-39] Although the NCD does not request information on the width of gastric conduit, the rate of reconstruction using a whole stomach should be very low (about 1%) according to the comprehensive registry of esophageal cancer in Japan.[6]

Regarding pneumonia, there was no significant difference between the PM and RS routes in previous studies.[21,23-27] Therefore, for the first time, the present study showed the lower risks of pneumonia in the RS route over the PM route after esophagectomy followed by gastric conduit reconstruction using a Japanese nationwide database. In this study, the slightly higher rate of elderly patients ≥70 y in the PM group than the RS group (43.1% vs 41.1%) may explain the cause of higher incidence of pneumonia; however, multivariable analyses identified the PM route as an independent risk factor for pneumonia. In the PM group, the posterior mediastinum could be massively occupied by the pulled-up stomach and omentum, depending on the size of the gastric conduit and the abdominal visceral fat volume; this may compress the trachea and bronchus, and cause pulmonary atelectasis and pneumonia. In addition, there may be a difference between the PM and RS groups with regard to the incidence of gastroesophageal reflux, which may also cause pneumonia.[40] Because anastomotic leak may be one of the multiple causes of postoperative pneumonia, a possible higher impact of anastomotic leak on the development of pneumonia in the PM group may explain the higher incidence of pneumonia in the PM group than in the RS group. However, it is difficult to differentiate which complication occurred first in patients with a coincidence of anastomotic leak and pneumonia, and the causal relationship between these two complications remain unclear in this study using the NCD. These hypothetical mechanisms need to be verified in future studies, including more detailed data, such as body fat percentage, acid reflux, and the onset time of complications.

Regarding mortality after esophagectomy, there was no significant difference in either 30-d or operative mortality rates between the PM and RS groups. Although the effects of the reconstruction route on the long-term outcomes were not evaluated, the difference in the major morbidity rates between the PM and RS routes in the present study suggest an impact of the reconstruction route on the oncological outcomes after esophagectomy. Indeed, previous studies on esophageal SCC and adenocarcinoma showed an association of postoperative complications such as pneumonia with poor oncological outcomes.[41-43] Therefore, the reconstruction route following esophagectomy may impact survival by affecting the risks of postoperative morbidities.

The limitations of the current study include a lack of anastomotic procedures, such as hand-suture and stapling anastomosis, and a lack of long-term outcomes over 3 mo and quality of life after surgery. In addition, our study did not capture known short- and long-term complications, such as anastomotic stenosis, gastroesophageal reflux, and malnutrition because the NCD did not collect these data. The raw data outcomes of anastomotic leak and SSI could be underestimated, and those of pneumonia could be overestimated by hospital volume, which may be associated with postoperative complications, as speculated by its impact on risk-adjusted mortality following esophagectomy[44] and the preference of the RS route for reconstruction in hospitals with a higher esophagectomy case volume per year (Table 1). Training status and compliance, and the certification status of the institute and surgeon could also influence the outcomes.[45] However, these factors were included in the multivariable analysis as a hospital esophagectomy case volume in this study, and the outcomes shown in Table 2 were further supported by the multivariable analysis.

A major strength of this study is that this is a large-scale comparison report based on a nationwide database. In contrast to RCTs, which generally enroll patients below a certain age limit, without serious comorbidities, in limited institutions the NCD registered almost all surgical cases in Japan. The present study analyzed a large number of patients who underwent esophagectomy in the whole of Japan using the NCD, and unveiled the current status of reconstruction route choice after esophagectomy. Moreover, we examined the impact of the reconstruction route on postoperative morbidities after esophagectomy, without excluding elderly patients or those with serious comorbidities.

In conclusion, the present study first analyzed the impact of the reconstruction route on postoperative morbidities using the nationwide clinical database of patients undergoing esophagectomy for esophageal cancer. The RS route was identified as a risk factor for anastomotic leak and SSI, and the PM route was identified as a risk factor for pneumonia after esophagectomy. Although there may be some bias in the indication of reconstruction route based on the patients' condition and tumor stage, risk-adjusted models in the present study provided important information about the risks of major morbidities, which should be considered for the indication of reconstruction route preoperatively.

ACKNOWLEDGMENTS

We thank all data managers and hospital staff who participated in this National Clinical Database project for their efforts in data entry. We also thank Drs. Nao Ichihara, MD, MPH, PhD, and Yoshihiro Hiramatsu MD, PhD, and Kinji Kamiya MD, PhD for their advice.

REFERENCES

1. Bray F, Ferlay J, Soerjomataram I, Siegel RL, Torre LA, Jemal A. Global cancer statistics 2018: GLOBOCAN estimates of incidence and mortality worldwide for 36 cancers in 185 countries. CA Cancer J Clin. 2018;68(6):394–424.
2. Enzinger PC, Mayer RJ. Esophageal cancer. N Engl J Med. 2003;349(23):2241–52.
3. van Hagen P, Hulshof MC, van Lanschot JJ, et al. Preoperative chemoradiotherapy for esophageal or junctional cancer. N Engl J Med. 2012;366(22):2074–84.
4. Pennathur A, Gibson MK, Jobe BA, Luketich JD. Oesophageal carcinoma. Lancet. 2013;381(9864):400–12.
5. Arnold M, Ferlay J, van Berge Henegouwen MI, Soerjomataram I. Global burden of oesophageal and gastric cancer by histology and subsite in 2018. Gut. 2020;69(9):1564–71.
6. Tachimori Y, Ozawa S, Numasaki H, et al. Comprehensive registry of esophageal cancer in Japan, 2011. Esophagus. 2018;15(3): 127–52.
7. Akiyama H, Tsurumaru M, Udagawa H, Kajiyama Y. Radical lymph node dissection for cancer of the thoracic esophagus. Ann Surg. 1994;220(3):364–72.
8. Ando N, Ozawa S, Kitagawa Y, Shinozawa Y, Kitajima M. Improvement in the results of surgical treatment of advanced squamous esophageal carcinoma during 15 consecutive years. Ann Surg. 2000;232(2):225–32.
9. Findlay JM, Gillies RS, Millo J, Sgromo B, Marshall RE, Maynard ND. Enhanced recovery for esophagectomy: a systematic review and evidence-based guidelines. Ann Surg. 2014;259(3):413–31.
10. Takeuchi H, Miyata H, Gotoh M, et al. A risk model for esophagectomy using data of 5354 patients included in a Japanese nationwide web-based database. Ann Surg. 2014;260(2):259–66.
11. Ohkura Y, Miyata H, Konno H, et al. Development of a model predicting the risk of eight major postoperative complications after esophagectomy based on 10826 cases in the Japan National Clinical Database. J Surg Oncol. 2020;121(2):313–21
12. Kikuchi H, Miyata H, Konno H, et al. Development and external validation of preoperative risk models for operative morbidities after total gastrectomy using a Japanese web-based nationwide registry. Gastric Cancer. 2017;20(6):987–97.
13. Kakeji Y, Takahashi A, Hasegawa H, et al. Surgical outcomes in gastroenterological surgery in Japan: Report of the National Clinical Database 2011–2018. Ann Gastroenterol Surg. 2020;4(3):250–74.
14. Kakeji Y, Yamamoto H, Ueno H, et al. Development of gastroenterological surgery over the last decade in Japan: analysis of the National Clinical Database. Surg Today. 2021;51(2):187–93.
15. Shiloach M, Frencher SK Jr, Steeger JE, et al. Toward robust information: data quality and inter-rater reliability in the American College of Surgeons National Surgical Quality Improvement Program. J Am Coll Surg. 2010;210(1):6–16.
16. Marubashi S, Liu JY, Miyata H, et al. Surgical quality improvement programs in Japan and USA: Report from the collaborative projects between Japanese Society of Gastroenterological Surgery and American College of Surgeons National Surgical Quality Improvement Program. Ann Gastroenterol Surg. 2019;3(4):343–51.
17. Yoshida N, Yamamoto H, Baba H, et al. Can minimally invasive esophagectomy replace open esophagectomy for esophageal cancer? Latest analysis of 24,233 esophagectomies from the Japanese National Clinical Database. Ann Surg. 2020;272(1):118–24.

18. Li SJ, Wang ZQ, Li YJ, et al. Diabetes mellitus and risk of anastomotic leakage after esophagectomy: a systematic review and meta-analysis. Dis Esophagus. 2017;30(6):1–12.
19. Ojima T, Iwahashi M, Nakamori M, et al. Atrial fibrillation after esophageal cancer surgery: an analysis of 207 consecutive patients. Surg Today. 2014;44(5):839–47.
20. Sohda M, Kuriyama K, Kumakura Y, et al. Evaluation of surgical procedures that affect the hemodynamics using the FloTrac system in esophageal cancer patients. Vivo. 2019;33(4):1221–6.
21. Wong AC, Law S, Wong J. Influence of the route of reconstruction on morbidity, mortality and local recurrence after esophagectomy for cancer. Dig Surg. 2003;20(3):209–14.
22. Takeuchi H, Miyata H, Ozawa S, et al. Comparison of short-term outcomes between open and minimally invasive esophagectomy for esophageal cancer using a nationwide database in Japan. Ann Surg Oncol. 2017;24(7):1821–7.
23. van Lanschot JJ, van Blankenstein M, Oei HY, Tilanus HW. Randomized comparison of prevertebral and retrosternal gastric tube reconstruction after resection of oesophageal carcinoma. Br J Surg. 1999;86(1):102–8.
24. Wang H, Tan L, Feng M, Zhang Y, Wang Q. Comparison of the short-term health-related quality of life in patients with esophageal cancer with different routes of gastric tube reconstruction after minimally invasive esophagectomy. Qual Life Res. 2011;20(2):179–89.
25. Chan ML, Hsieh CC, Wang CW, Huang MH, Hsu WH, Hsu HS. Reconstruction after esophagectomy for esophageal cancer: retrosternal or posterior mediastinal route? J Chin Med Assoc. 2011;74(11):505–10.
26. Zheng YZ, Dai SQ, Li W, et al. Comparison between different reconstruction routes in esophageal squamous cell carcinoma. World J Gastroenterol. 2012;18(39):5616–21.
27. Yamasaki M, Miyata H, Yasuda T, et al. Impact of the route of reconstruction on post-operative morbidity and malnutrition after esophagectomy: a multicenter cohort study. World J Surg. 2015;39(2):433–40.
28. Ngan SY, Wong J. Lengths of different routes for esophageal replacement. J Thorac Cardiovasc Surg. 1986;91(5):790–2.
29. Coral RP, Constant-Neto M, Silva IS, et al. Comparative anatomical study of the anterior and posterior mediastinum as access routes after esophagectomy. Dis Esophagus. 2003;16(3):236–8.
30. Chen H, Lu JJ, Zhou J, et al. Anterior versus posterior routes of reconstruction after esophagectomy: a comparative anatomic study. Ann Thorac Surg. 2009;87(2):400–4.
31. Hu H, Ye T, Tan D, Li H, Chen H. Is anterior mediastinum route a shorter choice for esophageal reconstruction? A comparative anatomic study. Eur J Cardiothorac Surg. 2011;40(6):1466–9.
32. Mine S, Watanabe M, Okamura A, Imamura Y, Kajiyama Y, Sano T. Superior thoracic aperture size is significantly associated with cervical anastomotic leakage after esophagectomy. World J Surg. 2017;41(10):2598–604.
33. Sato S, Nakatani E, Higashizono K, et al. Size of the thoracic inlet predicts cervical anastomotic leak after retrosternal reconstruction after esophagectomy for esophageal cancer. Surgery. 2020;168(3):558–66.
34. Inoue S, Yoshida T, Nishino T, et al. The sterno-tracheal distance is an important factor of anastomotic leakage of retrosternal gastric tube reconstruction after esophagectomy. Esophagus. 2020;17(3):264–9.
35. Collard JM, Tinton N, Malaise J, Romagnoli R, Otte JB, Kestens PJ. Esophageal replacement: gastric tube or whole stomach? Ann Thorac Surg. 1995;60(2):261–6.
36. Shu YS, Sun C, Shi WP, Shi HC, Lu SC, Wang K. Tubular stomach or whole stomach for esophagectomy through cervico-thoraco-abdominal approach: a comparative clinical study on anastomotic leakage. Ir J Med Sci. 2013;182(3):477–80.
37. Zhang R, Wang P, Zhang X, Zhang L, Li C. Gastric tube reconstruction prevents postoperative recurrence and metastasis of esophageal cancer. Oncol Lett. 2016;11(4):2507–9.
38. Tabira Y, Sakaguchi T, Kuhara H, Teshima K, Tanaka M, Kawasuji M. The width of a gastric tube has no impact on outcome after esophagectomy. Am J Surg. 2004;187(3):417–21.
39. Zhang C, Wu QC, Hou PY, et al. Impact of the method of reconstruction after oncologic oesophagectomy on quality of life–a prospective, randomised study. Eur J Cardiothorac Surg. 2011;39(1):109–14.
40. Katsoulis IE, Robotis I, Kouraklis G, Yannopoulos P. Duodenogastric reflux after esophagectomy and gastric pull-up: the effect of the route of reconstruction. World J Surg. 2005;29(2):174–81.
41. Booka E, Takeuchi H, Nishi T, et al. The impact of postoperative complications on survivals after esophagectomy for esophageal cancer. Medicine (Baltimore). 2015;94(33):e1369.
42. Kataoka K, Takeuchi H, Mizusawa J, et al. Prognostic impact of postoperative morbidity after esophagectomy for esophageal cancer: exploratory analysis of JCOG9907. Ann Surg. 2017;265(6):1152–7.
43. Luc G, Durand M, Chiche L, Collet D. Major post-operative complications predict long-term survival after esophagectomy in patients with adenocarcinoma of the esophagus. World J Surg. 2015;39(1):216–22.
44. Nishigori T, Miyata H, Okabe H, et al. Impact of hospital volume on risk-adjusted mortality following oesophagectomy in Japan. Br J Surg. 2016;103(13):1880–6.
45. Motoyama S, Yamamoto H, Miyata H, et al. Impact of certification status of the institute and surgeon on short-term outcomes after surgery for thoracic esophageal cancer: evaluation using data on 16,752 patients from the National Clinical Database in Japan. Esophagus. 2020;17(1):41–9.

25

Dislocation of the gastric conduit reconstructed via the posterior mediastinal route is a significant risk factor for anastomotic disorder after McKeown esophagectomy

Masanobu Nakajima[1] | Hiroto Muroi[1] | Maiko Kikuchi[1] | Junki Fujita[1] | Keisuke Ihara[1] | Masatoshi Nakagawa[1] | Shinji Morita[1] | Takatoshi Nakamura[1] | Satoru Yamaguchi[2] | Kazuyuki Kojima[1]

[1]First Department of Surgery, Dokkyo Medical University, Shimotsugagun, Japan

[2]Department of Surgery, Dokkyo Medical University Nikko Medical Center, Nikko, Japan

Correspondence
Masanobu Nakajima, First Department of Surgery, Dokkyo Medical University, 880 Kitakobayashi, Mibu, Shimotsuga-gun, Tochigi 321-0293, Japan.
Email: mnakajim@dokkyomed.ac.jp

Abstract

Background: Anastomotic disorder of the reconstructed gastric conduit is a life-threating morbidity after thoracic esophagectomy. Although there are various reasons for anastomotic disorder, the present study focused on dislocation of the gastric conduit (DGC).

Methods: The study cohort comprised 149 patients who underwent transthoracic esophagectomy. The relationships between DGC and peri- and postoperative morbidities were analyzed retrospectively. Data were analyzed to determine whether body mass index (BMI) and extension of the gastric conduit were related to DGC. Uni- and multivariate Cox regression analyses were performed to identify the factors associated with anastomotic disorder.

Results: DGC was significantly related to anastomotic leakage ($P < .001$), anastomotic stricture ($P = .018$), and mediastinal abscess/empyema ($P = .031$). Compared with the DGC-negative group, the DGC-positive group had a significantly larger mean preoperative BMI (23.01 ± 3.26 kg/m^2 vs. 21.22 ± 3.13 kg/m^2, $P = .001$) and mean maximum cross-sectional area of the gastric conduit (1024.75 ± 550.43 mm^2 vs. 619.46 ± 263.70 mm^2, $P < .001$). Multivariate analysis revealed that DGC was an independent risk factor for anastomotic leakage (odds ratio: 4.840, 95% confidence interval: 1.770-13.30, $P < .001$). Body weight recovery tended to be better in the DGC-negative group than in the DGC-positive group, although this intergroup difference was not significant.

Conclusion: DGC reconstructed via the posterior mediastinal route is a significant cause of critical morbidities related to anastomosis. In particular, care is required when performing gastric conduit reconstruction via the posterior mediastinal route in patients with a high BMI.

KEYWORDS
anastomotic leak, esophageal neoplasms, esophagectomy, morbidity, quality of life

1 | INTRODUCTION

Esophageal cancer is the seventh most common type of cancer and the sixth leading cause of overall mortality worldwide.[1] Despite recent developments in surgical technique and perioperative management, esophagectomy for esophageal cancer is one of the most invasive gastroenterological surgeries with a very high morbidity rate.[2-5] Anastomotic disorder of the reconstructed organs, especially the gastric conduit, is a common, severe, and life-threatening complication of esophagectomy.[6,7]

Esophageal reconstruction with a gastric conduit is typically performed via the subcutaneous, retrosternal, or posterior mediastinal (PM) route.[8-10] Among these three routes, the PM route is considered the most physiological.[11,12] However, PM reconstruction carries a risk of severe morbidities such as mediastinal abscess, empyema, and tracheobronchial fistula.[13-16] Therefore, it is important to identify the risk factors for anastomotic disorder of the gastric conduit reconstructed through the PM route.

Previous studies have reported that anastomotic disorder, especially anastomotic leakage, results from ischemia of the gastric conduit,[17,18] compression[19] or tension[20,21] of the anastomotic site, or poor anastomotic technique.[22] However, dislocation of the gastric conduit (DGC) is rarely discussed.

DGC is often seen after esophagectomy and has an unfavorable effect on postoperative quality of life (QOL) in patients who have undergone esophagectomy in clinical practice. However, this seems to be an empirical finding. Despite a thorough search, we could not find any previous reports on the relationship between esophagectomy and DGC.

In this study, we investigated the risk of post-esophagectomy anastomotic disorder of the gastric conduit reconstructed through the PM route, focusing on DGC.

2 | METHODS

2.1 | Patients

We retrospectively reviewed the medical records of 273 patients with esophageal cancer who underwent radical thoracic esophagectomy and gastric conduit reconstruction between January 2009 and December 2018 at Dokkyo Medical University Hospital. We excluded patients who underwent transhiatal esophagectomy (28 cases) and salvage esophagectomy after definitive chemoradiotherapy (nine cases) or laryngopharyngoesophagectomy (four cases). We also excluded 69 cases of retrosternal reconstruction and one of subcutaneous reconstruction. Thus, data from 163 patients who underwent McKeown esophagectomy with gastric conduit reconstruction via the PM route were extracted. Of these 163 patients, we excluded nine who underwent hand-sewn anastomosis and five who underwent mechanical anastomosis using a linear stapler because we performed these anastomoses on rare occasions in unfavorable condition, such as in patients with a short gastric conduit or short remnant esophagus.

The final study cohort comprised 149 patients who underwent thoracoscopic or transthoracic subtotal esophagectomy and open or hand-assisted laparoscopic esophageal reconstruction with a gastric conduit via the PM route and cervical stapled anastomosis using a circular stapler.

The patients were staged using the TNM classification (8th edition) of the American Joint Committee on Cancer and the International Union Against Cancer. Informed consent for surgery was obtained from all patients in accordance with our institutional guidelines. The study was approved by the Medical Ethics Committee of Dokkyo Medical University (approval number: R-20-7J).

2.2 | Esophageal reconstruction

After subtotal esophagectomy, abdominal lymphadenectomy and gastric conduit reconstruction was started with the patient in the supine position. The open method was used in 122 cases, while hand-assisted laparoscopic surgery (HALS) was performed in 27 cases. Gastrectomy was performed to remove the mobilized esophagus, with lymphadenectomy around the left gastric artery and celiac artery. After mobilization of the full stomach and esophagus, a gastric conduit with a width of 3.5-4 cm was created by dividing the lesser curvature of the stomach. The right gastric artery and right gastroepiploic artery provided the vascular supply to the created gastric conduit. The gastric conduit was pulled up via the PM route. The esophagogastrostomy was performed in the neck by end-to-side stapled anastomosis. A 21-mm or 25-mm intraluminal circular stapler was used as the stapling device (CDH21, CDH25, Ethicon Ltd.; EEA21, EEA25, Medtronic). The inserted part of the gastric conduit was closed using a linear stapling device (ECHELON FLEX 60, Powered ECHELON FLEX 60, ECR60D, Ethicon Ltd.; Endo GIA tristaple, EGIA60AMT, Medtronic).

2.3 | Definition of DGC

We focused on DGC as a risk factor for anastomotic leakage because DGC results in tension at the anastomotic site. In cases where the gastric conduit is reconstructed via the PM route, the gastric conduit usually dislocates to the right pleural cavity because the mediastinal pleura is resected with the thoracic esophagus. DGC was defined as dislocation of more than 2/3 of the width of the gastric conduit to the right side from the line on the edge of the sternum and thoracic vertebral body (Figure 1).

Imaging assessment

DGC was assessed on the axial view of the first computed tomography (CT) scan. If there were no symptoms of postoperative morbidity, we routinely performed CT 3 months after esophagectomy. When postoperative morbidity was suspected, we immediately performed CT. The earliest CT among this series was performed

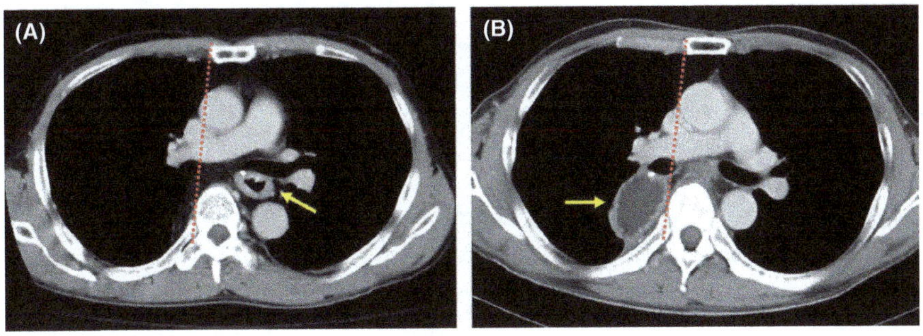

FIGURE 1 Computed tomography images of the gastric conduit. (A) DGC-negative case. The gastric conduit (arrow) is in the usual posterior mediastinal space. (B) DGC-positive case. The gastric conduit (arrow) is located outside of the line on the right edge of the sternum and thoracic vertebral body (dotted line) on the axial view. DGC, dislocation of the gastric conduit

on postoperative day 1. The maximum cross-sectional area of the gastric conduit was measured by setting the region of interest with Nazca View ver. 3.2.10000.20 (AstroStage Inc).

2.4 | Definitions of peri- and postoperative morbidities

Peri- and postoperative morbidities were defined as complications that seemed to be related to the reconstruction procedure. Complications were assessed in accordance with the Clavien-Dindo classification, and complications of grade II or above were regarded as significant.

2.5 | Comparison between preoperative body mass index and DGC

Patients with a high body mass index (BMI) may have a small PM space after esophagectomy and a large volume of greater omentum associated with the gastric conduit. As a result, DGC may occur more easily in patients with a high BMI than in patients with a normal BMI. Therefore, we compared the preoperative BMI between the DGC-positive and DGC-negative groups.

2.6 | Examination of the relationship between extension and DGC

We noticed that the gastric conduits that had dislocated to the pleural cavity tended to be more extended than the non-dislocated gastric conduits. Therefore, we examined the relationship between the maximum cross-sectional area of the gastric conduit and DGC.

2.7 | Examination of body weight change

Body weight change was examined as an indicator of long-term QOL.

2.8 | Statistical analysis

The chi-squared test and Fisher's exact test were used for statistical comparisons of nominal variables where appropriate. Continuous data were compared with the Student's *t*-test or analyzed by repeated measures one-way analysis of variance. Multivariate analysis was performed using logistic regression. Differences were considered significant if the *P* value was $<.05$. All statistical analyses were carried out using EZR (version 1.54) (Saitama Medical Center, Jichi Medical University), which is a graphical user interface for R (The R Foundation for Statistical Computing).

3 | RESULTS

3.1 | Patients' characteristics and DGC

The characteristics of the eligible patients are described in Table 1. In summary, the population was typical for Japanese patients with esophageal cancer. The mean age was 65.15 years, and the main histologic type was squamous cell carcinoma (91.9%). Sixty-seven cases (45.0%) were node-positive clinically, and 35 patients (23.5%) received neoadjuvant chemotherapy using the cisplatin and 5-fluorouracil regimen or the docetaxel, cisplatin, and 5-fluorouracil regimen. Thoracoscopic esophagectomy was performed in 77 patients (51.7%), while HALS was performed in 27 patients (18.1%). The mean BMI was 21.91 kg/m^2. DGC was detected in 57 patients (38.3%). Although we did not decide on the level of measurement, the maximally dislocated level was just below the bifurcation in almost all patients.

3.2 | DGC and peri- and postoperative morbidities

Compared with the DGC-negative group, the DGC-positive group had significantly higher incidences of anastomotic leakage ($P < .001$) and anastomotic stricture ($P = .018$). Mediastinal abscess and empyema occurred in six patients, five (83.3%) of whom were in the DGC-positive group ($P = .031$) (Figure 2). Among the 29 cases

TABLE 1 Characteristics of the 149 eligible patients who underwent esophagectomy

Variable	Value
Age in years, mean ± SD	65.15 ± 8.45
Sex (male/female)	120/29
Tumor location (upper/middle/lower)	17/79/53
Histology (SCC/AC/other)	132/10/7
T (1/2/3/4)	60/18/65/6
N (0/1/2/3)	82/31/20/16
M (0/1)	142/7
Stage (I/II/III/IVA/IVB)	53/35/46/8/7
NAC (yes/no)	35/114
Preoperative BMI in kg/m^2, mean ± SD	21.91 ± 3.29
TTE/TSE	72/77
Laparotomy/HALS	122/27
Operation time in minutes, mean ± SD	461.41 ± 73.24
Blood loss in g, median [range]	350 [30-2090]
Circular stapler size (21 mm/25 mm)	19/130
DGC (yes/no)	57/92

Abbreviations: AC, adenocarcinoma; BMI, body mass index; DGC, distension of the gastric conduit; HALS, hand-assisted laparoscopic surgery; M, distant metastasis; N, lymph node metastasis; NAC, neoadjuvant chemotherapy; SCC, squamous cell carcinoma; SD, standard deviation; T, depth of tumor invasion; TSE, thoracoscopic esophagectomy; TTE, transthoracic open esophagectomy.

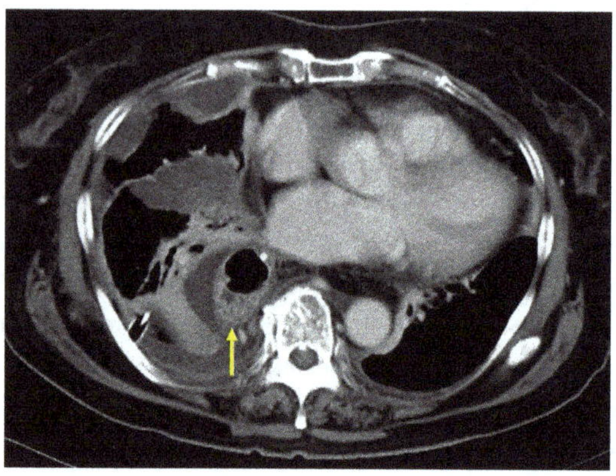

FIGURE 2 A case of empyema. The dislocated gastric conduit (arrow) with pleural fluid collection and pulmonary atelectasis is seen in the right pleural cavity

of stricture, 12 cases (41.4%) had anastomotic leakage. Meanwhile, five patients (83.3%) had anastomotic leakage among six patients with mediastinal abscess and empyema. The incidence of pneumonia, which may be caused by pulmonary atelectasis due to DGC, was not increased in the DGC-positive group. Delayed gastric emptying (DGE) is a typical postoperative disorder of esophagectomy. In this study, DGE tended to be more frequent in the DGC-positive group although the increase in frequency was not significant (*P* = .070; Table 2).

TABLE 2 Relationship between dislocation of the gastric conduit and anastomosis-related postoperative morbidities

	DGC		
Morbidity	Negative	Positive	*P* value
Anastomotic leakage			
No	85	39	<.001
Yes	7	18	
Anastomotic stricture			
No	80	40	.018
Yes	12	17	
Mediastinal abscess/empyema			
No	91	52	.031
Yes	1	5	
Pneumonia			
No	86	51	.537
Yes	6	6	
Delayed gastric emptying			
No	81	43	.070
Yes	11	14	

Abbreviation: DGC, distension of the gastric conduit.

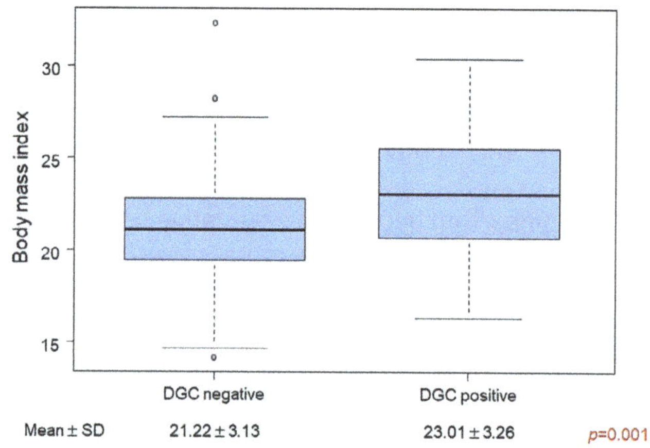

FIGURE 3 Relationship between DGC and BMI. The BMI of the DGC-positive group is significantly larger than that of the DGC-negative group. BMI, body mass index; DGC, dislocation of the gastric conduit; SD, standard deviation

3.3 | Preoperative BMI and DGC

The mean preoperative BMI in the DGC-negative group (21.22 ± 3.13 kg/m^2) was significantly smaller than that in the DGC-positive group (23.01 ± 3.26 kg/m^2, *P* = .00108; Figure 3).

3.4 | Relationship between extension and DGC

The mean maximum cross-sectional area of the gastric conduit was significantly smaller in the DGC-negative group (619.46 ± 263.70

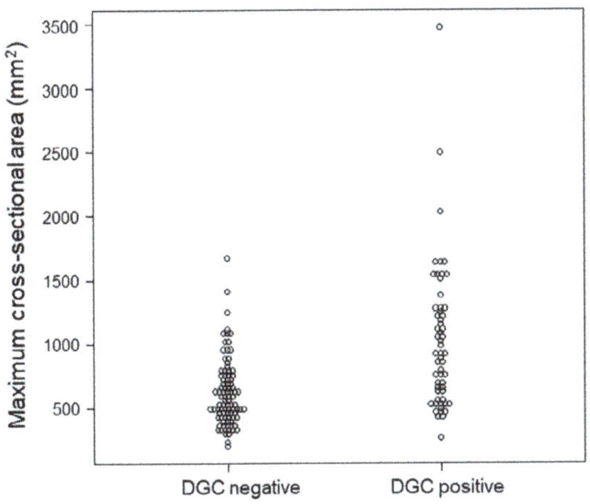

FIGURE 4 Relationship between dislocation and extension of the gastric conduit. The maximum cross-sectional area is significantly larger in DGC-positive patients than in DGC-negative patients. DGC, dislocation of the gastric conduit; SD, standard deviation

mm^2) than in the DGC-positive group (1024.75 ± 550.43 mm^2, $P < .001$) (Figure 4).

3.5 | Factors associated with anastomotic disorder

Univariate Cox regression analysis revealed that the factors significantly associated with anastomotic leakage were the preoperative BMI, thoracoscopic esophagectomy, HALS, and DGC (all $P < .05$). These factors were entered in the multivariate model. Multivariate analysis revealed that DGC was an independent risk factor for anastomotic leakage (odds ratio: 4.840, 95% confidence interval: 1.770-13.30, $P < .001$) (Table 3). Uni- and multivariate analyses were also performed to identify the factors associated with anastomotic stricture, mediastinal abscess/empyema, and entire anastomotic disorders. However, no independent risk factors were identified (data not shown).

3.6 | Body weight change and DGC

Among the 149 eligible patients, the patients who survived more than 2 years without recurrence were selected. As a result, the postoperative body weight change of 101 patients was analyzed (58 in the DGC-negative group and 43 in the DGC-positive group). The body weight recovery tended to be better in the DGC-negative group than in the DGC-positive group; however, this intergroup difference was not significant (Figure 5).

4 | DISCUSSION

The present study is the first to demonstrate that DGC is an independent risk factor for anastomotic leakage and is closely related to other anastomotic disorders.

Anastomotic leakage is one of the most frequent and life-threatening complications that often results in mediastinitis, mediastinal abscess, and empyema, especially in patients who undergo PM reconstruction.[13] To improve peri- and postoperative QOL, it is very important to investigate the cause of anastomotic leakage and identify preventative measures. Although previous studies have reported that the causes of anastomotic leakage are tension, compression, ischemia, hyperemia, and an unskilled anastomotic technique, we focused on DGC because we had subjectively noticed that DGC was common in cases with anastomotic leakage.

Even in cases without anastomotic leakage, the gastric conduit is sometimes dislocated to the right pleural cavity after reconstruction via the PM route. Such dislocation may occur because of the weight of the gastric conduit itself or a mismatch between the volume of the gastric conduit and the mediastinal space after esophagectomy. The gastric conduit may be increasingly pulled toward the pleural cavity and distended by the negative breathing pressure. As seen in the present study, the dislocated gastric conduits became distended. However, distension of the gastric conduit was not found in the patients without DGC. Therefore, gastric distension must be partly a result of DGC. In many cases, the extension of gastric conduit was transient. It might be optimized according to the recovery of gastric motility from postoperative disorder.

The anastomosis was under strong tension, which may have caused the anastomotic leakage. The tension pulls the anastomotic site into the mediastinum, and pus pools in the mediastinum or pleural cavity. This phenomenon was more common in patients with a high BMI because of the large weight and volume of the gastric conduit due to the fatty greater omentum and the small mediastinal space due to the thick mediastinal fat tissue. Anastomotic leakage also leads to anastomotic stricture.

We often experienced the phenomenon that we could not pull the gastric conduit up to the level that we estimated in advance, and we could not avoid anastomosing at a more distal site than that we had planned. In such cases, we observed a finding suggestive of DGC (bending nasogastric tube to the right side) on X-ray images just after the operation. However, there were cases where the finding suggestive of DGC was first observed on postoperative day 1 or later. In the cases where DGC occurs earliest, DGC must be the first cause of anastomotic disorder because the anastomotic site is strongly tensioned and more distal and ischemic due to bending. However, among the cases of DGC that occur after postoperative day 1, a gastric conduit that is too long may be the cause of anastomotic disorder and DGC. The anastomotic site of a gastric conduit that is too long must be ischemic, and the too long gastric conduit may be gradually pulled into the right pleural cavity. Thus, even though DGC may not be a cause of anastomotic disorder in every case, there is a significant relationship between DGC and anastomotic disorder.

DGE is a well-known postoperative morbidity of esophagectomy. The incidence of clinically relevant DGE is in the range of 10%-20%.[23] In our study, 16.8% of all patients received medication for DGE. Although it was not significant, patients with DGC tended to have DGE. DGE might be influenced by the bend of

TABLE 3 Cox regression analysis to identify the factors associated with anastomotic leakage

	Univariate analysis			Multivariate analysis		
Factors	OR	95% CI	*P* value	OR	95% CI	*P* value
Age						
<65 years/≥65 years	1.120	0.473-2.640	.798			
Sex						
Female/male	3.200	0.710-14.40	.130			
Tumor location						
Middle or lower/upper	1.630	0.483-5.480	.432			
Stage						
I-II/III-IV	0.396	0.148-1.060	.065			
NAC						
No/yes	0.285	0.063-1.280	.102			
Preoperative BMI						
<21.9 kg/m^2/≥21.9 kg/m^2	4.240	1.590-11.40	.004	2.290	0.774-6.750	.134
TSE						
No/yes	3.600	1.350-9.630	.011	2.750	0.942-8.000	.064
HALS						
No/yes	2.920	1.140-7.540	.026	0.180	0.637-5.400	.257
Operation time						
<461.4 min/≥461.4 min	2.020	0.831-4.920	.121			
Blood loss						
<350 g/≥350 g	0.923	0.391-2.180	.855			
Blood transfusion						
No/yes	0.683	0.145-3.210	.630			
Circular stapler size						
21 mm/25 mm	0.509	0.165-1.570	.240			
DGC						
No/yes	5.600	2.160-14.50	<.001	4.840	1.770-13.30	<.001
EGC						
<650 mm^2/≥650 mm^2	1.340	0.563-3.170	.511			

Abbreviations: BMI, body mass index; CI, confidence interval; DGC, distension of the gastric conduit; EGC, extension of the gastric conduit; HALS, hand-assisted laparoscopic surgery; NAC, neoadjuvant chemotherapy; OR, odds ratio; TSE, thoracoscopic esophagectomy.

the gastric conduit or negative pressure of the pleural cavity. Moreover, DGE probably affected postoperative body weight. According to the examination of body weight change, body weight recovery tended to be poorer in the DGC-positive group. DGC may indirectly impair body weight recovery via DGE. However, the body weight recovery in patients with high BMI was poorer than that in patients with low BMI (data not shown). There is a possibility that the preoperative BMI was related to the difference in body weight recovery between the DGC-positive and -negative group because the DGC rate was higher in patients with high preoperative BMI.

As mentioned above, DGC certainly has some unfavorable effects on patients who have undergone esophagectomy. Therefore, the strategy to prevent DGC is important. We usually pull the gastric conduit down to the abdominal cavity after esophago-gastric anastomosis. In fatty cases, we attenuate the greater omentum accompanying the gastric conduit. However, very often the gastric conduit will not stay in the mediastinal space after esophagectomy. Because a strong upward vertical force may lead to straightening of the gastric conduit and avoid dislocation, we examined the effect of tumor location and anastomotic level on DGC. However, both were found to be unrelated. Nevertheless, we might not be able to avoid DGC using only a strong upward vertical force.

Numerous studies have evaluated the peri- and postoperative QOL of patients who have undergone PM vs retrosternal reconstruction after esophagectomy.[8,9,12,18,24,25] However, the optimal reconstruction route remains controversial, and the variation between studies may be due to the interstudy differences in the outcomes being evaluated. Regarding the frequency of anastomotic leakage, many studies have shown the superiority of the PM route.[26-28] In

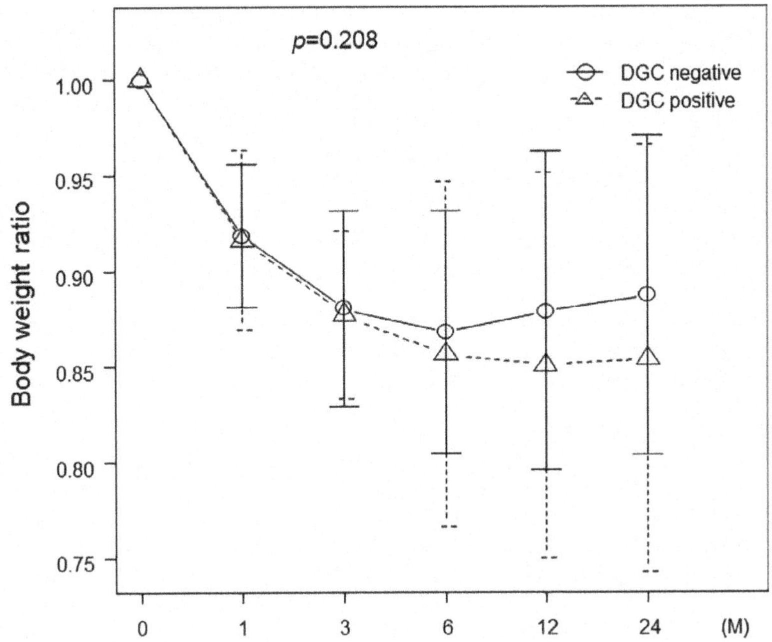

FIGURE 5 Relationship between DGC and postoperative body weight change. The body weight recovery of the DGC-negative group tends to be better than that of the DGC-positive group, although this intergroup difference was not significant. DGC, dislocation of the gastric conduit; SD, standard deviation

		0	1	3	6	12	24
Mean ± SD	DGC negative	1	0.921 ± 0.043	0.881 ± 0.051	0.868 ± 0.066	0.881 ± 0.087	0.888 ± 0.085
	DGC positive	1	0.922 ± 0.047	0.881 ± 0.044	0.861 ± 0.080	0.858 ± 0.100	0.863 ± 0.112
p-value		0.907	0.907	0.949	0.662	0.270	0.258

the present study, we evaluated the incidences of anastomotic leakage and related morbidities, especially mediastinal abscess and empyema. PM reconstruction is reportedly inferior to retrosternal reconstruction regarding the incidences of mediastinal abscess, empyema, and mediastinal fistula.[14,29] However, the retrosternal route is a newly formed space that is separate to the pleural cavity, so it is less affected by negative pressure in the pleural cavity and by DGC. Thus, retrosternal reconstruction may result in less tension at the anastomotic site than PM reconstruction. Particularly in patients with a high BMI, gastric conduit reconstruction via the retrosternal route should be considered to avoid severe anastomosis-related morbidities.

The mediastinal pleura is preserved when transhiatal esophagectomy is performed, resulting in a low risk of DGC. However, classical transhiatal esophagectomy does not allow the surgeon to perform adequate mediastinal lymphadenectomy. Therefore, to keep the oncological radicality, advanced methods such as mediastinoscope-assisted transhiatal esophagectomy are required.[30]

The present study had some limitations. First, these operations were performed in a single institution. In such a situation, there is some possibility of continuing inadequate procedures. Second, this was a retrospective study, and the patients may have had various comorbidities that affected the incidences of postoperative morbidities. The present findings require confirmation in a multicenter prospective study that includes patients who undergo retrosternal reconstruction. Further studies will aid in the identification of the best reconstruction method in consideration of not only short-term morbidity but also long-term QOL.

5 | CONCLUSIONS

DGC after reconstruction via the PM route is a significant cause of critical morbidities related to anastomosis. In particular, care is required when performing PM reconstruction in patients with a high BMI.

ACKNOWLEDGEMENTS

We thank Kelly Zammit, BVSc, and John Holmes, MSc, from Edanz Group for editing a draft of this manuscript.

REFERENCES

1. Bray F, Ferlay J, Soerjomataram I, Siegel RL, Torre LA, Jemal A. Global cancer statistics 2018: GLOBOCAN estimates of incidence and mortality worldwide for 36 cancers in 185 countries. CA Cancer J Clin. 2018;68(6):394–424.
2. Watanabe M, Okamura A, Toihata T, et al. Recent progress in perioperative management of patients undergoing esophagectomy for esophageal cancer. Esophagus. 2018;15(3):160–4.

3. Takeuchi H, Miyata H, Gotoh M, Kitagawa Y, Baba H, Kimura W, et al. A risk model for esophagectomy using data of 5354 patients included in a Japanese nationwide web-based database. Ann Surg. 2014;260(2):259–66.
4. Ozawa S, Koyanagi K, Ninomiya Y, Yatabe K, Higuchi T. Postoperative complications of minimally invasive esophagectomy for esophageal cancer. Ann Gastroenterol Surg. 2020;4(2):126–34.
5. Kitagawa Y, Matsuda S. Prevention of postoperative pulmonary complication is desired to reduce mortality and improve long-term survival after esophagectomy for esophageal cancer. Ann Gastroenterol Surg. 2020;4(5):478–9.
6. Gooszen JAH, Goense L, Gisbertz SS, Ruurda JP, van Hillegersberg R, van Berge Henegouwen MI. Intrathoracic versus cervical anastomosis and predictors of anastomotic leakage after oesophagectomy for cancer. Br J Surg. 2018;105(5):552–60.
7. Morita M, Ikeda K, Sugiyama M, Saeki H, Egashira A, Yoshinaga K, et al. Repair using the pectoralis major muscle flap for anastomotic leakage after esophageal reconstruction via the subcutaneous route. Surgery. 2010;147(2):212–8.
8. Yamasaki M, Miyata H, Yasuda T, Shiraishi O, Takahashi T, Motoori M, et al. Impact of the route of reconstruction on post-operative morbidity and malnutrition after esophagectomy: a multicenter cohort study. World J Surg. 2015;39(2):433–40.
9. Nakajima M, Kato H, Miyazaki T, Fukuchi M, Manda R, Masuda N, et al. Comprehensive investigations of quality of life after esophagectomy with special reference to the route of reconstruction. Hepatogastroenterology. 2007;54(73):104–10.
10. Chung JH, Lee SH, Yi E, Jung JS, Han JW, Kim TS, et al. A nonrandomized retrospective observational study on the subcutaneous esophageal reconstruction after esophagectomy: is it feasible in high-risk patients? J Thorac Dis. 2017;9(3):675–84.
11. Hirahara N, Yamamoto T, Tanaka T. A method of gastric conduit elevation via the posterior mediastinal pathway in thoracoscopic subtotal esophagectomy. World J Surg Oncol. 2012;10:20.
12. Park SY, Jung I, Heo SJ, Byun GE, Lee EY, Kim DJ. Comparison of QoL Between Substernal and Posterior Mediastinal Routes in Esophagogastrostomy. J Gastrointest Surg. 2021;25(3):635–40.
13. Shuto K, Kono T, Akutsu Y, Uesato M, Mori M, Matsuo K, et al. Naso-esophageal extraluminal drainage for postoperative anastomotic leak after thoracic esophagectomy for patients with esophageal cancer. Dis Esophagus. 2017;30(3):1–9.
14. Yasuda T, Sugimura K, Yamasaki M, Miyata H, Motoori M, Yano M, et al. Ten cases of gastro-tracheobronchial fistula: a serious complication after esophagectomy and reconstruction using posterior mediastinal gastric tube. Dis Esophagus. 2012;25(8):687–93.
15. Morita M, Saeki H, Okamoto T, Oki E, Yoshida S, Maehara Y. Tracheobronchial fistula during the perioperative period of esophagectomy for esophageal cancer. World J Surg. 2015;39(5):1119–26.
16. Tsukamoto T, Inoue K, Osugi H, Yamamoto T, Kakinoki E, Kinoshita H, et al. Refractory empyema caused by an intraoperative rib fracture sustained during esophagectomy: report of a case. Surg Today. 2003;33(4):290–3.
17. Briel JW, Tamhankar AP, Hagen JA, DeMeester SR, Johansson J, Choustoulakis E, et al. Prevalence and risk factors for ischemia, leak, and stricture of esophageal anastomosis: gastric pull-up versus colon interposition. J Am Coll Surg. 2004;198(4):536–41; discussion 541–2.
18. Urschel JD. Esophagogastrostomy anastomotic leaks complicating esophagectomy: a review. Am J Surg. 1995;169(6):634–40.
19. Liebermann-Meffert DM, Meier R, Siewert JR. Vascular anatomy of the gastric tube used for esophageal reconstruction. Ann Thorac Surg. 1992;54(6):1110–5.
20. Allaix ME, Long JM, Patti MG. Hybrid Ivor Lewis Esophagectomy for Esophageal Cancer. J Laparoendosc Adv Surg Tech A. 2016;26(10):763–7.
21. Cui Y, Chen H. The effect of tension on esophagogastric anastomotic wound healing in rats. J Cardiovasc Surg (Torino). 2003;44(6):775–8.
22. Mitchell JD. Anastomotic leak after esophagectomy. Thorac Surg Clin. 2006;16(1):1–9.
23. Konradsson M, Nilsson M. Delayed emptying of the gastric conduit after esophagectomy. T Thorac Dis. 2019;11(suppl5):S835–44.
24. Moremen JR, Ceppa DP, Rieger KM, Birdas TJ. Substernal reconstruction following esophagectomy: operation of last resort? J Thorac Dis. 2017;9(12):5040–5.
25. Katsoulis IE, Robotis I, Kouraklis G, Yannopoulos P. Duodenogastric reflux after esophagectomy and gastric pull-up: the effect of the route of reconstruction. World J Surg. 2005;29(2):174–81.
26. Kunisaki C, Makino H, Akiyama H, Kojima Y, Takagawa R, Kosaka T, et al. Appropriate routes of reconstruction following transthoracic esophagectomy. Hepatogastroenterology. 2007;54(79):1997–2002.
27. Chan ML, Hsieh CC, Wang CW, Huang MH, Hsu WH, Hsu HS. Reconstruction after esophagectomy for esophageal cancer: retrosternal or posterior mediastinal route? J Chin Med Assoc. 2011;74(11):505–10.
28. Akiyama Y, Iwaya T, Endo F, Shioi Y, Chiba T, Takahara T, et al. Stability of cervical esophagogastrostomy via hand-sewn anastomosis after esophagectomy for esophageal cancer. Dis Esophagus. 2017;30(5):1–7.
29. Schweigert M, Dubecz A, Beron M, Muschweck H, Stein HJ. Management of anastomotic leakage-induced tracheobronchial fistula following oesophagectomy: the role of endoscopic stent insertion. Eur J Cardiothorac Surg. 2012;41(5):e74–80.
30. Fujiwara H, Shiozaki A, Konishi H, Kosuga T, Komatsu S, Ichikawa D, et al. Perioperative outcomes of single-port mediastinoscope-assisted transhiatal esophagectomy for thoracic esophageal cancer. Dis Esophagus. 2017;30(10):1–8.

26

Current status and perspectives of the future of pancreatic surgery: Establishment of evidence by integration of "art" and "science"

Mee Joo Kang | Sun-Whe Kim

Department of Surgery, Center for Liver and Pancreato-Biliary Cancer, National Cancer Center, Goyang-si, Korea

Correspondence
Sun-Whe Kim, Department of Surgery, Center for Liver and Pancreato-Biliary Cancer, National Cancer Center, 323 Ilsan-ro, Ilsan-dong, Goyang-si, Gyunggi-do 10408, Korea.
Email: sunkim@ncc.re.kr

Abstract

Pancreatic cancer surgery continues to be associated with a high operative morbidity rate, poor long-term survival outcomes, and various challenges in obtaining high-level evidence. Not only is the early postoperative morbidity rate high, but also late morbidity involves lifelong nutritional support for long-term survivors. Due to poor survival outcomes even after curative surgery, pancreatic surgeons have doubts about the role of surgery as the definitive treatment for pancreatic cancer. Additionally, conducting clinical trials to obtain high-level evidence in the field of pancreatic surgery is difficult, and the results have only had a moderate impact on clinical practice due to skepticism regarding their quality. Therefore, quality evidence regarding the extent of resection, mode of approach to dissection, reconstruction methods for pancreatico-enteric anastomosis, determination of resectability, timing of surgery, and the definition of the resection margin is lacking. However, numerous innovative pancreatic surgical procedures have been developed, which may aptly have been called "art" when they were first introduced, regardless of whether they subsequently were supported by scientific evidence. In this review, we provide recent examples of the integration of art and science in the field of pancreatic surgery, which illustrate how the creative ideas of pancreatic surgeons evolved into generally accepted clinical practice. Pancreatic surgeons should be considered "surgical artists," "surgical scientists," and "surgical practitioners." We look forward to more "surgical artists" educating future "surgical artists and scientists" to create a richer "spirit of innovation," leading to a more beautiful integration of art and science in the field of pancreatic surgery.

KEYWORDS
evidence-based medicine, inventions, neoplasms, pancreas, pancreatectomy

1 | INTRODUCTION

Compared to other malignancies of the gastrointestinal tract, pancreatic cancer surgery is unique in terms of its associated high operative morbidity rate, poor long-term survival outcomes, and challenges in terms of obtaining high-level evidence based on randomized clinical trials (RCTs). Until recently, the pancreas has been referred to as "no man's land," which may explain why even the brightest thinkers in the East and West did not describe the pancreas in their anatomical diagrams (Figure 1).

After pancreatectomy, early morbidity is associated with pancreatic leakage, bleeding, delayed gastric emptying, and local sepsis, which often result from complex surgical procedures requiring multiple anastomoses.[1-3] In addition, surgery-related and systemic complications are more frequent due to the long operation time and, compared to other gastrointestinal malignancies, the general preoperative condition of patients with pancreatic cancer is worse. Late operative morbidity consists of exocrine and endocrine pancreatic insufficiency due to the loss of pancreatic parenchyma and marginal ulcers or the development of afferent loop syndrome attributable to gastrointestinal tract reconstruction.[4] These late complications give rise to nutritional disorders demanding lifelong nutritional support in long-term survivors.[5] Therefore, the history of pancreatectomy procedures and treatments lead to the constant efforts currently made to reduce postoperative complications.

Moreover, survival outcomes for pancreatic cancer remain low and have not improved significantly over the past few decades.[6] Only 20%-30% of patients at the time of pancreatic cancer diagnosis are considered candidates for surgery, while 70%-80% of patients eventually fail to receive curative treatment mainly due to systemic metastasis.[6] Moreover, due to poor survival outcomes even after curative resection, pancreatic surgeons have doubts about the role of surgery as the definitive treatment for pancreatic cancer. For these reasons, pancreatic cancer is considered a systemic disease; however, surgeons should also focus on achieving safer and more complete local control of the tumor through surgery.

Nevertheless, there is a lack of high-level evidence in the field of pancreatic surgery. Consequently, we do not yet have detailed guidelines for pancreatic surgical procedures, partly due to limitations in conducting RCTs, especially those focused on pancreatic cancer. Despite a noticeable increase in the quantity and quality of RCTs focused on pancreatic surgery, many are limited in their design and reporting, including selective reporting, limited assessment of long-term effects, and the risk of small sample bias.[7,8] Specifically, given small differences in the expected effect of pancreatic surgery, the sample size can be "prohibitively large" while the number of pancreatic cancer patients is insufficient for case recruitment.[9] Moreover, standardization of surgical techniques is difficult due to the complexity of the procedures.[10] As a result of deep-rooted skepticism, RCTs for pancreatic surgery have had only a moderate impact on daily clinical practice. For this reason, neither a synthesis of evidence nor a systematic review of filtered evidence is easily obtainable for pancreatic cancer surgery.[11]

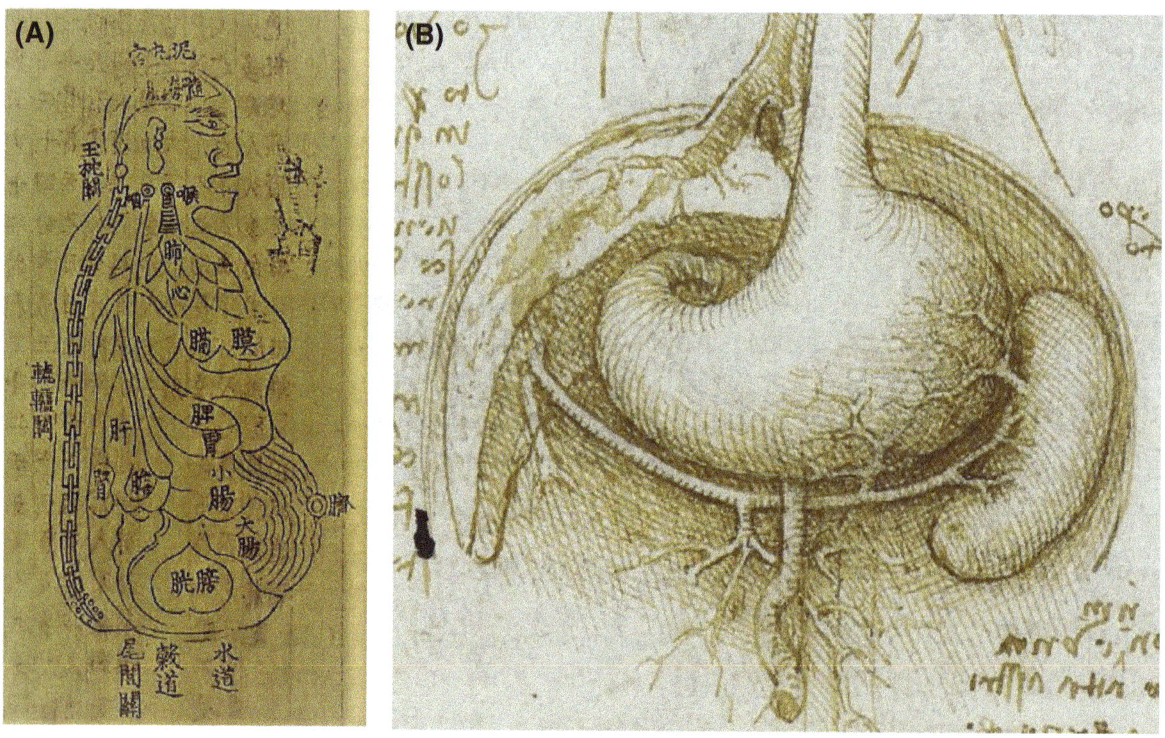

FIGURE 1 Understanding abdominal viscera as represented in classics from the Orient and the Occident. A. Drawing of the overall body, viscera, and bowel (Sinhyeongjangbudo) in Donguibogam. B. Abdominal anatomy according to Leonardo da Vinci

2 | CURRENT ISSUES IN PANCREATIC SURGERY

As previously mentioned, a number of issues regarding pancreatic surgical procedures, especially those for pancreatic cancer, still need to be addressed (Table 1). However, authoritative in-depth guidelines, including those from the National Comprehensive Cancer Network (NCCN),[12]American Society of Clinical Oncology (ASCO),[13] European Society for Medical Oncology (ESMO),[14] Japan Pancreas Society (JPS),[15] and the International Study Group for Pancreatic Surgery (ISGPS),[16] have yet to be provided for pancreatic surgery. Each of the current issues in pancreatic surgery will be discussed below.

First, there is much debate regarding the appropriate extent of resection, which includes observation vs surgery, excision vs partial pancreatectomy, partial vs total pancreatectomy, the extent of gastric resection during pancreaticoduodenectomy ([PD]; standard Whipple operation, pylorus preservation, or pylorus resection), and organ preservation (duodenum, spleen, or splenic vessels; detailed in the "spleen-preserving distal pancreatectomy" section), depending on the nature and extent of the disease.[17, 18] Additionally, the extent of lymphadenectomy, resection of major vessels, and nerve plexus dissection can be controversial for several reasons; for example, whether to include the resection or dissection of remote site lymph nodes, the portomesenteric vein, and major arteries including the celiac axis (detailed in the "modified Appleby operation for advanced pancreatic body cancer" section), superior mesenteric artery (SMA), and hepatic arteries. Previous RCTs have confirmed that prophylactic hemi-circumferential peri-SMA nerve plexus dissection was not beneficial for survival gain.[19-22] However, even though R0 resection can be achieved by adjusting the dissection level, no consensus has been achieved on the systematic criteria for the extent of resection according to the extent of the patient's primary disease.[23] Finally, although the definition remains controversial, the mesopancreas should also be considered when determining the extent of surgery (detailed in the "meso-pancreas excision" section).[24]

Second, the various modes of approaching dissection require further discussion, which include different types of SMA (first) approaches mainly for pancreatic head cancer,[25-31] radical antegrade modular pancreato-splenectomy for pancreatic body and tail cancer,[32, 33] the no-touch isolation technique,[28] *en bloc* dissection,[34, 35] and minimally invasive surgery.[36-38] Recently, the Miami International Evidence-based Guidelines strongly recommended minimally invasive distal pancreatectomy for benign and low-grade malignant tumors over open surgery; however, data on the advantages of minimally invasive PD over open surgery are insufficient. Minimally invasive pancreatectomy is recommended in high-volume centers, and the requirement for a structured training program for minimally invasive pancreatectomy must also be emphasized.[38]

Third, a major factor contributing to morbidity after pancreatectomy is the leakage of pancreatic juice from the pancreaticoenterostomy or pancreatic stump. Therefore, pancreatic surgeons are continuously searching for the best techniques for anastomosis and stump closure, which include various methods of reconstruction, the site and route of anastomosis, the use and type of stent or surgical drain, the use of surgical tissue adhesives, and other innovative techniques to restore pancreatico-enteric continuity.[39, 40]

Fourth, the criteria and tools for determining resectability are constantly evolving. To date, several resectability criteria have been proposed by various institutions and academic societies. Since its first introduction in 2002, the NCCN resectability criteria have been the most widely adopted.[12] Particularly, diagnostic criteria for borderline resectable pancreatic cancer have primarily evolved with a focus on technical resectability.[16] However, the concept of this disease entity includes oncological curability supported by neoadjuvant treatment.[41] Consequently, the criteria for determining tumor resectability are expanding beyond only anatomical or technical perspectives. Recently, the biological criteria proposed by the MD Anderson Cancer Center and the International Association of Pancreatology (IAP) have been validated.[42, 43] Criteria for imaging and non-anatomical criteria such as tumor markers, patient condition, and genetic profiling are also being developed.[44] In particular, establishing criteria for biological markers and morphological and functional imaging after neoadjuvant therapy is challenging.[45] Furthermore, the appropriate timing of surgery (upfront or after neoadjuvant therapy) and conversion surgery is fiercely debated.[46]

Lastly, the appropriate definition and assessment of the resection margin of the surgical specimen is controversial. PD specimens for pancreatic cancer have the most resection margins among the gastrointestinal malignancies, with seven margin evaluations recommended, including transection (pancreatic neck, proximal and distal gastrointestinal tract, bile duct, and vessel segment [if present]) and circumferential margins (portomesenteric groove, SMA margin [or retroperitoneal margin], posterior margin, and anterior surface).[12] In addition, a consensus regarding the definition of "positive resection margin" has not been reached. In 1977, the American Joint Committee on Cancer defined a positive resection margin as the presence of tumor cells on the margin.[47] However, the alternative definition presented in 2006 by the Royal College of Pathologists included the presence of tumor cells within 1 mm of the resection margin.[48,49] Since this new definition was introduced, the prognostic implications and real-world practicality have been debated.[50,51]

3 | WHAT IS "ART," "SCIENCE," AND THEIR INTEGRATION?

Some of the abovementioned current issues have reached some level of consensus, while others are still under debate. As evidence accumulates over time, the level of consensus will likely increase in the future. However, by reflecting on past experiences, we can speculate on how this process will unfold in the future; the process required not only the mechanical accumulation of evidence, but also innovation and imagination that could be described as "art" beyond the boundaries of science.

TABLE 1 Current issues in pancreatic surgery

Current issues in pancreatic surgery
Extent of surgery
Organ
Observation vs surgery
Excision vs pancreatectomy
Partial vs total pancreatectomy
Pancreaticoduodenectomy: standard Whipple vs pylorus preservation vs pylorus resection
Organ preservation (duodenum, spleen, or splenic vessels)
Lymph node dissection: standard vs extended
Nerve plexus dissection: preservation vs half-circumferential removal vs 360° removal
Major vessels resection
Portal vein or superior mesenteric vein: technical amenability in relation to the first or second jejunal vein and duodenal inferior margin
Superior mesenteric artery: under trials in some centers
Common hepatic artery
Celiac artery: distal pancreatectomy with celiac artery resection (DPCAR)
Meso-pancreas excision
Definition of the area
Level of dissection
Mode of approach for dissection
Various superior mesenteric artery first approach
Infra-colic (mesenteric) vs supra-colic
Right or left vs supra-pancreatic
Radical ante-grade modular pancreato-splenectomy (RAMPS): anterior and posterior
No touch isolation technique
En bloc dissection
Minimally invasive surgery
Reconstruction method (pancreatic anastomosis)
Pancreaticojejunostomy vs pancreaticogastrostomy
Dunking/invaginating method vs duct-to-mucosa anastomosis
Internal vs external vs no stent
Many innovative modifications of pancreatic restoration
Usage and duration of surgical drain
Transection and stump management
Stapling vs hand sewing
With or without use of sealant, type of sealant
With or without use of somatostatin
Determination of resectability
Criteria
Various criteria: National Comprehensive Cancer Network (NCCN) criteria, etc.
International Association of Pancreatology (IAP) consensus criteria (+ biologic/conditional criteria)
Tools and their reliability: CT, MRI, PET, cytology, etc.

(Continues)

TABLE 1 (Continued)

Determination after neoadjuvant treatment
Response evaluation by CT tumor marker, PET, etc.
Timing of Surgery
Upfront surgery, surgery after neoadjuvant therapy
Timing and indication of conversion surgery
Resection margin and residual tumor
Significance of multiple margins
Concept of residual tumor (tumor at the margin vs 1-mm margin)

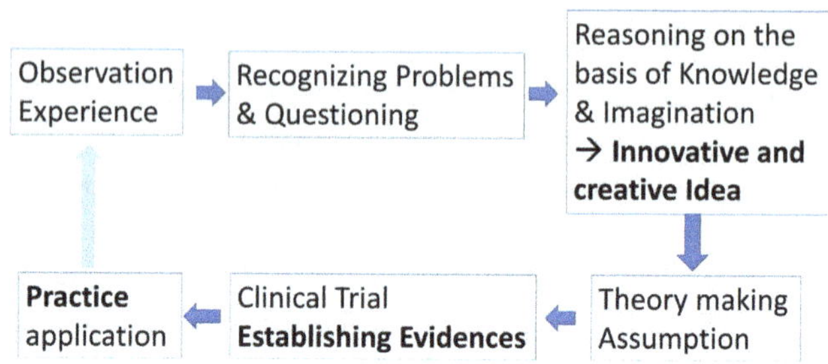

FIGURE 2 A sample diagram of the integration of art and science in the field of surgery

Based on these concepts, a sample diagram integrating "art" and "science" in the field of surgery is presented in Figure 2. Surgeons recognize problems and raise questions based on their observations and experiences in clinical practice. Surgeons' reasoning based on their knowledge and imagination can lead to the development of innovative and creative ideas, which result in theories and hypotheses that enable surgeons to conduct RCTs to establish evidence for future clinical applications. This process exists as an iterative cycle because new practice cannot be perfect.

Most surgeons would claim they know what science is; however, what is art? The following are representative quotes about art that set it apart from science: "Art is not based on evidence, but on experience. Art does not confine to logic, it is an expression of feeling. Art does not work with hypothesis and does not need evidence and hence art is separate from science"[52] and "art is the solution of a problem which cannot be expressed explicitly until it is solved. Art is the creative process and it goes through all fields."[53]

There have been numerous creative and innovative surgical procedures in the history of pancreatic surgery that deserve to be called "art." Most of the procedures belong to the realm of "art" when they are first introduced, regardless of whether they have been supported by scientific evidence or have become general practice. Likewise, there are many concepts and techniques applied to pancreatic surgery that are still considered "art." Consequently, a few recent examples of "art, science, and their integration" are presented below. The first example demonstrates an experience in which an innovative technique, introduced by a need derived from clinical experience, continued to evolve through the integration of art and science. The second example illustrates how an innovative procedure adopted from other surgical disciplines overcame problems specific to pancreatic surgery. The third example shows the continuous integration of art and science regarding the meso-pancreas, whose concept has not yet been fully established; the innovative concept, along with the development of a variety of surgical approaches in the area, is being evidenced through ongoing trials. The last example describes the integration of physiology and pancreatic surgery, which goes beyond the limits of the anatomical or technical perspective of surgery, often overlooked by surgeons.

3.1 | Spleen-preserving distal pancreatectomy

Overwhelming post-splenectomy infection (OPSI) is a rare but fatal complication after distal pancreatectomy with splenectomy (Figure 3a).[54] The first solution introduced to manage this problem was the Warshaw procedure, in which the spleen is preserved (though not the splenic vessels) during distal pancreatectomy.[55] However, many surgeons had concerns about splenic infarction and gastric varix, which can develop after splenic vessel resection.[55,56] Therefore, the Kimura procedure, which involves the preservation of both the spleen and splenic vessels, was proposed.[57] Many surgeons have attempted both the Warshaw and Kimura procedures and have demonstrated their feasibility in clinical practice. Although initial reports appealed for improved technical reliability and safety compared to traditional distal pancreatectomy with splenectomy,[57] a recent systematic review and meta-analysis have revealed that the incidence of splenic infarction and secondary splenectomy associated with the Kimura procedure is significantly lower than that of the Warshaw procedure.[58]

However, OPSI were discovered to be more rare and preventable than expected, and splenic infarction and gastric varices were also rare, with little clinical significance.[59, 60] Moreover, the benefits of splenic vessel preservation are not clear, since long-term patency of the preserved vessels is uncertain.[61] As a result, surgeons are currently performing all three procedures (conventional splenectomy and spleen preservation with or without splenic vessel preservation) based on clinical experience and value judgments regarding the risk of complications. As "practitioners," surgeons can choose between these options based on their own experience, their feasibility, and on evidence provided by the "surgical scientists."

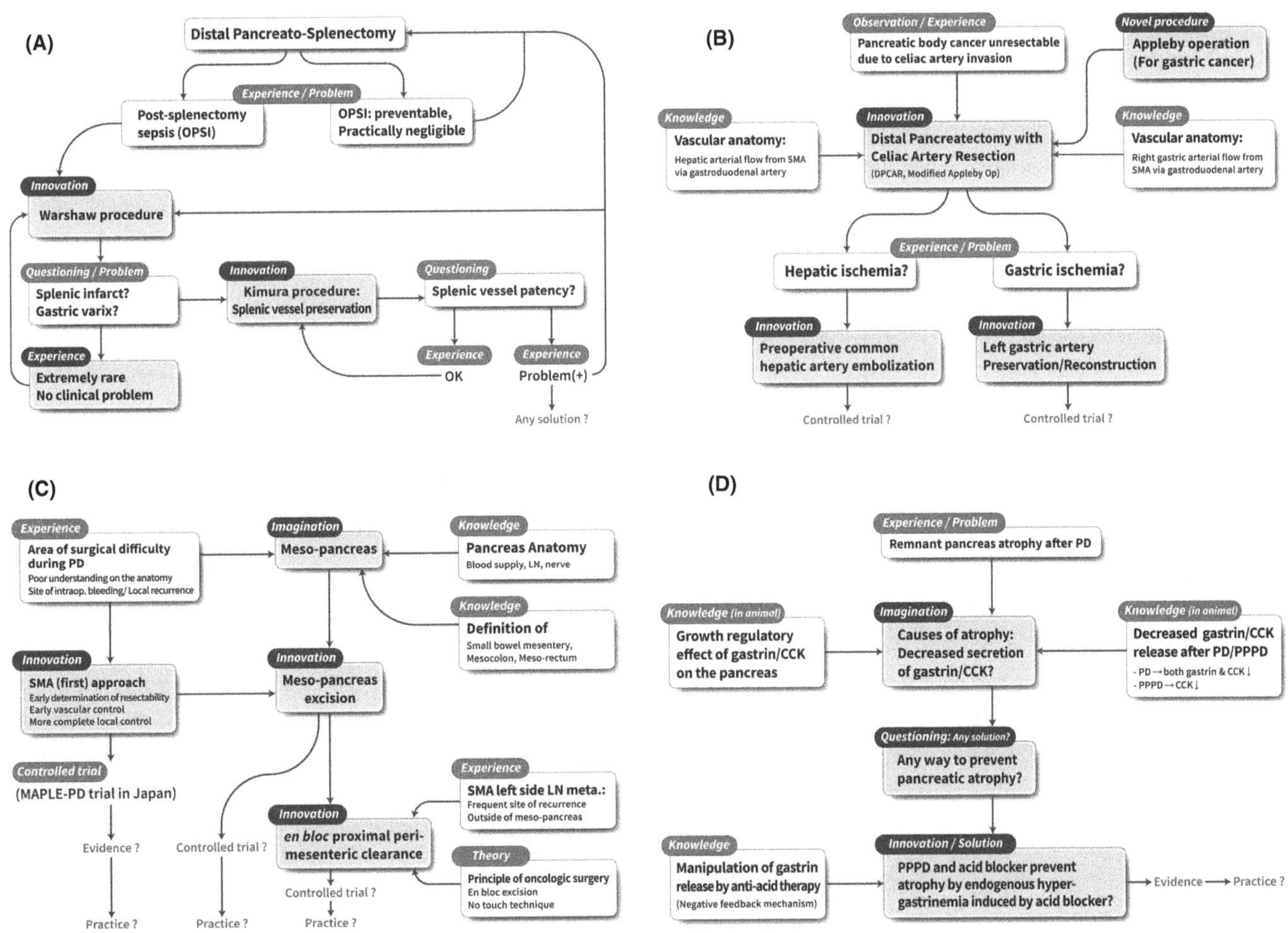

FIGURE 3 Cascade of knowledge, experience, questioning, hypothesis, and building evidence triggered by imagination and innovation. A. Spleen-preserving distal pancreatectomy. B. Modified Appleby operation for advanced pancreatic body cancer. C. Meso-pancreas excision. D. Preventing atrophy of the remnant pancreas after pancreatic head resection

3.2 | Modified Appleby operation for advanced pancreatic body cancer

Pancreatic body cancers frequently infiltrate the celiac artery due to its proximity to the tumor. Originally designed for advanced gastric cancer, the Appleby operation includes a total gastrectomy and celiac artery resection (Figure 3-b).[62] The modified Appleby procedure, which involves preserving the right gastric artery and right gastroepiploic vessel to preserve the entire stomach, has been proposed and shown to be technically feasible as a treatment for pancreatic body cancer.[63, 64] Additionally, hepatic and gastric blood flow is expected to be preserved by collateral blood flow from the SMA through the gastroduodenal and pancreaticoduodenal arteries after celiac and common hepatic artery resections. However, understandably, many pancreatic surgeons are concerned about hepatic and gastric ischemia, which have been reported but are extremely rare.[65] Therefore, innovative procedures have been developed to address these issues, including preoperative common hepatic artery embolization to ensure hepatic blood flow[34, 66] and the preservation or reconstruction of the left gastric artery to prevent gastric ischemia.[67, 68] Since these innovative techniques have only been reported in a limited number of cases, RCTs are required to confirm their technical feasibility and safety.

3.3 | Meso-pancreas excision

Based on our understanding of pancreatic anatomy and the definition of the mesentery, meso-colon, and meso-rectum, the concept of the meso-pancreas has emerged (Figure 3-c).[69] Although the anatomical concept of the meso-pancreas is still controversial, some surgeons perform meso-pancreas excision during PD for pancreatic head cancer to remove all soft tissue from this area since tumor involvement of retroperitoneal resection margin (R1 resection) and local recurrence is frequently reported after surgery.[70, 71] In addition, innovative SMA-first approaches that emphasize the principles of oncological surgery have been introduced to facilitate meso-pancreas excision. One example is the MAPLE-PD (mesenteric approach versus conventional approach for pancreatic cancer during Pancreaticoduodenectomy) trial currently in progress in Japan.[72] Another example is the concept of "*en bloc* proximal peri-mesenteric clearance," which was proposed due to cancer recurrence at the SMA left-side lymph node, located outside of the meso-pancreas, and for which RCT-based evidence is expected in the future.[35] Through the above process, we can speculate how art and science are integrated to refine the establishment of innovative surgical procedures. All surgeons who have proposed this concept and attempted meso-pancreas excision should be considered "surgical artists" as well as "surgical scientists."

3.4 | Preventing atrophy of the remnant pancreas after pancreatic head resection

Atrophy of the distal remnant pancreas is a frequently observed phenomenon after PD due to pancreaticojejunostomy stricture, postoperative radiation therapy, or the presence of an altered route for food passage, among others (Figure 3-d).[73] Additionally, the physiological change in gastrin/cholecystokinin (CKK) secretion has emerged as another potential cause of atrophy. This is based on the understanding that gastrin/CCK secretion is reduced after PD or pylorus-preserving PD (PPPD) and through the growth-stimulating effect that gastrin/CCK has on the pancreas that has clearly been identified in animal models.[74] Therefore, it has been theorized that one of the causes of remnant pancreatic atrophy after PD/PPPD could be a decrease in gastrin/CCK secretion after PD and a decrease in CCK secretion after PPPD. Gastrin is secreted from the gastric antrum, and CCK is secreted from the duodenum; therefore, a consequence of both PD and PPPD is the removal of the source of these hormones.[75]

Therefore, we wondered if there was any way to prevent pancreatic atrophy. The extent of post-PPPD atrophy was hypothesized to be less than that of post-PD atrophy because PPPD preserves the gastrin secretion zone. In addition, a significant level of preserved gastrin/CCK response was observed in post-PPPD patients but not in post-PD patients.[76, 77] Based on the knowledge that gastrin secretion can be manipulated by acid blockers through physiological negative feedback mechanisms,[78] an innovative idea emerged; it was hypothesized that acid blockers may prevent or reduce the extent of atrophy of the remnant pancreas after PPPD by stimulating endogenous gastrin secretion. Subsequently, an RCT of patients after PPPD with induced hypergastrinemia showed a significant reduction in the extent of atrophy of the distal pancreas, along with an increased level of stool elastase.[73] Although long-term administration of acid blockers after PD has not become general practice due to potential side effects, it was an innovation that should be considered an "art," since a solution was proposed from a new perspective based on the surgeon's observation and experience. Pancreatic exocrine insufficiency that occurs immediately after PD/PPPD in association with pancreatic tissue loss and gastrin/CCK regulation gradually returns to normal functional levels within 6 months.[4,79] Therefore, the current version of the ISGPS position paper recommends that pancreatic enzyme replacement therapy should be routinely initiated and continued for at least 6 months postoperatively in patients who undergo PD.[5]

4 | CONCLUSION

This review illustrates how the creative ideas of pancreatic surgeons have evolved into generally accepted clinical practice. Surgeons should be considered "surgical artists," "surgical scientists," and "surgical practitioners" due to their capacity to combine art and science in clinical practice. We look forward to witnessing more "surgical artists" educating future "surgical artists and scientists" to continue the rich "spirit of innovation" in pancreatic surgery, which will lead to more innovative ideas and the development of more efficient methods of establishing high levels of evidence, and, thus, a more beautiful integration of art and science in the field of pancreatic surgery.

ACKNOWLEDGMENTS

The figure work was supported by the Creative Media Service of the National Cancer Center Korea. We would like to thank Editage (www.editage.co.kr) for English language editing.

DISCLOSURE

Author Contribution: Mee Joo Kang: conceptualization (supporting), formal analysis (supporting), methodology (supporting), visualization (equal), writing - original draft preparation (equal), writing - review & editing (equal). Sun-Whe Kim: conceptualization (lead), formal analysis (lead), methodology (lead), supervision (lead), visualization (equal), writing - original draft preparation (equal), writing - review & editing (equal).

REFERENCES

1. Bassi C, Marchegiani G, Dervenis C, Sarr M, Abu Hilal M, Adham M, et al. The 2016 update of the International Study Group (ISGPS) definition and grading of postoperative pancreatic fistula: 11 Years After. Surgery. 2017;161:584–91.
2. Wente MN, Veit JA, Bassi C, Dervenis C, Fingerhut A, Gouma D, et al. Postpancreatectomy hemorrhage (PPH): an International Study Group of Pancreatic Surgery (ISGPS) definition. Surgery. 2007;142:20–5.
3. Wente MN, Bassi C, Dervenis C, Fingerhut A, Gouma DJ, Izbicki JR, et al. Delayed gastric emptying (DGE) after pancreatic surgery: a suggested definition by the International Study Group of Pancreatic Surgery (ISGPS). Surgery. 2007;142:761–8.
4. Park JW, Jang JY, Kim EJ, Kang MJ, Kwon W, Chang YR, et al. Effects of pancreatectomy on nutritional state, pancreatic function and quality of life. Br J Surg. 2013;100:1064–70.
5. Gianotti L, Besselink MG, Sandini M, Hackert T, Conlon K, Gerritsen A, et al. Nutritional support and therapy in pancreatic surgery: A position paper of the International Study Group on Pancreatic Surgery (ISGPS). Surgery. 2018;164:1035–48.
6. Mizrahi JD, Surana R, Valle JW, Shroff RT. Pancreatic cancer. Lancet. 2020;395:2008–20.
7. Huttner FJ, Capdeville L, Pianka F, Ulrich A, Hackert T, Büchler MW, et al. Systematic review of the quantity and quality of randomized clinical trials in pancreatic surgery. Br J Surg. 2019;106:23–31.
8. Kaido T. Recent randomized controlled trials in pancreaticoduodenectomy. Pancreas. 2006;33:228–32.
9. Pawlik TM, Abdalla EK, Barnett CC, Ahmad SA, Cleary KR, Vauthey JN, et al. Feasibility of a randomized trial of extended lymphadenectomy for pancreatic cancer. Arch Surg. 2005;140(6):589–91;discussion 589–591.
10. Katz MH, Merchant NB, Brower S, Branda M, Posner MC, William Traverso L, et al. Standardization of surgical and pathologic variables is needed in multicenter trials of adjuvant therapy for pancreatic cancer: results from the ACOSOG Z5031 trial. Ann Surg Oncol. 2011;18:337–44.
11. Probst P, Huttner FJ, Meydan O, Kalkum E, Kretschmer R, Jensen K, et al. Evidence map of pancreatic surgery: protocol for a living systematic review and meta-analysis. BMJ Open. 2019;9:e032353.
12. National Comprehensive Cancer Network. NCCN Clinical Practice Guidelines in Oncology: Pancreatic Adenocarcinoma, Version 2.2021 [Internet]. Plymouth Meeting, PA: National Comprehensive Cancer Network; c2021 [cited 2021 Apr 7]. Available from: https://www.nccn.org/professionals/physician_gls/pdf/pancreatic.pdf
13. Khorana AA, McKernin SE, Berlin J, Hong TS, Maitra A, Moravek C, et al. Potentially curable pancreatic adenocarcinoma: ASCO clinical practice guideline update. J Clin Oncol. 2019;37:2082–8.
14. Ducreux M, Cuhna AS, Caramella C, Hollebecque A, Burtin P, Goéré D, et al. Cancer of the pancreas: ESMO Clinical Practice Guidelines for diagnosis, treatment and follow-up. Ann Oncol. 2015;26(Suppl 5):v56–68.
15. Japan Pancreas Society. Classification of pancreatic carcinoma (4th edn). Tokyo: Kanehara & Co., Ltd.; 2017.
16. Bockhorn M, Uzunoglu FG, Adham M, Imrie C, Milicevic M, Sandberg AA, et al. Borderline resectable pancreatic cancer: a consensus statement by the International Study Group of Pancreatic Surgery (ISGPS). Surgery. 2014;155:977–88.
17. Klaiber U, Probst P, Strobel O, Michalski CW, Dörr-Harim C, Diener MK, et al. Meta-analysis of delayed gastric emptying after pylorus-preserving versus pylorus-resecting pancreatoduodenectomy. Br J Surg. 2018;105:339–49.
18. Yang DJ, Xiong JJ, Liu XT, Li J, Dhanushka Layanthi Siriwardena KM, Hu WM. Total pancreatectomy compared with pancreaticoduodenectomy: a systematic review and meta-analysis. Cancer Manag Res. 2019;11:3899–908.
19. Kang MJ, Jang JY, Kim SW. Surgical resection of pancreatic head cancer: What is the optimal extent of surgery? Cancer Lett. 2016;382:259–65.
20. Jang JY, Kang MJ, Heo JS, Choi SH, Choi DW, Park SJ, et al. A prospective randomized controlled study comparing outcomes of standard resection and extended resection, including dissection of the nerve plexus and various lymph nodes, in patients with pancreatic head cancer. Ann Surg. 2014;259:656–64.
21. Inoue Y, Saiura A, Yoshioka R, Ono Y, Takahashi M, Arita J, et al. Pancreatoduodenectomy with systematic mesopancreas dissection using a supracolic anterior artery-first approach. Ann Surg. 2015;262:1092–101.
22. Yamada S, Satoi S, Takami H, Yamamoto T, Yoshioka I, Sonohara F, et al. Multicenter randomized phase II trial of prophylactic right-half dissection of superior mesenteric artery nerve plexus in pancreatoduodenectomy for pancreatic head cancer. Ann Gastroenterol Surg. 2021;5:111–8.
23. Inoue Y, Saiura A, Oba A, Kawakatsu S, Ono Y, Sato T, et al. Optimal extent of superior mesenteric artery dissection during pancreaticoduodenectomy for pancreatic cancer: balancing surgical and oncological safety. J Gastrointest Surg. 2019;23:1373–83.
24. Ramia JM, De-la-Plaza R, Manuel-Vazquez A, Lopez-Marcano A, Morales R. Systematic review of the mesopancreas: concept and clinical implications. Clin Transl Oncol. 2018;20:1385–91.
25. Nakao A, Takagi H. Isolated pancreatectomy for pancreatic head carcinoma using catheter bypass of the portal vein. Hepatogastroenterology. 1993;40:426–9.
26. Pessaux P, Varma D, Arnaud JP. Pancreaticoduodenectomy: superior mesenteric artery first approach. J Gastrointest Surg. 2006;10:607–11.
27. Shukla PJ, Barreto G, Pandey D, Kanitkar G, Nadkarni MS, Neve R, et al. Modification in the technique of pancreaticoduodenectomy: supracolic division of jejunum to facilitate uncinate process dissection. Hepatogastroenterology. 2007;54:1728–30.
28. Hirota M, Kanemitsu K, Takamori H, Chikamoto A, Tanaka H, Sugita H, et al. Pancreatoduodenectomy using a no-touch isolation technique. Am J Surg. 2010;199:e65–8.
29. Weitz J, Rahbari N, Koch M, Buchler MW. The "artery first" approach for resection of pancreatic head cancer. J Am Coll Surg. 2010;210:e1–4.
30. Kurosaki I, Minagawa M, Takano K, Takizawa K, Hatakeyama K. Left posterior approach to the superior mesenteric vascular pedicle in pancreaticoduodenectomy for cancer of the pancreatic head. JOP. 2011;12:220–9.
31. Sanjay P, Takaori K, Govil S, Shrikhande SV, Windsor JA. 'Artery-first' approaches to pancreatoduodenectomy. Br J Surg. 2012;99:1027–35.

32. Mitchem JB, Hamilton N, Gao F, Hawkins WG, Linehan DC, Strasberg SM. Long-term results of resection of adenocarcinoma of the body and tail of the pancreas using radical antegrade modular pancreatosplenectomy procedure. J Am Coll Surg. 2012;214:46–52.
33. Chun YS. Role of radical antegrade modular pancreatosplenectomy (RAMPS) and pancreatic cancer. Ann Surg Oncol. 2018;25:46–50.
34. Hirano S, Kondo S, Hara T, Ambo Y, Tanaka E, Shichinohe T, et al. Distal pancreatectomy with en bloc celiac axis resection for locally advanced pancreatic body cancer: long-term results. Ann Surg. 2007;246:46–51.
35. Kang MJ, Kim SW. En bloc proximal peri-mesenteric clearance for pancreatic head cancer surgery. Ann Hepatobiliary Pancreat Surg. 2020;24:389–95.
36. de Rooij T, van Hilst J, van Santvoort H, Boerma D, van den Boezem P, Daams F, et al. Minimally Invasive Versus Open Distal Pancreatectomy (LEOPARD): A Multicenter Patient-blinded Randomized Controlled Trial. Ann Surg. 2019;269:2–9.
37. van Hilst J, de Rooij T, Bosscha K, Brinkman DJ, van Dieren S, Dijkgraaf MG, et al. Laparoscopic versus open pancreatoduodenectomy for pancreatic or periampullary tumours (LEOPARD-2): a multicentre, patient-blinded, randomised controlled phase 2/3 trial. Lancet Gastroenterol Hepatol. 2019;4:199–207.
38. Asbun HJ, Moekotte AL, Vissers FL, Kunzler F, Cipriani F, Alseidi A, et al. The Miami International Evidence-based Guidelines on Minimally Invasive Pancreas Resection. Ann Surg. 2020;271:1–14.
39. Kawaida H, Kono H, Hosomura N, Amemiya H, Itakura J, Fujii H, et al. Surgical techniques and postoperative management to prevent postoperative pancreatic fistula after pancreatic surgery. World J Gastroenterol. 2019;25:3722–37.
40. Jang JY, Chang YR, Kim SW, Choi SH, Park SJ, Lee SE, et al. Randomized multicentre trial comparing external and internal pancreatic stenting during pancreaticoduodenectomy. Br J Surg. 2016;103:668–75.
41. Kang MJ, Jang JY, Kwon W, Kim SW. Clinical significance of defining borderline resectable pancreatic cancer. Pancreatology. 2018;18:139–45.
42. Katz MH, Pisters PW, Evans DB, Sun CC, Lee JE, Fleming JB, et al. Borderline resectable pancreatic cancer: the importance of this emerging stage of disease. J Am Coll Surg. 2008;206(5):833–46;discussion 846–838.
43. Isaji S, Mizuno S, Windsor JA, Bassi C, Fernández-del Castillo C, Hackert T, et al. International consensus on definition and criteria of borderline resectable pancreatic ductal adenocarcinoma 2017. Pancreatology. 2018;18:2–11.
44. Kato H, Horiguchi A, Ito M, Asano Y, Arakawa S. Essential updates 2019/2020: Multimodal treatment of localized pancreatic adenocarcinoma: Current topics and updates in survival outcomes and prognostic factors. Ann Gastroenterol Surg. 2021;5:132–51.
45. Wang ZJ, Arif-Tiwari H, Zaheer A, Ameli S, Bhosale PR, Do RK, et al. Therapeutic response assessment in pancreatic ductal adenocarcinoma: society of abdominal radiology review paper on the role of morphological and functional imaging techniques. Abdom Radiol (NY). 2020;45:4273–89.
46. Satoi S, Yamamoto T, Yamaki S, Sakaguchi T, Sekimoto M. Surgical indication for and desirable outcomes of conversion surgery in patients with initially unresectable pancreatic ductal adenocarcinoma. Ann Gastroenterol Surg. 2020;4:6–13.
47. American Joint Committee for Cancer Staging and End Results Reporting. Manual for Staging of Cancer 1977. Chicago, Ill: American Joint Committee on Cancer; 1977.
48. Verbeke CS, Leitch D, Menon KV, McMahon MJ, Guillou PJ, Anthoney A. Redefining the R1 resection in pancreatic cancer. Br J Surg. 2006;93:1232–7.
49. The Royal College of Pathologists. Standards and minimum datasets for reporting cancers. Minimum dataset for the histopathological reporting of pancreatic, ampulla of Vater and bile duct carcinoma. 2002. The Royal College of Pathologists.
50. Campbell F, Smith RA, Whelan P, Sutton R, Raraty M, Neoptolemos JP, et al. Classification of R1 resections for pancreatic cancer: the prognostic relevance of tumour involvement within 1 mm of a resection margin. Histopathology. 2009;55:277–83.
51. DemirIE,JagerC,SchlitterAM,KonukiewitzB,StecherL,SchornS,etal. R0 Versus R1 Resection Matters after Pancreaticoduodenectomy, and Less after Distal or Total Pancreatectomy for Pancreatic Cancer. Ann Surg. 2018;268:1058–68.
52. Chandra R. Being at Home. Lulu.com. 2014.
53. Hein P. [Quoted in] Duane Preble. Man creates art creats man 1973:14.
54. Waghorn DJ, Mayon-White RT. A study of 42 episodes of overwhelming post-splenectomy infection: is current guidance for asplenic individuals being followed? J Infect. 1997;35:289–94.
55. Warshaw AL. Conservation of the spleen with distal pancreatectomy. Arch Surg. 1988;123:550–3.
56. Miura F, Takada T, Asano T, Kenmochi T, Ochiai T, Amano H, et al. Hemodynamic changes of splenogastric circulation after spleen-preserving pancreatectomy with excision of splenic artery and vein. Surgery. 2005;138:518–22.
57. Kimura W, Inoue T, Futakawa N, Shinkai H, Han I, Muto T. Spleen-preserving distal pancreatectomy with conservation of the splenic artery and vein. Surgery. 1996;120:885–90.
58. Nakata K, Shikata S, Ohtsuka T, Ukai T, Miyasaka Y, Mori Y, et al. Minimally invasive preservation versus splenectomy during distal pancreatectomy: a systematic review and meta-analysis. J Hepatobiliary Pancreat Sci. 2018;25:476–88.
59. Malleo G, Damoli I, Marchegiani G, Esposito A, Marchese T, Salvia R, et al. Laparoscopic distal pancreatectomy: analysis of trends in surgical techniques, patient selection, and outcomes. Surg Endosc. 2015;29:1952–62.
60. Yoon YS, Lee KH, Han HS, Cho JY, Ahn KS. Patency of splenic vessels after laparoscopic spleen and splenic vessel-preserving distal pancreatectomy. Br J Surg. 2009;96:633–40.
61. Yoon YS, Lee KH, Han HS, Cho JY, Jang JY, Kim S-W, et al. Effects of laparoscopic versus open surgery on splenic vessel patency after spleen and splenic vessel-preserving distal pancreatectomy: a retrospective multicenter study. Surg Endosc. 2015;29:583–8.
62. Appleby LH. The coeliac axis in the expansion of the operation for gastric carcinoma. Cancer. 1953;6:704–7.
63. Hishinuma S, Ogata Y, Matusui J, et al. Two cases of cancer of the pancreatic body undergoing gastric preservation with distal pancreatectomy combined with resection of the celiac axis. Jpn J Gastroenterol Surg. 1991;24:2782–6.
64. Nagino M, Nimura Y, Hayakawa N, Kamiya J, Kondo S. Appleby's operation for pancreas cancer. Tan to Sui. 1991;12:1361–8.
65. Mollberg N, Rahbari NN, Koch M, Hartwig W, Hoeger Y, Büchler MW, et al. Arterial resection during pancreatectomy for pancreatic cancer: a systematic review and meta-analysis. Ann Surg. 2011;254:882–93.
66. Kondo S, Katoh H, Shimizu T, Omi M, Hirano S, Ambo Y, et al. Preoperative embolization of the common hepatic artery in preparation for radical pancreatectomy for pancreas body cancer. Hepatogastroenterology. 2000;47:1447–9.
67. Kimura A, Yamamoto J, Aosasa S, Hatsuse K, Nishikawa M, Nishiyama K, et al. Importance of maintaining left gastric arterial flow at Appleby operation preserving whole stomach for central pancreatic cancer. Hepatogastroenterology. 2012;59:2650–2.
68. Sato T, Saiura A, Inoue Y, Takahashi Y, Arita J, Takemura N. Distal Pancreatectomy with En Bloc Resection of the Celiac Axis with Preservation or Reconstruction of the Left Gastric Artery in Patients with Pancreatic Body Cancer. World J Surg. 2016;40:2245–53.
69. Gockel I, Domeyer M, Wolloscheck T, Konerding MA, Junginger T. Resection of the mesopancreas (RMP): a new surgical classification of a known anatomical space. World J Surg Oncol. 2007;5:44.

70. Peparini N, Chirletti P. Mesopancreas: a boundless structure, namely R1 risk in pancreaticoduodenectomy for pancreatic head carcinoma. Eur J Surg Oncol. 2013;39:1303–8.
71. Kawabata Y, Tanaka T, Ishikawa N, Hayashi H, Tajima Y. Modified total meso-pancreatoduodenum excision with pancreaticoduodenectomy as a mesopancreatic plane surgery in borderline resectable pancreatic cancer. Eur J Surg Oncol. 2016;42:698–705.
72. Hirono S, Kawai M, Okada KI, Fujii T, Sho M, Satoi S, et al. MAPLE-PD trial (Mesenteric Approach vs. Conventional Approach for Pancreatic Cancer during Pancreaticoduodenectomy): study protocol for a multicenter randomized controlled trial of 354 patients with pancreatic ductal adenocarcinoma. Trials. 2018;19(1):613.
73. Jang JY, Kim SW, Han JK, Park S-J, Park Y-C, Joon Ahn Y, et al. Randomized prospective trial of the effect of induced hypergastrinemia on the prevention of pancreatic atrophy after pancreatoduodenectomy in humans. Ann Surg. 2003;237:522–9.
74. Kim SW, Kim KH, Park SJ, Her HH, Jang JY, Park YH. Endogenous gastrin stimulates regeneration of remnant pancreas after partial pancreatectomy. Dig Dis Sci. 2001;46:2134–9.
75. Kim SW, Kim KH, Han JK, Park YH. Pylorus-preservation decreases the extent of atrophy of the remnant pancreas after pancreatoduodenectomy. HPB. 1999;1:65–70.
76. Takada T, Yasuda H, Shikata J, Watanabe S, Shiratori K, Takeuchi T. Postprandial plasma gastrin and secretin concentrations after a pancreatoduodenectomy. A comparison between a pylorus-preserving pancreatoduodenectomy and the Whipple procedure. Ann Surg. 1989;210:47–51.
77. Tangoku A, Nishikawa M, Adachi A, Suzuki T. Plasma gastrin and cholecystokinin response after pylorus-preserving pancreatoduodenectomy with Billroth-I type of reconstruction. Ann Surg. 1991;214:56–60.
78. Xu G, Sumi S, Koike M, Tanigawa K, Nio Y, Tamura K. Role of endogenous hypergastrinemia in regenerating endocrine pancreas after partial pancreatectomy. Dig Dis Sci. 1996;41:2433–9.
79. Ohtsuka T, Yamaguchi K, Chijiiwa K, Kinukawa N, Tanaka M. Quality of life after pylorus-preserving pancreatoduodenectomy. Am J Surg. 2001;182:230–6.

Permissions

All chapters in this book were first published by Wiley Online Library; hereby published with permission under the Creative Commons Attribution License or equivalent. Every chapter published in this book has been scrutinized by our experts. Their significance has been extensively debated. The topics covered herein carry significant findings which will fuel the growth of the discipline. They may even be implemented as practical applications or may be referred to as a beginning point for another development.

The contributors of this book come from diverse backgrounds, making this book a truly international effort. This book will bring forth new frontiers with its revolutionizing research information and detailed analysis of the nascent developments around the world.

We would like to thank all the contributing authors for lending their expertise to make the book truly unique. They have played a crucial role in the development of this book. Without their invaluable contributions this book wouldn't have been possible. They have made vital efforts to compile up to date information on the varied aspects of this subject to make this book a valuable addition to the collection of many professionals and students.

This book was conceptualized with the vision of imparting up-to-date information and advanced data in this field. To ensure the same, a matchless editorial board was set up. Every individual on the board went through rigorous rounds of assessment to prove their worth. After which they invested a large part of their time researching and compiling the most relevant data for our readers.

The editorial board has been involved in producing this book since its inception. They have spent rigorous hours researching and exploring the diverse topics which have resulted in the successful publishing of this book. They have passed on their knowledge of decades through this book. To expedite this challenging task, the publisher supported the team at every step. A small team of assistant editors was also appointed to further simplify the editing procedure and attain best results for the readers.

Apart from the editorial board, the designing team has also invested a significant amount of their time in understanding the subject and creating the most relevant covers. They scrutinized every image to scout for the most suitable representation of the subject and create an appropriate cover for the book.

The publishing team has been an ardent support to the editorial, designing and production team. Their endless efforts to recruit the best for this project, has resulted in the accomplishment of this book. They are a veteran in the field of academics and their pool of knowledge is as vast as their experience in printing. Their expertise and guidance has proved useful at every step. Their uncompromising quality standards have made this book an exceptional effort. Their encouragement from time to time has been an inspiration for everyone.

The publisher and the editorial board hope that this book will prove to be a valuable piece of knowledge for researchers, students, practitioners and scholars across the globe.

List of Contributors

Hiroomi Ogawa, Makoto Sohda, Ken Shirabe and Hiroshi Saeki
Department of General Surgical Science, Graduate School of Medicine, Gunma University, Maebashi, Japan

Toshiki Yajima
Department of General Surgical Science, Graduate School of Medicine, Gunma University, Maebashi, Japan
Department of Innovative Cancer Immunotherapy, Graduate School of Medicine, Gunma University, Maebashi, Japan

Ryota Nakanishi, Yuichi Hisamatsu, Tomonori Nakanoko, Koji Ando, Mitsuhiko Ota, Yasue Kimura, Eiji Oki and Tomoharu Yoshizumi
Department of Surgery and Science, Graduate School of Medical Sciences, Kyushu University, Fukuoka, Japan

Yoshiaki Fujimoto and Masahiko Sugiyama
Department of Gastroenterological Surgery, National Hospital Organization Kyushu Cancer Center, Fukuoka, Japan

Yoshiko Ando
Department of Nursing, Japanese Red Cross Osaka Hospital, Osaka, Japan
Department of Health Science, Graduate School of Medicine, Osaka University, Osaka, Japan

Tetsuya Tajima
Department of Health Science, Graduate School of Medicine, Osaka University, Osaka, Japan

Arata Takahashi
NCD Data Quality Management Subcommittee, The Japanese Society of Gastroenterological Surgery, Tokyo, Japan
Department of Health Policy and Management, School of Medicine, Keio University, Tokyo, Japan
Department of Healthcare Quality Assessment, Graduate School of Medicine, The University of Tokyo, Tokyo, Japan

Hiroyuki Yamamoto and Hiroaki Miyata
Department of Health Policy and Management, School of Medicine, Keio University, Tokyo, Japan
Department of Healthcare Quality Assessment, Graduate School of Medicine, The University of Tokyo, Tokyo, Japan
Department of Healthcare Quality Assessment, Graduate School of Medicine, University of Tokyo, Bunkyo-ku, Japan
Department of Healthcare Quality Assessment, The University of Tokyo, Tokyo, Japan

Hiroshi Hasegawa and Toshimoto Kimura
Project Management Subcommittee, The Japanese Society of Gastroenterological Surgery, Tokyo, Japan

Yukio Nishiguchi
Department of Surgery, Osaka City Juso Hospital, Osaka, Japan

Yoshihiro Kakeji
Database Committee, The Japanese Society of Gastroenterological Surgery, Tokyo, Japan
Division of Gastrointestinal Surgery, Department of Surgery, Graduate School of Medicine, Kobe University, Kobe, Japan
Database Committee, The Japanese Society of Gastroenterological Surgery, Minato-ku, Japan

Hideaki Obara, Gaku Shimane, Hirofumi Kawakubo, Minoru Kitago and Koji Okabayashi
Department of Surgery, Keio University School of Medicine, Tokyo, Japan

Yasunori Sato
Department of Preventive Medicine and Public Health, Keio University School of Medicine, Tokyo, Japan

Jun Okui
Department of Surgery, Keio University School of Medicine, Tokyo, Japan
Department of Preventive Medicine and Public Health, Keio University School of Medicine, Tokyo, Japan

Yi-Ming Shyr, Shin-E Wang, Shih-Chin Chen, Bor-Uei Shyr and Bor-Shiuan Shyr
Division of General Surgery, Department of Surgery, Taipei Veterans General Hospital and School of Medicine, National Yang Ming University, Taipei, Taiwan

Michinori Matsumoto, Kyohei Abe, Yasuro Futagawa, Takanori Kurogochi, Nana Takeuchi and Tomoyoshi Okamoto
Department of Surgery, The Jikei University Daisan Hospital, Komae, Japan

Kenei Furukawa, Koichiro Haruki, Shinji Onda and Toru Ikegami
Department of Surgery, The Jikei University School of Medicine, Minato-ku, Japan

Kohei Ogawa, Kei Tamura, Katsunori Sakamoto, Akihiro Takai and Yasutsugu Takada
Department of Hepato-Biliary- Pancreatic and Breast Surgery, Ehime University Graduate School of Medicine, Shitsukawa, Toon, Japan

Jota Watanabe and Hiromi Ohtani
Department of Surgery, Ehime Prefectural Central Hospital, Matsuyama, Japan

Masahiko Honjo
Department of Hepato-Biliary- Pancreatic and Breast Surgery, Ehime University Graduate School of Medicine, Shitsukawa, Toon, Japan
Department of Surgery, Ehime Prefectural Central Hospital, Matsuyama, Japan

Taiji Tohyama
Department of Hepato-Biliary- Pancreatic and Breast Surgery, Ehime University Graduate School of Medicine, Shitsukawa, Toon, Japan
Department of Surgery, Kurashiki Medical Center, Kurashiki, Japan

Norikatsu Miyoshi, Hidekazu Takahashi, Mamoru Uemura, Hirofumi Yamamoto and Hidetoshi Eguchi
Department of Gastroenterological Surgery, Osaka University Graduate School of Medicine, Suita, Japan

Takayuki Ogino and Tsunekazu Mizushima
Department of Therapeutics for Inflammatory Bowel Diseases, Osaka University Graduate School of Medicine, Suita, Japan
Department of Gastroenterological Surgery, Osaka University Graduate School of Medicine, Osaka, Japan
Department of Therapeutics for Inflammatory Bowel Diseases, Osaka University Graduate School of Medicine, Osaka, Japan

Yu Saito, Mitsuo Shimada, Yuji Morine and Shinichiro Yamada
Department of Surgery, Tokushima University, Tokushima, Japan

Maki Sugimoto
Department of Surgery, Tokushima University, Tokushima, Japan
Okinaga Research Institute, Teikyo University, Chiyoda-ku, Japan

Hiroharu Shinozaki and Tadashi Matsuoka
Department of Surgery, Saiseikai Utsunomiya Hospital, Tochigi, Japan

Momoko Ichihara and Naotsugu Haraguchi
Department of Gastroenterological Surgery, Osaka University Graduate School of Medicine, Osaka, Japan

Makoto Fujii
Division of Health Science, Osaka University Graduate School of Medicine, Osaka, Japan
Department of Health Science, Graduate School of Medicine, Osaka University, Osaka, Japan

Daichi Nomoto, Takahiko Akiyama, Kazuo Okadome, Masaaki Iwatsuki, Shiro Iwagami, Yuji Miyamoto and Naoya Yoshida
Department of Gastroenterological Surgery, Graduate School of Medical Sciences, Kumamoto University, Kumamoto, Japan

Yoshifumi Baba
Department of Gastroenterological Surgery, Graduate School of Medical Sciences, Kumamoto University, Kumamoto, Japan
Department of Next-Generation Surgical Therapy Development, Graduate School of Medical Sciences, Kumamoto University, Kumamoto, Japan

Masayuki Watanabe
Department of Gastroenterological Surgery, Cancer Institute Hospital, Japanese Foundation for Cancer Research, Tokyo, Japan

Hideo Baba
Department of Gastroenterological Surgery, Graduate School of Medical Sciences, Kumamoto University, Kumamoto, Japan
Center for Metabolic Regulation of Healthy Aging, Kumamoto University, Kumamoto, Japan

Motonari Ri, Koshi Kumagai, Shinichiro Atsumi, Masaru Hayami, Rie Makuuchi, Satoshi Ida, Manabu Ohashi, Takeshi Sano and Souya Nunobe
Department of Gastroenterological Surgery, Cancer Institute Hospital, Japanese Foundation for Cancer Research, Tokyo, Japan

Ken Namikawa
Department of Gastroenterology, Cancer Institute Hospital, Japanese Foundation for Cancer Research, Tokyo, Japan

Ryusei Yamamoto, Teiichi Sugiura, Ryo Ashida, Katsuhisa Ohgi, Mihoko Yamada, Shimpei Otsuka and Katsuhiko Uesaka
Division of Hepato-Biliary- Pancreatic Surgery, Shizuoka Cancer Center, Shizuoka, Japan

Masaki Kaibori and Kosuke Matsui
Department of Surgery, Kansai Medical University, Osaka, Japan

Shoji Kubo
Department of Hepato-Biliary- Pancreatic Surgery, Osaka City University Graduate School of Medicine, Osaka, Japan

Kiyoshi Hasegawa
Hepato-Biliary- Pancreatic Surgery Division, Department of Surgery, Graduate School of Medicine, The University of Tokyo, Tokyo, Japan

Hirotoshi Kikuchi, Kinji Kamiya and Hiroya Takeuchi
The Japanese Society of Gastroenterological Surgery, Minato-ku, Japan
Department of Surgery, Hamamatsu University School of Medicine, Hamamatsu, Japan

Yoshihiro Hiramatsu
The Japanese Society of Gastroenterological Surgery, Minato-ku, Japan
Department of Surgery, Hamamatsu University School of Medicine, Hamamatsu, Japan
Department of Perioperative Functioning Care and Support, Hamamatsu University School of Medicine, Hamamatsu, Japan

Hiraku Kumamaru and Shiyori Usune
Department of Healthcare Quality Assessment, Graduate School of Medicine, University of Tokyo, Bunkyo-ku, Japan

Hiroyuki Konno
The Japanese Society of Gastroenterological Surgery, Minato-ku, Japan
Hamamatsu University School of Medicine, Hamamatsu, Japan

Tatsunori Miyata, Yo-ichi Yamashita, Kota Arima, Takaaki Higashi, Hiromitsu Hayashi, Katsunori Imai and Akira Chikamoto
Department of Gastroenterological Surgery, Graduate School of Life Sciences, Kumamoto University, Kumamoto, Japan

Hidetoshi Nitta
Department of Surgery, Saiseikai Kumamoto Hospital, Kumamoto, Japan

Toru Beppu
Department of Gastroenterological Surgery, Graduate School of Life Sciences, Kumamoto University, Kumamoto, Japan
Department of Surgery, Yamaga City Medical Center, Kumamoto, Japan

Hideya Kashihara, Kozo Yoshikawa, Jun Higashijima, Takuya Tokunaga, Masaaki Nishi, Chie Takasu and Toshiaki Yoshimoto
Department of Surgery, Tokushima University, Tokushima, Japan

Yasuyuki Fukami, Takuya Saito, Takaaki Osawa, Takaaki Hanazawa, Takehiro Kurahashi, Shintaro Kurahashi, Tatsuki Matsumura, Shunichiro Komatsu, Kenitiro Kaneko and Tsuyoshi Sano
Division of Gastroenterological Surgery, Department of Surgery, Aichi Medical University, Nagakute, Japan

Hiroshi Sawayama, Katsuhiro Ogawa and Rikako Kato
Department of Gastroenterological Surgery, Graduate School of Medical Sciences, Kumamoto University, Kumamoto, Japan

Yukiharu Hiyoshi and Yuki Kiyozumi
Department of Gastroenterological Surgery, Cancer Institute Hospital of Japanese Foundation for Cancer Research, Tokyo, Japan

Atsushi Ishihara, Shogo Tanaka, Hiroji Shinkawa, Shigekazu Takemura, Ryosuke Amano, Kenjiro Kimura, Go Ohira and Kohei Nishio
Department of Hepato-Biliary- Pancreatic Surgery, Osaka City University Graduate School of Medicine, Osaka, Japan

Hisako Yoshida
Department of Medical Statistics, Osaka City University Graduate School of Medicine, Osaka, Japan

Ryota Mori, Yuki Sekido and Tsuyoshi Hata
Department of Gastroenterological Surgery, Graduate School of Medicine, Osaka University, Osaka, Japan
Department of Surgery, Osaka Police Hospital, Osaka, Japan

Hideki Endo
Department of Healthcare Quality Assessment, The University of Tokyo, Tokyo, Japan

Soji Ozawa
Department of Gastroenterological Surgery, Tokai University School of Medicine, Isehara, Japan
Department of Gastroenterological Surgery, Tokai University School of Medicine, Kanagawa, Japan

Hisahiro Matsubara
Department of Frontier Surgery, Chiba University Graduate School of Medicine, Chiba, Japan
The Japan Esophageal Society, Tokyo, Japan

Yuichiro Doki
The Japan Esophageal Society, Tokyo, Japan
Department of Gastroenterological Surgery, Osaka University Graduate School of Medicine, Osaka, Japan

Yuko Kitagawa
Department of Surgery, Keio University School of Medicine, Tokyo, Japan
The Japanese Society of Gastroenterological Surgery, Minato-ku, Japan
The Japanese Society of Gastroenterological Surgery, Tokyo, Japan

Masanobu Nakajima, Hiroto Muroi, Maiko Kikuchi, Junki Fujita, Keisuke Ihara, Masatoshi Nakagawa, Shinji Morita, Takatoshi Nakamura and Kazuyuki Kojima
First Department of Surgery, Dokkyo Medical University, Shimotsugagun, Japan

Satoru Yamaguchi
Department of Surgery, Dokkyo Medical University Nikko Medical Center, Nikko, Japan

Mee Joo Kang and Sun-Whe Kim
Department of Surgery, Center for Liver and Pancreato-Biliary Cancer, National Cancer Center, Goyang-si, Korea

Index

www.ingramcontent.com/pod-product-compliance
Lightning Source LLC
LaVergne TN
LVHW082127200926
848484LV00008B/2017